ANNALS OF
THE NEW YORK ACADEMY
OF SCIENCES

Volume 1031

EDITORIAL STAFF

Director, Publishing and New Media
SARAH GREENE

Managing Editor
JUSTINE CULLINAN

The New York Academy of Sciences
2 East 63rd Street
New York, New York 10021

THE NEW YORK ACADEMY OF SCIENCES
(Founded in 1817)

BOARD OF GOVERNORS, September 2004 – September 2005

TORSTEN N. WIESEL, *Chairman of the Board*
GERALD D. FISCHBACH, *Vice Chairman*
MICHAEL SCHMERTZLER, *Treasurer*
ELLIS RUBINSTEIN, *Chief Executive Officer* [ex officio]

Honorary Life Governors
WILLIAM T. GOLDEN   JOSHUA LEDERBERG

Governors

KAREN E. BURKE	VIRGINIA W. CORNISH	PETER B. CORR
R. BRIAN FERGUSON	RONALD L. GRAHAM	MARNIE IMHOFF
WENDY EVANS JOSEPH	JACQUELINE LEO	RODERT W. LUCKY
PAUL MARKS	BRUCE McEWEN	RONAY MENSCHEL
JOHN T. MORGAN	JOHN F. NIBLACK	SANDRA PANEM
PETER RINGROSE	DAVID D. SABATINI	JOHN SEXTON
	DEBORAH WILEY	

VICTORIA BJORKLUND, *Counsel* [ex officio]   LARRY R. SMITH, *Secretary* [ex officio]

VITAMIN E AND HEALTH

ANNALS OF THE NEW YORK ACADEMY OF SCIENCES
Volume 1031

VITAMIN E AND HEALTH

Edited by Frank Kelly, Mohsen Meydani, and Lester Packer

The New York Academy of Sciences
New York, New York
2004

Copyright © 2004 by the New York Academy of Sciences. All rights reserved. Under the provisions of the United States Copyright Act of 1976, individual readers of the Annals are permitted to make fair use of the material in them for teaching or research. Permission is granted to quote from the Annals provided that the customary acknowledgment is made of the source. Material in the Annals may be republished only by permission of the Academy. Address inquiries to the Permissions Department (editorial@nyas.org) at the New York Academy of Sciences.

Copying fees: For each copy of an article made beyond the free copying permitted under Section 107 or 108 of the 1976 Copyright Act, a fee should be paid through the Copyright Clearance Center, Inc., 222 Rosewood Drive, Danvers, MA 01923 (www.copyright.com).

♾ The paper used in this publication meets the minimum requirements of the American National Standard for Information Sciences—Permanence of Paper for Printed Library Materials, ANSI Z39.48-1984.

Library of Congress Cataloging-in-Publication Data

Vitamin E and health / edited by Frank Kelly, Mohsen Meydani, and Lester Packer.
    p. ; cm. — (Annals of the New York Academy of Sciences ; v. 1031)
    Based on a conference held May 22-24, 2004, in Boston, Mass.
    Includes bibliographical references and index.
    ISBN 1-57331-527-3 (cloth : alk. paper) — ISBN 1-57331-528-1 (pbk. : alk. paper)
    1. Vitamin E—Health aspects—Congresses.
    [DNLM: 1. Vitamin E—physiology—Congresses. 2. Vitamin E—therapeutic use—Congresses.] I. Kelly, Frank J. II. Meydani, Mohsen. III. Packer, Lester. IV. Series.
    Q11.N5 vol. 1031
    [QP772.T6]
    500 s—dc22
    [612.3/
                            2004028983

GYAT/PCP
Printed in the United States of America
ISBN 1-57331-527-3 (cloth)
ISBN 1-57331-528-1 (paper)
ISSN 0077-8923

ANNALS OF THE NEW YORK ACADEMY OF SCIENCES

Volume 1031
December 2004

VITAMIN E AND HEALTH

Editors
FRANK KELLY, MOHSEN MEYDANI, AND LESTER PACKER

This volume is the result of the conference entitled **Vitamin E and Health** held by the New York Academy of Sciences with the co-sponsorship of Cognis Nutrition and Health and BASF Aktiengesellschaft on May 22–24, 2004 in Boston Massachusetts.

CONTENTS

Preface. *By* FRANK KELLY, MOHSEN MEYDANI, AND LESTER PACKER......... xi

Part I. Bioavailability and Biokinetics of Vitamin E

Vitamin E Trafficking. *By* MARET G. TRABER, GRAHAM W. BURTON, AND ROBERT L. HAMILTON... 1

Discovery, Characterization, and Significance of the Cytochrome P450 ω-Hydroxylase Pathway of Vitamin E Catabolism. *By* ROBERT S. PARKER, TIMOTHY J. SONTAG, JOY E. SWANSON, AND CHARLES C. MCCORMICK.. 13

Inter- and Intra-Individual Vitamin E Uptake in Healthy Subjects Is Highly Repeatable across a Wide Supplementation Dose Range. *By* FRANK J. KELLY, ROSALIND LEE, AND IAN S. MUDWAY...................... 22

The Effect of Age on Vitamin E Status, Metabolism, and Function.: Metabolism as Assessed by Labeled Tocopherols. *By* REGINA BRIGELIUS-FLOHÉ, JOHANNES M. ROOB, BEATE TIRAN, SANDRA WUGA, JOSEP RIBALTA, EDMOND ROCK, AND BRIGITTE M. WINKLHOFER-ROOB.. 40

Part II. Antioxidant Functions of Vitamin E

Molecular Mechanisms of Vitamin E Transport. *By* ACHIM STOCKER........ 44

Physiological Factors Influencing Vitamin E Biokinetics. *By* JOHN K. LODGE, WENDY L. HALL, YVONNE M. JEANES, AND ANNA R. PROTEGGENTE.... 60

α-Tocopherol and Endothelial Nitric Oxide Synthesis. *By* REGINE HELLER, GABRIELE WERNER-FELMAYER, AND ERNST R. WERNER 74

Part III. Cell Regulatory Functions of Vitamin E

Vitamin E Mediates Cell Signaling and Regulation of Gene Expression. *By* ANGELO AZZI, RENÉ GYSIN, PETRA KEMPNÁ, ADELINA MUNTEANU, YESIM NEGIS, LUIS VILLACORTA, THERESA VISARIUS, AND JEAN-MARC ZINGG 86

Vitamin E and Gene Expression in Immune Cells. *By* SUNG NIM HAN, OSKAR ADOLFSSON, CHEOL-KOO LEE, TOMAS A. PROLLA, JOSE ORDOVAS, AND SIMIN NIKBIN MEYDANI 96

Modulation of Hepatic Gene Expression by α-Tocopherol in Cultured Cells and *in Vivo*. *By* GERALD RIMBACH, ALEXANDRA FISCHER, ELISABETH STOECKLIN, AND LUCA BARELLA 102

α-Tocopherol Transfer Protein Deficiency in Mice Causes Multi-Organ Deregulation of Gene Networks and Behavioral Deficits with Age. *By* KISHORCHANDRA GOHIL, ROY GODZDANKER, ERIN O'ROARK, BETTINA C. SCHOCK, RAMESH R. KAINI, LESTER PACKER, CARROLL E. CROSS, AND MARET G.TRABER 109

Tocotrienol: The Natural Vitamin E to Defend the Nervous System? *By* CHANDAN K. SEN, SAVITA KHANNA, AND SASHWATI ROY 127

Tocotrienol-Rich Fraction from Palm Oil and Gene Expression in Human Breast Cancer Cells. *By* KALANITHI NESARETNAM, ROBERTO AMBRA, KANGA RANI SELVADURAY, AMMU RADHAKRISHNAN, RAFFAELLA CANALI, AND FABIO VIRGILI 143

Part IV. Protection from Oxidative Stress and Injury

Vitamin E and the Oxidative Stress of Exercise. *By* M.J. JACKSON, M. KHASSAF, A. VASILAKI, F. MCARDLE, AND A. MCARDLE 158

Effect of Vitamin E on Gene Expression Changes in Diet-Related Carcinogenesis. *By* JOSEPH LUNEC, EUGENE HALLIGAN, NALINI MISTRY, AND KATHERINE KARAKOULA 169

Oral Supplementation with *All-Rac-* and *RRR*-α-Tocopherol Increases Vitamin E Levels in Human Sebum after a Latency Period of 14–21 Days. *By* SWARNA EKANAYAKE-MUDIYANSELAGE, KLAUS KRAEMER, AND JENS J. THIELE 184

Part V. Vitamin E and Vascular Networks

Anti-inflammatory Effects of α-Tocopherol. *By* UMA SINGH AND ISHWARLAL JIALAL 195

Oxidative Stress and Antioxidant Treatment in Diabetes. *By* JOSHUA A. SCOTT AND GEORGE L. KING 204

Part VI. Prevention, Protection, and Treatment of Diseases

Vitamin E and Respiratory Infection in the Elderly. *By* SIMIN NIKBIN MEYDANI, SUNG NIM HAN, AND DAVIDSON H. HAMER 214

Tocopherols and the Treatment of Colon Cancer. *By* WILLIAM L. STONE, KOYAMANGALATH KRISHNAN, SHARON E. CAMPBELL, MIN QUI, SARAH G. WHALEY, AND HONGSONG YANG 223

Selenium and Vitamin E Cancer Prevention Trial. *By* ERIC A. KLEIN 234

Vitamin E in Preeclampsia. *By* LUCILLA POSTON, MAARTEN RAIJMAKERS, AND FRANK KELLY 242

Vitamin E in Neurodegenerative Disorders: Alzheimer's Disease. *By* ANATOL KONTUSH AND SVETLANA SCHEKATOLINA 249

Vitamin E in Neural and Visual Function. *By* S.M. HAYTON AND D.P.R. MULLER 263

Part VII. Epidemiological and Intervention Studies

Vitamin E Modulation of Cardiovascular Disease. *By* MOHSEN MEYDANI 271

Vitamin E and Cardiovascular Disease: Observational Studies. *By* J. MICHAEL GAZIANO 280

Vitamin E for the Treatment of Cardiovascular Disease: Is There a Future? *By* FRANCESCO VIOLI, ROBERTO CANGEMI, GIUSEPPE SABATINO, AND PASQUALE PIGNATELLI 292

Part VIII. Round-Table Discussions

Future Directions in Preclinical Vitamin E Research: Panel Discussion A. LESTER PACKER, *Moderator*; ANGELO AZZI, KLAUS KRAEMER, NESRIN OZER, HELMUT SIES, ETSUO NIKI, FRANCESCO VIOLI, AND GOVIND VATASSERY, *Panel*.. 305

Future Directions in Clinical Vitamin E Research: Panel Discussion B. LESTER PACKER, *Moderator*; JEFFREY BLUMBERG, ISHWARLAL JIALAL, JOE LUNEC, SIMIN MEYDANI, FRANCESCO VIOLI, AND WALTER WILLETT, *Panel*.. 313

Part IX. Short Papers

Fluorescent Tocopherols as Probes of Inter-Vesicular Transfer Catalyzed by the α-Tocopherol Transfer Protein. *By* JEFFREY K. ATKINSON, PHILLIP NAVA, GRANT FRAHM, VALERIE CURTIS, AND DANNY MANOR 324

Gene–Nutrient Interactions Exemplified by the α-Tocopherol Content of Tissues from α-Tocopherol Transfer Protein–Null Mice Fed Different Dietary Vitamin E Concentrations. *By* YUNSOOK LIM, BETTINA C. SCHOCK, KISHORCHANDRA GOHIL, SCOTT W. LEONARD, LESTER PACKER, CARROLL E. CROSS, AND MARET G. TRABER 328

Intracellular Localization of α-Tocopherol Transfer Protein and α-Tocopherol. *By* JINGHUI QIAN, KATHLEEN WILSON, PHIL NAVA, SAMANTHA MORLEY, JEFFREY ATKINSON, AND DANNY MANOR 330

Structure–Function Relationship in the Tocopherol Transfer Protein. *By* S. MORLEY, C. PANAGABKO, A. STOCKER, J. ATKINSON, AND D. MANOR . 332

α-Tocopherol Affects Androgen Metabolism in Male Rat. *By* LUCA BARELLA, CRISTINA ROTA, ELISABETH STÖCKLIN, AND GERALD RIMBACH 334

The Transcriptional Signature of Vitamin E. *By* AMY JOHNSON AND
DANNY MANOR 337

α- and γ-Tocopherol Plasma and Urinary Biokinetics following α-Tocopherol
Supplementation. *By* JUDITH C.P. EICHHORN, ROSALIND LEE,
CHRISTINA DUNSTER, SAMAR BASU, AND FRANK J. KELLY 339

Oxidized Vitamin E and Ubiquinone: Competition for Binding Sites of the
Mitochondrial Cytochrome bc_1 Complex? *By* LARS GILLE, WOLFGANG
GREGOR, KATRIN STANIEK, AND HANS NOHL 341

Antioxidant Properties of Chromanols Derived from Vitamin E and
Ubiquinone. *By* WOLFGANG GREGOR, CHRISTIAN ADELWÖHRER,
THOMAS ROSENAU, GOTTFRIED GRABNER, AND LARS GILLE 344

Vitamin E in Uremia and Dialysis Patients. *By* FRANCESCO GALLI,
UMBERTO BUONCRISTIANI, CARMELA CONTE, CRISTINA AISA, AND
ARDESIO FLORIDI. 348

Oxidative Stress and Changes in α- and γ-Tocopherol Levels during
Coronary Artery Bypass Grafting. *By* A.T. ULUS, A. AKSOYEK,
M. OZKAN, S.F. KATIRCIOGLU, B. VESSBY, AND S. BASU 352

Cigarette Smoking Increases Human Vitamin E Requirements as Estimated by
Plasma Deuterium-Labeled CEHC. *By* SCOTT W. LEONARD,
RICHARD S. BRUNO, RAJASEKHAR RAMAKRISHNAN, TAMMY BRAY,
AND MARET G. TRABER 357

Effects of Vitamin E Depletion/Repletion on Biomarkers of Oxidative Stress
in Healthy Aging. *By* BRIGITTE M. WINKLHOFER-ROOB, ANDREAS
MEINITZER, MICHAELA MARITSCHNEGG, JOHANNES M. ROOB,
GHOLAMALI KHOSCHSORUR, JOSEP RIBALTA, ISABELLA SUNDL,
SANDRA WUGA, WILLIBALD WONISCH, BEATE TIRAN, AND
EDMOND ROCK FOR THE VITAGE STUDY GROUP 361

Consumption of Sesame Oil Muffins Decreases the Urinary Excretion of
γ-Tocopherol Metabolites in Humans. *By* JAN FRANK, AFAF
KAMAL-ELDIN, AND MARET G. TRABER 365

Characterization of Cellular Uptake and Distribution of Vitamin E. *By*
YOSHIRO SAITO, YASUKAZU YOSHIDA, KEIKO NISHIO, MIEKO
HAYAKAWA, AND ETSUO NIKI 368

Vitamin E Exhibits Concentration- and Vitamer-Dependent Impairment of
Microsomal Enzyme Activities. *By* T.J. SONTAG AND R.S. PARKER 376

The Decrease in γ-Tocopherol in Plasma and Lipoprotein Fractions Levels Off
within Two Days of Vitamin E Supplementation. *By* ISABELLA SUNDL,
ULRIKE RESCH, ANDREAS R. BERGMANN, JOHANNES M. ROOB, AND
BRIGITTE M. WINKLHOFER-ROOB 378

Does Aging Affect the Response of Vitamin E Status to Vitamin E Depletion
and Supplementation? *By* BRIGITTE M. WINKLHOFER-ROOB, JOHANNES
M. ROOB, MICHAELA MARITSCHNEGG, GRETE SPRINZ, DORIS HILLER,
ELISABETH MARKTFELDER, MELANIE PREINSBERGER, SANDRA WUGA,
ISABELLA SUNDL, BEATE TIRAN, NICOLAS CARDINAULT, JOSEP RIBALTA,
AND EDMOND ROCK FOR THE VITAGE STUDY GROUP 381

The Maximal Amount of α-Tocopherol Intake from Foods Alone in U.S.
Adults (1994–1996 CSFII): An Analysis by Linear Programming. *By*
XIANG GAO, PARKE E. WILDE, JANICE E. MARAS, ODILIA I. BERMUDEZ,
AND KATHERINE L. TUCKER 385

Current Status of Vitamin E Nutriture. *By* JASPREET K.C. AHUJA, JOSEPH D. GOLDMAN, AND ALANNA J. MOSHFEGH 387

γ-Tocotrienol Metabolism and Antiproliferative Effect in Prostate Cancer Cells. *By* CARMELA CONTE, ALESSANDRO FLORIDI, CRISTINA AISA, MARTA PIRODDI, ARDESIO FLORIDI, AND FRANCESCO GALLI 391

In Utero Origins of Cancer: Maternal Dietary Vitamin E, Fetal Oxidative DNA Damage, and Postnatal Carcinogenesis in p53 Knockout Mice. *By* CONNIE SHIHSIN CHEN AND PETER G. WELLS 395

γ-Tocopherol Induces Apoptosis in Androgen-Responsive LNCaP Prostate Cancer Cells via Caspase-Dependent and Independent Mechanisms. *By* QING JIANG, JEFF WONG, AND BRUCE N. AMES 399

Antiangiogenic Potency of Vitamin E. *By* TERUO MIYAZAWA, TSUYOSHI TSUZUKI, KIYOTAKA NAKAGAWA, AND MIKI IGARASHI 401

Modulation of Cell Proliferation and Gene Expression by α-Tocopheryl Phosphates: Relevance to Atherosclerosis and Inflammation. *By* ESRA OGRU, ROKSAN LIBINAKI, ROBERT GIANELLO, SIMON WEST, ADELINA MUNTEANU, JEAN-MARC ZINGG, AND ANGELO AZZI 405

Vitamin E Supplementation Reverses the Age-Associated Decrease in Effective Immune Synapse Formation in $CD4^+$ T Cells. *By* TANVIR AHMED, MELISSA MARKO, DAYONG WU, HEEKYUNG CHUNG, BRIGITTE HUBER, AND SIMIN NIKBIN MEYDANI 412

Synergistic Effect of Vitamin E and β-Carotene on the Suppression of Ovalbumin-Specific Immunoglobulin E Production in Mice. *By* NORIKO BANDO, MASAMI YAMAMOTO, RINTARO YAMANISHI, AND JUNJI TERAO 415

The Effect of Vitamin E on Secondary Bacterial Infection after Influenza Infection in Young and Old Mice. *By* RAINA GAY, SUNG NIM HAN, MELISSA MARKO, SARAH BELISLE, RODERICK BRONSON, AND SIMIN NIKBIN MEYDANI 418

Effect of Concomitant Consumption of Fish Oil and Vitamin E on Production of Inflammatory Cytokines in Healthy Elderly Humans. *By* DAYONG WU, SUNG NIM HAN, MOHSEN MEYDANI, AND SIMIN NIKBIN MEYDANI 422

Effect of Vitamin E on Prostacyclin (PGI_2) and Prostaglandin (PG) E_2 Production by Human Aorta Endothelial Cells: Mechanism of Action. *By* DAYONG WU, LIPING LIU, MOHSEN MEYDANI, AND SIMIN NIKBIN MEYDANI 425

Long-Term Vitamin E Deficiency in Mice Decreases Superoxide Radical Production in Brain. *By* SARAH L. CUDDIHY, ERIK S. MUSIEK, JASON D. MORROW, AND LAURA L. DUGAN 428

Tocopherol in Lipoproteins and Blood Cells after Cardiac Surgery. *By* M. HACQUEBARD, A. DUCART, D. SCHMARTZ, N. TEMBO, AND Y.A. CARPENTIER 432

Is *All-Rac*-α-Tocopherol Different from RRR-α-Tocopherol Regarding Cardiovascular Efficacy? A Meta-Analysis of Clinical Trials. *By* K. KRAEMER, W. KOCH, AND P.P. HOPPE 435

Evolution of Serum α-Tocopherol in the Postprandial and Postabsorptive Phases in Type 1 Diabetes Mellitus. *By* BEGOÑA MANUEL-Y-KEENOY, ANN VAN CAMPENHOUT, JAN VERTOMMEN, LUC VAN GAAL, AND IVO DE LEEUW 439

Topical α-Tocopherol Acetate in the Bulk Phase: Eight Years of Experience in Skin Treatment. *By* GIORGIO PANIN, RENATA STRUMIA, AND FULVIO URSINI 443

Appendix

Vitamin E and Health: Background and Objectives. *By* KAREN HOPKIN 449

Overview: New Roles for a Familiar Nutrient. *By* KAREN HOPKIN 455

Index of Contributors 461

Financial assistance was received from:

Cosponsors
- COGNIS NUTRITION AND HEALTH
- BASF AKTIENGESELLSCHAFT

Major Funders
- NATIONAL INSTITUTES OF HEALTH
  NATIONAL INSTITUTE OF DIBETES AND DIGESTIVE AND KIDNEY DISEASE, OFFICE OF DIETARY SUPPLEMENTS
- NATIONAL RESEARCH INITIATIVE, CSREES, UNITED STATES DEPARTMENT OF AGRICULTURE

Supporters
- ARCHER DANIELS MIDLAND
- DSM NUTRITIONAL PRODUCTS, INC.
- GLENN FOUNDATION FOR MEDICAL RESEARCH
- JEAN MAYER USDA HUMAN NUTRITION RESEARCH CENTER ON AGING AT TUFTS UNIVERSITY
- PHARMAVITE LLC
- PFIZER INC.
- ROSS INITIATIVE ON AGING AT TUFTS UNIVERSITY

Contributors
- DANONE VITAPOLE
- ENEREX BOTANICALS, LTD.
- HULKA S.R.L.
- JARROW FORMULAS/ JARROW INDUSTRIES
- JOHNSON & JOHNSON
- OXYGEN CLUB OF CALIFORNIA
- PHARMANEX

The New York Academy of Sciences believes it has a responsibility to provide an open forum for discussion of scientific questions. The positions taken by the participants in the reported conferences are their own and not necessarily those of the Academy. The Academy has no intent to influence legislation by providing such forums.

Vitamin E and Health
Preface

The last major conference devoted entirely to vitamin E was the New York Academy of Sciences' meeting held in 1988 and recorded in Volume 570 of the *Annals*, entitled *Vitamin E: Biochemistry and Health Implications* ([1989] edited by Anthony T. Diplock, Lawrence J. Machlin, Lester Packer, and William A. Pryor). This extremely successful meeting and subsequent volume set the scene in the 1990s for a number of novel functions to be identified in the family of vitamin E molecules. New information emerged regarding the role of vitamin E in the regulation of cellular signaling and gene activity. Proteins were identified that specifically bind and guide α-tocopherol to (sub)cellular destinations. In addition, the metabolism of individual tocopherols was elucidated. Tissue-specific functions of vitamin E, which could not have been predicted from the known functions of α-tocopherol, were identified by high-density oligonucleotide microarrays (GeneChips). Furthermore, information continues to emerge on the role of vitamin E in the prevention and treatment of diseases associated with oxidative stress and aging. Given all these advances in vitamin E research, we thought the time was right to convene another meeting to re-examine the present understanding of the bioavailability, metabolism, and mechanisms of action of vitamin E.

To achieve this aim, we sought to build upon the four cornerstones apparent in vitamin E research: (1) the biological importance of vitamin E in reproduction and its essentiality as a micronutrient; (2) the unique role of vitamin E as a lipophilic antioxidant in lipoproteins and cell membranes; (3) its antioxidant and non-antioxidant effects on cell signaling and gene expression; and (4) the identification of vitamin E–deficiency diseases and the recognition of the beneficial effects of vitamin E in human health and disease prevention. With these four cornerstones in mind, we invited experts from around the world to contribute to this meeting on **Vitamin E and Health**.

The first cornerstone has been appreciated for some time and was covered in detail in the 1988 meeting on vitamin E. Since then, there has been a much better appreciation of how the uptake and distribution of vitamin E is regulated in humans. To address these questions the first section of this volume, **Part I: Bioavailability and Biokinetics of Vitamin E,** reviews advances in understanding the uptake and availability of vitamin E. The second cornerstone was also covered in detail in the 1988 meeting, but since then vitamin E has been no longer thought to act alone, but rather as an important component of the antioxidant network. **Part II: Antioxidant Functions of Vitamin E** therefore deals with this concept and reviews data supporting it. **Part III: Cell Regulatory Functions of Vitamin E** relays recently obtained information on the third cornerstone. **Part IV: Protection from Oxidative Stress and Injury,** **Part V: Vitamin E and Vascular Networks,** and **Part VI: Prevention,**

Protection, and Treatment of Diseases review the action of vitamin E across a range of clinical conditions. **Part VII: Epidemiological and Intervention Studies** covers one of the most uncertain areas of vitamin E research.

On completing this formal series of papers, our aim was to synthesize an overall view on the multifunctional effects of vitamin E as an essential micronutrient. To achieve this, we held two round table discussions (**Part VIII**) with a range of eminent researchers present at the meeting. These discussions were concerned with the future directions in vitamin E research, Panel A covering preclinical research and Panel B discussing clinical research. Each of these panel discussions was used to draw together the various insights that were revealed during the conference and to formulate a plan for future activities in the field of vitamin E research. Panel A, which focused on basic research, reviewed such questions as: What does vitamin E do in the body? What is its active form? What biomarkers should researchers measure to track oxidative stress, inflammation, and the progression of disease? Panel B, which focused on clinical trials, continued the discussion of biomarkers. In addition, panelists in this session addressed whether vitamin E should be studied in combination with other supplements, reviewed the status of ongoing clinical trials, and pondered the question of whether the research community is ready to accept a study that demonstrates that vitamin E can prevent human disease. We believe that both sessions achieved their goals and we extend our thanks to all the panel members involved.

Just prior to the publication of this volume, E.R. Miller and colleagues (Ann. Intern. Med. **142:** 37–46 [2005]) published a meta-analysis in which they concluded that use of greater than 400 IU vitamin E supplements was associated with increased patient mortality. This publication has already incurred much comment, including a plethora of letters to the same journal, many of which question possible selection bias and the statistical approach. Given the seriousness of this issue, it now needs to be examined in detail by other groups and an independent panel of experts. Whatever the outcome, it is clear that there are still many challenges and unanswered questions in the vitamin E research arena. Indeed we are looking forward to the next New York Academy of Sciences meeting on this important micronutrient.

We would like to thank BASF Aktiengesellschaft and Cognis Nutrition and Health for co-sponsoring the meeting along other contributors including the National Institutes of Health; the National Research Initiative, CSREES; Archer Daniels Midland; Danone Vitapole; DSM Nutritional Products, Inc.; Enerex Botanicals, Ltd.; Glenn Foundation for Medical Research; HULKA S.R.L.; Jarrow Formulas, Jarrow Industries; Johnson & Johnson; the Oxygen Club of California; Pharmanex; Pharmavite LLC; and the Ross Initiative on Aging at Tufts University. We are grateful for the warm hospitality extended to us by our hosts, the Jean Mayer USDA Human Nutrition Research Center on Aging at Tufts University and the staff of the New York Academy of Sciences who helped to organize the meeting, to prepare an early eBriefing so that much of the material would be available on the web within weeks of the conference, and to see this publication—the complete record of the proceedings—through the press. Finally, our thanks are extended to the colleagues and friends who attended the meeting, contributed to the vigorous discussions that led to critical insights of vitamin E research, and provided manuscripts for this volume.

Finally, as an appendix to this volume, we've included Karen Hopkin's journalistic report on the conference, which includes background material for the nonspecialist. We also invite you to visit the eBriefing posted for this meeting <http://www.nyas.org/vite> for additional material from the conference, including Open Questions, complete audio and slides of many speakers' presentations, audio of the culminating round-table discussions on future directions of preclinical and clinical research, and links to web and print resources on the subject.

—FRANK KELLY
—MOHSEN MEYDANI
—LESTER PACKER

Vitamin E Trafficking

MARET G. TRABER,[a] GRAHAM W. BURTON,[b] AND ROBERT L. HAMILTON[c]

[a]Linus Pauling Institute, Oregon State University, Corvallis, Oregon 97331, USA

[b]Occell, Inc., Ottawa, Ontario K1B 5B0, Canada

[c]Department of Anatomy, Cardiovascular Research Institute, University of California, San Francisco, California 94143, USA

ABSTRACT: The α-tocopherol transfer protein (α-TTP) is required to prevent vitamin E deficiency in humans and in α-TTP null mice. Whereas α-TTP is not required to facilitate intestinal absorption of vitamin E, it is required to maintain normal α-tocopherol concentrations in plasma and extrahepatic tissues. α-Tocopherol secretion from the liver in very low density lipoproteins (VLDLs) is impaired in humans with a defect in the α-TTP gene. In perfusions of isolated cynomolgus monkey livers, VLDLs were preferentially enriched in RRR-α-tocopherol. The mechanism by which α-TTP incorporates α-tocopherol into nascent VLDLs is the topic of this report. VLDL assembly is a multistep secretory process that occurs within the membrane compartments of the endoplasmic reticulum and Golgi apparatus. Thus, we postulated that α-TTP might transfer α-tocopherol onto nascent VLDLs either in the endoplasmic reticulum or in the Golgi apparatus. To test these possibilities, we isolated nascent VLDLs from highly purified RER and Golgi apparatus membrane fractions from livers of rats fed equimolar ratios of RRR- and SRR-α-tocopherols labeled with different amounts of deuterium. Although the plasma was enriched in RRR-α-tocopherol 14 hours after the dose, no enrichment of nascent VLDL precursors from either of the secretory compartments was detected, indicating that VLDL enrichment with α-tocopherol may occur as a post-VLDL secretory process. Therefore, we hypothesize that α-TTP may facilitate movement of α-tocopherol to the hepatocyte plasma membrane (by unknown mechanisms) where newly secreted, nascent VLDLs could acquire both α-tocopherol and unesterified cholesterol while within the space of Disse. Clearly, critical information is lacking in our understanding of the mechanism by which α-TTP facilitates the preferential enrichment of VLDLs with α-tocopherol.

KEYWORDS: α-tocopherol transfer protein; very low density lipoproteins; endoplasmic reticulum; Golgi apparatus; liver

INTRODUCTION

Vitamin E transport in circulating plasma lipoproteins was described more than 40 years ago.[1,2] Because vitamin E readily exchanges and equilibrates between lipoproteins,[3] it was not obvious that a specific protein was required for the incorpora-

Address for correspondence: Maret G. Traber, Ph.D., Linus Pauling Institute, Oregon State University, Corvallis, OR 97331-6512. Voice: 541-737-7977; fax: 541-737-5077.
maret.traber@oregonstate.edu

tion of vitamin E into lipoproteins. Subsequently, the α-tocopherol transfer protein (α-TTP) was demonstrated to be necessary for maintaining plasma α-tocopherol concentrations based on studies in α-TTP null mice.[4,5] In humans after oral administration of deuterium-labeled vitamin E homologues, intestinal absorption and chylomicron secretion, all of the forms of vitamin E appeared similarly in plasma and were distributed to all of the circulating lipoproteins.[6–9] Less than 12 hours after the oral dose, the plasma became enriched in *RRR*–α-tocopherol, the naturally occurring vitamin E homologue with the highest biologic activity. Importantly, the first lipoprotein that that was preferentially enriched in *RRR*–α-tocopherol was nascent very low density lipoprotein (VLDL).[6,8]

HEPATIC α-TTP

The hepatic mechanism for the preferential secretion of *RRR*–α-tocopherol compared with other dietary vitamin E forms, or with synthetic α-tocopherol, is also a result of the function of the hepatic α-TTP. Human subjects with an abnormality in the gene for α-TTP (the disorder is termed "ataxia with vitamin E deficiency"[AVED])[10] or mice generated to lack α-TTP[4,11] are vitamin E–deficient. Studies in α-TTP null mice also demonstrated that they were unable to distinguish between natural and synthetic vitamin E (*RRR* and *all-rac*–α-tocopherols).[11] Moreover, AVED patients were unable to distinguish between *RRR* and *SRR*–α-tocopherols; two forms of α-tocopherol that only differ in chirality at the C2 position of α-tocopherol, where the tail and rings meet. Preferential enrichment of plasma lipoproteins with *RRR*–α-tocopherol has been consistently observed in rats,[12–14] guinea pigs,[15] salmon,[16] monkeys,[17] and in humans, both in normal subjects [8,9,18] and in patients with genetic abnormalities of lipoprotein metabolism.[9]

In studies of humans consuming deuterated vitamin E, chylomicrons have been shown to transport both d_6-*RRR*- and d_3-*SRR*–α-tocopherols.[8,9] Ingold *et al.*[12] demonstrated, that after long-term feeding of these two different isotopic forms to rats, the serum and all other tissues were preferentially enriched in *RRR*–α-tocopherol. However, the liver was exceptional in that the *RRR*/*SRR* ratio equaled approximately 1. Interestingly, the liver, which is the organ involved in the preferential enrichment of plasma and tissues with *RRR*–α-tocopherol, does not become enriched itself with *RRR*–α-tocopherol. Indeed, α-TTP null mice have plasma and tissue α-tocopherol concentrations 5–20% of wild-type littermates but have liver α-tocopherol concentrations that are approximately 50% of wild types.[4,11] These data emphasize that α-TTP is not required for delivery of dietary vitamin E to the liver, but it is required for α-tocopherol secretion from the liver into the plasma for maintenance of normal plasma and extrahepatic tissue α-tocopherol concentrations.

α-TTP has been purified to homogeneity from rat[19,20] and human liver,[21,22] and their amino acid sequences have been reported.[22,23] All of the following features of vitamin E are required for recognition and transfer by α-TTP:)1) the fully methylated, intact chromanol ring with a free 6-OH group; (2) the presence of the phytyl side chain; and (3) the stereochemical configuration of the phytyl tail in the 2*R*-position.[19] α-TTP transfers α-tocopherol in preference to other vitamin E forms between liposomes and microsomes.[19] These structural requirements have now been documented using mutant α-TTP [24] and using coordinates from the α-TTP crystal structure.[25,26]

In vitro, purified α-TTP transfers α-tocopherol from liposomes to microsomes.[19,22,27] In addition, Burton and Ingold[28] reported that partially purified α-TTP is preferentially enriched with *RRR*–α-tocopherol when isolated from rats fed differently deuterium-labeled *RRR*- and *SRR*–α-tocopherols. This ability to recognize and to transfer α-tocopherol suggests that α-TTP is likely responsible for the incorporation of *RRR*–α-tocopherol into VLDLs. Indeed, when cynomolgus monkeys were fed differently deuterium-labeled γ- and *RRR*– and *SRR*–α-tocopherols, the VLDLs isolated from their liver perfusates were preferentially enriched in *RRR*–α-tocopherol.[17]

BILIARY VITAMIN E EXCRETION

Vitamin E that is not secreted into the plasma is likely excreted because the liver does not accumulate "toxic" amounts of vitamin E. The consensus of opinion is that

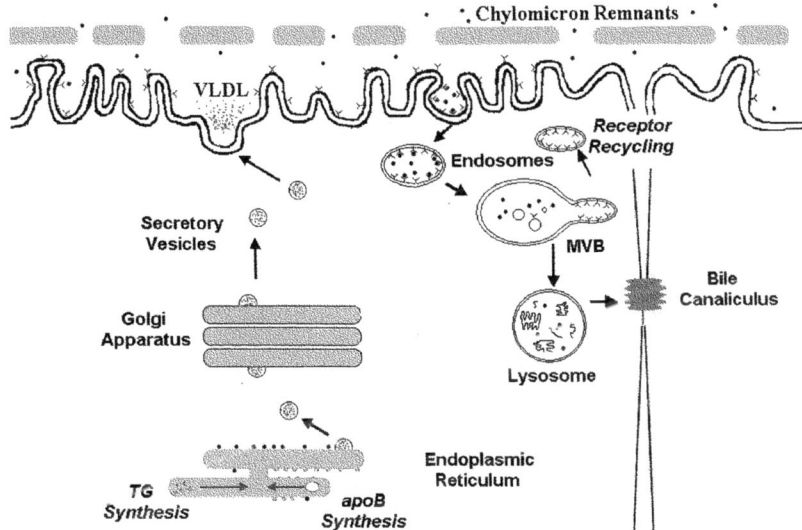

FIGURE 1. Scheme of chylomicron remnant uptake and hydrolysis and VLDL synthesis. Dietary vitamin E enters hepatocytes in chylomicron remnants through a receptor-mediated process, and the receptors return to the plasma membrane, while the contents of the endosomes are digested. If "excess α-tocopherol" or other dietary vitamin E forms are delivered to the liver, apparently the default pathway for hepatic vitamin E trafficking is into the endosomal/lysosomal pathway with ultimate vitamin E excretion from the lysosomes into bile. The newly acquired dietary lipids released from the chylomicrons are repackaged into VLDL. Synthesis of both triacyglycerides (TG) and apoB occurs in the endoplasmic reticulum; these nascent particles are exported to the Golgi apparatus and then to the plasma membrane. There are several potential locations where VLDLs could become enriched with *RRR*–α-tocopherol, but two of these have been ruled out. α-TTP does not appear to transfer α-tocopherol into nascent VLDLs during assembly at (1) the RER with apo B or with triacylglycerides, as core lipids are assembled, or (2) the Golgi apparatus, as the nascent VLP are further modified.

dietary vitamin E enters hepatocytes in chylomicron remnants through a receptor-mediated process that ultimately delivers the remnants to lysosomes (see FIG. 1).[29] The receptors involved in remnant uptake include the LDL receptor and the LDL receptor–related protein (LRP).[29] Studies in rats using LDL conjugated with colloidal gold to follow the intrahepatic catabolic pathway showed evidence that secondary lysosomes slowly empty their contents into bile.[30] Similarly, ^{14}C-labeled α-tocopherol was used to show that approximately 14% of the dose was excreted into bile.[31] Moreover, studies in humans examining the vitamin E content of bile showed that both α- and γ-tocopherol were excreted in bile.[32] Mustacich et al.[33] demonstrated that a member of the ATP (adenosine triphosphate) binding cassette family of transporters (ABCB4), *p*-glycoprotein (the gene product of human MDR3, or mouse mdr2), mediates the simultaneous secretion of both phospholipids and tocopherols into bile. Thus, if "excess α-tocopherol" or other dietary vitamin E forms are delivered to the liver via chylomicron remnants, apparently the default pathway for hepatic vitamin E trafficking is into the endosomal/lysosomal pathway with ultimate vitamin E excretion from the lysosomes into bile. Additionally, vitamin E may be metabolized to carboxyethyl hydroxychromans (CEHCs) by hepatocytes,[34] but discussion of metabolism is beyond the scope of this review.

VLDL ENRICHMENT WITH *RRR*–α-TOCOPHEROL

Mechanisms for VLDL Lipidation

Because VLDL apparently is the lipoprotein that is involved in α-tocopherol transport from the liver, it is important to consider how VLDL might acquire α-tocopherol. Whereas VLDL assembly is recognized as a multistep process, it has been hypothesized that the "core lipids" (triacylglycerides and cholesteryl esters) are combined with apolipoprotein B (apoB) by a "two-step mechanism" in the endoplasmic reticulum (see FIG. 1).[35,36] This model of nascent VLDL assembly proposes that initially small amounts of core lipids become associated with RER membrane-bound apoB, facilitating its dissociation from the membrane to release a small "first-step" particle within the RER lumenal compartment. Independently, a larger full-sized triglyceride-rich particle is assembled within the ribosomal-free smooth terminal ends of the RER (smooth ER). The microsomal triglyceride transfer protein (MTP) appears to be important for both "first- and second-step" particle formation.[37] Subsequently, the separately synthesized particles then coalesce to form nascent VLDLs. These completed nascent VLDLs are transported from the RER to the Golgi apparatus. Subsequently, Golgi secretory vesicles containing nascent VLDL exocytose at the plasma membrane, where VLDL is released into the space of Disse.

The mechanism by which VLDL become enriched with *RRR*–α-tocopherol is unknown. VLDL assembly does not depend on vitamin E incorporation; however, the importance of vitamin E function as an antioxidant to protect polyunsaturated lipids from oxidation support the need for identifying the mechanism for incorporation of vitamin E in VLDL. Clearly, α-TTP is necessary for this process, but where and how VLDL acquires vitamin E remains a mystery.

To localize the site of VLDL enrichment with *RRR*–α-tocopherol, we sought to determine where the subcellular paths of α-tocopherol trafficking and VLDL assembly become coincident. There are several potential intracellular locations where VLDL could become enriched with *RRR*–α-tocopherol. α-TTP could transfer α-tocopherol into nascent VLDL from the endosome/multivesicular bodies/lysosome: (1) in the RER with apo B or with triacylglycerides, as core lipids are assembled, or (2) in the Golgi apparatus, as the VLDLs are further modified. To investigate these possibilities, we isolated nascent VLDL particles at various stages of maturation from rats fed equimolar ratios of d_6-*RRR*–α- and d_3-*SRR*–α-tocopherols.

Deuterated Tocopherols and Their Analysis

SRR–α-5-(C^2H_3) tocopheryl (d_3-*SRR*–α-tocopheryl) and *RRR*–α-5,7-(C^2H_3)$_2$tocopheryl (d_6-*RRR*–α-tocopheryl) acetates were prepared at the NRC Canada. The internal standard used for α-T analysis, 2-*ambo*-α-5,7,8-(C^2H_3)$_3$ α-T (d_9-α-T), was synthesized previously.[12,14,38,39] The d_6-*RRR*- and d_3-*SRR*–α-tocopheryl acetates (1:1 ratio) were dissolved in tocopherol-stripped corn oil (Dyets, Bethlehem, PA).

Plasma, liver homogenate, and organelle labeled and unlabeled α-tocopherols were extracted and analyzed by gas chromatography/mass spectrometry as described previously.[40] Concentrations of d_0-, d_3-, and d_6-α- tocopherols were calculated from the peak areas of the corresponding parent ions in the mass spectrum relative to that of the d_9-α-tocopherol internal standard, after making corrections for the isotopic purities of each deuterated α-tocopherol. The initial *RRR/SRR* molar ratio was determined to be 0.96 ± 0.007.

Animals

The animal care, handling, and experimental procedures were conducted in accordance with the protocol approved by Animal Care and Use Committee of the University of California, San Francisco. Male Sprague Dawley rats (approximately 350 g) were fasted 24 h and then hand-fed bread with 100 μl of tocopherol stripped corn oil containing deuterated vitamin E (d_6-*RRR*- and d_3-*SRR*–α-tocopheryl acetates; approximately 2.5 mg total vitamin E; or 50 mg/kg body weight). Rats then were allowed food and water *ad libitum* after vitamin E administration. This protocol ensured that the rats ate the vitamin E when it was presented to them. No anesthesia was required. Approximately 7 or 14 h later, the rats were exsanguinated under ether anesthesia, and their livers were removed for homogenization. Note that we conducted a feeding study rather than to incorporate the labeled vitamin E into an intravenous emulsion because the mode of delivery of vitamin E in chylomicron remnants may be critical for its subsequent packaging into lipoproteins.[41] The rats were fed the deuterated tocopherols and killed either 7 or 14 h later for RER VLDL isolation or 14 h later for Golgi isolation.

RER VLDL Enrichment with d_6-RRR–α-Tocopherol

Hepatocytic rat liver RER membranes and nascent pre-VLDL particles were isolated as described previously.[42] This method uses rapid calcium precipitation to isolate a ribosomal-rich membrane fraction by a nonultracentrifugal technique.[36] The isolated RER fraction is highly enriched in ER markers such as glucose-6-phosphatase, acylCoA cholesterol acyltransferase (ACAT), diacylglycerol acyltrans-

TABLE 1. Rat serum and liver homogenate vitamin E concentrations after a 1:1 dose of d_6-RRR-/d_3-SRR-α-tocopheryl acetates

	Experiment 1 RER Isolation (n = 3)		Experiment 2 RER Isolation (n = 3)		Experiment 3 Golgi Isolation (n = 24)	
	Serum	Liver Homogenate	Serum	Liver Homogenate	Serum	Liver Homogenate
Time after dosing (h)	7	7	14	14	14	14
d_0-α-tocopherol (nmol/ml)	12.9 ± 1.5	14.8 ± 3.6	16.2 ± 1.9	26.2 ± 2.2	16.1 ± 3.2	24.4 ± 5.3
d_3-SRR-α-tocopherol (nmol/ml)	1.46 ± 0.11	5.74 ± 1.12	0.97 ± 0.23	2.21 ± 0.17	0.61 ± 0.25	2.44 ± 1.62
d_6-RRR-α-tocopherol (nmol/ml)	5.00 ± 0.62	4.35 ± 0.98	2.90 ± 0.21	2.21 ± 0.47	2.80 ± 1.16	2.37 ± 1.03
d_6-RRR/d_3-SRR	3.60 ± 0.17	0.79 ± 0.03	3.21 ± 0.47	1.06 ± 0.24	4.64 ± 0.98	1.06 ± 0.23

ferase (DGAT), and MTP activities but only contains small quantities of markers for plasma membranes, endosomes, mitochondria, and Golgi membranes.[35] ApoB100 and apoB48 (identified by Western blotting with rat apoB antisera) are present in this RER fraction, as components of putative apoB-containing "first-step" small (~15–25 nm diameter) lipoprotein particles mixed with apoB-free triglyceride-rich "second-step" larger (~35-85nm) particles together with completed nascent VLDL particles (R. L. Hamilton *et al.*, unpublished studies).

In rats, the extent of enrichment of serum, liver, and RER lipid-containing particles with d_6-RRR–α-tocopherol after administration of a single dose of d_6-RRR- and d_3-SRR tocopheryl acetates (1:1) was measured. In one experiment, the rats were killed 7 h after dosing with deuterated vitamin E, and in a second experiment they were killed after 14 h. In both of these experiments, rat serum was similarly enriched with RRR–α-tocopherol (d_6-RRR:d_3-SRR ratio >3), whereas the liver d_6-RRR: d_3-SRR ratio was ~1 (TABLE 1). Similar results regarding the d_6-RRR:d_3-SRR ratio in the RER and its contents were obtained in both experiments; the data from the 14-h experiment (n = 3 rats per experiment) is shown in FIGURE 2. Although the nascent VLDL (d < 1.006) and the pre-VLDL particles (d = 1.024 and 1.053) were enriched with RRR compared with the liver homogenate, the d_6-RRR:d_3-SRR ratio was less than the ratio found in the serum. We anticipated that the precursors of serum vitamin E should have a higher ratio than in serum; therefore, we examined subsequent steps in the assembly of VLDL.

Golgi VLDL Enrichment with d_6-RRR–α-Tocopherol

Golgi apparatus membranes were isolated from rat livers virtually free of endosomal contamination as described previously.[43] Golgi membranes were isolated as "intact" stacks of cisternae and secretory vesicles. Golgi membrane contents were released using a French pressure cell followed by isolation of nascent VLDL particles by ultracentrifugation as described.[43]

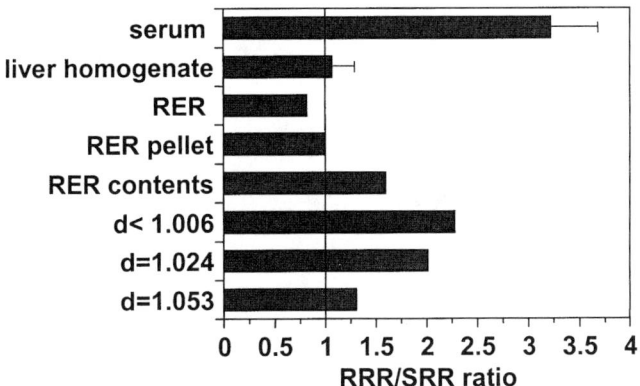

FIGURE 2. Lack of preferential incorporation of *RRR*–α-tocopherol in RER VLDL. Rats ($n = 3$ rats) were killed 14 h after a single dose of deuterated vitamin E (d_6-*RRR*:d_3*SRR* tocopheryl acetates, 1:1 ratio, total of 50 mg/kg body weight) administered orally with food. The extent of d_6-*RRR*–α-tocopherol-enrichment of serum, liver, and RER lipid-containing particles was evaluated. Although the nascent VLDL ($d < 1.006$) and the pre-VLDL particles ($d = 1.024$ and 1.053) were enriched with *RRR*-, the d_6-*RRR*: d_3*SRR* ratio was less than that of the serum compared with the liver homogenate. Thus, the data do not demonstrate preferential enrichment of VLDL with *RRR* as compared with *SRR*, as would be expected if α-TTP loaded VLDL precursors with d_6-*RRR*–α-tocopherol.

Using the same feeding protocol as described above, rats ($n = 24$) were fed a single dose of 1:1 d_6-*RRR*:d_3-*SRR* tocopheryl acetates and then were killed 14 h later to examine nascent VLDL isolated from the Golgi apparatus. As shown in FIGURE 3, the liver homogenate and Golgi VLDL had d_6-*RRR*:d_3-*SRR* ratios nearly equal to 1. These experiments also demonstrate that the serum, but not the liver homogenate or the Golgi VLDL is enriched in the d_6-*RRR*–α-tocopherol. The serum contained five times as much d_6-*RRR*–α-tocopherol, whereas nascent VLDL isolated from either RER or Golgi were not enriched with d_6-*RRR*- compared with d_3-*SRR*–α-tocopherol. Thus, it is clear that α-TTP facilitated preferential enrichment of the serum with d_6-*RRR*-α-tocopherol, but without enrichment of Golgi VLDL. Importantly, Arita *et al.*[44] demonstrated that overexpression of α-TTP in McArH7777 rat tumor cells increased α-tocopherol secretion. They used brefeldin A, at concentrations which completely disrupted the ER/Golgi secretory pathway, to prevent triglyceride secretion and found that α-tocopherol secretion was unimpaired. Their tissue culture data, when taken together with the studies presented here of the α-tocopherol content of ER and Golgi nascent VLDL precursors, strongly suggest that α-tocopherol must be secreted from liver independently from VLDL. However, neither of these studies eliminates postsecretory nascent VLDL as the physiologic α-tocopherol acceptor.

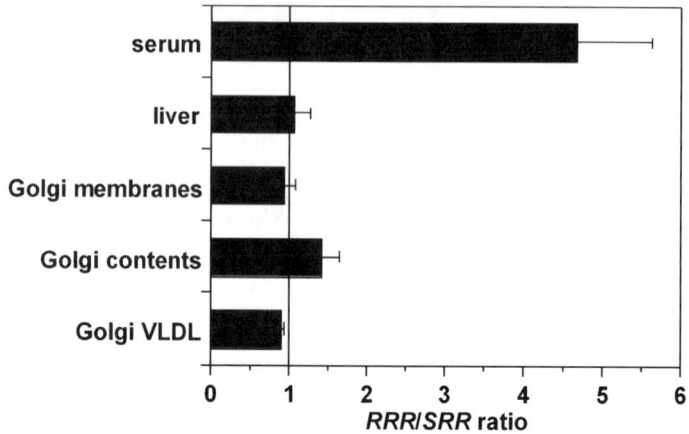

FIGURE 3. Lack of preferential incorporation of RRR–α-tocopherol in Golgi VLDL. Rats ($n = 24$ rats) were killed 14 h after a single dose of deuterated vitamin E (d_6-*RRR*: d_3-*SRR*–α-tocopheryl acetates, 1:1 ratio, total of 50 mg/kg body weight) administered orally with food. The extent of d_6-*RRR*–α-tocopherol enrichment of serum, liver, and Golgi lipid-containing particles was evaluated. The data do not demonstrate preferential enrichment of Golgi VLDL with d_6-*RRR*–α-tocopherol.

VLDL ENRICHMENT WITH α-TOCOPHEROL ACQUIRED FROM THE PLASMA MEMBRANE

It remains to be elucidated how the α-TTP–dependent mechanism results in VLDL enrichment with *RRR*–α-tocopherol. One possibility is that α-tocopherol and free cholesterol are incorporated into nascent VLDL by an analogous mechanism. It has been shown, for example, that nascent Golgi VLDLs differ from those of plasma (and perfused liver VLDLs) in that Golgi VLDLs contain one-fifth as much unesterified cholesterol compared with plasma VLDLs, but twice as much phospholipid, whereas Golgi VLDLs and plasma VLDLs contained virtually the same amounts of cholesteryl esters and triacylglycerides.[41] These findings strongly suggest that the bulk of unesterified cholesterol in plasma VLDLs is acquired after exocytosis of nascent VLDLs from the liver has occurred. Similarly, α-TTP may facilitate movement of α-tocopherol to the hepatocyte plasma membrane where newly secreted, nascent VLDL could acquire both α-tocopherol and unesterified cholesterol. Certainly, both α-tocopherol and unesterified cholesterol spontaneously transfer from membranes to lipoproteins.[3] Alternatively, the ATP binding cassette transporter, ABCA1, not only transfers cholesterol from membranes to apoAI (HDL),[45] but also has been shown to enrich HDL with vitamin E.[46] It is plausible that HDL then could spontaneously transfer α-tocopherol to VLDL because more α-tocopherol is transferred from HDL to VLDL than the reverse direction.[47] In addition, the transfer of vitamin E between HDL and apoB-containing lipoproteins could be potentiated by the plasma phospholipid transfer protein (PLTP).[48] However, studies from PLTP null mice[49] and PLTP overexpressing mice[50] suggest that PLTP serves to move α-tocopherol from VLDL to HDL; thus, it is unlikely to be involved in VLDL α-tocopherol enrichment.

Although membrane α-tocopherol might spontaneously enrich VLDL, the problem remains as to "how does the plasma membrane become enriched with α-tocopherol?"

INTRAENDOSOMAL α-TOCOPHEROL TRAFFICKING

Recently, Horiguchi et al.[51] reported that α-TTP is most abundant as a cytosolic protein in hepatocytes. However, after chloroquine treatment, which is known to disrupt the acidic pH of the endosomal organelles, significant amounts of α-TTP became associated with the cytosolic surface of late endosomes. They suggest that α-TTP translocates from the cytosol to late endosomes to acquire α-tocopherol and then α-TTP–α-tocopherol moves to the plasma membrane where α-TTP releases α-tocopherol to the membrane.[51] These findings suggest that chylomicron remnant– or LDL–α-tocopherol, after receptor-mediated uptake, could be released from the lipoprotein during hydrolysis in an early endosomal compartment and could remain with the sorting endosome as it matures into a late endosome. However, release of α-tocopherol from lipoproteins would most likely enrich the inner leaflet of the membrane. Zha et al.[52] have reported that ABCA1 in the endosomal compartment also plays a role in endocytosis by acting as a flippase to translocate phosphatidyl serine to the outer membrane and potentiate membrane budding. Because ABCA1 can also transfer α-tocopherol,[46] ABCA1 could enrich the outer membrane of the endocytic vesicles with both *RRR*– and *SRR*–α-tocopherols; α-TTP could then preferentially remove *RRR*–α-tocopherol from the outer leaflet of the endosomal membrane for transfer to the plasma membrane, where again it would need a flippase to transfer to the outer leaflet of the membrane. Clearly, the ordered cholesterol domains of both the endosomal and plasma membranes[53] suggest that a flippase is needed to orient α-tocopherol to the appropriate sides for uptake by α-TTP and nascent VLDL, respectively. The *p*-glycoprotein MDR3/mdr2 (ABCB4) has been shown to play this role in secretion of vitamin E into bile.[33] It remains to be clarified as to whether ABCA1 participates in α-tocopherol transfer directly to and from α-TTP, as was suggested by Horiguchi et al.,[51] or if some other transporters/flippases are also involved in α-tocopherol trafficking.

CONCLUSION

It is apparent that after receptor-mediated endocytosis of chylomicron remnants by the liver, there is vitamin E release from lipoproteins within the endocytic compartment. In the absence of α-TTP, α-tocopherol is not secreted back into the plasma. Excess vitamin E is not accumulated in the liver, but is excreted, mostly in bile, via a *p*-glycoprotein (ABCB4)–mediated process. In the presence of α-TTP, *RRR*–α-tocopherol ultimately is transferred to nascent VLDL. Based on the available evidence, the most likely mechanism for *RRR*–α-tocopherol secretion from the liver requires the specific function of α-TTP to transfer *RRR*–α-tocopherol from the endosomal membranes (by a pathway as yet undefined) to the plasma membrane. Once RRR-α-tocopherol is on the outer leaflet of the plasma membrane, nascent VLDLs within the space of Disse could spontaneously acquire α-tocopherol. Clearly, critical information is lacking in our understanding of precisely how α-TTP facilitates the preferential enrichment of VLDL with α-tocopherol. Because vitamin E deficiency occurs if the secretion of α-tocopherol facilitated by hepatic α-TTP does not occur, the elucidation of this pathway is critical for our understanding of human vitamin E nutrition.

ACKNOWLEDGMENTS

Shoshana Walcott and Malgorzata Daroszewski provided excellent technical assistance. This study was supported in part by gifts from the NSVEA and Henkel.

REFERENCES

1. LEWIS, L.A., M.L. QUAIFE & I.H. PAGE. 1954. Lipoproteins of serum, carriers of tocopherol. Am. J. Physiol. **178:** 221–222.
2. MCCORMICK, E.C., D.G. CORNWELL & J.B. BROWN. 1960. Studies on the distribution of tocopherol in human serum lipoproteins. J. Lipid Res. **1:** 221–228.
3. BJORNSON, L.K., C. GNIEWKOWSKI & H.J. KAYDEN. 1975. Comparison of exchange of α-tocopherol and free cholesterol between rat plasma lipoproteins and erythrocytes. J. Lipid Res. **16:** 39–53.
4. TERASAWA, Y., Z. LADHA, S.W. LEONARD, *et al.* 2000. Increased atherosclerosis in hyperlipidemic mice deficient in alpha-tocopherol transfer protein and vitamin E. Proc. Natl. Acad. Sci. USA **97:** 13830–13834.
5. YOKOTA, T., K. IGARASHI, T. UCHIHARA, *et al.* 2001. Delayed-onset ataxia in mice lacking alpha-tocopherol transfer protein: model for neuronal degeneration caused by chronic oxidative stress. Proc. Natl. Acad. Sci. USA **98:** 15185–15190.
6. TRABER, M.G., K.U. INGOLD, G.W. BURTON, *et al.* 1988. Absorption and transport of deuterium-substituted 2R,4'R,8'R-α-tocopherol in human lipoproteins. Lipids **23:** 791–797.
7. TRABER, M.G., R.J. SOKOL, G.W. BURTON, *et al.* 1990. Impaired ability of patients with familial isolated vitamin E deficiency to incorporate alpha-tocopherol into lipoproteins secreted by the liver. J. Clin. Invest. **85:** 397–407.
8. TRABER, M.G., G.W. BURTON, K.U. INGOLD, *et al.* 1990. RRR- and SRR-alpha-tocopherols are secreted without discrimination in human chylomicrons, but RRR-alpha-tocopherol is preferentially secreted in very low density lipoproteins. J. Lipid Res. **31:** 675–685.
9. TRABER, M.G., G.W. BURTON, L. HUGHES, *et al.* 1992. Discrimination between forms of vitamin E by humans with and without genetic abnormalities of lipoprotein metabolism. J. Lipid Res. **33:** 1171–1182.
10. CAVALIER, L., K. OUAHCHI, H.J. KAYDEN, *et al.* 1998. Ataxia with isolated vitamin E deficiency: heterogeneity of mutations and phenotypic variability in a large number of families. Am. J. Hum. Genet. **62:** 301–310.
11. LEONARD, S.W., Y. TERASAWA, R.V. FARESE, JR., *et al.* 2002. Incorporation of deuterated *RRR*- and *all rac* α–tocopherols into plasma and tissues of α–tocopherol transfer protein deficient mice. Am. J. Clin. Nutr. **75:** 555–560.
12. INGOLD, K.U., G.W. BURTON, D.O. FOSTER, *et al.* 1987. Biokinetics of and discrimination between dietary RRR- and SRR-alpha-tocopherols in the male rat. Lipids **22:** 163–172.
13. CHENG, S.C., G.W. BURTON, K.U. INGOLD, *et al.* 1987. Chiral discrimination in the exchange of α-tocopherol stereoisomers between plasma and red blood cells. Lipids **22:** 469–473.

14. BURTON, G.W., K.U. INGOLD, D.O. FOSTER, et al. 1988. Comparison of free alpha-tocopherol and alpha-tocopheryl acetate as sources of vitamin E in rats and humans. Lipids 23: 834–840.
15. BURTON, G.W., U. WRONSKA, L. STONE, et al. 1990. Biokinetics of dietary RRR-α-tocopherol in the male guinea pig at three dietary levels of vitamin C and two levels of vitamin E. Evidence that vitamin C does not "spare" vitamin E in vivo. Lipids 25: 199–210.
16. PARAZO, M.P., S.P. LALL, J.D. CASTELL, et al. 1998. Distribution of alpha- and gamma-tocopherols in Atlantic salmon (Salmo salar) tissues. Lipids 33: 697–704.
17. TRABER, M.G., L.L. RUDEL, G.W. BURTON, et al. 1990. Nascent VLDL from liver perfusions of cynomolgus monkeys are preferentially enriched in RRR- compared with SRR-α tocopherol: studies using deuterated tocopherols. J. Lipid Res. 31: 687–694.
18. TRABER, M.G., R.J. SOKOL, A. KOHLSCHÜTTER, et al. 1993. Impaired discrimination between stereoisomers of α-tocopherol in patients with familial isolated vitamin E deficiency. J. Lipid Res. 34: 201–210.
19. SATO, Y., K. HAGIWARA, H. ARAI, et al. 1991. Purification and characterization of the alpha-tocopherol transfer protein from rat liver. FEBS Lett. 288: 41–45.
20. YOSHIDA, H., M. YUSIN, I. REN, et al. 1992. Identification, purification, and immunochemical characterization of a tocopherol-binding protein in rat liver cytosol. J. Lipid Res. 33: 343–350.
21. KUHLENKAMP, J., M. RONK, M. YUSIN, et al. 1993. Identification and purification of a human liver cytosolic tocopherol binding protein. Protein Expr. Purif. 4: 382–389.
22. ARITA, M., Y. SATO, A. MIYATA, et al. 1995. Human alpha-tocopherol transfer protein: cDNA cloning, expression and chromosomal localization. Biochem. J. 306: 437–443.
23. SATO, Y., H. ARAI, A. MIYATA, et al. 1993. Primary structure of alpha-tocopherol transfer protein from rat liver. Homology with cellular retinaldehyde-binding protein. J. Biol. Chem. 268: 17705–17710.
24. MORLEY, S., C. PANAGABKO, D. SHINEMAN, et al. 2004. Molecular determinants of heritable vitamin E deficiency. Biochemistry 43: 4143–4149.
25. MIN, K.C., R.A. KOVALL & W.A. HENDRICKSON. 2003. Crystal structure of human α-tocopherol transfer protein bound to its ligand: implications for ataxia with vitamin E deficiency. Proc. Natl. Acad. Sci. USA 100: 14713–14718.
26. MEIER, R., T. TOMIZAKI, C. SCHULZE-BRIESE, et al. 2003. The molecular basis of vitamin E retention: structure of human alpha-tocopherol transfer protein. J. Mol. Biol. 331: 725–734.
27. HOSOMI, A., M. ARITA, Y. SATO, et al. 1997. Affinity for alpha-tocopherol transfer protein as a determinant of the biological activities of vitamin E analogs. FEBS Lett. 409: 105–108.
28. BURTON, G.W. & K.U. INGOLD. 1993. Biokinetics of vitamin E using deuterated tocopherols. In Vitamin E in Health and Disease. L. Packer & J. Fuchs, Eds.: 329–344. Marcel Dekker. New York.
29. HAVEL, R.J. & R.L. HAMILTON. 2004. Hepatic catabolism of remnant lipoproteins: where the action is. Arterioscler. Thromb. Vasc. Biol. 24: 213–215.
30. RENAUD, G., R.L. HAMILTON & R.J. HAVEL. 1989. Hepatic metabolism of colloidal gold-low-density lipoprotein complexes in the rat: evidence for bulk excretion of lysosomal contents into bile. Hepatology 9: 380–392.
31. BJORNEBOE, A., G.E. BJORNEBOE & C.A. DREVON. 1987. Serum half-life, distribution, hepatic uptake and biliary excretion of alpha-tocopherol in rats. Biochim. Biophys. Acta 921: 175–181.
32. TRABER, M.G. & H.J. KAYDEN. 1989. Preferential incorporation of alpha-tocopherol vs gamma-tocopherol in human lipoproteins. Am. J. Clin. Nutr. 49: 517–526.
33. MUSTACICH, D.J., J. SHIELDS, R.A. HORTON, et al. 1998. Biliary secretion of alpha-tocopherol and the role of the mdr2 P-glycoprotein in rats and mice. Arch. Biochem. Biophys. 350: 183–192.
34. BRIGELIUS-FLOHÉ, R. & M.G. TRABER. 1999. Vitamin E: function and metabolism. FASEB J. 13: 1145–1155.
35. HAMILTON, R.L., S.K. ERICKSON & R.J. HAVEL. 1995. Nascent VLDL assembly occurs in two steps in the endoplasmic reticulum (ER) of hepatocytes. In Atherosclerosis X. F.P. Woodford, J. Davignon & A. Sniderman, Eds. Elsevier Science B.V. Amsterdam.

36. HAMILTON, R.L., J.S. WONG, C.M. CHAM, *et al.* 1998. Chylomicron-sized particles are formed in the setting of apolipoprotein B deficiency. J. Lipid Res. **39:** 1543–1557.
37. WETTERAU, J.R., L.P. AGGERBECK, M.E. BOUMA, *et al.* 1992. Absence of microsomal triglyceride transfer protein in individuals with abetalipoproteinemia. Science **258:** 999–1001.
38. INGOLD, K.U., L. HUGHES, M. SLABY, *et al.* 1987. Synthesis of 2R,4'R,8'R-α-tocopherols selectively labelled with deuterium. J. Labelled Comp. Radiopharm. **24:** 817–831.
39. HUGHES, L., M. SLABY, G.W. BURTON, *et al.* 1990. Synthesis of alpha- and gamma-tocopherols selectively labelled with deuterium. J. Labelled Comp. Radiopharm. **28:** 1049–1057.
40. BURTON, G.W., A. WEBB & K.U. INGOLD. 1985. A mild, rapid, and efficient method of lipid extraction for use in determining vitamin E/lipid ratios. Lipids **20:** 29–39.
41. HAVEL, R.J. & R.L. HAMILTON. 1988. Hepatocytic lipoprotein receptors and intracellular lipoprotein catabolism. Hepatology **8:** 1689–1704.
42. HAMILTON, R.L., A. MOOREHOUSE, S.L. LEAR, *et al.* 1999. A rapid precipitation method of recovering large amounts of highly pure rough endoplasmic reticulum. J. Lipid Res. **40:** 1140–1147.
43. HAMILTON, R.L., A. MOOREHOUSE & R.J. HAVEL. 1991. Isolation and properties of nascent lipoproteins from highly purified rat hepatocytic Golgi fractions. J. Lipid Res. **32:** 529–543.
44. ARITA, M., K. NOMURA, H. ARAI, *et al.* 1997. alpha-tocopherol transfer protein stimulates the secretion of alpha-tocopherol from a cultured liver cell line through a brefeldin A-insensitive pathway. Proc. Natl. Acad. Sci. USA **94:** 12437–12441.
45. ORAM, J.F. & R.M. LAWN. 2001. ABCA1. The gatekeeper for eliminating excess tissue cholesterol. J. Lipid Res. **42:** 1173–1179.
46. ORAM, J.F., A.M. VAUGHAN & R. STOCKER. 2001. ATP-binding cassette transporter A1 mediates cellular secretion of alpha-tocopherol. J. Biol. Chem. **276:** 39898–39902.
47. TRABER, M.G., J.C. LANE, N. LAGMAY, *et al.* 1992. Studies on the transfer of tocopherol between lipoproteins. Lipids **27:** 657–663.
48. KOSTNER, G.M., K. OETTL, M. JAUHIAINEN, *et al.* 1995. Human plasma phospholipid transfer protein accelerates exchange/transfer of alpha-tocopherol between lipoproteins and cells. Biochem. J. **305:** 659–667.
49. JIANG, X.C., A.R. TALL, S. QIN, *et al.* 2002. Phospholipid transfer protein deficiency protects circulating lipoproteins from oxidation due to the enhanced accumulation of vitamin E. J. Biol. Chem. **277:** 31850–31856.
50. YANG, X.P., D. YAN, C. QIAO, *et al.* 2003. Increased atherosclerotic lesions in apoE mice with plasma phospholipid transfer protein overexpression. Arterioscler. Thromb. Vasc. Biol. **23:** 1601–1607.
51. HORIGUCHI, M., M. ARITA, D.E. KAEMPF-ROTZOLL, *et al.* 2003. pH-dependent translocation of alpha-tocopherol transfer protein (alpha-TTP) between hepatic cytosol and late endosomes. Genes Cells **8:** 789–800.
52. ZHA, X., J. GENEST, JR. & R. MCPHERSON. 2001. Endocytosis is enhanced in Tangier fibroblasts: possible role of ATP-binding cassette protein A1 in endosomal vesicular transport. J. Biol. Chem. **276:** 39476–39483.
53. POMORSKI, T., J.C. HOLTHUIS, A. HERRMANN, *et al.* 2004. Tracking down lipid flippases and their biological functions. J. Cell Sci. **117:** 805–813.

Discovery, Characterization, and Significance of the Cytochrome P450 ω-Hydroxylase Pathway of Vitamin E Catabolism

ROBERT S. PARKER, TIMOTHY J. SONTAG, JOY E. SWANSON, AND CHARLES C. McCORMICK

Division of Nutritional Sciences, Cornell University, Ithaca, New York 14853, USA

ABSTRACT: Tocopherols are known to undergo metabolism to phytyl chain-shortened metabolites excreted in urine. We sought to characterize the pathway, including associated enzymes, involved in this biotransformation. We previously found that human hepatoblastoma (HepG2) cultures metabolized tocopherols to their corresponding short-chain carboxychromanols. Putative metabolites of γ-tocopherol that contained intact chromanol moieties were structurally identified using HepG2 cultures and electron impact gas chromatography–mass spectrometry. A microsomal assay for synthesis of the initial ω-oxidation metabolites was developed and used to screen several recombinant human liver cytochrome P450 isozymes for ω-hydroxylase activity. Seven metabolites of γ-tocopherol were identified in HepG2 cultures, including 13'-hydroxy-γ-TOH and all six carboxychromanols predicted by sequential ω-oxidation truncation. Rat and human liver microsomes catalyzed synthesis of 13'-OH- and 13'-COOH-γ-TOH, but not other metabolites, in the presence of NADPH. Inclusion of NAD favored synthesis of the 13'-COOH metabolite. Recombinant CYP4F2, but not other major human liver CYP isoforms (including CYP3A4 and 3A7), exhibited tocopherol-ω-hydroxylase activity. Liver microsomes and recombinant CYP4F2 both exhibited substrate preference for γ-TOH over α-TOH, and recent studies show that tocotrienols are catabolized more extensively than the corresponding tocopherols. Comparative rates of ω-oxidation of tocochromanols in hepatocytes are inversely related to biopotency and directly related to cytotoxicity of these substances in macrophages. The liver contains a cytochrome P450–mediated pathway that preferentially catabolizes "non-α" tocochromanols to excretable metabolites. This metabolic pathway appears central to the optimization of tissue tocochromanol status.

KEYWORDS: tocopherols; vitamin E; omega-oxidation; metabolism; cytochrome P450; hepatocytes; microsomes; macrophage; cytotoxicity

INTRODUCTION

Vitamin E is consumed in several forms as tocopherols and tocotrienols, yet only one form, α-tocopherol, occurs in appreciable concentrations in blood and tissues.

Address for correspondence: Robert S. Parker, Division of Nutritional Sciences, 113 Savage Hall, Cornell University, Ithaca, NY 14853. Voice: 607-255-2661; fax: 607-255-1033.
rsp3@cornell.edu

In the United States, the major dietary forms of vitamin E are γ-tocopherol, δ-tocopherol, and α-tocopherol, in that order. In contrast, α-tocopherol represents more than 90% of tocopherols in plasma and tissues. Because all forms of vitamin E (the "tocochromanols") appear to be absorbed with similar efficiency, the selective deposition of α-tocopherol apparently results from postabsorptive vitamer-selective processes. We hypothesized that the elimination mechanisms exhibit selectivity that result in the preferential postabsorptive elimination of forms of vitamin E other than α-tocopherol. A vitamer-selective pathway of elimination could well underlie the superior bioactivity of α-tocopherol over other forms of vitamin E in the rat gestation-resorption assay and other whole-organism bioassays of vitamin E bioactivity in mammals.

CHARACTERIZATION OF THE ω-OXIDATION PATHWAY OF PHYTYL TAIL TRUNCATION

We initially reported that a substantial proportion of ingested γ-tocopherol, but not α-tocopherol, was eliminated in the urine as its 3'-carboxychromanol (γ-CEHC) metabolite.[1] This observation provided compelling evidence that phytyl tail truncation represented a major route of catabolism of at least certain forms of vitamin E that were consumed in appreciable quantities but did not accumulate. To investigate the mechanism of catabolism in a systematic fashion, we developed a cell culture model, the human hepatoblastoma line HepG2, which we demonstrated metabolized tocopherols to the same urinary metabolites excreted by humans.[2] Using this model, we identified the 5'-carboxychromanol metabolite of γ-tocopherol (FIG. 1). We fur-

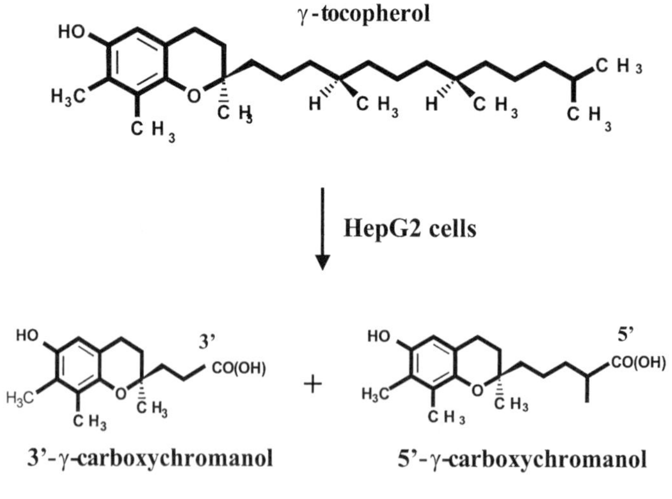

FIGURE 1. Metabolism of γ-tocopherol to its 3'- and 5'-γ-carboxychromanol metabolites by HepG2 cultures. HepG2 cultures were incubated with γ-tocopherol (25 mM) for 48 h and the medium was extracted and analyzed by GC-MS for putative metabolites possessing an intact γ-chromanol ring as indicated by the presence of m/z 223 ion.

ther found that these hepatocyte cultures metabolized γ- and δ-tocopherols to short-chain carboxychromanols much more extensively than α-tocopherol, mimicking the biology of tocopherol retention in humans and the relative bioactivity of tocopherols in the rat gestation-resorption assay.

Employing γ-tocopherol as a suitable substrate of this metabolic process, we further utilized its characteristic mass fragmentation pattern in gas chromatography–mass spectrometry (GC-MS) to probe extracts of HepG2 cultures for additional metabolites containing intact γ-chromanol ring moieties. This investigation resulted in the identification of all theoretical carboxychromanol intermediates of γ-tocopherol, including the 13'-, 11'-, 9'-, and 7'-carboxychromanols,[3] as shown in FIGURE 2. These metabolites represent sequential truncation of the phytyl tail of γ-tocopherol by either two-carbon moieties (in the absence of a branch methyl) or three-carbon moieties (in the presence of a branch methyl). The identification of a phytyl-terminal-carboxychromanol strongly suggested but did not prove that the initial oxidation event occurred at either of the two terminal methyl groups of the phytyl tail. The carboxy derivitives of these methyl groups are indistinguishable in our GC-MS assay, and we currently consider that both are formed.

More compelling evidence of an initial terminal (ω) oxidation event was provided by the identification of a terminal methyl-hydroxyl metabolite, but no hydroxyl metabolites of shortened tail length. Identified hydroxylated metabolites included a terminal methyl-OH metabolite,[3] arising from hydroxylation of either of the two terminal methyl moieties, and a 12'-OH metabolite (FIG. 3). The latter, representing ω-1 hydroxylation, cannot be oxidized to a carboxylic acid and therefore is consid-

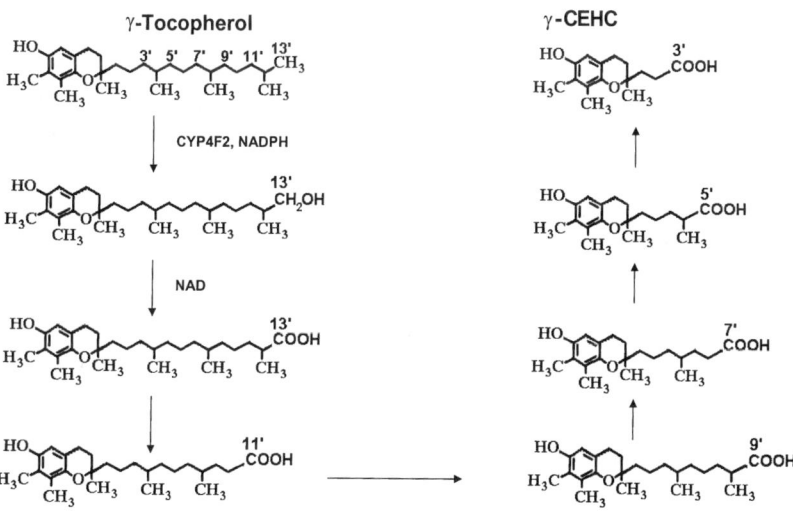

FIGURE 2. Pathway of metabolism of γ-tocopherol to phytyl tail shortened carboxychromanol metabolites. All indicated compounds were identified by GC-MS in HepG2 cultures incubated with γ-tocopherol.

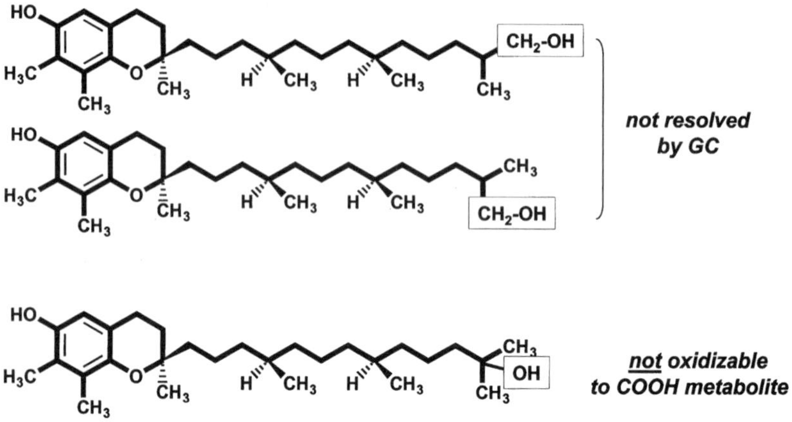

FIGURE 3. Hydroxychromanol metabolites of γ-tocopherol identified by GC-MS in HepG2 cultures incubated with γ-tocopherol. The two methyl-terminal metabolites are indistinguishable by GC-MS; both are anticipated to be formed.

ered not to be further metabolized to shorter carboxychromanols. The fate of the 12′-OH metabolite is currently a matter of investigation. In agreement with the report of Birringer et al.,[4] we have found that the tocotrienols are also catabolized to short-chain carboxychromanol by HepG2 cultures via this same ω-oxidation pathway.

IDENTIFICATION OF MICROSOMAL ω-HYDROXYLATION AS THE INITIATING EVENT IN THE TOCOPHEROL–ω-OXIDATION PATHWAY

Investigations in HepG2 cultures strongly suggested that the initial oxidation product of γ-tocopherol was a hydroxylation of one or both of the terminal methyl groups of the phytyl tail. We undertook to ascertain the nature of this biotransformation. Terminal (ω) hydroxylation reactions are commonly catalyzed by microsomal NADPH-dependent cytochrome P450 isozymes, which reside predominantly in the liver. Because we had shown that human hepatocyte cultures exhibited this activity, we probed rat and human liver microsomes for the ability to form the phytyl terminal hydroxyl or carboxyl metabolites of γ-tocopherol. Liver microsomes from both rat and human were shown to catalyze this reaction,[3] which was dependent on the presence of NADPH. Furthermore, the yield of the ω-carboxychromanol metabolite was enhanced in the presence of NAD+, indicating a precursor–product relationship between the ω-hydroxyl and the ω-carboxy metabolites, and the involvement of a microsomal dehydrogenase. The nature of the latter is under investigation. In microsomal systems containing NADPH and NAD+, no other tocopherol metabolites have yet been identified. This suggests either the involvement of other organelles in the phytyl tail truncation process or the requirement for other cofactors.

IDENTIFICATION OF CYP4F2 AS AN ENZYME RESPONSIBLE FOR TOCOPHEROL–ω-HYDROXYLASE ACTIVITY

The major cytochrome P450 in human liver is CYP3A4, for which ketoconazole was described as a selective inhibitor.[5] We observed that ketoconazole was a potent inhibitor of tocopherol–ω-hydroxylase activity in HepG2 cells and therefore suggested that this CYP isoform was responsible for the observed enzymatic activity.[6] However, this prediction, based primarily on the assumption of ketoconazole specificity, proved incorrect. Subsequent testing of recombinant human CYP3A4 (and CYP3A7), individually expressed in insect cell microsomes, showed no activity toward either γ- or α-tocopherol.[3] Numerous other CYP isoforms were tested for tocopherol–ω-hydroxylase activity, particularly the major human liver CYP enzymes, with emphasis on those with previously demonstrated ω-hydroxylase activity toward fatty acids or eicosanoids. Of the nearly two dozen human CYP enzymes tested to date, only one, CYP4F2, has exhibited appreciable tocopherol–ω-hydroxylase activity. This hepatic CYP isoform originally was reported as catalyzing the ω-hydroxylation of leukotriene B4.[7] The two other characterized members of the 4F family, 4F3A (neutrophil), and 4F3B (liver) exhibit little or no tocopherol-ω-hydroxylase activity, despite substantial sequence homology. However, of the three human 4F isoforms, 4F2 exhibits the highest K_m for LTB4,[7] and the *in vivo* relevance of this isoform to LTB4 catabolism is uncertain.

Recent studies of tocopherol-ω-hydroxylase in our laboratory have focused on the determination of kinetic constants (K_m, V_{max}) of the various tocopherols and tocotrienols. These investigations have been complicated by observations of substantial differences in the rates of membrane association of the various vitamers and suggest that *in vivo* the rates of catabolism are determined by the combination of substrate–enzyme interactions and substrate–membrane interactions (Sontag and Parker, unpublished observations). We have observed that in both microsomal systems and in cell cultures, the RRR form of α-tocopherol is metabolized to a greater extent than the all-racemic form, that is, the opposite of what is observed *in vivo*. It is likely that the hepatic tocopherol transfer protein is responsible for sparing RRR–α-tocopherol *in vivo* by facilitating its transport out of the liver, the principal site of tocopherol-ω oxidation.

INHIBITION OF THE TOCOPHEROL–ω-HYDROXYLASE PATHWAY BY NATURAL PRODUCTS

We are currently investigating the extent to which activity of the tocopherol–ω-hydroxylase pathway may be modulated by tocochromanol substrates or by other nonvitamin E dietary constituents. To date, we have identified two inhibitors of this pathway, in addition to the antifungal drug ketoconazole. The most potent dietary inhibitor found to date is sesamin, a benzofuran lignan in sesame seed oil,[6] with an IC_{50} of less than 0.5 mM in cultured hepatocytes. Sesamin has also been reported to inhibit certain fatty acid desaturases,[8,9] but with K_m or IC_{50} values of 155–280 mM in microsomes or cell cultures; *in vivo* effects of sesamin on fatty acid composition have not been investigated, but such kinetic constants render any effects unlikely. Cereal alkylresorcinols, and specifically 5-pentadecylresorcinol, also inhibits toco-

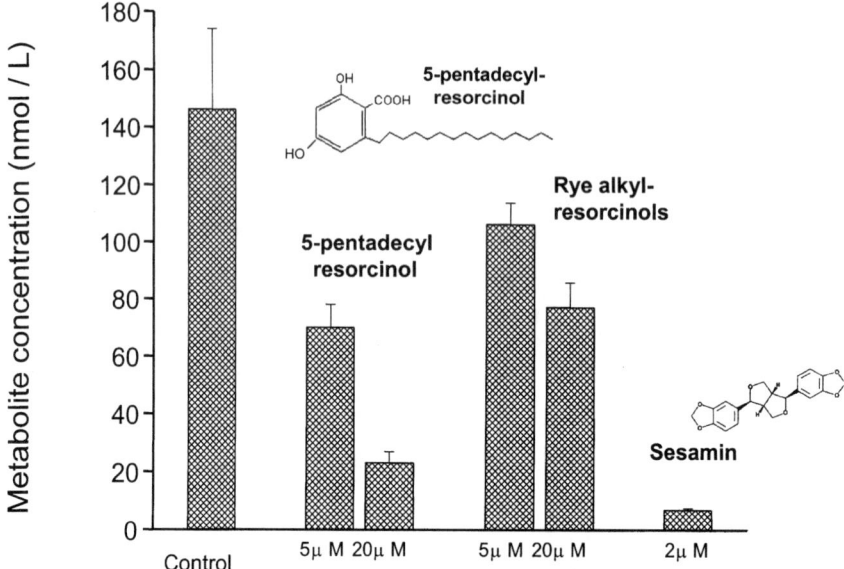

FIGURE 4. Inhibition of metabolism of γ-tocopherol by sesamin and rye alkylresorcinols in HepG2(C3A) cultures.

pherol–ω-oxidation in HepG2 cells and elevates γ-tocopherols levels in rats,[10] although not as potently as sesamin (FIG. 4). Sesamin consumption by rats and humans results in elevated plasma or tissue levels of γ-tocopherol,[11,12] demonstrating both the physiological importance of the tocopherol–ω-oxidation pathway to vitamin E (tocochromanol) status and that vitamin E status can be modulated by dietary factors other than vitamin E intake. Because α-tocopherol is a poor substrate for this pathway, neither sesamin nor alkylresorcinols affected α-tocopherol status.

INTERACTIONS AMONG SUBSTRATES OF THE TOCOPHEROL–ω-HYDROXYLASE PATHWAY

α-Tocopherol is widely consumed in supplement form, and supplement use is commonly associated with reduced plasma and tissues levels of other forms of vitamin E. We investigated whether α-tocopherol could influence the metabolism of γ-tocopherol, either in hepatocyte culture or in microsomes. In HepG2 cultures, coincubation of γ-tocopherol with increasing amounts of α-tocopherol resulted in a modest inhibition of metabolism of γ-tocopherol (FIG. 5). Interestingly, in microsomes supplemental α-tocopherol enhances ω-oxidation of γ-tocopherol (Sontag and Parker, unpublished observations). The apparently contradictory nature of these observations is under investigation.

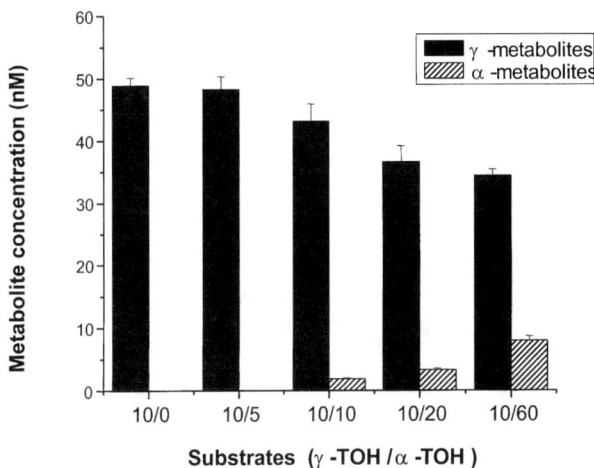

FIGURE 5. Effect of increasing concentrations of α-tocopherol on the metabolism of γ-tocopherol in HepG2(C3A) cultures. Hepatocytes were cultured for 24 h in the presence of 10 mM γ-tocopherol and various concentrations of α-tocopherol as indicated. Carboxychromanol metabolites (sum of 3′- and 5′-carboxychromanols) of γ-tocopherol were quantified by GC-MS.

BIOLOGICAL SIGNIFICANCE OF THE TOCOPHEROL–ω-OXIDATION PATHWAY OF VITAMER-SELECTIVE CATABOLISM AND ELIMINATION OF TOCOPHEROLS AND TOCOTRIENOLS

Evidence to date indicates that the tocopherol–ω-hydroxylase pathway, combined with the hepatic tocopherol transfer protein, strongly influences vitamin E status. The former is particularly responsible for the catabolism and elimination of the non–α-tocopherol tocochromanols. However, all tocopherols and tocotrienols are effective membrane-associated antioxidants, and as such the biological rationale for the remarkably effective catabolism and elimination of most dietary forms of vitamin E is not readily apparent. A plausible hypothesis is that certain tocochromanols, if allowed to accumulate, may cause detrimental effects. Such effects could be manifested via the physical nature of the cellular membranes in which they reside, or on radical-mediated events that cells rely on for normative function. Recent studies in our laboratories utilizing various cell culture models, including primary cells, support this hypothesis, which is additionally supported by other *in vivo* observations in animals. For example, murine macrophages (primary or RAW264 cells) exhibit remarkable vitamer-selective cytotoxicity in which δ-tocopherol and δ-tocotrienol are quite cytotoxic, α-tocopherol is relatively noncytotoxic, and γ-tocopherol exhibits intermediate cytotoxicity (FIG. 6). The relative cytotoxicity of these vitamers is directly correlated with their rates of catabolism in hepatocytes such that those vitamers that are most cytotoxic are most rapidly catabolized via the tocopherol-ω-oxidation pathway. These findings suggest that the tocopherol–ω-oxidation pathway

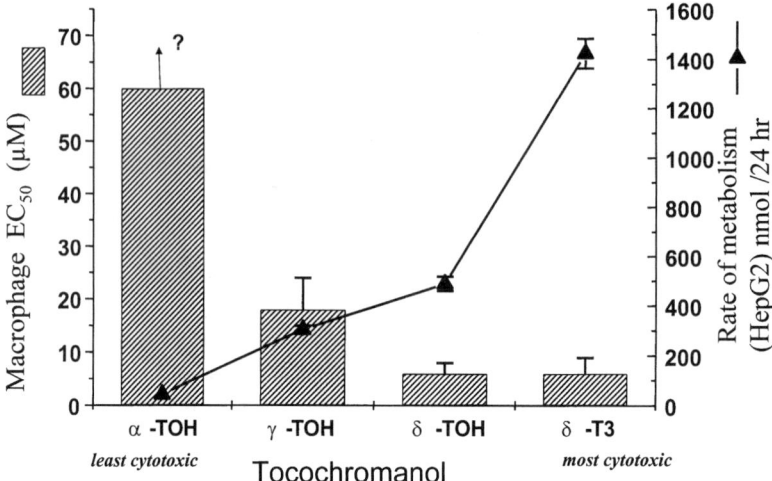

FIGURE 6. Relationship between cytotoxicity of various tocochromanols in RAW264 macrophage cell cultures and the rates of metabolism of the same tocochromanols in HepG2 cultures. Cytotoxicity studies were conducted in lipoprotein-free serum for 24 h, and cell viability was assessed using the MTT assay. The EC_{50} is the concentration required to achieve a 50% reduction in cell viability; data are mean and standard deviation of three independent experiments. Metabolism studies were conducted in 48-h HepG2(C3A) cultures using 25 mM substrate concentrations, and metabolite production is the sum of the 3'- and 5'-γ-carboxychromanol metabolites, the only metabolites produced in appreciable quantities under these conditions.

may have evolved to effectively eliminate tocochromanols that exhibit detrimental effects if allowed to accumulate. The molecular nature of the vitamer-specific cytotoxicity of the tocochromanols is currently under investigation. These investigations are rendered more important by recent findings of potential advantageous effects of tocochromanols other than α-tocopherol and the growing availability of these substances in supplement form.

SUMMARY

The cytochrome P450 pathway of ω-oxidation of tocochromanols serves a physiologically important role in mediating the concentrations and relative proportions of the various dietary forms of vitamin E. The initial microsomal ω-hydroxylation event in human tissues is catalyzed by CYP4F2, the tissue distribution of which will determine the sites of tocopherol catabolism. Currently, the liver is considered the primary site of this pathway, the products of which are transported in blood to the kidney for elimination in the urine. This pathway may serve to effectively prevent the accumulation of certain tocochromanols that are cytotoxic to some cell types for reasons that are not yet understood.

REFERENCES

1. SWANSON, J., R. BEN, G. BURTON & R. PARKER. 1999. Measurement of the 2,7,8-trimethyl-2-(β-carboxyethyl)-6-hydroxychroman metabolite of γ-tocopherol in human urine: evidence for urinary excretion as a major route of elimination of γ-tocopherol. J. Lipid Res. **40:** 665–671.
2. PARKER, R. & J. SWANSON. 2000. A novel 5′-carboxychroman metabolite of γ-tocopherol secreted by HepG2 cells and excreted in human urine. Biochem. Biophys. Res. Commun. **269:** 580–583.
3. SONTAG, T. & R. PARKER. 2002. Cytochrome P450 w-hydroxylase pathway of tocopherol catabolism: novel mechanism of regulation of vitamin E status. J. Biol. Chem. **277:** 25290–25296.
4. BIRRINGER, M., P. PFLUGER, D. KLUTH, et al. 2002. Identities and differences in the metabolism of tocotrienols and tocopherols in HepG2 cells. J. Nutr. **132:** 31113–31118.
5. PELKONEN, O., J. MAENPAA, P. TAAVITSAINEN, et al. 1998. Inhibition and induction of human cytochrome P450 (CYP) enzymes. Xenobiotica **28:** 1203–1253.
6. PARKER, R., T. SONTAG & J. SWANSON. 2000. Cytochrome P4503A-dependent metabolism of tocopherols and inhibition by sesamin. Biochem. Biophys. Res. Commun. **277:** 531–534.
7. KIKUTA, Y., E. KUSUNOSE & M. KUSONOSE. 2002. Prostaglandin and leukotriene ω-hydroxylases. Prostaglandins Other Lipid Mediat. **68–69:** 345–362.
8. SHIMIZU, S., K. AKIMOTO, Y. SHINMEN, et al. 1991. Sesamin is a potent and specific inhibitor of Δ5 desaturase in polyunsaturated fatty acid biosynthesis. Lipids **26:** 512–516.
9. UMEDA-SAWADA, R., Y. FUJIWARA, H. ABE & Y. SEYAMA. 2003. Effects of sesamin and capsaicin on the mRNA expressions of D6 and D5 desaturases in rat primary cultured hepatocytes. J. Nutr. Sci. Vitaminol. **49:** 442–446.
10. ROSS, A., Y. CHEN, J. FRANK, et al. 2004. Cereal alkylresorcinols elevate γ-tocopherol levels in male Sprague-Dawley rats and inhibit γ-tocopherol metabolism in vitro. J. Nutr. **143:** 506–510.
11. YAMASHITA, K., Y. LIZUKA, T. IMAI & M. NAMIKI. 1995. Sesame seed and its lignans produce marked enhancement of vitamin E activity in rats fed a low α-tocopherol diet. Lipids **30:** 1019–1028.
12. KAMAL-ELDIN, A, D. PETTERSSON & L.-A. APPELQUIST. 1995. Sesamin (a compound from sesame oil) increases tocopherol levels in rats fed *ad libitum*. Lipids **30:** 499–505.

Inter- and Intra-Individual Vitamin E Uptake in Healthy Subjects Is Highly Repeatable across a Wide Supplementation Dose Range

FRANK J. KELLY, ROSALIND LEE, AND IAN S. MUDWAY

School of Health and Life Sciences, King's College London, London SE1 9NH, United Kingdom

ABSTRACT: Vitamin E uptake after supplementation varies widely in the healthy population, and preliminary studies have indicated that individual responses are relatively stable over periods in excess of 1 year. This phenotypic stability suggests a genetic basis to this observed variation. To examine this issue further, we examined the repeatability of both baseline plasma α-tocopherol and urinary α-tocopherol metabolite concentrations, as well as individual responses of these parameters after vitamin E supplementation. In the first study, 65 subjects (33 males, 32 females, aged 30.7 ± 7.4 years) provided three plasma and urine samples for α-tocopherol and metabolite analysis with each collection separated by at least 2 weeks. Plasma α-tocopherol concentrations were found to be highly repeatable over this short interval (intraclass correlation coefficient [ICC] = 0.85), although the association deteriorated once values were corrected for plasma cholesterol (ICC = 0.64). Similarly, urinary α-tocopherol metabolites 2(2′-carboxyethyl)-6-hydroxychroman acid (α-CEHC) and quinone lactone (QL) concentration were found to display a moderate degree of intra-subject repeatability: ICC = 0.65 and 0.58, respectively. In a second study, plasma α-tocopherol and urinary metabolite responses were investigated in 18 healthy, nonsmoking subjects (12 males, 6 females, aged 33.1 ± 9.1 years) after successive 6-week periods of vitamin E (RRR–α-tocopherol acetate) supplementation at 15, 100, 200, and 400 mg/day. Plasma and urine samples were obtained on days 0, 7, 14, 21, and 28 (7 days after the final supplement) of each dosing period and the strength of the underlying association between responses determined using Kendall's tau_b test. Individual plasma α-tocopherol responses at the 100, 200, and 400 mg/day doses were found to be highly associated: τ, 0.51, $P = 0.02$ [100 vs. 200] and τ, 0.49, $P = 0.03$ [100 vs. 400] and τ, 0.56, $P = 0.005$ [200 vs. 400]. Together these data support the contention that α-tocopherol uptake is a stable individual phenotype under genetic regulation.

KEYWORDS: α-tocopherol; variability; bioavailability; metabolism; biokinetics

Address for corrrespondence: Professor Frank J. Kelly, School of Health and Life Sciences, King's College London, London SE1 9NN, United Kingdom. Voice: 4420-7848-4004; fax: 44-20-7848-3891.
frank.kelly@kcl.ac.uk

BACKGROUND

Epidemiological evidence suggests that antioxidants, in particular, vitamin E, are negative risk factors for heart disease.[1,2] Vitamin E's chain-breaking antioxidant activity has been reported to underlie this benefit.[3,4] Conversely, intervention studies in humans have failed to consistently improve outcome of diseased patients based on administration of vitamin E supplements.[5,6] In addition, intervention studies have shown variable outcomes when examining the effects of vitamin E supplements on lipid peroxidation, with some showing no effect and others showing an increase or decrease in oxidation of lipids.[7] In many of these studies, it is not clear to what extent vitamin E supplementation has been successful in raising blood/tissue vitamin E concentrations because these measurements are often not made. Recently, using a stable isotope approach, we demonstrated that vitamin E uptake in response to supplementation varies widely in the healthy population,[8] confirming similar earlier observations.[9] Variation in individual uptake responses implies not all individuals will benefit from supplementation strategies to an equal extent. This underlying variation may explain, in part, the ambiguous results obtained during recent supplement trials in subjects with cardiovascular disease.[10,11]

Variability in response to any given stimulus or intervention is a universal phenomenon in biological systems. Although a proportion of this variation can be attributed to measurement error and the influence of external factors, time-stable characteristics are more likely to reflect genetic background. Recently, we reported preliminary evidence indicating that individual responses to vitamin E supplementation are relatively stable over periods in excess of one year.[8] This observation, obtained using a stable isotope of α-tocopherol, although based on a limited number of subjects, implies that a genetic basis underlies the inter-subject variation in responses seen in the healthy population. Moreover, it suggests that in any clinical trial involving vitamin E supplementation there will be a wide range of vitamin E uptake within the treatment group. This difference alone, if not appreciated, could lead to difficulties in interpreting outcome to treatment. To investigate this phenomenon in greater detail, we designed the current study to examine both baseline stability in plasma α-tocopherol and urinary α-tocopherol metabolite (α-CEHC and QL) concentrations over short intervals to assess measurement error issues, as well as individual stability in vitamin E uptake and excretion responses across a wide range of supplemental doses.

METHODS

Subjects and Protocol

Study 1

Sixty-five subjects (33 males/32 females) with a mean age of 30.7 years (range, 21–51 years), BMI 23.6 ± 3.2 were recruited into Study 1 after providing written consent. Subjects were all healthy nonsmokers and were asked to refrain from antioxidant supplements or other medications for the duration of the study. Subjects visited the hospital on three separate occasions, each separated by a 2-week interval.

On each visit, subjects provided a first-morning-void urine sample, as well as a blood sample for determination of plasma α-tocopherol and urinary tocopherol metabolites. The St. Thomas' Hospital Research Ethics Committee approved this study.

Study 2

Eighteen healthy, nonsmoking subjects (12 males, 6 females) aged 33.1 years (range, 22.1–50.2 years), BMI 24.7 ± 3.4, underwent four 6-week periods of vitamin E (RRR–α-tocopherol acetate) supplementation (15, 100, 200, and 400 mg/day). Each period of supplementation was followed by a 3-week washout period. Plasma and urine samples were obtained on days 0, 7, 14, 21, and 28 (7 days after the final supplement) of each supplementation period for α-tocopherol (plasma) and α-tocopherol metabolites (urine) determinations. The study was approved by the St. Thomas' Hospital Research Ethics Committee.

Sample Collection

Blood (10 mL) was collected in lithium heparin tubes, and the plasma was separated by centrifugation at 3,000 rpm for 15 minutes at 4°C. Plasma was stored at –80°C before analysis. First-morning urine samples were collected and aliquoted before storage at –20°C. One aliquot of urine (1 mL) was retained for creatinine analysis.

Plasma Tocopherol and Cholesterol Analysis

Plasma α-tocopherol content was determined using reverse-phase HPLC as previously described[12] and normalized for plasma cholesterol content. Plasma cholesterol levels were determined by enzymatic colorimetric test using CHOD/PAP methods and Unimate 5 Chol kits (Roche Diagnostic, East Sussex, UK).

Urine Tocopherol Metabolite Analysis

Internal standards of d^3-QL, d^9-CEHC were added to urine aliquots (4 mL) before enzymatic hydrolysis of the glucuronide metabolite conjugates with *Escherichia coli* β glucuronidase (EC: 3.2.1.31; Sigma, Dorset, UK). The resulting solution was acidified to pH 1.5 before extraction with hexane/*tert* butyl methyl ether (99:1, 10 mL). After centrifugation, the organic layer was removed and evaporated under nitrogen. The residue was dissolved in anhydrous pyridine and silylated at 65°C for 1 hour with 50 μL *N,O*-bis (trimethylsilyl) trifluoroacetamide (BSTFA) containing 1% trimethylchlorosilane (TMS; Pierce Chemical Co., Rockford, IL). The solvents were evaporated under nitrogen and the residue dissolved in hexane for GCMS analysis as previously described.[13] Urine creatinine concentrations were determined spectrophotometrically using the Sigma Diagnostics creatinine kit and following the manufacturer's instructions (Sigma, St. Louis, MO).

Data Analysis and Statistics

Study 1

Both plasma α-tocopherol and urinary metabolite concentrations were found to be nonparametric using the Shapiro–Wilk test for normality. Data therefore are summarized as medians with interquartile range. Comparison of biweekly median plasma α-tocopherol and urinary metabolite concentrations were performed using the Wilcoxon signed rank test, with associations between individual values examined using Kendall's tau_b test. Repeatability of baseline α-tocopherol and metabolite concentrations was examined by standard methods,[14] after data transformation to the log10 to remove the underlying association between individual mean values and their associated standard deviation.[15] The mean within-subject variance was determined from a one-way ANOVA, with subjects as the group, with the within-subject (geometric) standard deviation (σw) calculated as the antilog of the square root of the residual mean squares, Aσw.[15] The intra-class correlation coefficient (ICC) was calculated as the ratio between-subject and total variation.[16] Note that the ICC calculation given in the cited reference was subsequently amended to: ICC = (m*SSB − SST) / ([m − 1] * SST) to allow for an algebraic precedence error in the original article, where m is the number of observations per subject and SSB and SST the between-subject and total sum of squares, respectively. All statistical analyses were executed using SPSS version 11.0 for Windows (SPSS Inc., Chicago, IL).

Study 2

As in Study 1, all plasma and urinary data were found to be nonparametric. Comparison of the plasma α-tocopherol and urinary metabolite concentrations across time at each of the supplementation doses therefore were conducted using the Quade two-way ANOVA for nonparametric data, with post hoc multiple comparisons performed with the t distribution using the Unistat statistical package, version 4.53d. Overall responses across the 28-day experimental period at each supplement dose were summarized as the area under the curve (AUC) determined using Microcal Origin, version 5 and compared with the Kendall's tau_b test. Comparisons between responses seen at each dose and between responses and baseline concentrations were also performed using Kendall's tau_b test. Responses also were compared between supplementation doses by examining molar changes in α-tocopherol and metabolite concentrations at days 7, 14, 21, and 28 relative to baseline day 0 values.

RESULTS

Study 1

Plasma α-tocopherol concentrations did not differ across the three separate collection intervals with group median (IQR) concentrations of 21.1 (19.4–25.3), 23.1 (20.5–27.4), and 22.6 (20.3–25.5) μM for each biweekly sample (FIG. 1). Individual concentrations were highly correlated for each of visit (first vs. second, τ, 0.61, $P <$ 0.001, first vs. third, τ, 0.63, $P < 0.001$ second vs. third τ, 0.63, $P < 0.001$) and were found to be highly repeatable, with a within-subject (geometric) standard deviation (Aσw) of 1.08 based on the data transformed to the log10 and an intra-class coefficient (ICC) of 0.85. Similar results were obtained once the data had been corrected for plasma cholesterol concentrations (FIG. 2), although the repeatability was reduced: ICC = 0.64. Urinary α-CEHC concentrations also did not differ between the three biweekly samples: 3.23 (2.02–4.87), 3.54 (1.85–6.18), and 3.52 (2.37–5.81) μM/mM creatinine (FIG. 3) and were highly correlated between the three visits (first

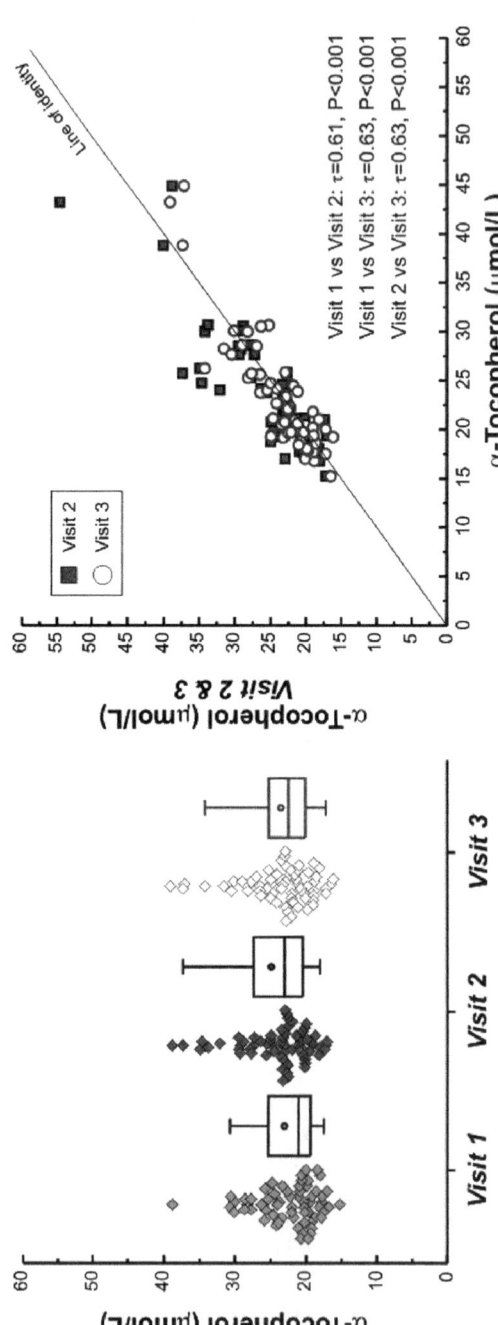

FIGURE 1. Repeat plasma α-tocopherol concentrations with individual samples collected at least 2 weeks apart. Data in the left-hand panel are presented as individual values and statistical boxplots. The central bar in the boxplots represents the median concentration, the open circle the mean, the upper and lower limits of the box the 75th and 25th percentile, respectively, and the whiskers the 95% confidence interval (CI), $n = 65$. The panel on the right shows the relationship between individual concentrations determined on visit 1 versus those obtained on the subsequent two visits relative to the line of identity. The strength of these associations was tested using Kendall's tau_b correlation. The results of these analyses are shown.

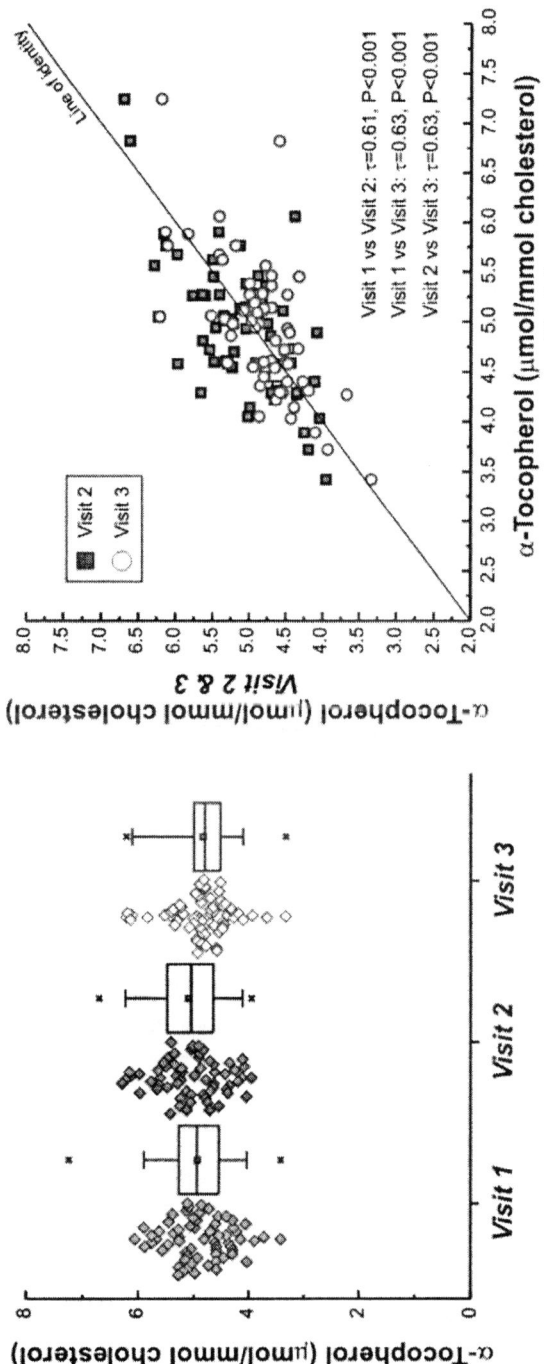

FIGURE 2. Repeat plasma α-tocopherol concentrations, corrected for plasma cholesterol, with individual samples collected at least 2 weeks apart. The format of this figure is as outlined in the legend to FIGURE 1.

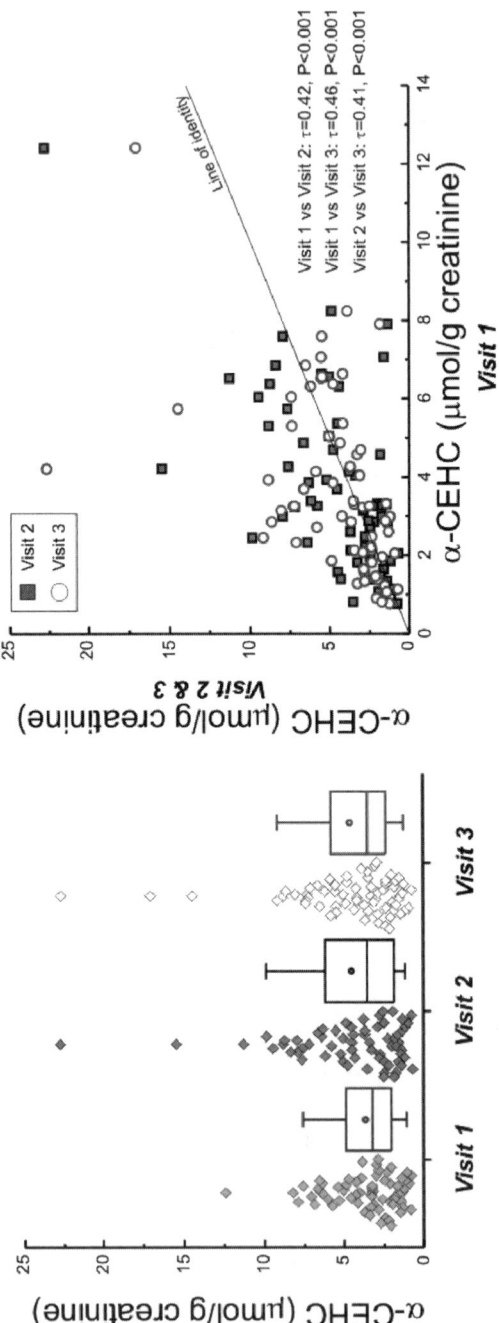

FIGURE 3. Repeat first-void urine α-CEHC concentrations with individual samples collected at least 2 weeks apart. The format of this figure is as outlined in the legend to FIGURE 1.

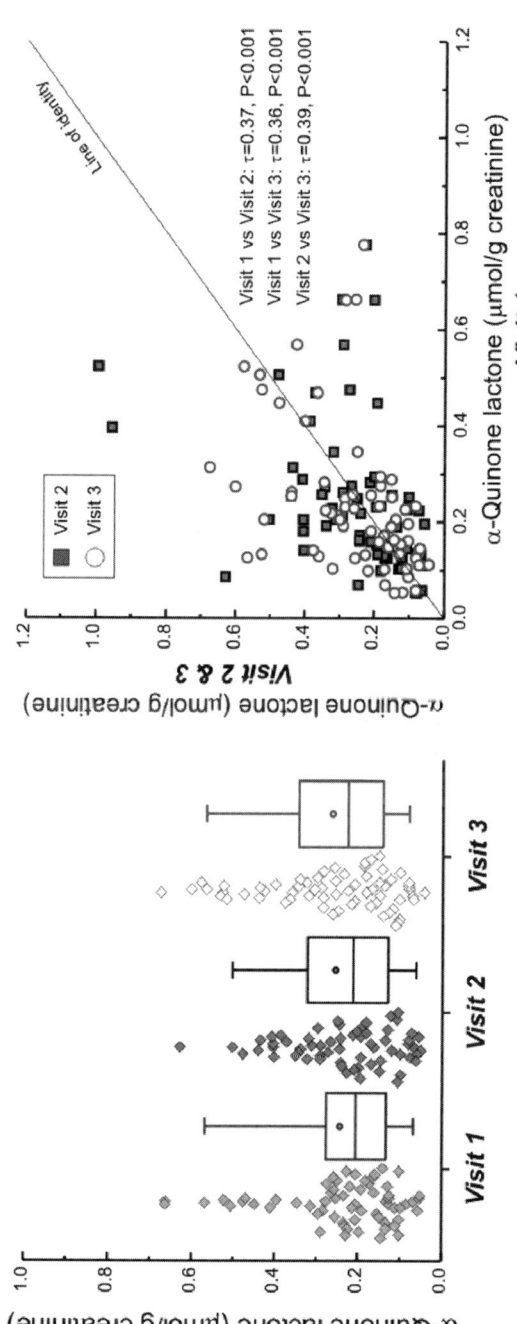

FIGURE 4. Repeat first-void urine QL concentrations in individual samples collected at least 2 weeks apart. The format of this figure is as outlined in the legend to FIGURE 1.

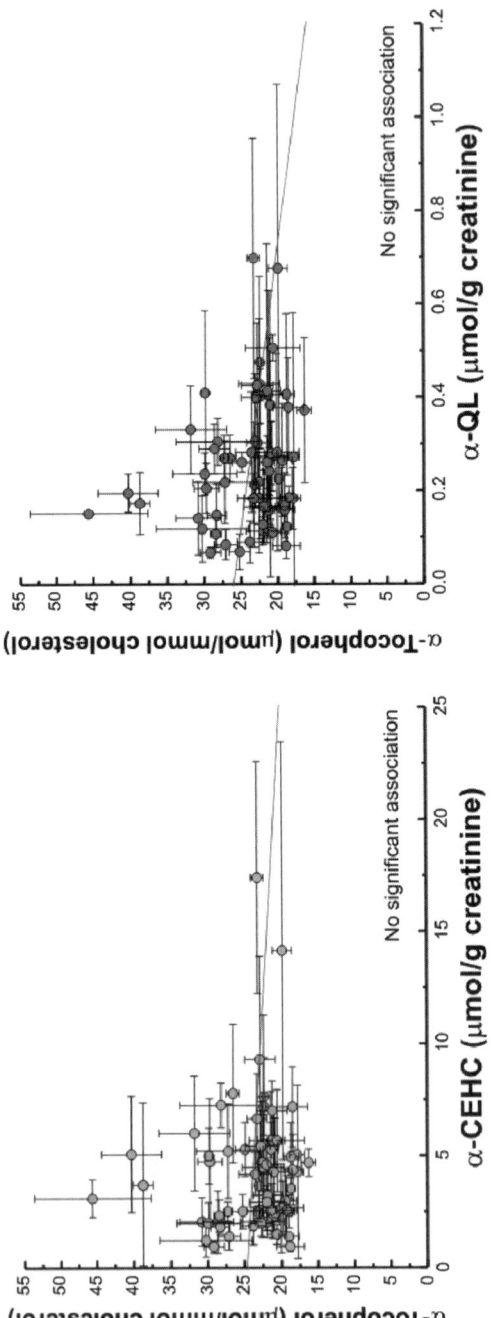

FIGURE 5. The lack of association between baseline α-tocopherol concentrations and the concentration of αCEHC and QL in first-void urine samples. The individual values shown are the mean and SD of the three repeat determinations.

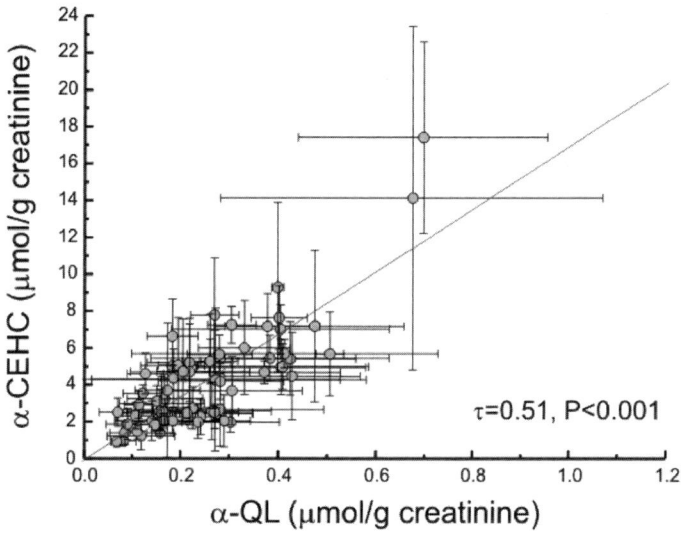

FIGURE 6. Significant association between baseline concentration of the urinary α-tocopherol metabolites αCEHC and QL. The individual values shown are the mean and SD of the three repeat determinations.

vs. second, τ, 0.42, $P < 0.001$, first vs. third, τ, 0.41, $P < 0.001$ second vs. third τ, 0.46, $P < 0.001$), with an ICC of 0.65 and a within-subject (geometric) standard deviation (Aσw) of 1.55. QL concentrations in the urine were significantly lower than α-CEHC concentrations, but again did not differ between the repeat measurements: 0.21 (0.13–0.28), 0.21 (0.13–0.33), and 0.23 (0.14–0.35) μM/mM creatinine (FIG. 4) and were significantly correlated (first vs. second, τ, 0.47, $P < 0.001$, first vs. third, τ, 0.43, $P < 0.05$, second vs. third τ, 0.63, $P < 0.001$). Only a moderate degree of repeatability was seen in QL determinations with an ICC of 0.58 and a Aσw of 1.54. It was notable that there was no simplistic association between individual plasma α-tocopherol concentrations and the concentration of urinary CEHC or QL (FIG. 5), although these two metabolites were strongly associated: τ, 0.51, $P < 0.001$ (FIG. 6).

Study 2

At the 15-mg/day supplementation dose we saw no increase in plasma α-tocopherol concentrations over the 28-day supplementation period (FIG. 7). In contrast, dose-dependant and significant increases in plasma α-tocopherol concentrations were observed during the 100-mg/day and 200-mg/day supplementation periods peaking at day 21 (8.91 [7.96–10.11]) and day 14 (9.96 [8.60–10.48] μM/mM cholesterol), respectively, before returning to baseline values 7 days after supplementation. The plasma α-tocopherol responses to the 400-mg/day supplementation were not statistically different from those seen at the 200-mg/day dose, with a peak again at day 14, 11.00 (9.52–11.95) μM/mM cholesterol. In accord with the results obtained from Study 1, we observed that the four baseline concentrations did not differ

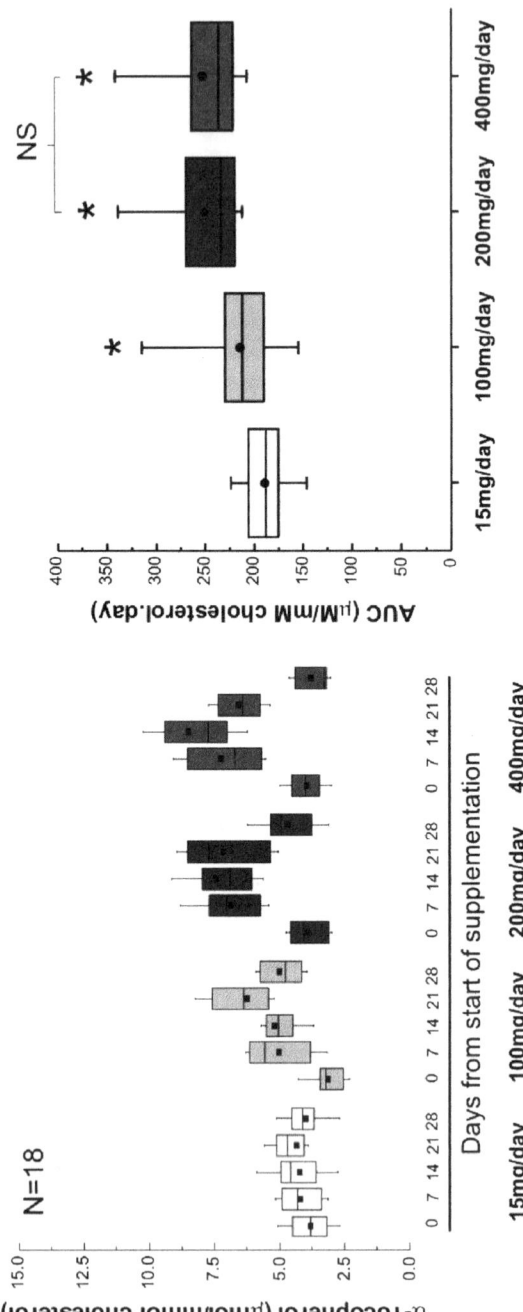

FIGURE 7. Plasma α-tocopherol concentrations after supplementation at four doses over a 21-day period. Concentration data in the left-hand panel are shown are mean (SD) of 18 subjects. The left-hand panel summarizes the overall response as an AUC at each of the supplementation levels using boxplots as described in FIGURE 1. Comparison of the AUC associated with each supplement level was performed using the Quade Two-Way ANOVA with post hoc tests using the t-distribution. Significant differences at the 5% level are indicated with asterisks.

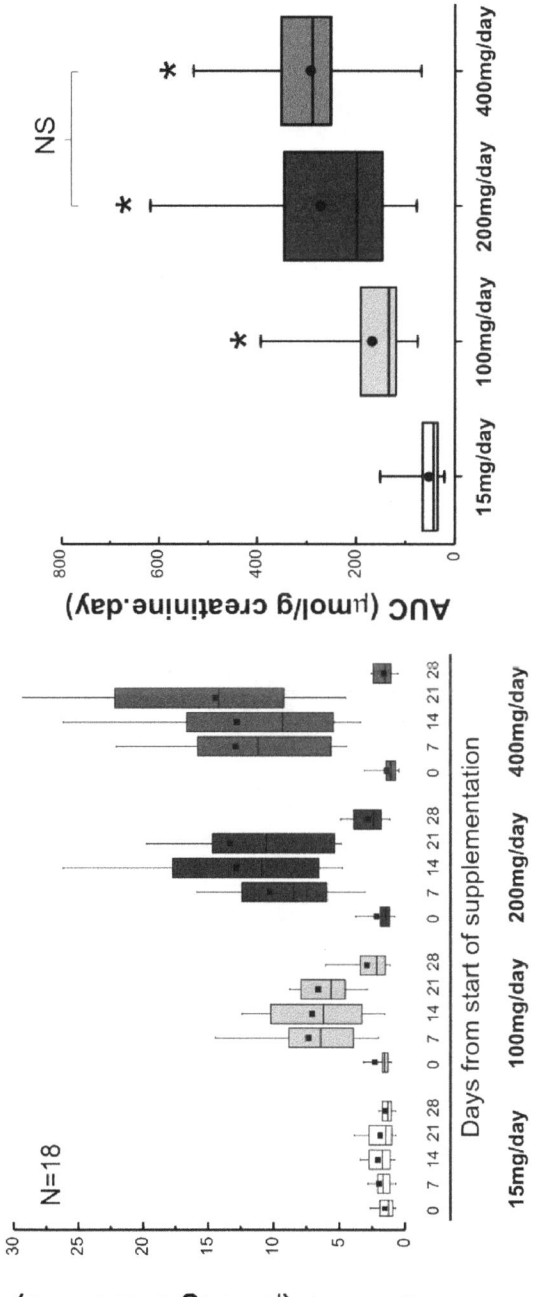

FIGURE 8. Urinary α-CEHC concentrations after supplementation at four doses over a 21-day period. The figure format is as outlined in the legend to FIGURE 7.

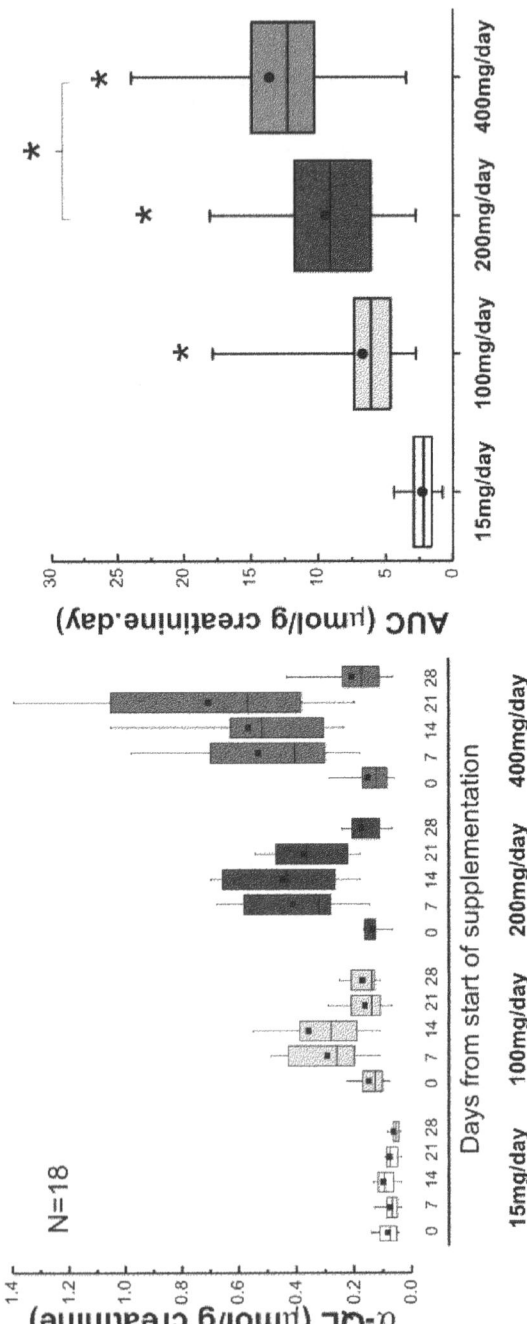

FIGURE 9. Urine α-QL concentrations after supplementation at four doses over a 21-day period. The figure format is as outlined in the legend to FIGURE 7.

significantly across the four supplementation periods: 6.32 (5.70–7.04) (15 mg/day), 5.63 (5.05–5.97) (100 mg/day), 6.55 (5.62–7.11) (200 mg/day), and 6.45 (5.97–7.04) (400 mg/day) µM/mM cholesterol.

To ascertain whether the magnitude of the individual responses to different α-tocopherol doses were related, we calculated the increase in concentration for each individual at each dose at days 7, 14, and 21, relative to the day 0 baseline. In addition, the decrease in α-tocopherol concentration observed across days 21 to 28 post supplementation was determined. The strength of any underlying association between these responses then was tested using Kendall's tau_b test. Using this approach, there was little evidence of response agreement between the supplementation doses. However, it was apparent that the day of the peak plasma concentration varied considerably for each subject. To overcome this, we calculated the total response, 0–28 days using the AUC for each individual at each dose. Using these data, we found that significant associations were apparent between individual responses at the 100-, 200-, and 400-mg/day doses: τ, 0.51, $P = 0.02$ [100 vs. 200] and τ, 0.49, $P = 0.03$ [100 vs. 400] and τ, 0.56, $P = 0.005$ [200 vs. 400]. It was also notable that the baseline α-tocopherol concentration (the mean of the four baselines) was highly associated with the magnitude of response: τ, 0.62, $P = 0.001$ [baseline vs. 15] and τ, 0.49, $P = 0.007$ [baseline vs. 100], τ, 0.54, $P = 0.007$ [baseline vs. 200] and τ, 0.52, $P = 0.005$ [baseline vs. 400]. Because the increase in plasma α-tocopherol concentrations seen after the 200- and 400-mg/day supplementation period were identical (242.68 [219.45–269.38] and 240.12 [223.17–267.49] µM/mM cholesterol/day, respectively], based on the AUC analysis, the intra-subject repeatability of these responses was examined using a one-way ANOVA on log10-transformed data. This revealed the individual responses at these two doses to be moderately repeatable, ICC = 0.58.

At the 15-mg/day dose, we saw no increase in urinary α-tocopherol metabolite (α-CEHC or α-QL) concentrations over the 28-day supplementation period (FIGS. 8 and 9). In contrast, dose-dependant and significant increases in urinary α-CEHC and α-QL concentrations were observed during the 100-, 200-, and 400-mg/day supplementation periods falling back to presupplementation values within 7 days of the end of the dosing protocol. Considering α-CEHC at the 100-mg/day dose, we found that urinary concentrations peaked between 7 and 14 days but shifted to 14–21 days at the 200- and 400-mg/day supplementation doses (FIG. 8). The overall urinary α-CEHC response to supplementation at 400 mg/day was not statistically different from that seen at the 200-mg/day dose. When the overall responses (AUC) were considered at each of the supplemental doses, only significant associations between urinary concentrations of α-CEHC were observed between the 100- and 200-mg/day doses: τ, 0.58, $P = 0.003$, with a trend toward an association at the 200- and 400-mg/day doses: τ, 0.44, $P = 0.05$. The low ICC of 0.53 reflected this later observation. Baseline urine α-CEHC concentrations were only predictive of the responses observed at the 400-mg/day dose: τ, 0.44, $P = 0.04$. QL concentrations at the 100- and 200-mg/day supplementation dose peaked between day 7 and 14, whereas the urine peak concentration occurred at day 21 at the highest dose (FIGURE 9). Notably, overall responses at the 200- and 400-mg/day dose differed significantly in contrast with the α-CEHC metabolite. As with α-CEHC, once supplementation was ceased, the excretion rate of α-QL fell rapidly back to control levels. Comparison of the responses (AUC) at each of the supplementation doses revealed that only the responses at 200 and 400 mg/day were significantly associated, τ, 0.43, $P = 0.03$. Baseline urine QL concentrations were predictive of the responses seen at the 100- and 200-mg/day doses: τ, 0.35, $P < 0.05$ and τ, 0.48, $P < 0.01$, respectively. We found, consistent with the observation that baseline α-CEHC and QL concentrations were significantly associated in Study 1, that overall responses also were associated at each of the supplementation levels: τ, 0.56, $P = 0.002$ [100 mg/day] and τ, 0.63, $P = 0.001$ [200 mg/day] and τ, 0.51, $P = 0.0125$ [400 mg/day].

DISCUSSION

Previously, we have demonstrated that α-tocopherol uptake, at a prescribed fat intake, varies widely in the healthy population.[8] In the current study we investigated whether individual baseline concentrations of plasma α-tocopherol and its associated urinary metabolites, α-CEHC and α-QL, were time-stable characteristics. In addition, we investigated whether there were consistent individual α-tocopherol uptake and excretion responses in healthy subjects over a wide range of supplementation doses: 15–400 mg/day. The aim of these studies was to establish whether there was sufficient temporal stability in the observed phenotypes to imply an underlying genetic basis to the observed differences between individuals. This concept was based, in part, on previous observations such as the concentration of vitamin E in plasma being tightly regulated and not increasing above certain concentrations in some individuals. A limit probably dictated by the saturation of hepatic α-TTP and hence the inability to incorporate further α-tocopherol into VLDLs.[17]

In the current study, plasma α-tocopherol concentrations were found to be within the normal published range, with both α-CEHC and α-QL metabolites present in all of the urine samples examined. In the α-CEHC metabolite, catabolism is confined to the phytl tail region of the molecule with the chroman ring remaining intact. It therefore has been argued that this metabolite arises from old α-tocopherol being displaced from the tissue by new, without the molecule's having participated in antioxidant reactions. Given this purported relationship, it was notable that we observed no underlying association between urinary concentrations of this metabolite and plasma α-tocopherol concentrations. In contrast, the presence of α-QL in the urine has been proposed to arise from the antioxidant function of the molecule, although this view remains contentious. We found the concentration of the α-QL metabolite to be 10-fold lower than α-CEHC, although both metabolites were highly correlated in individual urine samples. The presence of the α-QL in baseline urine samples from healthy subjects is at odds with the earlier findings of Schultz and colleagues[18] who suggested that the α-QL metabolite was an artefact arising from the oxidation of the chroman acid during the extraction protocol. Because the methodology used in these analyses included the use of d^9 α-CEHC as an internal control, if this later contention were true one might have expected to see the evolution of the d^9 α-QL metabolite during the sample workup. No such generation was noted. Furthermore, inclusion of butylated hydroxytoluene, duroquinone, and ascorbic acid during the extraction procedure did not influence the detection of the α-QL metabolite.

Plasma α-tocopherol showed a high degree of intrasubject repeatability over the studied intervals in Study 1, although it was notable that this deteriorated when the values were corrected for plasma cholesterol concentrations. In contrast, although baseline urinary α-CEHC and α-QL concentrations were strongly correlated for individuals between the three visits, the individual repeatability was substantially reduced, reflected by the large within-subject standard deviations. Note that because the within-subject standard deviations quoted in text are antilogs of the square root of the residual mean square obtained from the ANOVA on the log10 transformed data they are effectively dimensionless. Despite this, they can still be used to calculate a measure of the repeatability of the parameters using standard methods.[15]

In Study 2, we found that increasing intakes of vitamin E in the range 15–400 mg/day led to a range of responses within healthy individuals. At the 15-mg/day supplementation dose (i.e., an approximate one- to two-fold increase over dietary intake in the United Kingdom), we observed no change in circulating vitamin E concentrations over the 21-day supplementation period. Likewise, only small, but nonsignificant increases in α-tocopherol metabolite excretion were noted during this time. In contrast, supplementation with 100–400 mg vitamin E/day led to a marked increase in circulating vitamin E concentrations with no difference being seen between the 200- and 400-mg/day doses. Intake of these two large doses of vitamin E also led to increased excretion of two α-tocopherol metabolites in urine, namely, α-CEHC and α-QL. Underlying these general group responses to the various supplementation regimens, marked variation in individual responses were apparent. When individual responses to increasing vitamin E intake were examined in detail, strong evidence was obtained to indicate that individual responses to supplementation were time-stable characteristics. These findings confirm earlier reports of such individual variations by our group.[8,9]

Differences between individuals in how they acquire and metabolize vitamin E can arise for several reasons. First, they may simply absorb different amounts of this micronutrient. Vitamin E absorption in humans has been measured in only a few studies,[19,20] but it is generally agreed to be incomplete. It is not known why vitamin E is only partially absorbed, but individual variations in lipid absorption have been reported.[21] Efficient lipid absorption is dependent on the synchronization of several processes such as the secretion of bile and pancreatic lipases and the packaging of chylomicrons and their release into the systemic circulation. Within the enterocytes, polymorphisms in apoB or the microsomal transfer protein could influence the rate of chylomicron secretion and therefore appearance of dietary α-tocopherol in the systemic circulation.[22–24] Once present in the circulation, genetic polymorphisms in lipoprotein receptor genes could influence lipoprotein metabolism and therefore vitamin E tissue uptake and biokinetics.[25] Also, the requirement for vitamin E by different tissues may vary between individuals. Previously, we provided some evidence for this by showing that vitamin E uptake into erythrocytes varies markedly between healthy people, and it is not simply related to plasma concentrations of the vitamin.[8] It is evident therefore that there are several regulatory points in tocopherol uptake and processing pathways that could account for the inter-individual variations in response to vitamin E supplementation.

In conclusion, these data present further support for the contention that α-tocopherol uptake is genetically regulated. Furthermore, this mechanism also appears to regulate baseline plasma vitamin E concentration. Future intervention studies should take these differences into account, and further work is needed to gain a better understanding of the extent of inter-individual variation in vitamin E uptake in different population subgroups.

ACKNOWLEDGMENTS

This work was supported by project funding (NO 4014) from the UK Food Standards Agency.

REFERENCES

1. RIMM, E.B, M.J. STAMPFER, A. ASCHERIO, et al. 1993. Vitamin E consumption and the risk of coronary heart disease in men. N. Engl. J. Med. **328:** 1450–1456.
2. STAMPFER, M.J, C.H. HENNEKENS, J.E. MANSON, et al. 1993. Vitamin E consumption and the risk of coronary disease in women. N. Engl. J. Med. **328:** 1444–1449.
3. GEY, K.F., P. PUSKA, P. JORDAN & U.K. MOSER. 1991. Inverse correlation between plasma vitamin E and mortality from ischemic heart disease in cross-cultural epidemiology. Am. J. Clin. Nutr. **53:** 326S–334S.
4. YOCHUM, L.A., A.R. FOLSOM & L.H. KUSHI. 2000. Intake of antioxidant vitamins and risk of death from stroke in postmenopausal women. Am. J. Clin. Nutr. **72:** 476–483.
5. VIVEKANANTHAN, D.P., M.S. PENN, S.K. SAPP, et al. 2003. Use of antioxidant vitamins for the prevention of cardiovascular disease: meta-analysis of randomised trials. Lancet **361:** 2017–2023.
6. WATERS, D.D., E.L ALDERMAN, J. HSIA, et al. 2002. Effects of hormone replacement therapy and antioxidant vitamin supplements on coronary atherosclerosis in postmenopausal women: a randomized controlled trial. JAMA **288:** 2432–2440.
7. GRIFFITHS, H.R., L. MOLLER, G. BARTOSZ, et al. 2002. Biomarkers Mol. Aspects Med. **23:** 101–209.
8. ROXBOROUGH, H.E., G.W. BURTON & F.J. KELLY. 2000. Inter- and intra-individual variation in plasma and red blood cell vitamin E after supplementation. Free Radic. Res. **33:** 437–445.
9. CHEESEMAN, K.H., A.E. HOLLEY, F.J. KELLY, et al. 1995. Biokinetics in humans of RRR-alpha-tocopherol—the free phenol, acetate ester, and succinate ester forms of vitamin-E. Free Radic. Biol. Med. **19:** 591–598.
10. CLARKE, R. & ARMITAGE, J. 2002. Antioxidant vitamins and risk of cardiovascular disease. Review of large-scale randomised trials. Cardiovasc. Drugs Ther. **16:** 411–415.
11. SHEKELLE, P.G., S.C. MORTON, L.K. JUNGVIG, et al. 2004. Effect of supplemental vitamin E for the prevention and treatment of cardiovascular disease. J. Gen. Intern. Med. **19:** 380–389.
12. KELLY, F.J., W. RODGERS, J. HANDEL, et al. 1990. Time course of vitamin E repletion in the preterm infant. Br. J. Nutr. **63:** 631–638.
13. GALLI, F., R. LEE, J. ATKINSON, et al. 2003. γ-Tocopherol biokinetics and transformation in humans. Free Radic. Res. **37:** 1225–1233.
14. BLAND, J.M. & D.G. ALTMAN. 1996. Measurement error. BMJ **313:** 744.
15. BLAND, J.M. & D.G. ALTMAN. 1996. Measurement error proportional to the mean. BMJ **313:** 106.
16. BLAND, J.M. & D.G. ALTMAN. 1996. Measurement error and correlation coefficients. BMJ **313:** 41–42.
17. TRABER, M. 1994. Determinants of plasma vitamin E concentration. Free Radic. Biol. Med. **16:** 229–239.
18. SCHULTZ, M., M. LEIST, M. PETRZIKA, et al. 1995. Novel urinary metabolite of alpha-tocopherol, 2,5,7,8-tetramethyl-2(2'-carboxyethyl)-6-hydroxy chroman, as an indicator of an adequate vitamin E supply? Am. J. Clin. Nutr. **62:** 1527S–1534S.
19. BLOMSTRAND, R. & L. FORSGREN. 1968. Labelled tocopherols in man. Intestinal absorption and thoracic-duct lymph transport of DL-alpha-tocopheryl-3,4-14C2 acetate DL-alpha-tocopheramine-3,4-14C2 DL-alpha-tocopherol-(5-methyl-3H) and N-(methyl-3H)-DL-gamma-tocopheramine. Int. Z. Vitaminforsch. **38:** 328–344.
20. KELLEHER, J. & M.S. LOSOWSKY. 1970. The absorption of alpha-tocopherol in man. Br. J. Nutr. **24:** 1033–1047.

21. MCNAMARA, J.R., H. CAMPOS, J.M. ORDOVAS, et al. 1987. Effect of gender, age, and lipid status on low-density lipoprotein subfraction distribution. Results from the Framingham Offspring Study. Arteriosclerosis **7:** 483–490.
22. PEACOCK, R.E., F. KARPE, P.J. TALMUD, et al. 1995. Common variation in the gene for apolipoprotein B modulates postprandial lipoprotein metabolism: a hypothesis generating study. Atherosclerosis **116:** 135–145.
23. BERGERON, N. & R.J. HAVEL. 1997. Assessment of postprandial lipemia: nutritional influences. Curr. Opin. Lipidol. **8:** 43–52.
24. HUSSAIN, M.M. 2000. A proposed model for the assembly of chylomicrons. Atherosclerosis **148:** 1–15.
25. YE, S.Q. & P.O. KWITEROVICH. 2000. Influence of genetic polymorphisms on responsiveness to dietary fat and cholesterol. Am. J. Clin. Nutr. **72:** 1275S–1284S.

The Effect of Age on Vitamin E Status, Metabolism, and Function

Metabolism as Assessed by Labeled Tocopherols

REGINA BRIGELIUS-FLOHÉ,[a] JOHANNES M. ROOB,[b] BEATE TIRAN,[c] SANDRA WUGA,[d] JOSEP RIBALTA,[e] EDMOND ROCK,[f] AND BRIGITTE M. WINKLHOFER-ROOB[d]

[a]*German Institute of Human Nutrition, Potsdam-Rehbrücke, D-14558 Nuthetal, Germany*

[b]*Division of Clinical Nephrology, Department of Internal Medicine, Medical University, A8036 Graz, Austria*

[c]*Clinical Institute of Medicine and Chemical Laboratory Diagnostics, Medical University, A-8036 Graz, Austria*

[d]*Institute of Molecular Biosciences, Karl-Franzens University, A-8010 Graz, Austria*

[e]*Lipid Research Unit, University Rovira i Virgili, 43201 Reus, Spain*

[f]*UMMM, INRA-Theix, 63122 St. Genes Champanelle, France*

ABSTRACT: The effects of age on vitamin E metabolism were studied in 97 healthy 20–75-year-old male nonsmoking Austrian volunteers of the VITAGE project. After a single oral intake of 30 mg d_6-RRR-α- and d_2-RRR-γ-tocopheryl acetate, blood and 24-hour urine was collected. Deuterated tocopherols in plasma and deuterated urinary metabolites were analyzed by GC-MS. A first evaluation revealed a similar uptake of d_6-α- and d_2-γ-tocopherol during the first 6 hours, and then d_2-γ-tocopherol started to decrease. Urinary d_2-γ-carboxyethyl hydroxychroman metabolites (CEHCs) exceeded those of d_6-α-CEHCs by about 10 times. There was no effect of age. Thus, there might be no need for a higher vitamin E intake for healthy elderly nonsmoking men.

KEYWORDS: vitamin E; metabolism; absorption; α-tocopherol; γ-tocopherol; aging; α-CEHCs; γ-CEHCs

INTRODUCTION

The present study is part of the VITAGE project, which started in 2000 with funding from the European Union. The primary focus of this multidisciplinary and multicentric project was to characterize the putative changes in the status, the

Address for correspondence: Prof. Dr. Regina Brigelius-Flohé, German Institute of Human Nutrition, Potsdam-Rehbrücke, Arthur-Scheunert-Allee 114-116, D-14558 Nuthetal, Germany. Voice: +49-33200-88-353; fax: +49-33200-88-407.
  flohe@mail.dife.de

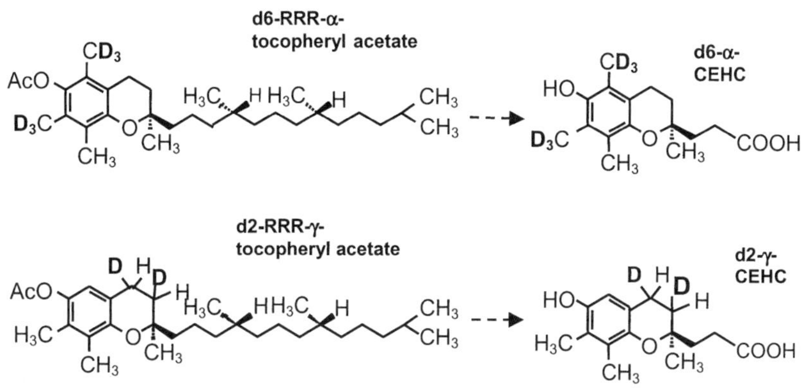

FIGURE 1. Structure of α- and γ-tocopheryl acetate, the final metabolites α- and γ-CEHC derived therefrom, and the positions of deuteration (D).

metabolism, and the functions of fat-soluble vitamins, including vitamin A, vitamin E, and carotenoids that may occur during nonpathological aging in humans.[1]

The topic of the study presented here is vitamin E and the aim was to investigate whether absorption and metabolism of α- and γ-tocopherol is similar or different and whether changes occur with age. Therefore equal amounts of deuterated α- and γ-tocopherol were taken by healthy volunteers and the changes in plasma levels thereof were measured. Vitamin E is not metabolically inert, but can be degraded and excreted into the urine.[2] Urinary metabolites have an intact chroman structure and a shortened side chain. Degradation starts with an ω-hydroxylation followed by β-oxidation.[3,4] The final products of all tocopherols and tocotrienols, the respective carboxyethyl hydroxychromans (CEHCs) (FIG. 1), are excreted as glucuronides and/or sulfates in the urine. Whereas the mechanism of side-chain degradation is the same for all forms of vitamin E, the rate by which individual tocopherols and tocotrienols are metabolized can differ tremendously.[5,6] Therefore the amount of urinary metabolites derived from d_6-α- and d_2-γ-tocopherol was estimated to determine whether α- and γ-tocopherol are metabolized to a different degree and whether metabolism changes with age.

STUDY DESIGN, SUBJECTS, AND METHODS

After an overnight fast, 97 healthy male nonsmoking Austrian volunteers were given a single oral dose of 30 mg each of d_6-RRR-α- and d_2-RRR-γ-tocopheryl acetate (synthesized by ORPHACHEM, Clermont-Ferrand, France) along with a standardized breakfast. Blood was drawn before and after 3, 6, 9, 12, 24, 48, 72, and 96 hours and 7, 11, and (in 45 volunteers only) 19 days after the test dose. Plasma concentrations of d_6-α- and d_2-γ-tocopherol were measured by gas chromatography/mass spectrometry as described.[7] In addition, 24-hr urine samples were collected before and daily during the first week and prior to day 11, and the final metabolites of d_6-α- and d_2-γ-tocopherol, the respective CEHCs, were determined.[7]

RESULTS

Deuterated α- and γ-Tocopherols in Plasma

Uptake of deuterated α-and γ-tocopherol was similar only during the first 6 hours. Thereafter γ-tocopherol started to decrease, whereas α-tocopherol increased up to 12 hours after application. d_2-γ-Tocopherol levels returned to baseline after 2 days, and d_6-α-tocopherol fell below 5% of the initial value only after 19 days. Thus, α-tocopherol is preferentially maintained in the circulation and γ-tocopherol is eliminated faster. These results on 97 volunteers confirm previous data obtained on only 4 subjects.[8] There was no effect of age in the plasma concentrations of d_6-α-tocopherol when standardized for cholesterol, demonstrating that the plasma concentrations of α-tocopherol rather depend on plasma lipid concentrations than on an age-related efficacy of absorption.

Urinary Vitamin E Metabolites Derived from Deuterated α- and γ-Tocopherol

The amounts of d_2-γ-CEHCs excreted during the first 6 days after the application were 1411 ± 754 µg; those of d_6-α-CEHC were 129 ± 89 µg. This shows that γ-CEHCs are about 10 times higher and confirms the reported higher metabolic rate of γ-tocopherol. Calculation of the percentage of tocopherols which can be found as CEHCs revealed that less than 1% of the applied d_6-α-tocopherol was degraded to α-CEHCs, whereas about 7.5% of d_2-γ-tocopherol appeared as γ-CEHCs in the urine. This is lower than the 50% suggested by Swanson et al.,[5] but nevertheless shows that metabolism and excretion of γ-tocopherol by far exceeds that of α-tocopherol. There was no effect of age on the amount of α- or γ-CEHCs released into the urine.

SUMMARY AND CONCLUSIONS

Although large individual variations were observed regarding the amount of deuterated α- and γ-tocopherol that were taken up and degraded by the 97 subjects, none of the variables measured was affected by the subjects' age. This indicates that there are no obvious changes in the absorption and degradation of α- and γ-tocopherol with age which would provide the scientific basis for specific recommendations of vitamin E intake for healthy elderly nonsmoking men. This might be different for smokers since the disappearance of vitamin E in the plasma has been shown to be increased in smokers.[9]

ACKNOWLEDGMENTS

This study was carried out with financial support from the Commission of the European Communities, specifically the RTD programme "Quality of Life and Management of Living Resources," QLK1-CT-1999-00830, VITAGE. It does not necessarily reflect its views and in no way anticipates the Commission's future policy in this area.

REFERENCES

1. ROCK, E., B.M. WINKLHOFER-ROOB, J. RIBALTA, et al. 2001. Vitamin A, vitamin E and carotenoid status and metabolism during ageing: functional and nutritional consequences (VITAGE PROJECT). Nutr. Metab. Cardiovasc. Dis. **11:** 70–73.
2. SCHULTZ, M., M. LEIST, M. PETRZIKA, et al. 1995. Novel urinary metabolite of alpha-tocopherol, 2,5,7,8-tetramethyl-2(2'-carboxyethyl)-6-hydroxychroman, as an indicator of an adequate vitamin E supply? Am. J. Clin. Nutr. **62:** 1527S–1534S.
3. BIRRINGER, M., P. PFLUGER, D. KLUTH, et al. 2002. Identities and differences in the metabolism of tocotrienols and tocopherols in HepG2 cells. J. Nutr. **132:** 3113–3118.
4. SONTAG, T.J. & R.S. PARKER. 2002. Cytochrome P450 omega-hydroxylase pathway of tocopherol catabolism. Novel mechanism of regulation of vitamin E status. J. Biol. Chem. **277:** 25290–25296.
5. SWANSON, J.E., R.N. BEN, G.W. BURTON & R.S. PARKER. 1999. Urinary excretion of 2,7, 8-trimethyl-2-(beta-carboxyethyl)-6-hydroxychroman is a major route of elimination of gamma-tocopherol in humans. J. Lipid Res. **40:** 665–671.
6. LODGE, J.K., J. RIDLINGTON, S. LEONARD, et al. 2001. Alpha-and gamma-tocotrienols are metabolized to carboxyethyl-hydroxychroman derivatives and excreted in human urine. Lipids **36:** 43–48.
7. TRABER, M.G., A. ELSNER & R. BRIGELIUS-FLOHÉ. 1998. Synthetic as compared with natural vitamin E is preferentially excreted as alpha-CEHC in human urine: studies using deuterated alpha-tocopheryl acetates. FEBS Lett. **437:** 145–148.
8. TRABER, M.G., G.W. BURTON, L. HUGHES, et al. 1992. Discrimination between forms of vitamin E by humans with and without genetic abnormalities of lipoprotein metabolism. J. Lipid Res. **33:** 1171–1182.
9. TRABER, M.G., B.M. WINKLHOFER-ROOB, J.M. ROOB, et al. 2001. Vitamin E kinetics in smokers and non-smokers. Free Radic. Biol. Med. **31:** 1368–1374.

Molecular Mechanisms of Vitamin E Transport

ACHIM STOCKER

Institute of Microbiology, Swiss Federal Institute of Technology, Zürich, Switzerland

ABSTRACT: Vitamin E is the most important lipid-soluble antioxidant in humans. Specific tocopherol-binding proteins favor the retention of the most potent vitamin E homologue, RRR-α-tocopherol (RRR-α-T) in man. The crystal structures of both the ligand-charged and the apo-forms of human α-tocopherol transfer protein (α-TTP) and of human supernatant protein factor (SPF) have been solved. The renewed interest in the biological function of tocopherol binders is based on the discovery of ataxia with vitamin E deficiency, a neurological disorder that is caused by genetic defects of the α-TTP gene and/ or vitamin E deficiency. The analysis of the crystal structure of α-TTP provides the molecular basis of vitamin E retention in man. SPF has been reported to enhance cholesterol biosynthesis by facilitating the conversion of squalene to lanosterol. Nevertheless, the physiological role of SPF as well as its ligand specificity is not known. Investigations on the substrate specificity of SPF have uncovered binding of RRR-α-tocopherylquinone (RRR-α-TQ). RRR-α-TQ represents the major physiological oxidation product of RRR-α-T. The three-dimensional overlay of the ligand-charged structures of SPF and α-TTP indicates that ligand specificity in both proteins is mostly modulated by side-chain variations rather than by the backbone. Recent reports point towards the *in vivo* reduction of RRR-α-TQ to RRR-α-TQH$_2$ and its protective role in low-density lipoprotein oxidation. On the basis of these reports, it is proposed that SPF may enhance cholesterol biosynthesis indirectly by mediating the transfer of RRR-α-TQ to low-density lipoprotein, thus reducing oxidation of low-density lipoprotein and its subsequent cellular uptake by scavenger receptors.

KEYWORDS: α-tocopherol transfer protein; squalene; α-tocopherylquinone; crystal structure; SEC14-like; CRAL_TRIO; ataxia; vitamin E deficiency

VITAMIN E HISTORY

The term "vitamin E" describes an essential nutrient factor that was introduced in 1922 by Evans and Bishop,[1] who observed that normal reproduction of female rats was abolished by feeding them with rancid fat. The animals developed a severe deficiency syndrome in which fetal resorption was the most characteristic symptom. Adding fresh salad to the diet was reversing the symptoms, and so they concluded that plants contain a specific factor responsible for the observations. Consequently, fetal resorption in rodents was further used for testing the biological activity of vitamin E.[2]

Address for correspondence: Dr. Achim Stocker, Institute of Microbiology, Swiss Federal Institute of Technology Zürich, Schmelzbergstr. 7, 8092 Zürich, Switzerland. Voice: +41-1-632-3322; fax: +41-1-632-5523.
achim.stocker@micro.biol.ethz.ch

The physicochemical properties of the factor began to appear in 1936 when two compounds with vitamin E activity were isolated and characterized from wheat germ oil.[3] These compounds were designated α- and β-tocopherol, deduced from the Greek *tokos* (childbirth) and *phorein* (to bring forth). In the following years, two additional tocopherols, γ- and δ-tocopherol, as well as the tocotrienols, were isolated from edible plant oils, so that today, a total of four tocopherols and four tocotrienols are known to occur in nature.[4–6]

CHEMISTRY OF TOCOPHEROLS AND TOCOTRIENOLS

The tocopherols, as well as the tocotrienols, are derivatives of 6-chromanol. The first group derives from tocol, which carries a saturated isoprenoid C_{-16} side chain and three chiral centers with configuration R at positions 2, 4', and 8'. The members of the second group have a triply unsaturated side-chain at positions 3', 7', and 11'. Within one group, the members are designated α, β, γ, and δ, depending on the number and the position of the methyl groups attached to the aromatic ring.[7]

Tocopherols are naturally occurring phenolic benzopyrans that display antioxidant activities *in vivo* and *in vitro*.[8] Since their initial discovery, they have been investigated in order to elucidate their mechanism of action and to identify potential metabolites. Much interest has been focused on their reactivity towards peroxyl radicals as well as on their remarkable regiospecificity towards oxidation and electrophilic substitution.[9–11] Burton and colleagues[12] have undertaken extensive studies on the effects of the chemical structure of phenolic compounds on their reactivity towards peroxyl radicals. By measuring the rate constant for hydrogen abstraction from tocopherols and related phenols, they found that α-tocopherol had the highest value ($k_1 = 2.35 \times 10^6$ M^{-1} s^{-1} at 30°C) of all compounds examined. It was concluded that the rate constant k_1 is determined primarily by the bond dissociation energy of the phenolic O-H bond, which is influenced by stereoelectronic effects as well as by constituent effects. They could demonstrate that the unpaired electron of the α-tocopheroxyl radical is resonance-stabilized over the heterocyclic chromanol ring and that the effect is increased by the electron-donating methyl groups.

Besides having radical trapping properties, α-tocopherol can act as a strong reductant and as an electrophilic agent in chemical reactions, depending on its environment. It has recently been shown that chemical oxidation of α-tocopherol (α-T) to α-tocopherylquinone (α-TQ) proceeds in two steps under retention of configuration R of the chiral center at the 2-position and is accompanied by the formation of a para-quinoid transition state and its mesomeric orthoquinone methide (FIG. 1).[11]

Investigations of the chemistry of the quinone methide indicate that the intermediate is reactive towards nucleophilic agents as well as towards protic solvents. Reactions of the orthoquinone methide that is formed by the phenolic OH group and a ring methyl group always occur in the 5-position, never by the 7-methyl group. The preference of the 5-position, the so-called Mills–Nixon Effect, has been calculated and ascribed to simple changes in conjugative effects, as discussed by Behan and colleagues.[13] Accordingly, tocopheryl quinones (TQs) can be divided in two classes, the nonarylating α-TQs and the arylating γ- and δ-TQs, the latter two lacking the 5-methyl group and being highly cytotoxic by stimulating apoptosis in mammalian cells.[14,15] The observation that partially substituted TQs form Michael adducts with

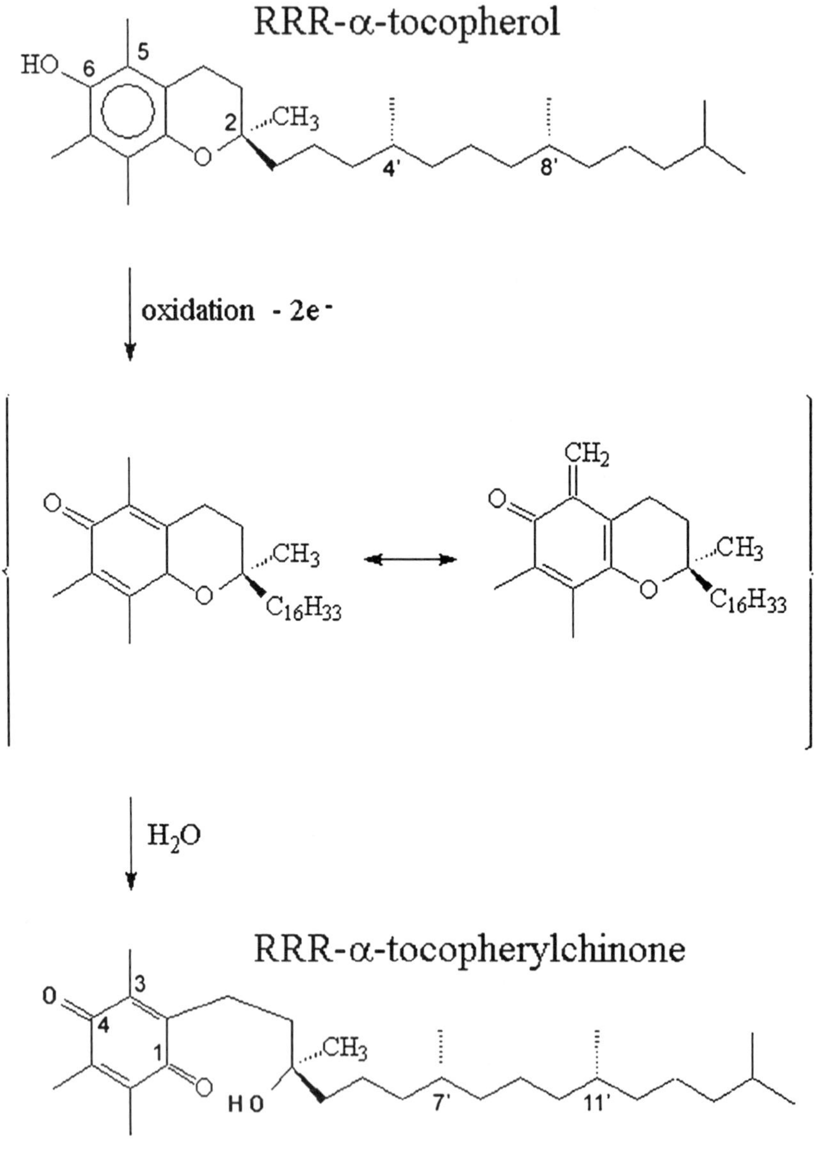

FIGURE 1. Flowchart describing the oxidation of RRR-α-T to RRR-α-TQ (atom numbering included).

high mutagenicity in mammalian cells has led to the hypothesis that the selective accumulation of RRR-α-T might represent an evolutionary advantage due to the relatively low toxicity of its corresponding oxidation product, RRR-α-TQ.[14] Consequently, alterations in the biological activity of tocopherols depend on specific structural alterations, including the presence or absence of ring methyl groups, the stereochemistry of the chiral carbon centers, and the branching or desaturation of the side-chain.

VITAMIN E METABOLISM

Post-absorptive elimination of the various forms of vitamin E appears to play a major role in regulating tissue tocopherol concentrations.[16] This pathway involves ω-hydroxylation of the tocopherol phytyl side-chain by cytochrome p450 enzymes such as CYP4F2 and CYP3A4,[17,18] followed by stepwise removal of two- or three-carbon moieties, ultimately yielding the carboxyethyl-hydroxychromane (CEHC) metabolite that is excreted largely as glucuronide conjugate in the urine.[19] In this way, the liver does not accumulate toxic levels of vitamin E. Administering high doses of RRR-α-T (335 mg/day) increases plasma RRR-α-T only to a threshold of 1.5–3.0-fold and instead increases plasma α-CEHC, the major metabolite of RRR-α-T, 15–30-fold.[20] Nevertheless, urinary α-CEHC excretion in normal control subjects is negligible, significant amounts being observed solely after supplementation of RRR-α-T at levels that exceed nutritional intake. In contrast, substantial proportions of estimated daily intake of all other vitamin E homologues such as RRR-γ-T are excreted in human urine as CEHC-glucuronide conjugates. All forms of vitamin E have been shown to activate gene expression via the pregnane X receptor.[21] This nuclear receptor is known to regulate drug-metabolizing enzymes such as CYP3A4. In conclusion, these findings again stress the importance of α-tocopherol transfer protein (α-TTP) in rescuing RRR-α-T from hepatic elimination by drug-metabolizing enzymes, a process that appears to be the "default" pathway of vitamin E in man.

RELATIONSHIP BETWEEN STRUCTURE AND BIOLOGICAL ACTIVITY OF VITAMIN E

Although the physiological process has remained obscure, vitamin E is thought to act mainly through its antioxidant properties in preventing damage caused by free radicals. Various independent studies confirm the outstanding role for RRR-α-T as the most potent chain-breaking antioxidant in membranes and the most biologically active of the eight vitamin E homologues.[22–26] Unlike naturally occurring RRR-α-tocopherol (RRR-α-T), the most common synthetic form of vitamin E, *all-rac*-α-tocopherol (*all-rac*-α-T), contains eight different stereoisomers arising from the three stereocenters of the tocopherol backbone. Although the *all-rac*-α-T form displays impaired biological activity, it is equally potent as an antioxidant.[27,28] This indicates that the stereochemistry of RRR-α-T is essential for its biological activity, but moreover that antioxidant activities of tocopherols do not necessarily match corresponding biological activities. Following uptake of dietary vitamin E, RRR-α-T is selectively retained in the body whereas other vitamin E homologues, including non-natural stereoisomers, encounter rapid clearance.[29,30] Thus, the outstanding biological potency of RRR-α-T seems to be associated with a bio-discrimination that modulates its extracellular and intracellular abundance.

ABSORPTION OF VITAMIN E

In man, vitamin E is taken up passively by micellar absorption together with dietary fats through the brush border membrane of the intestine.[31] A combination of triglycerides, phospholipids, cholesterol, vitamin E, and apolipoproteins is then reassembled to chylomicrons in the mucosa cells.[32] The chylomicrons are stored as secretory granula in the mucosa and eventually excreted by exocytosis to the lymphatic compartment from where they reach the blood stream via the ductus thoracicus.[33] The high clearance rate (24 hr) of a bolus of vitamin E from plasma makes it likely that the transformation of chylomicrons to remnants triggers receptor-mediated endocytotis of the latter by hepatic receptors for apo-E and apo-B.[34–36] Intravascular degradation of the chylomicrons to remnants by the endothelial lipoprotein lipase (LPL) as well as the apolipoprotein exchange between chylomicrons (types AI, AII, and B_{48}) and HDL (types C and E) seem to be instrumental for this process. The plasma lipoproteins are transported to the endosomal compartment, undergo hydrolysis, and release the vitamin E associated with them.[37] Several lines of evidence indicate that after it reaches the liver endosomal compartment, dietary vitamin E encounters rapid elimination, with the exception of RRR-α-T, which is re-secreted into plasma in conjunction with very-low-density lipoprotein (VLDL).[33,38] It has been known for some time that plasma and tissue RRR-α-T concentrations are remarkably stable. This stability suggests that protein factors are involved in its regulation.

REGULATION OF VITAMIN E BY TOCOPHEROL-BINDING PROTEINS

α-Tocopherol Transfer Protein

Hepatic RRR-α-T levels have been proven to be under the control of α-TTP, a cytosolic 32-kDa protein first described by Catignani.[39,40] α-TTP selectively binds to RRR-α-T (100%) relative to RRR-β-T (38%), RRR-γ-T (9%), and RRR-δ-T (2%).[41] Of these four naturally occurring analogues, RRR-β-T is found in negligible amounts in food, whereas RRR-δ-T, RRR-α-T, and RRR-γ-T are abundant in different ratios in most edible oils,[42] stressing the prominent role of α-TTP as a carrier for food-derived RRR-α-T.[43]

The crystal structure of human α-TTP has been solved in two distinct conformations at 1.9 Å resolution, shedding light on its transfer mechanism and its function as a physiological carrier for RRR-α-T (FIG. 2).[44]

In the closed RRR-α-T-charged form of α-TTP, a mobile helical surface segment seals its binding pocket. The conformation of this lid affects ligand access to the lipid-binding site. The RRR-α-T molecule is deeply buried in a hydrophobic pocket that is closed by the lid. The hydrophobic side of the lid helix lies on the entrance of the pocket, whereas the more polar one faces the solvent. In the presence of detergent, α-TTP adopts a conformation with an open lid most likely representing the

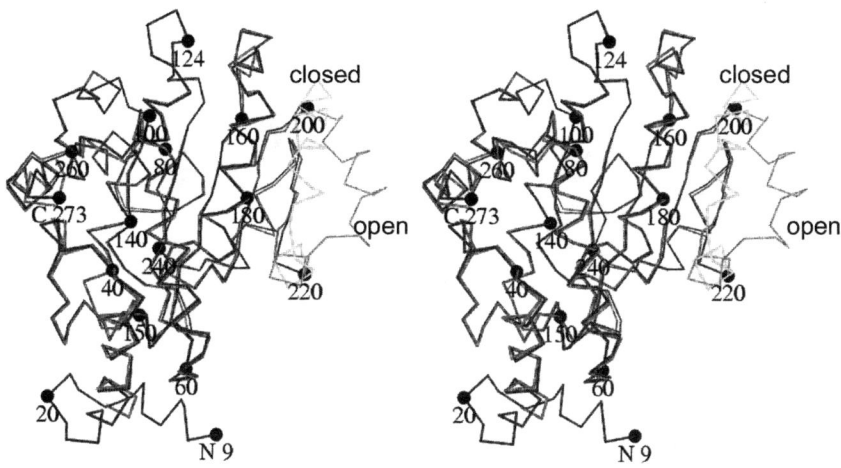

FIGURE 2. Stereoview of labeled Cα traces of the open end of the closed conformation of the α-TTP structure. Figures were prepared using the PYMOL program (Warren Delano, http://www.pymol.org).

membrane-bound form of the protein. The hydrophobic side of the lid helix now faces the solvent. The rotation of the lid by about 80° causes a shift of about 14 Å. The crystallographic evidence obtained from two distinct conformational states of α-TTP allows a rather precise prediction concerning the transfer mechanism of RRR-α-T.

In the closed conformation, a large hydrophobic area (Phe203, Val 206, Phe207, Ile210, and Leu214) of the lid is in direct contact with the side-chain of RRR-α-T. Opening of the lid shifts these residues towards the exterior, establishing new hydrophobic contacts with lipids, detergents, or hydrophobic surfaces. Bound tocopherol is then released into the membrane or, vice versa, is shuffled into the empty or water-filled binding pocket by lid closure. Water molecules in the cavity, if present, are probably squeezed out through a tunnel connecting the rear of the pocket with the hydrophilic solvent. The closed lid exposes a more polar face to the solvent, and the charged carrier–ligand complex can leave the membrane.

The preference of α-TTP for RRR-α-tocopherol can be explained semi-quantitatively from the observed van der Waals contacts in the lipid-binding pocket of the crystal structure (FIG. 3). The chromanol moiety of RRR-α-T is mostly surrounded by hydrophobic residues, with the exception of Ser 136, Ser140, and three water molecules. One of these connects the para hydroxyl group of the chromanol ring with the backbone carbonyl of Val182 through a hydrogen bond. The aromatic methyl group in 5-position of the chromanol moiety fits snugly into a niche formed by the side chains of residues Ile194, Val191, Ile154, and Leu183, the latter two being in van der Waals contact, with a distance of about 3.6 Å. On the other side of the chromanol ring, the two aromatic methyl groups in 7- and 8-position make contacts to Phe187, Phe133, and Leu137. The position and geometry of the pyran half-chair

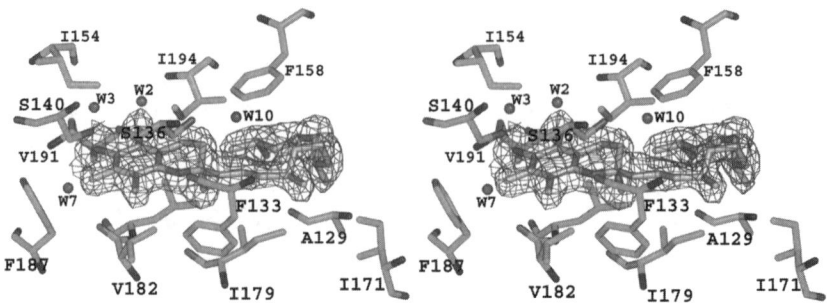

FIGURE 3. Stereoview of the ligand-binding pocket of α-TTP with electron density of bound RRR-α-tocopherol. Shown is a $2F_o$-F_c density map contoured at 1.0 sigma above the mean. The map was computed before the ligand was included in the model. RRR-α-T and residues within van der Waals distance are depicted as stick models, with internal water molecules shown as balls.

of the chromanol ring determine the relative positions of the substituents at the stereocenter in 2-position with the axial methyl group protruding into an indent of the cavity formed by residues Phe133, Val182, and Ile179. The prenyl side-chain is bent into a U-turn involving both stereocenters at the 4′- and at the 8′-position.

RRR-γ-T lacks one aromatic methyl group in 5-position and therefore fits into the cavity as well. However, the absence of one methyl group reduces the surface available for hydrophobic interactions and diminishes the packing density. Studies by Fersht and colleagues derived an average penalty of 1.3 ± 0.5 kcal/mol for the removal of a single methylene group from the hydrophobic main core of chymotrypsin inhibitor 2.[45] If this number is taken as a rough guide for the removal of a methyl group from the hydrophobic cavity of α-TTP, a binding ratio of 8.3 ± 6.7 (at 310 K) is obtained for $K^{\gamma-T}/K^{\alpha-T}$. This estimate fits the experimentally determined 10-fold reduction in RRR-γ-T binding.[41] Of course, the error is large because of the varying extent of hydrophobic contacts of a methyl group, which is reflected in the large uncertainty of the figure given by Fersht and colleagues. In the case of RRR-δ-T, where an additional methyl group is missing in 7-position, the computed ratio of $K^{\delta-T}/K^{\alpha-T}$ equals 92, a value that correlates reasonably well with the experimentally observed 50-fold reduction in binding, provided the large error is again considered.

The importance of RRR-α-T retention in man becomes evident by analyzing mutations in the gene of α-TTP in patients suffering from ataxia with vitamin E deficiency (AVED).[46,47] The AVED syndrome is characterized by deficient plasma vitamin E and by a progressive peripheral neuropathy with a specific dying back of the larger caliber axons and the sensory neurons, which finally results in ataxia.[48] Mapping the known AVED-causing amino acid substitutions onto the crystal structure indicates that the binding pocket is not affected in either case, indicating that these mutations seem to influence function rather by impairing the stability of the protein than by prohibiting ligand transfer (FIG. 4).

The six mutations (R59W, R221W, R192H, E141K, A120T, and H101Q) have been investigated by base substitution mutagenesis of recombinant wild-type α-TTP.[49] It was shown that variants associated with the severe version of AVED pa-

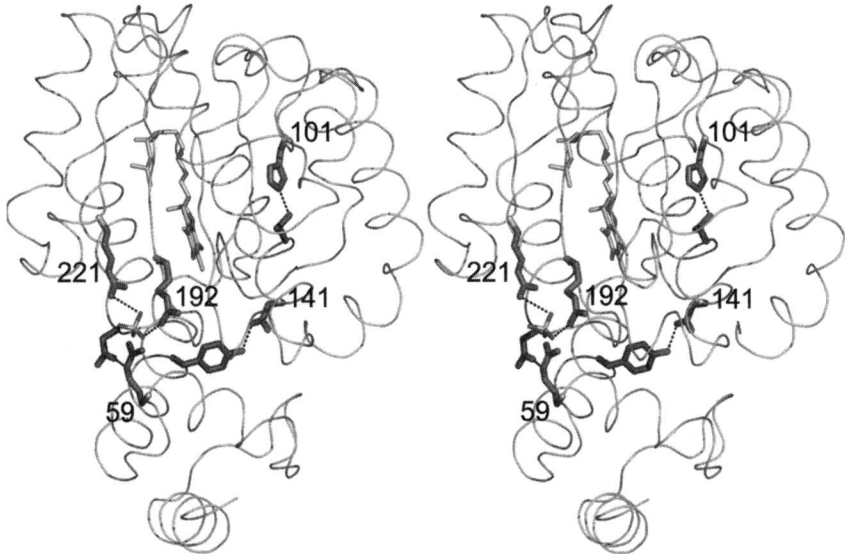

FIGURE 4. AVED-associated mutations in α-TTP. The clinically characterized mutations are mapped onto the three-dimensional structure. Residues undergoing mutation are depicted as stick models; the interacting amino acids described in the text are shown without labeling.

thology (R59W, E141K, and R221W) are impaired in both binding and transfer activities. On the other hand, variants associated with the milder forms of AVED (H101Q, A120T, and R192H) were strikingly similar to the wild-type protein. In accordance with these results, our preliminary attempts to overexpress in *Escherichia coli* and isolate the mutants R59W and R221W turned out to be unsuccessful because of the formation of insoluble protein aggregates. Only the mutant H101Q could be isolated as soluble protein. The comparison of the transfer activities, in accordance with the work of Hosomi and colleagues,[41] did not reveal significant differences between wild-type α-TTP and freshly prepared mutant H101Q, although the latter showed a rapid loss of transfer activity even when kept at 4°C. This indicates that helix 9 (residues 129–143) represents an important element of the α-TTP fold, forming one wall of the tocopherol-binding cavity. The hydrogen bond between T139 and the semi-conserved H101 most likely is not completely abolished by the replacement of histidine with glutamine and thus may explain why this mutation exhibits less severe phenotypes than, for example, the E141K mutation on the opposite site of helix 9.[50]

Not only does the liver express α-TTP (with a high expression rate), the mammalian brain seems to be able to express its own α-TTP. Accordingly, the neurological phenotype of α-TTP$^{-/-}$ mice has been found to be even more severe and shows an earlier onset than that of wild-type mice when maintained on an α-T-deficient diet,[51] the severe phenotype being unable to walk straight forward. Moreover, an uterine form of α-TTP has been reported to be essential for embryogenesis by supplying the

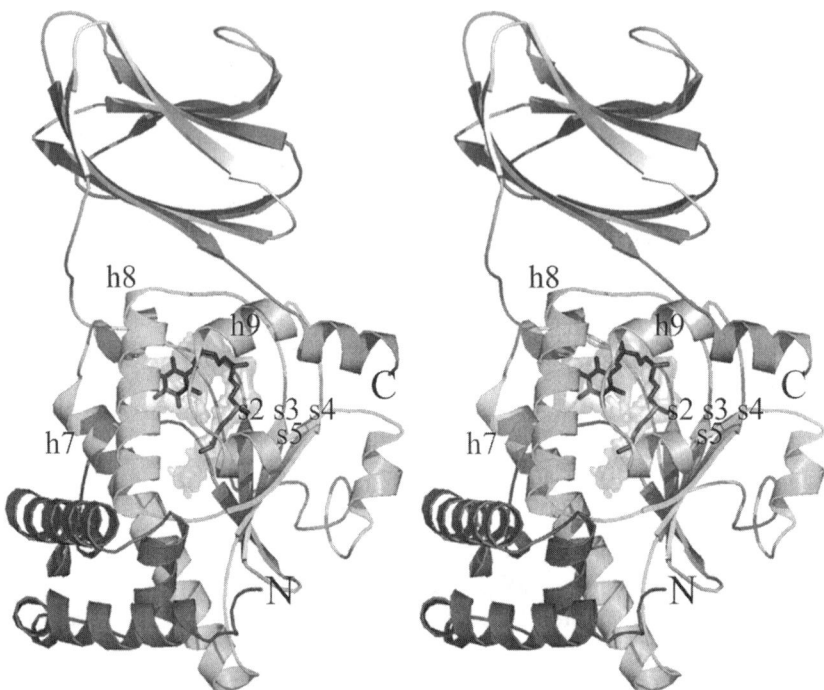

FIGURE 5. Stereoview of the SPF-RRR-α-TQ complex showing the three-helix coil (N-terminus), CRAL_TRIO lipid-binding domain with cavity, jellyroll (C-terminus).

labyrinth region of the placenta with RRR-α-T during development.[52] Both tissues are known to be exposed to high rates of oxidative stress and therefore seem to be specifically protected by α-TTP-mediated tocopherol delivery.

The function of α-TTP in mediating the incorporation of RRR-α-T into VLDL has remained elusive. Its re-secretion into plasma has been shown to be independent from Golgi-associated processes, and therefore seems not to depend on the secretion of VLDL into plasma. It has been suggested that the process of tocopherol re-secretion is linked to cellular cholesterol transport, which would implicate an involvement of the endosomal compartment.[53,54] The most recent report that α-TTP transiently localizes to late endosomes provides evidence for this hypothesis, showing that RRR-α-T is transiently removed by α-TTP from the endosomal compartment separating it from the other homologues of vitamin E that are destined for elimination.[37]

Supernatant Protein Factor

In 1999, a novel binder of vitamin E, termed tocopherol-associated protein (TAP), was discovered in the cytosol of bovine liver with the use of radioactively labeled α-tocopherol as tracer.[55] Subsequently, from the partial amino acid sequence of the bovine protein, its human homologue was identified. The human homologue

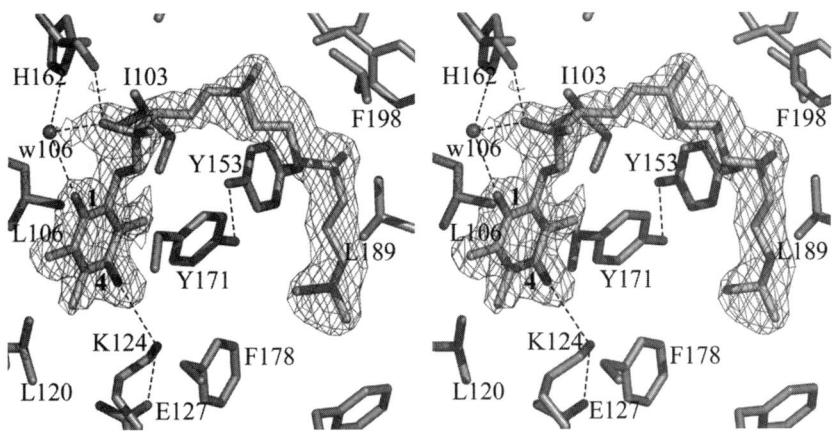

FIGURE 6. Electron density map of the RRR-α-TQ molecule embedded in the ligand-binding pocket of SPF. Shown is a $2F_o\text{-}F_c$ density map contoured at 1.0 sigma above the mean. The map was computed before RRR-α-TQ was included in the model. RRR-α-TQ and residues within van der Waals distance to the quinone molecule are depicted as stick models (atom numbering included), with internal water molecules shown as balls.

of bovine TAP (hTAP) was cloned into *E. coli*, and its tissue-specific expression was assessed by Northern blot analysis.[56] On the basis of dot-blot analysis, it was concluded that the major mRNA transcript of hTAP is widely expressed in human tissues, with the highest levels being found in liver, brain, and prostate. In order to establish if hTAP interacts directly with tocopherol, a biotinylated α-tocopherol derivative was synthesized and used as a ligand for binding measurements performed using an IASys-resonant mirror system. The measured dissociation constant of 4.6×10^{-7} M suggested that hTAP is expressed with a functional lipid-binding domain and that it is able to bind to biotinylated tocopherol well within physiological concentrations.

Recently, hTAP has been re-identified as Bloch's supernatant protein factor (SPF), which has been reported to stimulate the conversion of squalene to squalene-epoxide.[57] Therefore, the TAP designation has not been maintained. SPF is considered to be essential to human cholesterol production, though its precise function and ligand specificity have remained obscure.[57–59] The crystal structures of human apo-SPF and of its complex with RRR-α-TQ, the major physiological oxidation product of RRR-α-T, have been solved at resolutions of 1.90 Å and 1.95 Å, respectively.[60,61] The structure of apo-SPF consists essentially in two structural entities, an N-terminal CRAL_TRIO domain and a C-terminal jellyroll β fold (FIG. 5).

The N-terminal CRAL_TRIO lipid-binding motif defines SPF as a member of the family of SEC14-like lipid-transfer proteins, including phosphatidylinositol/phosphatidylcholine transfer protein (SEC14) from *Saccharomyces cerevisiae*, cellular retinaldehyde-binding protein (CRALBP), and α-TTP.[56] Database sequence analysis indicates that the jellyroll domain of SPF represents the structural prototype of the recently discovered GOLD (Golgi dynamics) domain.[62] The GOLD domain has been identified as an obligatory element of the widespread p24 protein superfamily serving as an anchor in protein recruitment and the formation of membrane-associated protein complexes at the Golgi apparatus. This hints towards an adaptor role of SPF in the assembly of membrane-associated complexes or in regulating assembly of cargo into membranous vesicles.

The structure of the complex reveals how SPF sequesters RRR-α-TP in its protein body and permits a comparison with the structure of human α-TTP in complex with RRR-α-TP. The overall structure of the SPF-RRR-α-TQ complex does not reveal significant differences compared with apo-SPF. The binding pocket of the SPF-RRR-α-TQ complex is mostly lined by hydrophobic amino acid side chains. The methyl groups at positions 5 and 6 of the quinone head group are in van der Waals distance to Val167, Val108, and Leu120, whereas the methyl group in position 3 at

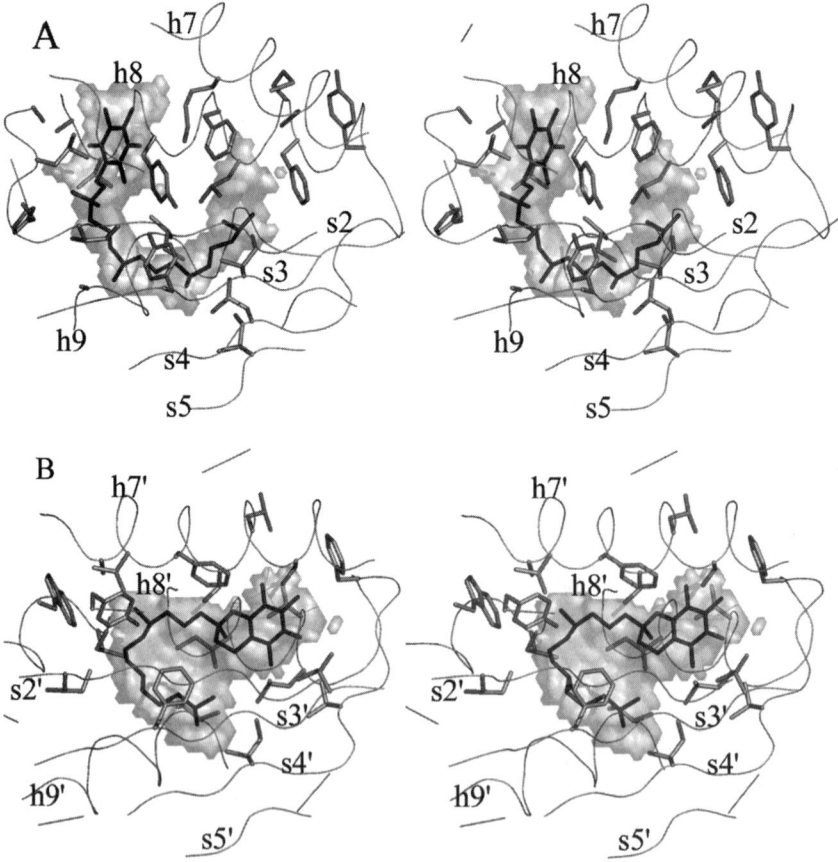

FIGURE 7. Stereoview of the ligand-binding pockets of (**A**) SPF with RRR-α-TQ and (**B**) α-TTP with RRR-α-T. Cavities are shown after least-squares superimposition of the Cα traces of the protein structures.

the opposite side of the ring forms van der Waals contacts to Leu106, Ile103, and Tyr171 (FIG. 6).

The side chain is embedded between Tyr153 and Phe198 and ends between Phe178 and Leu189. In contrast to the rather hydrophobic cavity of α-TTP that lacks charged residues, the RRR-α-TQ molecule of SPF is in vicinity to Lys124, which forms on one side a salt bridge (distance: 2.9 Å) with Glu127, and is on the other side hydrogen-bonded (distance: 3.4 Å) to the carbonyl oxygen in position 4 of the quinone head group. The second carbonyl oxygen in position 1 of the quinone forms a hydrogen bond via a water molecule to His162, the backbone carbonyl oxygen of which is hydrogen-bonded to the C3' hydroxyl group of the quinone, which itself forms a second hydrogen bond (distance: 2.4 Å) to the water molecule mentioned earlier (FIG. 6). In analogy to the complex of α-TTP with RRR-α-T, the RRR-α-TQ molecule is sitting in the cavity of SPF with the phytyl tail facing the cavity entrance and the quinone head pointing towards the interior, as can be expected for a lipid being pulled out of a micelle or bilayer (FIG. 7).

In contrast to the Cα-traces, the overall positions of α-TQ in SPF and α-T in TTP are grossly different in their respective binding pockets, which indicates that the ligand position in both proteins is mostly modulated by side-chain variations rather than by the backbone.

The physiologic role of RRR-α-TQ is not known yet. Nevertheless, RRR-α-TQ levels have been found to be remarkably low in the cerebrospinal fluid of patients with sporadic amyotrophic lateral sclerosis.[63] It has been reported by several groups that RRR-α-TQ is reduced *in vivo* to RRR-α-TQH$_2$.[64–67] In addition, oral supplementation of humans with RRR-α-T has been shown to result in micromolar plasma levels of both RRR-α-T and RRR-α-TQH$_2$.[68] Thus, plasma-bound RRR-α-TQH$_2$ has been proposed to serve together with other lipophilic antioxidants as a defense in blocking LDL (per)oxidation.[69] The concept that RRR-α-TQH$_2$ may act as co-antioxidant in LDL is based on the assumption that a specific carrier exists that mediates the transfer of RRR-α-TQ or RRR-α-TQH$_2$ to plasma lipoproteins in analogy to α-TTP that transfers RRR-α-T to plasma VLDL.[29,70] Blocking LDL oxidation by RRR-α-TQH$_2$ would diminish the uptake of oxidized LDL by the scavenger receptor CD36, with a resulting reduction in cellular cholesterol uptake.[71] Low levels of intracellular cholesterol would then subsequently induce cholesterol synthesis via known cellular feedback mechanisms.[72,73] Interestingly, recent studies from independent research groups have shown that overexpression of SPF in hepatoma cells increases cholesterol synthesis by two-fold and have suggested that SPF may have a role in regulating cholesterol synthesis *in vivo*.[57,74] Investigations on the role of RRR-α-TQH$_2$ as natural antioxidant[75] further support the idea of a putative link between the carrier function of SPF for RRR-α-TQ and its regulatory role in cellular cholesterol synthesis.

REFERENCES

1. EVANS, H.M. & K.S. BISHOP. 1922. On the existence of a hitherto unrecognized dietary factor essential for reproduction. Science **55**: 650–651.
2. LETH, T. & H. SONDERGAARD. 1977. Biological activity of vitamin E compounds and natural materials by the resorption-gestation test, and chemical determination of the vitamin E activity in foods and feeds. J. Nutr. **107**: 2236–2243.

3. EVANS, H.M., O.H. EMERSON & G.A. EMERSON. 1936. Isolation von tocopherolen. J. Biol. Chem. **113:** 319.
4. EMERSON, O.H., G.A. EMERSON, A. MOHAMMAD & H.M. EVANS. 1937. gamma-Tocopherol. J. Biol. Chem. **122:** 99.
5. STERN, M.H., R.C.D., L. WEISLER & J.G. BAXTER. 1947. delta-Tocopherol. J. Am. Chem. Soc. **69:** 869.
6. PENNOCK, J.F., F.W. HEMMING & J.D. KERR. 1964. A reassessment of tocopherol in chemistry. Biochem. Biophys. Res. Commun. **17:** 542–548.
7. KWIATKOWSKA, J. 1988. Nomenclature of tocopherols and related compounds. Postepy Biochem. **34:** 461–465.
8. BURTON, G.W. *et al.* 1983. Vitamin E as an antioxidant in vitro and in vivo. Ciba Found. Symp. **101:** 4–18.
9. ROSENAU, T. & W.D. HABICHER. 1997. "Vitamin CE," a novel prodrug form of vitamin E. Chem. Pharm. Bull. (Tokyo) **45:** 1080–1084.
10. ROSENAU T., C.-L. CHEN & W.D. HABICHER. 1995. A vitamin E derivative as a novel, extremely advantageous amino-protecting group. J. Org. Chem. **60:** 8120–8121.
11. ROSENAU T. & W.D. HABICHER. 1995. Novel tocopherol compounds. Tetrahedron **51:** 7917–7926.
12. BURTON, G.W., A. JOYCE & K.U. INGOLD. 1982. First proof that vitamin E is major lipid-soluble, chain-breaking antioxidant in human blood plasma [letter]. Lancet **2:** 327.
13. BEHAN J.M., F.M. DEAN & R.A.W. JOHNSTONE. 1976. Photoelectron spectra of cyclic aromatic ethers. Tetrahedron **32:** 167–171.
14. JONES, K.H. *et al.* 2002. Gamma-tocopheryl quinone stimulates apoptosis in drug-sensitive and multidrug-resistant cancer cells. Lipids **37:** 173–184.
15. CORNWELL, D.G. *et al.* 2002. Mutagenicity of tocopheryl quinones: evolutionary advantage of selective accumulation of dietary alpha-tocopherol. Nutr. Cancer. **43:** 111–118.
16. BRIGELIUS-FLOHE, R. 2003. Vitamin E and drug metabolism. Biochem. Biophys. Res. Commun. **305:** 737–740.
17. SONTAG, T.J. & R.S. PARKER. 2002. Cytochrome P450 omega-hydroxylase pathway of tocopherol catabolism: novel mechanism of regulation of vitamin E status. J. Biol. Chem. **277:** 25290–25296.
18. PARKER, R.S., T.J. SONTAG & J.E. SWANSON. 2000. Cytochrome P4503A-dependent metabolism of tocopherols and inhibition by sesamin. Biochem. Biophys. Res. Commun. **277:** 531–534.
19. SCHONFELD, A. *et al.* 1993. A novel metabolite of RRR-alpha-tocopherol in human urine. Nahrung **37:** 498–500.
20. SCHULTZ, M. *et al.* 1995. Novel urinary metabolite of alpha-tocopherol, 2,5,7,8-tetramethyl-2(2′- carboxyethyl)-6-hydroxychroman, as an indicator of an adequate vitamin E supply? Am. J. Clin. Nutr. **62:** 1527S–1534S.
21. LANDES, N. *et al.* 2003. Vitamin E activates gene expression via the pregnane X receptor. Biochem. Pharmacol. **65:** 269–273.
22. INGOLD, K.U. *et al.* 1987. Biokinetics of and discrimination between dietary RRR- and SRR-alpha-tocopherols in the male rat. Lipids **22:** 163–172.
23. KIYOSE, C. *et al.* 1997. Biodiscrimination of alpha-tocopherol stereoisomers in humans after oral administration. Am. J. Clin. Nutr. **65:** 785–789.
24. WEISER, H. & M. VECCHI. 1981. Stereoisomers of alpha-tocopheryl acetate: characterization of the samples by physico-chemical methods and determination of biological activities in the rat resorption-gestation test. Int. J. Vitam. Nutr. Res. **51:** 100–113.
25. WEISER, H., M. VECCHI & M. SCHLACHTER. 1986. Stereoisomers of alpha-tocopheryl acetate. IV. USP units and alpha-tocopherol equivalents of all-rac-, 2-ambo- and RRR-alpha-tocopherol evaluated by simultaneous determination of resorption-gestation, myopathy and liver storage capacity in rats. Int. J. Vitam. Nutr. Res. **56:** 45–56.
26. WEBER, P., A. BENDICH & L.J. MACHLIN. 1997. Vitamin E and human health: rationale for determining recommended intake levels. Nutrition **13:** 450–460.

27. WEISER, H., G. RISS & A.W. KORMANN. 1996. Biodiscrimination of the eight alpha-tocopherol stereoisomers results in preferential accumulation of the four 2R forms in tissues and plasma of rats. J. Nutr. **126:** 2539–2549.
28. BURTON, G.W. et al. 1998. Human plasma and tissue alpha-tocopherol concentrations in response to supplementation with deuterated natural and synthetic vitamin E. Am. J. Clin. Nutr. **67:** 669–684.
29. TRABER, M.G. & H.J. KAYDEN. 1989. Preferential incorporation of alpha-tocopherol vs. gamma-tocopherol in human lipoproteins. Am. J. Clin. Nutr. **49:** 517–526.
30. TRABER, M.G. & H.J. KAYDEN. 1989. Alpha-tocopherol as compared with gamma-tocopherol is preferentially secreted in human lipoproteins. Ann. N.Y. Acad. Sci. **570:** 95–108.
31. GALLO-TORRES, H.E. 1970. Obligatory role of bile for the intestinal absorption of vitamin E. Lipids **5:** 379–384.
32. BJORNEBOE, A., G.E. BJORNEBOE & C.A. DREVON. 1990. Absorption, transport and distribution of vitamin E. J. Nutr. **120:** 233–242.
33. BJORNSON, L.K. et al. 1976. The transport of alpha-tocopherol and beta-carotene in human blood. J. Lipid Res. **17:** 343–352.
34. BUTTRISS, J.L. & A.T. DIPLOCK. 1988. The alpha-tocopherol and phospholipid fatty acid content of rat liver subcellular membranes in vitamin E and selenium deficiency. Biochim. Biophys. Acta **963:** 61–69.
35. MATHIAS, P.M. et al. 1981. Studies on the in vivo absorption of micellar solutions of tocopherol and tocopheryl acetate in the rat: demonstration and partial characterization of a mucosal esterase localized to the endoplasmic reticulum of the enterocyte. J. Lipid Res. **22:** 829–837.
36. HANDELMAN, G.J. et al. 1985. Oral alpha-tocopherol supplements decrease plasma gamma-tocopherol levels in humans. J. Nutr. **115:** 807–813.
37. HORIGUCHI, M. et al. 2003. pH-dependent translocation of alpha-tocopherol transfer protein (alpha-TTP) between hepatic cytosol and late endosomes. Genes Cells **8:** 789–800.
38. PEAKE, I.R., H.G. WINDMUELLER & J.G. BIERI. 1972. A comparison of the intestinal absorption, lymph and plasma transport, and tissue uptake of tocopherols in the rat. Biochim. Biophys. Acta **260:** 679–688.
39. CATIGNANI, G.L. 1975. An alpha-tocopherol binding protein in rat liver cytoplasm. Biochem. Biophys. Res. Commun. **67:** 66–72.
40. SATO, Y. et al. 1991. Purification and characterization of the alpha-tocopherol transfer protein from rat liver. FEBS Lett. **288:** 41–45.
41. HOSOMI, A. et al. 1997. Affinity for alpha-tocopherol transfer protein as a determinant of the biological activities of vitamin E analogs. FEBS Lett. **409:** 105–108.
42. LEHMANN, J. et al. 1986. Vitamin E in foods from high and low linoleic acid diets. J. Am. Diet. Assoc. **86:** 1208–1216.
43. TRABER, M.G. & H. ARAI. 1999. Molecular mechanisms of vitamin E transport. Annu. Rev. Nutr. **19:** 343–355.
44. MEIER, R. et al. 2003. The molecular basis of vitamin E retention: structure of human alpha-tocopherol transfer protein. J. Mol. Biol. **331:** 725–734.
45. OTZEN, D.E., M. RHEINNECKER & A.R. FERSHT. 1995. Structural factors contributing to the hydrophobic effect: the partly exposed hydrophobic minicore in chymotrypsin inhibitor 2. Biochemistry **34:** 13051–13058.
46. OUAHCHI, K. et al. 1995. Ataxia with isolated vitamin E deficiency is caused by mutations in the alpha-tocopherol transfer protein. Nat. Genet. **9:** 141–145.
47. YOKOTA, T. et al. 1996. Retinitis pigmentosa and ataxia caused by a mutation in the gene for the alpha-tocopherol-transfer protein. N. Engl. J. Med. **335:** 1770–1771.
48. GOTODA, T. et al. 1995. Adult-onset spinocerebellar dysfunction caused by a mutation in the gene for the alpha-tocopherol-transfer protein (see comments). N. Engl. J. Med. **333:** 1313–1318.
49. MANOR, D. et al. 2003. Biochemical characterization of AVED causing mutations of a-TTP. Unpublished results.

50. YOKOTA, T. *et al.* 1997. Friedreich-like ataxia with retinitis pigmentosa caused by the His101Gln mutation of the alpha-tocopherol transfer protein gene. Ann. Neurol. **41:** 826–832.
51. YOKOTA, T. *et al.* 2001. Delayed-onset ataxia in mice lacking alpha-tocopherol transfer protein: model for neuronal degeneration caused by chronic oxidative stress. Proc. Natl. Acad. Sci. USA **98:** 15185–15190.
52. JISHAGE, K. *et al.* 2001. Alpha-tocopherol transfer protein is important for the normal development of placental labyrithine trophoblasts in mice. J. Biol. Chem. **276:** 1669–1672.
53. ARITA, M. *et al.* 1997. Alpha-tocopherol transfer protein stimulates the secretion of alpha-tocopherol from a cultured liver cell line through a brefeldin A-insensitive pathway. Proc. Natl. Acad. Sci. USA **94:** 12437–12441.
54. FRAGOSO, Y.D. & A.J. BROWN. 1998. In vivo metabolism of alpha-tocopherol in lipoproteins and liver: studies on rabbits in response to acute cholesterol loading. Rev. Paul. Med. **116:** 1753–1759.
55. STOCKER, A. *et al.* 1999. Identification of a novel cytosolic tocopherol-binding protein: structure, specificity, and tissue distribution. IUBMB Life **48:** 49–55.
56. ZIMMER, S. *et al.* 2000. A novel human tocopherol-associated protein: cloning, in vitro expression, and characterization. J. Biol. Chem. **275:** 25672–25680.
57. SHIBATA, N. *et al.* 2001. Supernatant protein factor, which stimulates the conversion of squalene to lanosterol, is a cytosolic squalene transfer protein and enhances cholesterol biosynthesis. Proc. Natl. Acad. Sci. USA **98:** 2244–2249.
58. FUKS-HOLMBERG, D. & K. BLOCH. 1983. Intermembrane transfer of squalene promoted by supernatant protein factor. J. Lipid Res. **24:** 402–408.
59. FRIEDLANDER, E.J. *et al.* 1980. Supernatant protein factor facilitates intermembrane transfer of squalene. J. Biol. Chem. **255:** 8042–8045.
60. STOCKER, A., *et al.* 2002. Crystal structure of the human supernatant protein factor. Structure (Cambridge) **10:** 1533–1540.
61. STOCKER, A. & U. BAUMANN. 2003. Supernatant protein factor in complex with RRR-alpha-tocopherylquinone: a link between oxidized vitamin E and cholesterol biosynthesis. J. Mol. Biol. **332:** 759–765.
62. ANANTHARAMAN, V. & L. ARAVIND. 2002. The GOLD domain, a novel protein module involved in Golgi function and secretion. Genome Biol. **3(5):** research0023.1–research0023.7.
63. TOHGI, H. *et al.* 1996. alpha-Tocopherol quinone level is remarkably low in the cerebrospinal fluid of patients with sporadic amyotrophic lateral sclerosis. Neurosci. Lett. **207:** 5–8.
64. HUGHES, P.E. & S.B. TOVE. 1980. Identification of an endogenous electron donor for biohydrogenation as alpha-tocopherolquinol. J. Biol. Chem. **255:** 4447–4452.
65. HUGHES, P.E. & S.B. TOVE. 1980. Synthesis of alpha-tocopherolquinone by the rat and its reduction by mitochondria. J. Biol. Chem. **255:** 7095–7097.
66. HAYASHI, T. *et al.* 1992. Reduction of alpha-tocopherolquinone to alpha-tocopherolhydroquinone in rat hepatocytes. Biochem. Pharmacol. **44:** 489–493.
67. NAKAMURA, M. & T. HAYASHI. 1994. One- and two-electron reduction of quinones by rat liver subcellular fractions. J. Biochem. (Tokyo) **115:** 1141–1147.
68. KOHAR, I. *et al.* 1995. Is alpha-tocopherol a reservoir for alpha-tocopheryl hydroquinone? Free Radic. Biol. Med. **19:** 197–207.
69. NEUZIL, J., P.K. WITTING & R. STOCKER. 1997. Alpha-tocopheryl hydroquinone is an efficient multifunctional inhibitor of radical-initiated oxidation of low density lipoprotein lipids. Proc. Natl. Acad. Sci. USA **94:** 7885–7890.
70. TRABER, M.G. *et al.* 1992. Studies on the transfer of tocopherol between lipoproteins. Lipids. **27:** 657–663.
71. KUNJATHOOR, V.V. *et al.* 2002. Scavenger receptors class A-I/II and CD36 are the principal receptors responsible for the uptake of modified low-density lipoprotein leading to lipid loading in macrophages. J. Biol. Chem. **277:** 49982–49988.
72. YANG, T. *et al.* 2002. Crucial step in cholesterol homeostasis: sterols promote binding of SCAP to INSIG-1, a membrane protein that facilitates retention of SREBPs in ER. Cell **110:** 489–500.

73. ATHANIKAR, J.N. & T.F. OSBORNE. 1998. Specificity in cholesterol regulation of gene expression by coevolution of sterol regulatory DNA element and its binding protein. Proc. Natl. Acad. Sci. USA **95:** 4935–4940.
74. SINGH, D.K. *et al.* 2003. Phosphorylation of supernatant protein factor enhances its ability to stimulate microsomal squalene monooxygenase. J. Biol. Chem. **278:** 5646–5651.
75. SIEGEL, D. *et al.* 1997. The reduction of alpha-tocopherolquinone by human NAD(P)H: quinone oxidoreductase: the role of alpha-tocopherolhydroquinone as a cellular antioxidant. Mol. Pharmacol. **52:** 300–305.

Physiological Factors Influencing Vitamin E Biokinetics

JOHN K. LODGE, WENDY L. HALL, YVONNE M. JEANES, AND ANNA R. PROTEGGENTE

Centre for Nutrition and Food Safety, School of Biomedical and Molecular Sciences, University of Surrey, Guildford, Surrey GU2 7XH, United Kingdom

ABSTRACT: Limited information is available on factors that can influence vitamin E bioavailability. In several studies we have investigated the influence of dietary, biochemical, and genetic factors on vitamin E biokinetics. In these studies, subjects ingested a capsule containing 150 mg deuterated *RRR*-α-tocopheryl acetate, blood was taken up to 48 hr, and tocopherols were analyzed by liquid chromatography and mass spectroscopy. There was significantly greater plasma-labeled α-tocopherol concentrations when the capsule was consumed with a high-fat meal (17.5 g) versus a low-fat meal (2.7 g), and there was also a difference between a high-fat toast and butter and a cereal with full-fat milk meal (both 17.5 g fat), indicating that both the amount of fat and food matrix is important for vitamin E absorption. Dyslipidemic subjects displayed a reduced plasma uptake of newly absorbed α-tocopherol, and differences were also apparent in individual lipoproteins. A decreased uptake of labeled α-tocopherol was also observed in erythrocytes, platelets, and lymphocytes of dyslipidemics. Following vitamin E supplementation (400 mg/day, 4 weeks), the uptake of newly absorbed α-tocopherol was decreased, presumably because of saturation of α-tocopherol transfer protein. We also found that apoE3 subjects displayed a considerably reduced uptake of newly absorbed labeled α-tocopherol compared to apoE4 subjects, which may be a consequence of the reduced low-density lipoprotein catabolic rate in these subjects. Taken together, these data show that several physiological factors influence the uptake of newly absorbed α-tocopherol, and that this is an important consideration in the design of future vitamin E supplementation studies.

KEYWORDS: deuterated; tocopherol; plasma; diet; dyslipidemia; apoE genotype; saturation

INTRODUCTION

Vitamin E is a group of eight compounds (α, γ, β, and δ tocopherols and α, β, δ, and γ tocotrienols) that differ in their methyl substitution and saturation. The predominant form in the body, constituting over 90% of vitamin E, is α-tocopherol.[1,2]

Address for correspondence: Dr. John K. Lodge, School of Biomedical and Molecular Sciences, University of Surrey, Guildford, Surrey GU2 7XH, United Kingdom. Voice: +44 (0)1483 879 702; fax: +44 (0)1483 879 702.
  j.lodge@surrey.ac.uk

Ann. N.Y. Acad. Sci. 1031: 60–73 (2004). © 2004 New York Academy of Sciences.
doi: 10.1196/annals.1331.006

This form has been widely researched owing to its antioxidant and non-antioxidant functions and to its putative cardioprotective role.

The absorption, transport, and distribution of vitamin E within the body are linked to those of dietary fat. Intestinal absorption requires the presence of bile salts, pancreatic enzymes, and adequate fat.[3] The process is similar for all the fat-soluble vitamins in that there is a prerequisite for the formation of micelles containing dietary lipids, emulsified in the presence of bile salts. The importance of bile salts and pancreatic secretions is demonstrated in subjects with either cholestatic liver disease or cystic fibrosis[4] who malabsorb vitamin E and become vitamin E– deficient. Once internalized, vitamin E is packaged into chylomicrons (CMs), along with the apolipoproteins apoB48, apoCII, and apoE, and enters the circulation via lymph. During circulation, CM triglycerides are hydrolyzed by endothelium-bound lipoprotein lipase (LPL), which is activated by apoCII. This process results in the transfer of lipids and vitamin E to peripheral tissues.[5] Excess CM surface area is consequently produced, and along with vitamin E, it is transferred to high-density lipoprotein (HDL). The resultant CM remnants are taken up into to the liver by way of the apoE receptor, and *RRR*-α-tocopherol is preferentially incorporated into very-low-density lipoprotein (VLDL) through an as yet unknown process that relies on the sorting of the various forms of vitamin E by the hepatic α-tocopherol transport protein (α-TTP). VLDL, containing apoB and apoE, is catabolized by LPL, forming VLDL remnants (IDL), 50% of which are taken up by the liver through the apoE receptor, while the rest are converted to low-density lipoprotein (LDL), which is the major carrier of vitamin E to the peripheral tissues. During the hydrolysis process, vitamin E can be transferred to HDL and tissues,[3] and there is also a constant flux of vitamin E between circulating lipoproteins,[6] with HDL reportedly a better vitamin E donor,[6] and presumably also between the vascular endothelium and blood components.

Using deuterium-labeled vitamin E, we have followed the uptake of newly absorbed α-tocopherol into plasma, erythrocytes, platelets, and lymphocytes of normolipidemic males ($n = 12$) following ingestion of a capsule containing 150 mg deuterated *RRR*-α-tocopheryl acetate (FIG. 1).[7] The uptake and distribution of newly absorbed vitamin E has previously been reported in plasma,[8–10] lipoproteins,[8] and erythrocytes.[11] In plasma, it has been shown that newly absorbed α-tocopherol rapidly displaces preexisting or "old" α-tocopherol in the circulation.[9] This can be observed by the extent of labeling. Plasma maximum concentrations (C_{max}) of newly absorbed α-tocopherol were reached between 9 and 12 hr, and up to 40% of the vitamin E was in the labeled form following this 150-mg dose (FIG. 1). This rapid turnover of newly absorbed α-tocopherol helps to explain the limitations in plasma vitamin E concentrations following supplementation, such that concentrations cannot be raised more than 3-fold no matter the supplementation regime.[8] Vitamin E uptake into erythrocytes was more gradual, with a maximum concentration after 24 hr. Erythrocytes contain vitamin E within their membranes, which is thought to be obtained via tocopherol-binding proteins.[12] An extensive turnover of α-tocopherol in erythrocytes was also apparent, as the percentage of labeling also reached 40% following a 150-mg dose. The labeled α-tocopherol uptake profile in platelets and in lymphocytes was very similar, and both contained a maximum of ~ 25% of labeled α-tocopherol following the 150-mg dose. This was significantly lower than that in plasma and erythrocytes, showing that the amount of newly absorbed α-tocopherol taken up into platelets and lymphocytes is limiting. It is not known how cells and tis-

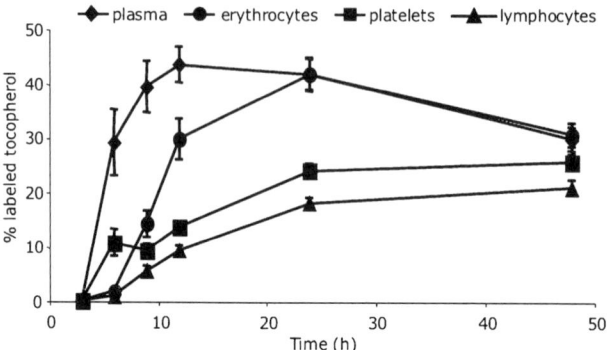

FIGURE 1. The percentage of labeled α-tocopherol in blood components over time following ingestion of a capsule containing 150 mg of deuterium-labeled RRR-α-tocopheryl acetate. Each values is a mean ± SEM.

sues obtain their vitamin E, but various mechanisms have been implicated.[13] These include uncontrolled transfer during LPL-mediated, triglyceride-rich lipoprotein hydrolysis,[5,14] uptake within lipoprotein particles via the LDL receptor,[15] and transfer via the scavenger receptor class B1 (SR-B1).[16,17] The latter mechanism involves transfer from HDL, whereas the others involve CMs and VLDL, and LDL respectively. Thus, vitamin E can be transferred to peripheral tissues from all lipoproteins by different mechanisms. Lymphocytes have LDL receptors and could obtain their vitamin E through the LDL receptor pathway. Similarly, the apoB moiety of LDL interacts with an unidentified receptor on platelet membranes that allows for the transfer of lipids to platelets.[18] As the profile of newly absorbed α-tocopherol uptake into lymphocytes and platelets is different from that for plasma and erythrocytes, then it is likely that different mechanisms are apparent, the uptake of α-tocopherol into lymphocytes and platelets appearing to occur through a more controlled mechanism.

α-Tocopherol inhibits platelet aggregation *in vitro* and *in vivo*,[19] and also influences lymphocyte proliferation *in vitro*.[20] Therefore, both platelets and lymphocytes are functionally affected by vitamin E, making these blood components useful markers of functional vitamin E status, as we have previously suggested.[21]

High vitamin E intakes have been associated with decreased risk of cardiovascular disease. Because of these observational studies, vitamin E has been the subject of many clinical trials. However, there is still limited data on factors influencing vitamin E bioavailability. Many studies are performed without any indication of the extent of absorption, and many neglect to account for genetic factors that could influence variation. Large inter-individual variation exists not only in steady-state plasma vitamin E levels, but also in the response to supplementation.[11,22] Sources of this variation could include efficiency of absorption and genetic factors that are known to influence dietary responsiveness. There is limited human data on factors that can influence vitamin E bioavailability. With this in mind, we have, in several studies, investigated physiological factors that can potentially influence bioavailability, and have studied this using stable-isotope (deuterium) labeled α-tocopherol biokinetics.

DIETARY FACTORS

It is widely accepted that dietary fat is required for the absorption of vitamin E; however, the amount of fat necessary for maximal vitamin E absorption in humans is currently undetermined.[23,24] There are only a few human studies that have investigated the influence of dietary fat on vitamin E absorption. Roodenburg and colleagues showed that plasma α-tocopherol levels were similar following 7 days of supplementation with 50 mg of vitamin E consumed with either a low-fat meal (<6.5 g fat/day) or high-fat meal (~45 g fat/day).[25] However, Dimitrov and colleagues reported significantly greater plasma uptake of α-tocopherol in humans fed a high-fat diet (~115 g fat/day) compared to a low-fat diet (~51 g fat/day) over 5 days of supplementation with 800 mg of synthetic vitamin E.[26] Similarly, greater plasma α-tocopherol levels were found after 15 days of supplementation with 300 mg of vitamin E when consumed with a meal compared to an "empty stomach."[27]

We have investigated the influence of dietary fat on plasma vitamin E uptake during the absorptive phase (FIG. 2).[28] In this randomized crossover study, 8 subjects (5 female, 3 male; mean age: 28 ± 6 years; mean body mass index: 23 ± 4 kg m^{-2}; fasting plasma cholesterol and TAG levels: 4.2 ± 0.7 and 0.95 ± 0.2 mmol/L, respectively) consumed a capsule containing 150 mg of deuterated RRR-α-tocopheryl acetate with a test meal of either toast and butter (17.5 g fat), cereal with full-fat milk and added single cream (17.5 g fat), cereal with semi-skimmed milk (2.7 g fat), or water (0 g fat). Blood was collected at time points up to 9 hr, and deuterium-labeled α-tocopherol was analyzed in plasma and CM fractions by liquid chromatography

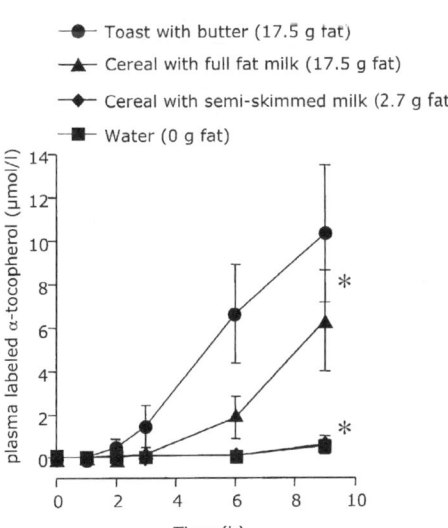

FIGURE 2. Influence of dietary fat on vitamin E biokinetics. Plasma deuterated α-tocopherol concentrations following ingestion of a capsule containing 150 mg of deutcrated RRR-α-tocopheryl acetate with various test meals as indicated. There was a significant difference over time ($P < 0.001$) and between test meals ($P < 0.001$) in deuterated α-tocopherol concentration. Each value is a mean ± SD. *: significant difference between high-fat and low-fat meals ($P < 0.05$).

and mass spectroscopy.[7] Significantly higher plasma concentrations of labeled α-tocopherol were found following meals containing 17.5 g fat compared to 2.7 g fat ($P < 0.05$) (FIG. 2).[28] There was no difference in labeled α-tocopherol concentration when the labeled vitamin E capsule was taken with the 2.5-g fat cereal meal or water, indicating that in this study 2.7 g of fat was not enough to promote sufficient vitamin E absorption from a capsule containing 150 mg of vitamin E. We also found that the food matrix influences vitamin E absorption, as differences were observed in the labeled α-tocopherol concentration:time profiles between the toast and butter, and the cereal with full-fat milk and cream meals, both of which contained 17.5 g of fat ($P = 0.065$).[28] A few studies have investigated the influence of the physical properties of the meal on vitamin E bioavailability. Hayes and colleagues[29] reported that milk enhanced vitamin E uptake, irrespective of fat content. A 3-week diet rich in unsaturated fat increased serum concentrations of α-tocopherol by 7%, whereas a diet rich in saturated fat decreased the α-tocopherol concentration by a similar amount.[30] More recently, Leonard and colleagues[24] found increased vitamin E bioavailability from a fortified breakfast cereal compared to that from a capsule when taken with fat-free milk. This study also found greater vitamin E bioavailability when a capsule is consumed with cereal and milk, rather than milk alone, also demonstrating that the physical properties of a meal influence absorption. The physical properties of food are known to influence gastric emptying,[31] providing a potential mechanism for this effect. As supplemental vitamin E is of major consumer interest, these data show that it is important to take into account both the amount of fat and the type of food, with respect to the consumption of vitamin E capsules.

PLASMA LIPID STATUS

Vitamin E biokinetics within the systemic circulation are governed by plasma lipoprotein metabolism[3]; hence, perturbations to the lipid status, such as dyslipidemias, would be expected to influence vitamin E status. However, vitamin E homeostasis in dyslipidemia is not well documented. Vitamin E concentration is closely correlated to that of cholesterol and total lipid,[32,33] so it is not surprising that individuals with hypercholesterolemia usually have increased concentrations of plasma vitamin E compared to normolipidemics.[34,35] The reverse situation is observed in hypocholesterolemia.[36] Similarly, subjects with raised triglycerides also appear to have higher plasma vitamin E,[37,38] sometimes even higher than in hypercholesterolaemia.[38] The implications of raised plasma vitamin E concentration on tissue vitamin E status are poorly understood. Erythrocyte vitamin E concentrations were found to be lower in hypercholesterolemics, even when plasma levels were similar.[34,39] These studies highlight the limitations of measuring plasma levels alone. More important, they also suggest that the transfer of vitamin E from plasma lipoproteins could be impaired in dyslipidemia. In order to ascertain whether the transfer of vitamin E is impaired in dyslipidemia, we have compared deuterium-labeled α-tocopherol uptake into plasma, lipoproteins, erythrocytes, platelets, and lymphocytes in normolipidemics and dyslipidemics. Subjects classified as either normolipidemic (N; total cholesterol < 5.5 mmol/L and TAG < 1.5 mmol/L), hypercholesterolemic (HC; total cholesterol > 6.5 mmol/L and TAG < 1.5 mmol/L), and combined hypercholesterolaemic and hypertriglyceridaemic (HCT; total cholesterol

> 6.5 mmol/L and TAG > 2.5 mmol/L) were recruited and consumed a capsule containing 150 mg of deuterium-labeled *RRR*-α-tocopheryl acetate with a standard meal containing 40 g of fat. Blood was collected at various times over 48 hr, blood components were isolated, and tocopherols were analyzed by standard methods.[7,21] Subject characteristics were as follows: N: $n = 9$ (6 male, 3 female); mean age: 43 ± 9 years; mean BMI: 26 ± 3 kg m^{-2}; plasma and LDL cholesterol: 4.7 ± 0.5 and 2.9 ± 0.3 mmol/L, respectively; plasma TAG: 1.2 ± 0.5 mmol/L. HC: $n = 10$ (7 male, 3 female); mean age: 50 ± 8 years; mean BMI: 25 ± 3 kg m^{-2}; plasma and LDL cholesterol: 6.9 ± 0.7 and 4.3 ± 0.6 mmol/L, respectively; plasma TAG: 1.2 ± 0.2 mmol/L. HCT: $n = 6$ (male); mean age: 50 ± 10 years; mean BMI: 26 ± 2 kg m^{-2}; plasma and LDL cholesterol: 7.0 ± 0.8 and 4.6 ± 0.6 mmol/L, respectively; plasma TAG: 2.3 ± 0.9 mmol/L.

The biokinetic profiles in blood components are shown in FIGURE 3. In plasma, there was a significant group and time effect in labeled α-tocopherol concentration ($P < 0.0005$), which was due to decreased plasma uptake in the HCT group, demonstrated as a lower C_{max} and delayed time for C_{max}, compared to the N and HC

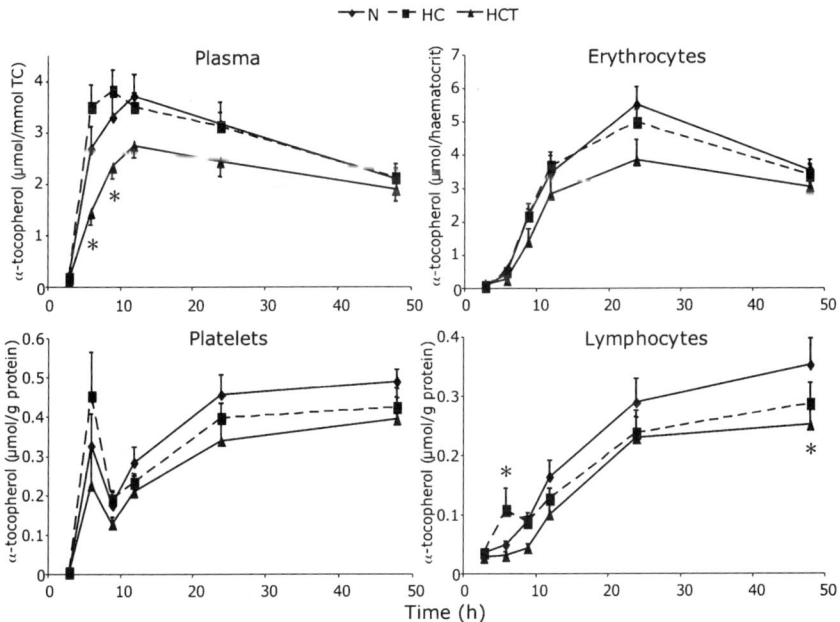

FIGURE 3. Influence of the plasma lipid status on vitamin E biokinetics. Deuterated α-tocopherol concentrations in blood components of normolipidemic (N), hypercholesterolemic (HC), and combined hypercholesterolemic and hypertriglyceridemic (HCT) subjects following ingestion of a capsule containing 150 mg of deuterated *RRR*-α-tocopheryl acetate. Each value is a mean ± SEM. In plasma and lymphocytes, there was a significant group and time interaction (plasma: $P < 0.0005$; lymphocytes: $P < 0.05$) in labeled α-tocopherol concentrations (significant at 6 and 9 hr and 6 and 48 hr in plasma and lymphocytes, respectively). TC: total cholesterol.

TABLE 1. Area under the curve analysis of labeled α-tocopherol in blood components between normolipidemic and dyslipidemic patients

Variable	N	HC	HCT
Plasma	134.59 ± 44.4	126.85 ± 35.4	97.94 ± 25.6
CM	177.23 ± 134.6	290.97 ± 115.8	175.65 ± 46.9
VLDL	1049.64 ± 185.8	656.28 ± 461.2	832.41 ± 125.8
LDL	534.12 ± 313.7	515.45 ± 80.7	357.77 ± 35.9
HDL	47.93 ± 4.9	48.21 ± 10.1	47.93 ± 17.5
Erythrocytes	174.09 ± 40.3	164.64 ± 59.0	130.27 ± 42.9
Platelets	18.12 ± 4.2	15.41 ± 5.4	13.34 ± 5.0
Lymphocyes	11.84 ± 3.7	9.28 ± 3.8	8.11 ± 2.9

groups. The HC group had a more rapid time for C_{max}, being between 6 and 9 hr compared to 12 hr in the N and HCT groups. Thus, differences in steady-state lipid status appear to influence the uptake of newly absorbed α-tocopherol into plasma. We then looked at labeled α-tocopherol uptake in the individual lipoproteins in each subject group, as the analysis of lipoprotein fractions can give further insights into the differing responses in plasma α-tocopherol uptake. This data is presented as the area under the curve (AUC) from labeled α-tocopherol concentration:time profiles in TABLE 1. In CMs, the largest AUC was found in the HC group, with no difference between the N and HCT groups. This was due to a significant group-by-time interaction in labeled α-tocopherol concentration, with a large C_{max} at 6 hr in the HC group ($P < 0.00005$), which reflected an approximately 4-fold higher concentration than in the N and HCT groups (data not shown). As with the AUC data, no differences were found between the N and HCT groups. Thus, the decreased plasma response in the HCT group was not caused by decreased absorption. In VLDL, the HC group had the lowest AUC, whereas in LDL, the HCT group had the lowest AUC. No differences were observed in HDL. Thus, the changes apparent in plasma (FIG. 3) are due to the α-tocopherol content of LDL. Hypertriglyceridemia is associated with decreased LPL activity and therefore a delayed postprandial response. Vitamin E biokinetics have been investigated in subjects who have genetic abnormalities of the LPL gene and lack LPL activity.[40] These subjects demonstrate a retention of newly absorbed α-tocopherol in their triglyceride-rich lipoproteins, which become the major carrier of vitamin E in the absence of LDL. However, in the present study, no retention of α-tocopherol in CMs and VLDL was observed in the HCT group. Thus, it appears that differences in the present study may be related to the transfer of α-tocopherol to/from LDL.

To see whether the differing responses in plasma could influence the delivery of vitamin E to cells, we looked at erythrocytes, platelets, and lymphocytes (FIG. 3). In each blood component, there was a reduced uptake of newly absorbed α-tocopherol over the time period in the order N > HC > HCT. The profile in platelets was particularly interesting, as there appeared to be a biphasic response characterized by an initial rise in labeled α-tocopherol concentration at 6 hr, which then decreased and was followed again by a more gradual increase from 12 hr. This peak corresponded to the C_{max} peak in CMs (data not shown). Thus platelets receive vitamin E from CMs, presumably during CM hydrolysis. This appears to be a function of the CM α-tocopherol concentration, as the extent of this response was related to the C_{max} peak in CMs. This phenomenon also occurred in the lymphocytes of the HC group only, demonstrating that when vitamin E-rich CMs are produced during LPL-mediated hydrolysis, excess α-tocopherol is distributed. It is interesting, though, that the erythrocytes of the HC group did not receive any α-tocopherol at this point; the reasons for this are unclear.

Thus, dyslipidemia is associated with differential plasma and lipoprotein uptake of newly absorbed α-tocopherol, and decreased uptake into blood components. The mechanism for these differences presumably originates in the transfer of α-tocopherol during hydrolysis and the formation of LDL.

VITAMIN E STATUS

Plasma vitamin E concentrations are limiting; they reach saturation biokinetics and cannot be raised more than 2- to 3-fold, no matter what the supplementation regime is.[8,26,41] The rapid displacement of existing α-tocopherol by newly absorbed α-tocopherol,[8] which can be demonstrated by the extent of labeling, helps to explain this phenomenon to a certain degree. We have also used a different approach to study this phenomenon. As part of an apoE genotyping study (also described in next section), male subjects ($n = 15$) carrying either the apoE3 or apoE4 genotype ($n = 5$ and $n = 10$, respectively; mean age: 45 ± 12 years; mean BMI: 27.2 ± 3.8 kg m^{-2}; plasma cholesterol: 6.75 ± 0.96 mmol/L; plasma TAG: 1.83 ± 0.6 mmol/L) underwent a 48-hr biokinetic protocol, ingesting a capsule containing 150 mg of deuterium-labeled *RRR*-α-tocopheryl acetate with a standard meal containing 20 g of fat, both prior to (pre) and following (post) supplementation with *RRR*-α-tocopheryl acetate (400 mg/day) for 4 weeks. This time period is enough to demonstrate steady-state plasma vitamin E concentrations following plasma vitamin E saturation, which reaches C_{max} following 5 half-lives (~50 hr) or 10–15 days.[42] FIGURE 4 shows the baseline (unlabeled) α-tocopherol concentration pre- and post-supplementation, the labeled α-tocopherol concentration during the 48-hr biokinetic protocols pre- and post-supplementation, and the AUC from the labeled α-tocopherol concentration:time profiles. Following supplementation, plasma α-tocopherol concentration was significantly increased by approximately 2-fold ($P < 0.005$). However, the bioavailability of the newly absorbed labeled α-tocopherol was decreased post-supplementation, as demonstrated by a decreased C_{max} from 9 hr, and a decreased AUC. These results show that following plasma saturation, the ability for the plasma to take up newly absorbed α-tocopherol is diminished. This effect, along with the rapid turnover of α-tocopherol in plasma,[8,9] would limit the maximum plasma concentration of vitamin E. Since much of the regulation of plasma vitamin E is governed by the hepatic α-tocopherol transfer protein (α-TTP), we can hypothesize that this reduced bioavailability is due to the saturation of α-TTP after high intakes of α-tocopherol over a prolonged period. It has been suggested that only following α-TTP saturation is there significant metabolism of α-tocopherol.[43] Thus, after chronic high intakes of vitamin E, a-TTP is saturated with α-tocopherol, less of the newly absorbed α-toco-

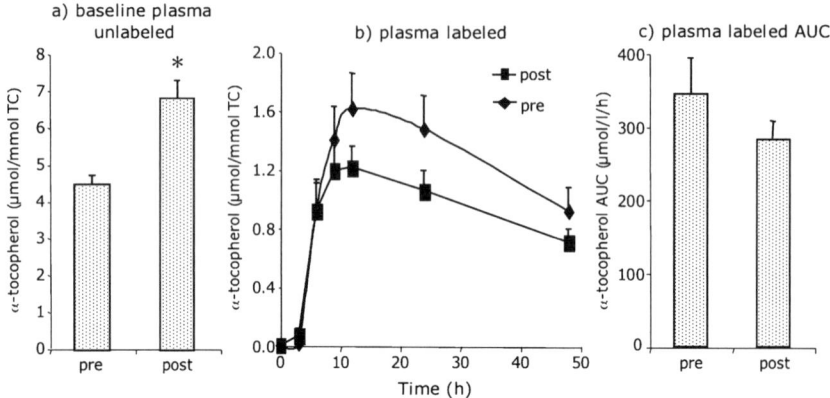

FIGURE 4. Influence of vitamin E supplementation on vitamin E biokinetics. Baseline plasma unlabeled α-tocopherol concentrations (**a**), plasma deuterated α-tocopherol concentrations over time following ingestion of a capsule containing 150 mg of deuterated *RRR*-α-tocopheryl acetate (**b**), and plasma deuterated α-tocopherol area under the curve (AUC) (**c**) in subjects (combined apoE3 and apoE4 carriers) pre- and post-supplementation with *RRR*-α-tocopheryl acetate (400 mg/day) for 4 weeks. Each value is a mean ± SEM. *: baseline unlabeled α-tocopherol concentration significantly increased following supplementation ($P < 0.005$). TC: total cholesterol.

pherol can be secreted into the plasma, and this α-tocopherol is metabolized and excreted. Another possibility is the influence of α-tocopherol on α-TTP expression. Tocopherols are known to influence the expression of α-TTP. In vitamin E-deficient rats, supplementation with both α- and δ-tocopherol increased hepatic levels of α-TTP mRNA.[44] However, no studies have yet demonstrated if vitamin E "overload" can downregulate α-TTP. Thus, vitamin E biokinetics are influenced by vitamin E status and become limiting following high vitamin E intakes, which reduce the ability of α-TTP to select newly absorbed α-tocopherol for systemic distribution.

GENETIC FACTORS

Considerable heterogeneity exists in lipid responses to dietary intervention, with certain genetic factors appearing to account for a proportion of inter-individual variation or response to diet.[45] ApoE is a multifunctional protein mainly produced by the liver (and secreted in triglyceride-rich lipoproteins), where it modulates the metabolism of these particles in both hepatic and non-hepatic tissues. ApoE is a polymorphic protein with three common alleles yielding apoE2 (Cys 112 Cys 158), apoE3 (Cys 112 Arg 158), and apoE4 (Arg 112 Arg 158). In northern Europe, approximately 55–60% of the population are homozygous for the E3 allele (E3/E3), with 12–15% being E2 carriers and the remaining 25–27% being either heterozygous or homozygous for the apoE4 isoform.[46] Population studies have shown that risk of diseases characterized by oxidative damage such as coronary heart disease, stroke, and Alzheimer's disease are significantly higher in apoE4 carriers. Although much of the increased cardiovascular risk is thought to be attributable to alterations in lipoprotein metabolism, with significantly higher LDL cholesterol,[47] and apoB levels[46] in E4 carriers, recent evidence suggests that the function of the apoE protein as a regulator of cellular oxidative status may also be a significant contributor to disease progression. A recent study[48] has demonstrated that cigarette smoking is an even greater risk factor for CHD in men carrying the apoE4 allele relative to homozygote E3 individuals, the greater risk being attributable to a lower antioxidant status in this subgroup.

Therefore, apoE is directly involved in processes that could influence vitamin E status, and as this represents a common polymorphism, it is worthy of investigation. We have investigated the influence of apoE genotype on vitamin E biokinetics. In this study, we screened[49] and recruited male subjects carrying the apoE3 ($n = 5$) and apoE4 ($n = 10$) allele, and they consumed a capsule containing 150 mg of deuterium-labeled *RRR*-α-tocopheryl acetate with a standard meal containing 20 g of fat. As described earlier, the subjects then underwent a 4-week supplementation regime of *RRR*-α-tocopheryl acetate (400 mg/day), followed again by a 48-hr biokinetics protocol as described. Plasma was isolated, and tocopherols were analyzed by liquid chromatography and mass spectroscopy.[7] The subjects were of similar age (E3: 44 ± 12 years; E4: 46 ± 11 years) and BMI (E3: 27.9 ± 4.3 kg m^{-2}; E4: 26.6 ± 3.4 kg m^{-2}). The apoE4 carriers had significantly higher total plasma cholesterol (E3: 5.82 ± 0.82 mmol/L; E4: 7.68 ± 1.1 mmol/L; $P = 0.007$) and higher triglyceride (E3: 1.49 ± 0.47 mmol/L; E4: 2.18 ± 0.75 mmol/L; $P = 0.065$) than the apoE3 carriers, as has been previously demonstrated.[47] FIGURE 5 shows the unlabeled (existing) and labeled α-tocopherol concentration over 48 hr, and the labeled α-tocopherol AUC. Baseline unlabeled α-tocopherol concentration was similar between the two groups (time: 0 hr). No influence of apoE genotype on steady-state vitamin A and E levels has been previously found.[50] However, plasma uptake of newly absorbed labeled α-tocopherol was significantly lower in the apoE3 carriers compared to the apoE4 carriers, as demonstrated by the lower concentration of labeled α-tocopherol at each time point, and the lower AUC. In the circulation, apoE is an important determinant of lipolytic activity and acts as a co-factor in the hepatic lipase (HL)-mediated conversion of VLDL to LDL[51] with significantly greater conversion of VLDL to LDL in apoE4 carriers (70–80%) relative to homozygous E3 controls (50–60%) in healthy volunteers. ApoE also acts as a high-affinity ligand for the binding of CMs and VLDL remnants to hepatic receptors,[52] influencing removal from the circulation. The E4 protein has a more than 25-fold-higher affinity for the LDL receptor (LDL-R) relative to LDL.[53] This competitive inhibition, in combination with the increased conversion of VLDL to LDL, leads to a reduced LDL fractional catabolic rate and hence increased LDL levels.[46,54] As LDL is the principal transport vehicle of α-tocopherol in the circulation, the increased newly absorbed α-tocopherol seen in the apoE4 individuals could represent the retention of vitamin E in LDL, as less LDL is delivered to peripheral tissues. It remains to be investigated if a defective vitamin E delivery system could contribute to the increased oxidative stress seen in apoE4 carriers. If so, these subjects could benefit from an antioxidant-rich diet.

ApoE genotype therefore influences the bioavailability of newly absorbed α-tocopherol. As this represents a common polymorphism in the population, this could be an important contributor to inter-individual variation in the response to vitamin E supplementation.

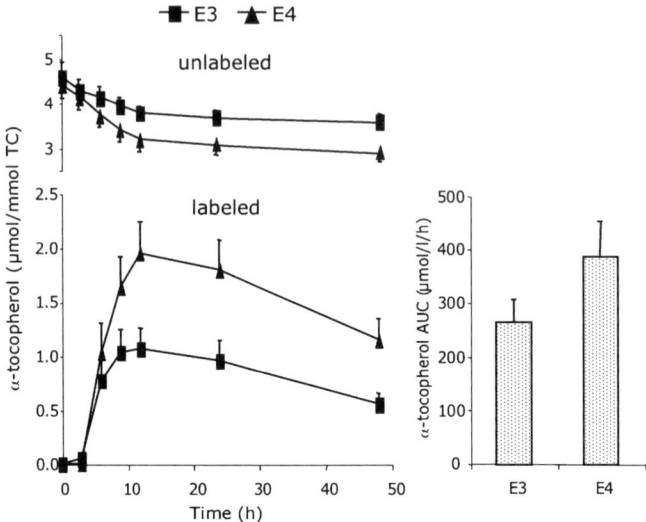

FIGURE 5. Influence of apoE genotype on vitamin E biokinetics. Plasma unlabeled and labeled α-tocopherol concentrations following ingestion of a capsule containing 150 mg of deuterated *RRR*-α-tocopheryl acetate in apoE3 and apoE4 subjects. The area under the curve from the labeled α-tocopherol concentration:time profile is also shown. Each value is a mean ± SEM. TC:total cholesterol.

CONCLUSIONS

Vitamin E biokinetics is associated with large inter-individual variation; subjects display a wide range of responses to newly absorbed vitamin E. This could be the result of a combination of factors that influence the absorption, transport, and distribution of vitamin E. In several studies, we have investigated dietary, biochemical, and genetic factors on the biokinetics of vitamin E using deuterium-labeled *RRR*-α-tocopheryl acetate. We have shown that the uptake of newly absorbed α-tocopherol is dependent not only on the amount of fat in a meal the capsule is taken with, but also on the food matrix. We have shown that the plasma lipid status influences uptake of α-tocopherol in that dyslipidemic subjects have a reduced uptake into plasma and lipoproteins, and a reduced uptake into erythrocytes, platelets, and lymphocytes. The vitamin E status itself also influences biokinetics, as less newly absorbed α-tocopherol is taken up into the plasma following saturation of the plasma, which followed 4 weeks of vitamin E supplementation. We also investigated the influence of apoE genotype, as apoE is involved in lipoprotein metabolism and antioxidant action. We have shown that apoE3 subjects take up less newly absorbed α-tocopherol into the plasma than apoE4 subjects. Therefore, many factors can influence vitamin E status and contribute to the inherent inter-individual variation in response to vitamin E supplementation. Previous vitamin E supplementation studies have had varied results, and many of these studies have no indication of relative bioavailability. Therefore, it is important to take into account the influence of dietary, biochemical, and genetic factors on vitamin E bioavailability in the design of future vitamin E clinical studies.

REFERENCES

1. BRIGELIUS-FLOHE, R. & M.G. TRABER. 1999. Vitamin E: function and metabolism. FASEB J. **13:** 1145–55.
2. BURTON, G.W. & M.G. TRABER. 1990. Vitamin E: antioxidant activity, biokinetics and bioavailability. Annu. Rev. Nutr. **10:** 357–382.
3. KAYDEN, H.J. & M.G. TRABER. 1993. Absorption, lipoprotein transport, and regulation of plasma concentrations of vitamin E in humans. J. Lipid Res. **34:** 343–358.
4. SOKOL, R.J., N. BUTLER-SIMON, J.E. HEUBI, et al. 1989. Vitamin E deficiency neuropathy in children with fat malabsorption: studies in cystic fibrosis and chronic cholestasis. Ann. N.Y. Acad. Sci. **570:** 156–69.
5. TRABER, M.G., T. OLIVECRONA & H.J. KAYDEN. 1985. Bovine milk lipoprotein lipase transfers tocopherol to human fibroblasts during triglyceride hydrolysis in vitro. J. Clin. Invest. **75:** 1729–1734.
6. TRABER, M.G., J.C. LANE, N. LAGMAY, et al. 1992. Studies on the transfer of tocopherol between lipoproteins. Lipids **27:** 657–663.
7. HALL, W.L., Y.M. JEANES, J. PUGH, et al. 2003. Development of a liquid chromatographic time-of-flight mass spectrometric method for the determination of unlabelled and deuterium-labelled alpha-tocopherol in blood components. Rapid Commun. Mass Spectrom. **17:** 2797–2803.
8. TRABER, M.G., D. RADER, R.V. ACUFF, et al. 1998. Vitamin E dose-response studies in humans with use of deuterated RRR-alpha-tocopherol. Am. J. Clin. Nutr. **68:** 847–853.
9. TRABER, M.G., R. RAMAKRISHNAN & K.J. KAYDEN. 1994. Human plasma vitamin E kinetics demonstrate rapid recycling of plasma *RRR*-alpha-tocopherol. Proc. Natl. Acad. Sci. USA **91:** 10005–10008.
10. ACUFF, R.V., S.S. THEDFORD, N.N. HIDIROGLOU, et al. 1994. Relative bioavailability of RRR- and all-rac-alpha-tocopheryl acetate in humans: studies using deuterated compounds. Am. J. Clin. Nutr. **60:** 397–402.
11. ROXBOROUGH, H.E., G.W. BURTON & F.J. KELLY. 2000. Inter- and intra-individual variation in plasma and red blood cell vitamin E after supplementation. Free Radic. Res. **33:** 437–445.
12. KITABCHI, A.E. & J. WIMALASENA. 1982. Specific binding sites for D-alpha-tocopherol on human erythrocytes. Biochim. Biophys. Acta **684:** 200–206.
13. MARDONES, P. & A. RIGOTTI. 2004. Cellular mechanisms of vitamin E uptake: relevance in alpha-tocopherol metabolism and potential implications for disease. J. Nutr. Biochem. **15:** 252–260.
14. GOTI, D., Z. BALAZS, U. PANZENBOECK, et al. 2002. Effects of lipoprotein lipase on uptake and transcytosis of low density lipoprotein (LDL) and LDL-associated alpha-tocopherol in a porcine in vitro blood-brain barrier model. J. Biol. Chem. **277:** 28537–28544.
15. TRABER, M.G. & H.J. KAYDEN. 1984. Vitamin E is delivered to cells via the high affinity receptor for low density lipoprotein. Am. J. Clin. Nutr. **40:** 747–751.
16. MARDONES, P., P. STROBEL, S. MIRANDA, et al. 2002. alpha-Tocopherol metabolism is abnormal in scavenger receptor class B type I (SR-BI)-deficient mice. J. Nutr. **132:** 443–449.
17. GOTI, D., A. HRZENJAK, S. LEVAK-FRANK, et al. 2001. Scavenger receptor class B, type I is expressed in porcine brain capillary endothelial cells and contributes to selective uptake of HDL-associated vitamin E. J. Neurochem. **76:** 498–508.
18. RELOU, I.A., C.M. HACKENG, J.W. AKKERMAN, et al. 2003. Low-density lipoprotein and its effect on human blood platelets. Cell Mol. Life Sci. **60:** 961–971.

19. FREEDMAN, J.E., J.H. FARHAT, J. LOSCALZO, *et al.* 1996. alpha-Tocopherol inhibits aggregation of human platelets by a protein kinase C-dependent mechanism. Circulation **94:** 2434–2440.
20. ROY, R.M., M. PETRELLA & W.M. ROSS. 1991. Modification of mitogen-induced proliferation of murine splenic lymphocytes by in vitro tocopherol. Immunopharmacol. Immunotoxicol. **13:** 531–550.
21. JEANES, Y.M., W.L. HALL, A.R. PROTEGGENTE, *et al.* 2004. Cigarette smokers have decreased lymphocyte and platelet alpha-tocopherol levels and increased excretion of the gamma-tocopherol metabolite gamma-carboxyethyl-hydroxychroman (gamma-CEHC). Free Radic. Res. **38:** 861–868.
22. GALLI, F., R. LEE, C. DUNSTER, *et al.* 2001. gamma-Tocopherol metabolism and its relationship with alpha-tocopherol in humans: a stable isotope supplementation study. Biofactors **15:** 65–69.
23. COHN, W. 1997. Bioavailability of vitamin E. Eur. J. Clin. Nutr. **51:** S80–S85.
24. LEONARD, S.W., C.K. GOOD, E.T. GUGGER, *et al.* 2004. Vitamin E bioavailability from fortified breakfast cereal is greater than that from encapsulated supplements. Am. J. Clin. Nutr. **79:** 86–92.
25. ROODENBURG, A.J., R. LEENEN, K.H. VAN HET HOF, *et al.* 2000. Amount of fat in the diet affects bioavailability of lutein esters but not of alpha-carotene, beta-carotene, and vitamin E in humans. Am. J. Clin. Nutr. **71:** 1187–1193.
26. DIMITROV, N.V., C. MEYER, D. GILLILAND, *et al.* 1991. Plasma tocopherol concentrations in response to supplemental vitamin E. Am. J. Clin. Nutr. **53:** 723–729.
27. IULIANO, L., F. MICHELETTA, M. MARANGHI, *et al.* 2001. Bioavailability of vitamin E as a function of food intake in healthy subjects: effects on plasma peroxide-scavenging activity and cholesterol-oxidation products. Arterioscler. Thromb. Vasc. Biol. **21:** E34–E37.
28. JEANES, Y.M., W.L. HALL, S. ELLARD, *et al.* 2004. The absorption of vitamin E is influenced by the amount of fat in a meal and the food matrix. Br. J. Nutr.: in press.
29. HAYES, K., A. PRONCZUK & D. PERLMAN. 2001. Vitamin E in fortified cow milk uniquely enriches human plasma lipoproteins. Am. J. Clin. Nutr. **74:** 211–218.
30. OHRVALL, M., I.B. GUSTAFSSON & B. VESSBY. 2001. The alpha and gamma tocopherol levels in serum are influenced by the dietary fat quality. J. Hum. Nutr. Diet **14:** 63–68.
31. LOW, A.G. 1990. Nutritional regulation of gastric secretion, digestion and emptying. Nutr. Res. Rev. **3:** 229–252.
32. HORWITT, M.K., C.C. HARVEY, C.H. DAHM, JR., *et al.* 1972. Relationship between tocopherol and serum lipid levels for determination of nutritional adequacy. Ann. N.Y. Acad. Sci. **203:** 223–236.
33. THURNHAM, D.I., J.A. DAVIES, B.J. CRUMP, *et al.* 1986. The use of different lipids to express serum tocopherol:lipid ratios for the measurement of vitamin E status. Ann. Clin. Biochem. **23**(5): 514–520.
34. SIMON, E., J.L. PAUL, T. SONI, *et al.* 1997. Plasma and erythrocyte vitamin E content in asymptomatic hypercholesterolemic subjects. Clin. Chem. **43:** 285–289.
35. LEONHARDT, W., M. HANEFELD & F. SCHAPER. 1999. Diminished susceptibility to in vitro oxidation of low-density lipoproteins in hypercholesterolemia: key role of alpha-tocopherol content. Atherosclerosis **144:** 103–107.
36. MULDOON, M.F., S.B. KRITCHEVSKY, R.W. EVANS, *et al.* 1996. Serum total antioxidant activity in relative hypo- and hypercholesterolemia. Free Radic. Res. **25:** 239–245.
37. VAN TITS, L.J., P.N. DEMACKER, J. DE GRAAF, *et al.* 2000. alpha-Tocopherol supplementation decreases production of superoxide and cytokines by leukocytes ex vivo in both normolipidemic and hypertriglyceridemic individuals. Am. J. Clin. Nutr. **71:** 458–464.
38. BARONI, S.S., M. AMELIO, A. FIORITO, *et al.* 1999. Monounsaturated diet lowers LDL oxidisability in type IIb and type IV dyslipidemia without affecting coenzyme Q10 and vitamin E contents. Biofactors **9:** 325–330.
39. SIMON, E., J.L. PAUL, V. ATGER, *et al.* 1998. Erythrocyte antioxidant status in asymptomatic hypercholesterolemic men. Atherosclerosis **138:** 375–381.
40. TRABER, M.G., G.W. BURTON, L. HUGHES, *et al.* 1992. Discrimination between forms of vitamin E by humans with and without genetic abnormalities of lipoprotein metabolism. J. Lipid Res. **33:** 1171–1182.

41. JIALAL, I., C.J. FULLER & B.A. HUET. 1995. The effect of alpha-tocopherol supplementation on LDL oxidation: a dose-response study. Arterioscler. Thromb. Vasc. Biol. **15:** 190–198.
42. HOPPE, P.P. & G. KRENNRICH. 2000. Bioavailability and potency of natural-source and all-racemic alpha-tocopherol in the human: a dispute. Eur. J. Nutr. **39:** 183–193.
43. SCHUELKE, M., A. ELSNER, B. FINCKH, et al. 2000. Urinary alpha-tocopherol metabolites in alpha-tocopherol transfer protein-deficient patients. J. Lipid Res. **41:** 1543–1551.
44. FECHNER, H., M. SCHLAME, F. GUTHMANN, et al. 1998. alpha- and delta-Tocopherol induce expression of hepatic alpha-tocopherol-transfer-protein mRNA. Biochem. J. **331**(2): 577–581.
45. MASSON, L.F., G. MCNEILL & A. AVENELL. 2003. Genetic variation and the lipid response to dietary intervention: a systematic review. Am. J. Clin. Nutr. **77:** 1098–1111.
46. DAVIGNON, J., R.E. CREGG & C.F. SING. 1988. Apolipoprotein E polymorphism and atherosclerosis. Arteriosclerosis **8:** 1–21.
47. MINIHANE, A.-M., S. KHAN, E.C. LEIGH-FIRBANK, et al. 2000. ApoE polymorphism and fish oil supplementation in subjects with an atherogenic lipoprotein phenotype. Arterioscler. Thromb. Vasc. Biol. **20:** 1990–1997.
48. HUMPHRIES, S.E., P.J. TALMUD, E. HAWE, et al. 2001. Apolipoprotein E4 and coronary heart disease in middle-aged men who smoke: a prospective study. Lancet **358:** 115–119.
49. HIXSON, J.E. & D.T. VERNIER. 1990. Restriction isotyping of human apolipoprotein E by gene amplification and cleavage with HhaI. J. Lipid Res. **31:** 545–548.
50. GOMEZ-CORONADO, D., A. ENTRALA, J.J. ALVAREZ, et al. 2002. Influence of apolipoprotein E polymorphism on plasma vitamin A and vitamin E levels. Eur. J. Clin. Invest. **32:** 251–258.
51. WELTY, F.K. et al. 2000. Effects of apoE genotype on apoB48 and apoB100 kinetics with stable isotopes in humans. Arterioscler. Thromb. Vasc. Biol. **20:** 1807–1810.
52. BEISIEGEL, U. et al. 1989. The LDL-receptor-related protein, LRP, is an apolipoprotein E-binding protein. Nature **341:** 162–164.
53. MAHLEY, R.W. & Y. HUANG. 1999. Apolipoprotein E: from atherosclerosis to Alzheimer's disease and beyond. Curr. Opin. Lipidol. **10:** 207–217.
54. CATTIN, L., M. FISICARO, M. TONIZZO, et al. 1997. Polymorphism of the apolipoprotein E gene and early carotid atherosclerosis defined by ultrasonography in asymptomatic adults. Arterioscler. Thromb. Vasc. Biol. **17:** 91–94.

α-Tocopherol and Endothelial Nitric Oxide Synthesis

REGINE HELLER,[a] GABRIELE WERNER-FELMAYER,[b] AND ERNST R. WERNER[b]

[a]*Institute of Molecular Cell Biology, Friedrich-Schiller-University of Jena, D-99089 Erfurt, Germany*

[b]*Institute of Medical Chemistry and Biochemistry, University of Innsbruck, A-6020 Innsbruck, Austria*

ABSTRACT: Nitric oxide (NO), a central regulator of vascular tone and homeostasis, is generated upon activation of endothelial NO synthase (eNOS), which is mediated by an increase of intracellular calcium and/or by eNOS phosphorylation. A reduction of NO bioavailability leads to endothelial dysfunction that has been shown to be improved by α-tocopherol in certain conditions. The underlying mechanisms, however, are not completely clarified. The present study was performed to investigate whether α-tocopherol is able to affect endothelial NO synthesis. The formation of NO was measured in human umbilical vein endothelial cells using citrulline (coproduct) and cGMP (product of the NO-activated soluble guanylate cyclase) as indicator molecules. α-Tocopherol (10–200 μM, 24 hr) increased ionomycin-induced citrulline and cGMP formation in intact cells in a concentration-dependent manner. In parallel, ionomycin-stimulated phosphorylation of eNOS at serine 1177, known to support enzyme activation, was increased by α-tocopherol, suggesting that this was the mechanism responsible for enhanced NO formation. The effect of α-tocopherol was dependent on its hydrophobic structure because it was mimicked by γ-tocopherol but not by trolox, a hydrophilic derivative of α-tocopherol. Coincubation with ascorbic acid (100 μM, 24 hr) amplified the effects of α-tocopherol on eNOS phosphorylation and NO formation, which is possibly related to the regeneration of oxidized α-tocopherol by ascorbate. Our data suggest that vasoprotective effects of α-tocopherol *in vivo* may be related to an increase of NO formation. The effect of α-tocopherol seems to be dependent on tissue saturation with ascorbic acid, and both vitamins may act synergistically to provide optimal conditions for endothelial NO formation.

KEYWORDS: nitric oxide synthase; phosphorylation; endothelium; α-tocopherol; ascorbic acid.

Address for correspondence: Dr. Regine Heller, Institute of Molecular Cell Biology, Friedrich-Schiller-University of Jena, Nordhäuser Str. 78, 99089 Erfurt, Germany. Voice: +49-361-741 1437; fax: +49-361-741 1336.
heller@zmkh.ef.uni-jena.de

INTRODUCTION

Endothelium-derived nitric oxide (NO) was originally discovered as a vasodilator product and is now known as a central regulator of vascular homeostasis and as a potent antiatherosclerotic molecule. NO is generated from the conversion of L-arginine to L-citrulline by the enzymatic action of an NADPH-dependent NO synthase (NOS).[1] NOS consists of a C-terminal reductase domain containing binding sites for NADPH and the flavin cofactors FAD (flavin-adenine dinucleotide) and FMN (flavin mononucleotide) and an N-terminal oxygenase domain with binding sites for heme, tetrahydrobiopterin, and L-arginine. Both domains are linked by a recognition site for calmodulin (CaM). The endothelial NOS isoform (eNOS) is activated upon an increase of intracellular Ca^{2+}. The binding of the subsequently formed Ca^{2+}/CaM complex to eNOS releases the enzyme from its inhibitory complex with caveolin-1 and permits intradomain and interdomain electron flux, which is required for NO generation.[2] Importantly, the cofactor tetrahydrobiopterin acts as a one-electron donor in this reaction to couple oxygen reduction to L-arginine oxidation.[3] Further activities of tetrahydrobiopterin include the ability to shift the heme iron to its high-spin state, the promotion of arginine binding, and the stabilization of the active dimeric form of the enzyme.[3]

Recent evidence suggests that eNOS can also be activated through the phosphorylation of the amino acid residue serine 1177, which reduces the Ca^{2+} requirement of the enzyme and enhances the rate of electron flux from the reductase to the oxygenase domain.[1] Several protein kinases, including protein kinase Akt/protein kinase B (PKB), protein kinase A (PKA), AMP-dependent protein kinase, and CaM-dependent kinase II (CaMKII), have been shown to phosphorylate eNOS at serine 1177.[4–8] In contrast, constitutive phosphorylation at threonine 495, most probably by protein kinase C (PKC),[9] reduces eNOS activity by increasing Ca^{2+}/CaM dependence. Dephosphorylation of this residue in response to bradykinin has been shown to result in increased eNOS activity.[8,10]

Loss of NO bioavailability due to decreased production and/or increased NO scavenging by oxidized low-density lipoprotein (LDL) or reactive oxygen species is a key feature of endothelial dysfunction, an early event in atherosclerosis.[11] NO bioavailability can be measured experimentally in isolated vessels or in clinical studies as agonist-induced or flow-mediated vasorelaxation. Early studies found an impaired vasorelaxation in vessels prepared from vitamin E-deficient rats, an impairment that was improved when these animals were supplemented with vitamin E.[12–14] Similar results were obtained in arteries and aortas from cholesterol-fed rabbits.[15–19] Supplementation with vitamin E or α-tocopherol, the predominating form of vitamin E in human plasma and tissues, did not only improve acetylcholine-induced vasorelaxation but also increased resistance of LDL against oxidation[15–18] and reduced biomarkers[19] of oxidative stress, suggesting that protection of NO from inactivation by oxidized LDL or oxygen radicals was the responsible mechanism. However, preservation of NO bioactivity was not always correlated with inhibition of LDL oxidation,[16] suggesting that additional activities of α-tocopherol might play a role. Indeed, α-tocopherol has been shown to modulate cell signaling via inhibition of PKC[20,21] and might counteract the activation of PKC by oxidized LDL in endothelial cells.[22] Thus, the α-tocopherol content of the vascular wall seems to be important for the protection of endothelial function as well. Recent studies convincingly demonstrated that α-tocopherol was able to alter the redox state of the vascular wall through decreasing NADPH oxidase and increasing superoxide dismutase activities in aortas of spontaneously hypertensive rats.[23,24] This effect led to an improvement of endothelium-dependent vasorelaxation, most probably due to protection of NO from inactivation, and prevented progression of hypertension.

α-Tocopherol plasma levels are correlated with an index of endothelial function in healthy humans as well[25,26]; accordingly, several clinical studies investigated whether vitamin E supplementation was able to improve vasorelaxation in patients with hypercholesterolemia,[27–34] diabetes,[35–40] or coronary artery disease[41–43] and in smokers.[44–46] The studies varied with respect to the investigated vascular bed, the chemical form and dose of the applied vitamin E, and the duration of the treatment. Morever, most study groups were small (7 to 25 subjects). Some of the human studies confirmed positive findings seen in animal trials,[29–31,33,34,36–40,42,45,46] whereas others were negative for effects of α-tocopherol on NO bioactivity.[27,28,32,35,41,43,44] The reason for these discrepancies is not clear and might be related to differences of the study design. It might be that α-tocopherol is more effective when given at an earlier time point in the development of endothelial dysfunction. This possibility has been raised because two studies performed in hyperlipidemic children found an improvement of vasorelaxation by a combined vitamin E plus vitamin C therapy.[29,34] In addition, certain subjects, including hypercholesterolemic smokers[31] or patients with diabetes type I,[36,37,40] seem to be more susceptible to vitamin E treatment of endothelial dysfunction than others. To better understand this apparent selectivity and to identify patients who may benefit from α-tocopherol, it seems necessary to fully characterize the mechanisms underlying the amelioration of endothelial dysfunction by α-tocopherol, especially as this was not always correlated with a decrease of biomarkers of oxidative stress. Against this background, we designed a study to investigate whether α-tocopherol was able to directly affect NO synthesis in endothelial cells and to reveal underlying mechanisms.

MATERIALS AND METHODS

Cell Culture and Experimental Incubation

Human umbilical vein endothelial cells (HUVECs) were grown in medium 199 (M199) as described previously.[47,48] Preincubation of HUVECs with test compounds was performed in culture medium. In experiments investigating the phosphorylation of eNOS, a 6-hr incubation period in serum-free M199 containing 0.25% human serum albumin (HSA) was included. Stock solutions of RRR-α-, RRR-δ-, and RRR-γ-tocopherol; rac-β-tocopherol; and trolox (Sigma-Aldrich Chemie GmbH, Taufkirchen, Germany) were prepared in ethanol. Preincubations with KN-93 (30 µM, 30 min; Merck Biosciences GmbH, Schwalbach, Germany) as well as stimulation of cells with ionomycin (2 µM, 15 min) were performed in the absence of test compounds in Hepes buffer (10 mM Hepes (pH 7.4), 145 mM NaCl, 5 mM KCl, 1 mM $MgSO_4$, and 10 mM glucose, 1.5 mM $CaCl_2$) containing 0.25% HSA (Hepes/HSA).

Determination of Citrulline and cGMP Formation

NO was assayed upon cell stimulation (2 µM ionomycin, 15 min) with the help of two indicator molecules, citrulline (coproduct of NO) and cGMP (product of the

NO-activated soluble guanylate cyclase). For citrulline measurement, cell stimulation was performed in the presence of 10 µM L-[^{3}H]arginine (0.33 Ci/mmol; Amersham Biosciences, Freiburg, Germany). The generated [^{3}H]citrulline was separated by cation exchange chromatography and quantified by liquid scintillation counting.[47,48] cGMP was measured by radioimmunoassay (Amersham) as described previously.[47,48]

Measurement of Intracellular Tetrahydrobiopterin

HUVECs were detached with trypsin/EDTA (0.05%/0.02%, v/v) and oxidized with 0.02 M KI/I$_2$ under acidic or alkaline conditions to detect total biopterin or 7,8-dihydrobiopterin plus biopterin, respectively. Quantification of biopterin in supernatants was performed by high-performance liquid chromatography as described previously.[48] The amount of 5,6,7,8-tetrahydrobiopterin was calculated from the difference of total biopterin and 7,8-dihydrobiopterin plus biopterin.

Immunoblotting

Cell homogenates for eNOS expression studies were prepared in Hepes/sorbitol buffer (10 mM Hepes (pH 7.4), 340 mM sorbitol, 1 mM EDTA, and 2 mM dithiothreitol (DTT)) containing protease inhibitors. For preparation of membrane and cytosolic fractions, cell suspensions were sonicated and centrifuged for 1 hr at 100,000 × g and 4°C. Lysates for eNOS phosphorylation studies were prepared in Tris buffer (50 mM Tris (pH 7.4), 2 mM EDTA, and 1 mM EGTA) containing phosphatase and protease inhibitors. Proteins were separated by sodium dodecyl sulfate-polyacrylamide gel electrophoresis (SDS-PAGE) and subjected to Western blot analysis with a monoclonal antibody against human eNOS (BD Transduction Laboratories, BD Biosciences, Heidelberg, Germany) or polyclonal antibodies against eNOS phosphorylated at serine 1177 (Cell Signaling Technologies, Beverly, MA) or threonine 495 (Upstate Biotechnology, Lake Placid, NY).

Statistical Analysis

All data are given as means ± SEM of three to six independent experiments performed in duplicate. To determine the statistical significance, Student's t-test for paired or unpaired data or analysis of variance (ANOVA) for repeated measurements followed by the Newman–Keuls test were performed. A P value of below 0.05 was accepted as statistically significant.

RESULTS AND DISCUSSION

α-Tocopherol Increases Citrulline and cGMP Formation in Endothelial Cells

When HUVECs were pretreated with α-tocopherol (10–200 µM, 24 hr) and stimulated with ionomycin, they generated up to 1.5-fold and 1.4-fold more citrulline and cGMP than control cells, respectively, suggesting that NO synthesis was enhanced under these conditions (FIG. 1). These data are in line with previous observations on an increased eNOS activity in aortas of vitamin E-treated hypertensive rats[24,49] and

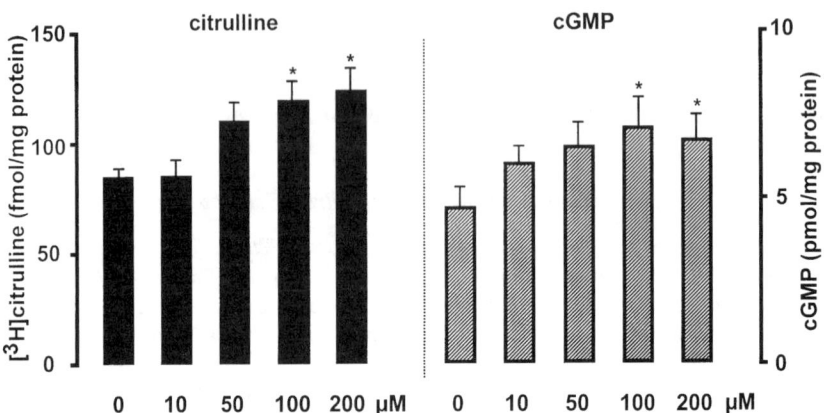

FIGURE 1. Influence of α-tocopherol on citrulline and cGMP formation in endothelial cells. Cells were preincubated for 24 hr with α-tocopherol, stimulated with ionomycin (2 μM, 15 min) and processed for either citrulline or cGMP measurement. The presented data were calculated from differences between stimulated and unstimulated cells (mean ± SEM; $n = 4$; *$P < 0.05$ vs. untreated control cells).

in human platelets supplemented with vitamin E.[50,51] The effect of α-tocopherol alone was moderate in our study, but interestingly, it was augmented by coincubation with ascorbic acid. FIGURE 2 shows that the combination of ascorbate (1–100 μM, 24 hr) with α-tocopherol (100 μM, 24 hr) led to an up to 4.3-fold increase of ionomycin-stimulated citrulline and cGMP formation, which was considerably higher than the effects of α-tocopherol or ascorbate alone. The potentiating effect of ascorbic acid on NO synthesis has been demonstrated in earlier studies from our group and from other groups,[47,48,52–54] and has been related to an increased availability of the eNOS cofactor tetrahydrobiopterin because of its protection from irreversible oxidation.[48] The data presented here suggest that ascorbate may affect NO formation not only by providing saturated cofactor conditions, but also by promoting effects of α-tocopherol. Ascorbate has been shown to recycle oxidized α-tocopherol back to its native form[55] and might protect endothelial cells from prooxidant effects of the α-tocopheroxyl radical. Interestingly, coenzyme Q, another α-tocopherol-recycling agent, was also able to amplify the effects of α-tocopherol on eNOS activation (data not shown), thus confirming the importance of α-tocopherol regeneration. Our data suggest that the combination of vitamin E and vitamin C may be of particular benefit for the amelioration of endothelial dysfunction. Accordingly, several studies[29,34,39,40,46] (although not all[28,43]) in which individuals with coronary risk factors were supplemented with α-tocopherol plus ascorbic acid showed an improved vasoreactivity.

α-Tocopherol Does Not Affect eNOS Expression or Tetrahydrobiopterin Availability

To investigate whether the increased NO formation was due to an enhanced eNOS expression, a Western blot analysis with lysates from HUVECs pretreated with α-

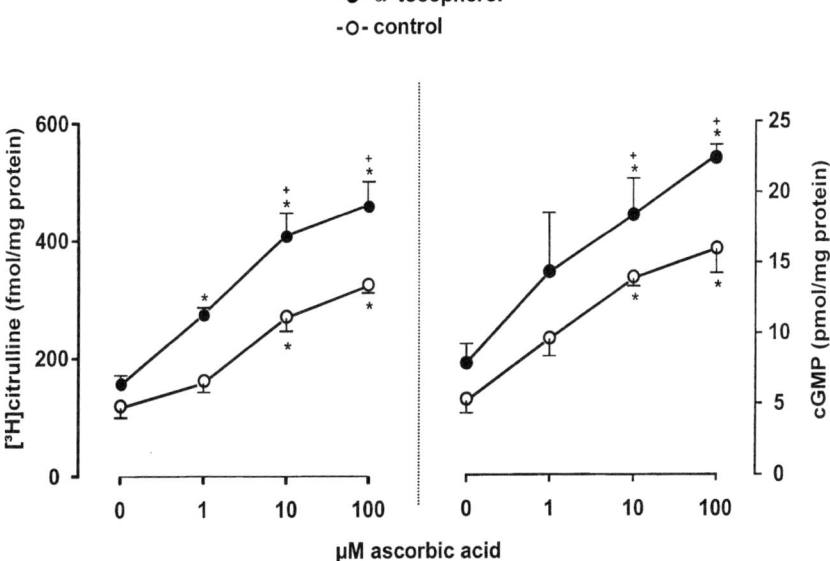

FIGURE 2. Influence of ascorbic acid on α-tocopherol-induced increase of citrulline and cGMP formation. Cells were preincubated for 24 hr with ascorbic acid in the absence or presence of 100 μM α-tocopherol, stimulated with ionomycin (2 μM, 15 min), and processed for either citrulline or cGMP measurement. Data were calculated from the difference between stimulated and unstimulated cells (mean ± SEM; $n = 4$; *$P < 0.05$ vs. untreated controls; +$p < 0.05$ vs. cells pretreated with ascorbic acid alone). (From Heller et al.[56] Reprinted by permission.)

tocopherol (100 μM, 24 hr) in the absence or presence of ascorbic acid (100 μM) was performed. FIGURE 3 shows that neither eNOS expression nor its distribution between cytosolic and particulate subcellular fractions was changed after experimental incubations.

Because the effect of α-tocopherol was maintained in the presence of 100 μM ascorbate, which is known to saturate intracellular tetrahydrobiopterin levels,[48] we did not expect that it was mediated via tetrahydrobiopterin. Indeed, intracellular tetrahydrobiopterin levels were comparable in control cells and cells pretreated with α-tocopherol (100 μM, 24 hr) (0.28 ± 0.046 and 0.32 ± 0.150 pmol/mg protein, respectively). Similarly, α-tocopherol did not induce a further increase of tetrahydrobiopterin levels in ascorbate-treated cells (100 μM each, 24 hr) (1.02 ± 0.095 and 1.02 ± 0.200 pmol/mg protein, with and without tocopherol, respectively). These data are in line with an *in vivo* study in mice where vitamin E did not affect the metabolism of tetrahydrobiopterin[54] and indicate that a hydrophilic structure of antioxidants may be required to interfere with oxidative degradation of tetrahydrobiopterin. Interestingly, trolox, a water-soluble derivative of α-tocopherol that is lacking the phytyl side-chain, was able to increase intracellular tetrahydrobiopterin levels and to potentiate endothelial NO formation.[56]

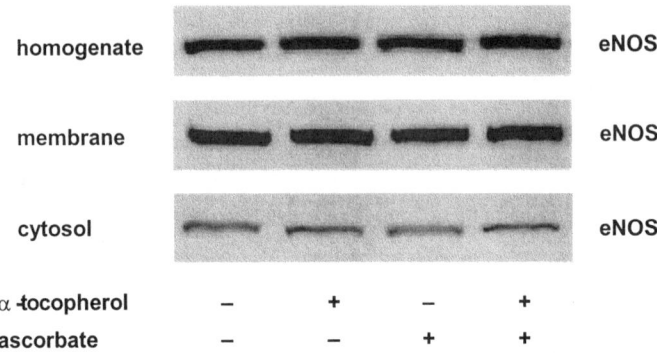

FIGURE 3. Effect of α-tocopherol on the expression of endothelial NO synthase (eNOS). HUVECs were preincubated for 24 hr with 100 μM α-tocopherol, 100 μM ascorbate, or a combination of both. Cell homogenates and subcellular fractions prepared by ultracentrifugation were separated by SDS-PAGE, and Western blotting analysis was performed using a monoclonal antibody against human eNOS. A representative figure out of three is shown.

α-Tocopherol Increases eNOS Activity via Increasing Phosphorylation at Serine 1177

Because phosphorylation at key regulatory sites plays an important role in the regulation of eNOS activity, we investigated whether α-tocopherol preincubation of HUVECs affects the phosphorylation state of the enzyme. The Ca^{2+}-ionophore ionomycin used as an agonist in our study induced phosphorylation of eNOS at serine 1177 in a time-dependent manner, but did not change threonine 495 phosphorylation (data not shown). Serine 1177 phosphorylation has originally been thought to activate eNOS upon stimulation with shear stress or growth factors in the absence of a sustained increase of intracellular calcium, but recent studies have also revealed its involvement in Ca^{2+}-dependent eNOS activation.[8] Importantly, when HUVECs were preincubated with α-tocopherol (100 μM, 24 hr), ionomycin-induced phosphorylation of the eNOS residue serine 1177 was increased, suggesting that this was the mechanism responsible for the observed potentiation of NO formation (FIG. 4). Accordingly, when added simultaneously, ascorbic acid was not only able to amplify the effect of α-tocopherol on NO formation (FIG. 2), it was also able to amplify its effect on serine 1177 phosphorylation, whereas no change of eNOS phosphorylation was observed with ascorbic acid alone (FIG. 4). The results presented here agree with a previous report showing that α-tocopherol as well as γ- and δ-tocopherol enhanced NO production and modified eNOS phosphorylation in platelets, although the residue serine 1177 was not investigated.[51] In contrast, phorbol ester-mediated overall eNOS phosphorylation in platelets was inhibited by α-tocopherol,[50] suggesting that PKC-mediated phosphorylation of the eNOS residue threonine 495 was reduced, which was, however, not confirmed in our experiments.[56]

After ionomycin stimulation, serine 1177 was mainly phosphorylated through CAMKII because inhibition of this enzyme by KN-93 (30 μM, 30 min preincuba-

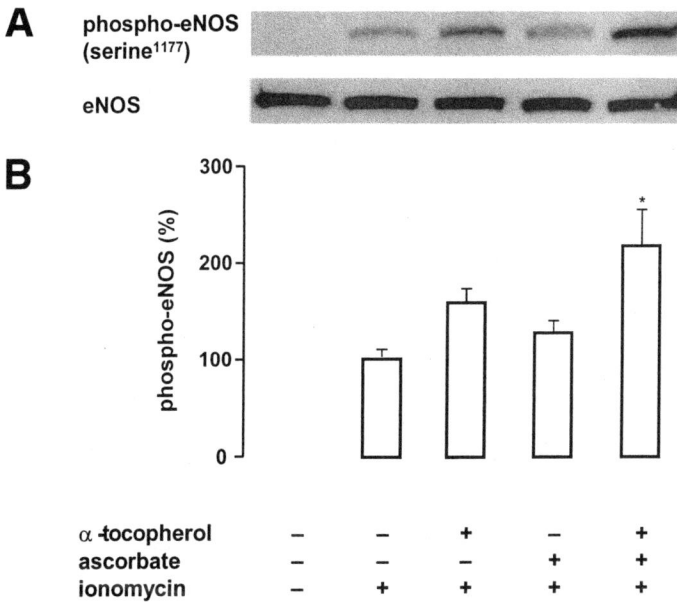

FIGURE 4. Effect of α-tocopherol on the phosphorylation of endothelial NO synthase (eNOS). HUVECs were preincubated with α-tocopherol or ascorbic acid as indicated (100 μM each, 24 hr), stimulated with ionomycin (2 μM, 15 min) and lysed in Tris buffer (pH 7.4) containing 1% Triton X-100 and 0.1% SDS. Immunoblotting was performed using antibodies against eNOS phosphorylated at serine 1177 and an anti-eNOS antibody for counterstaining. (**A**) Representative experiment. (**B**) Densitometric analysis (values are normalized to the staining of the untreated control) (mean ± SEM; $n = 5$; *$P < 0.05$ vs. untreated controls). (From Heller et al.[56] Reprinted by permission.)

tion) reduced the phosphorylation signal by 80 ± 3.2% (densitometric analysis, $n = 4$) and the formation of citrulline by 48% (285 ± 13.03 and 138 ± 20.11 fmol [^{3}H]citrulline/mg protein in control and inhibitor-treated cells, respectively, $n = 6$). Interestingly, when we inhibited CaMKII in α-tocopherol/ascorbate-pretreated cells with KN-93, the reduction of ionomycin-induced serine 1177 phosphorylation of eNOS was lower than in control cells (57 ± 5.9%, $n = 4$), and citrulline formation was not significantly decreased (391 ± 29.94 vs. 326 ± 20.48 fmol [^{3}H]citrulline/mg protein without and with KN-93, respectively, $n = 6$). These data let us suggest that stimulation of other protein kinases or inhibition of protein phosphatases may be involved in the effect of α-tocopherol on eNOS phosphorylation. We found, however, that inhibition of either PKA or the PI3K/Akt pathway, both known to mediate serine 1177 phosphorylation, did not suppress the amplifying effect of α-tocopherol.[56] Moreover, protein phosphatase 2A, known to be responsible for the dephosphorylation of serine 1177, has been shown to be activated rather than inhibited by α-tocopherol.[57]

In order to know whether the observed activities were specific to α-tocopherol, we investigated the effects of the isoforms β-, γ-, and δ-tocopherol, which all contain the hydrophobic side chain, and of the hydrophilic analogue trolox on eNOS phosphorylation. We found that mainly γ-tocopherol and to a lesser extent β- and δ-tocopherol were able to increase ionomycin-stimulated serine 1177 phosphorylation, whereas trolox had no effect (densitometric ratios compared to control cells: 1.72 ± 3.63,* 1.54 ± 3.04, 2.04 ± 2.98,* 1.49 ± 1.17, and 1.15 ± 1.62 for α-, β-, γ-, and δ-tocopherol and trolox, respectively, $n = 3$, *$P < 0.05$). These data suggest that effects specifically attributed to α-tocopherol such as PKC inhibition[20] were most probably not involved, whereas the appropriate membrane incorporation of α-tocopherol via the phytyl chain seemed to be essential to increase eNOS phosphorylation. Interestingly, α-tocopherol is known to alter membrane properties by increasing microviscosity, which has been shown to cause an increased binding of signaling molecules to membranes.[58] Thus, α-tocopherol might be involved in the colocalization of eNOS and its regulating protein kinases in membranes and might support the activation of phosphorylating enzymes such as CaMKII and its interaction with eNOS.

Our data underline the importance of serine 1177 phosphorylation as a regulatory target for eNOS activation even at saturated cofactor levels. Interestingly, a decreased phosphorylation of serine 1177 has been seen with hyperglycemia or pulmonary hypertension[59,60]; conversely, regular physical activity has been shown to improve endothelial function in patients by increasing serine 1177 phosphorylation of eNOS.[61] Thus, although not yet proven *in vivo*, our results may help to define vascular disease states that might benefit from α-tocopherol supplementation.

ACKNOWLEDGMENTS

Experimental work was supported by the Interdisziplinäres Zentrum für Klinische Forschung, Klinikum der Friedrich-Schiller-Universität Jena (project B, 378-01040, to R.H.), the Austrian research funds "Zur Förderung der wissenschaftlichen Forschung" (project P16059, to G.W.-F.), and the "Jubiläumsfonds" of the Austrian National Bank (project 9918, to E.R.W.). We thank Gunda Guhr, Elke Teuscher, and Petra Loitzl for their excellent technical assistance.

REFERENCES

1. FLEMING, I. & R. BUSSE. 2003. Molecular mechanisms involved in the regulation of the endothelial nitric oxide synthase. Am. J. Physiol. **284:** R1–R12.
2. ALDERTON, W.K., C.E. COOPER & R.G. KNOWLES. 2001. Nitric oxide synthases: structure, function and inhibition. Biochem. J. **357:** 593–615.
3. WERNER, E.R., A.C.F. GORREN, R. HELLER, *et al.* 2003. Tetrahydrobiopterin and nitric oxide: mechanistical and pharmacological aspects. Exp. Biol. Med. **228:** 1291–1302.
4. FULTON, D., J.-P. GRATTON, T.J. MCCABE, *et al.* 1999. Regulation of endothelium-derived nitric oxide production by the protein kinase Akt. Nature **399:** 597–601.
5. DIMMELER, S., I. FLEMING, B. FISSLTHALER, *et al.* 1999. Activation of nitric oxide synthase in endothelial cells by Akt-dependent phosphorylation. Nature **399:** 601–605.
6. BOO, Y.C., G. SORESCU, N. BOYD, *et al.* 2002. Shear stress stimulates phosphorylation of endothelial nitric-oxide synthase at Ser1179 by Akt-independent mechanisms: role of protein kinase A. J. Biol. Chem. **277:** 3388–3396.
7. CHEN, Z.P., K.I. MITCHELHILL, B.J. MICHELL, *et al.* 1999. AMP-activated protein kinase phosphorylation of endothelial NO synthase. FEBS Lett. **443:** 285–289.
8. FLEMING, I., B. FISSLTHALER, S. DIMMELER, *et al.* 2001. Phosphorylation of Thr(495) regulates Ca(2+)/calmodulin-dependent endothelial nitric oxide synthase activity. Circ. Res. **88:** e68–e75.

9. MICHELL, B.J., Z.-P. CHEN, T. TIGANIS, et al. 2001. Coordinated control of endothelial nitric-oxide synthase phosphorylation by protein kinase C and the cAMP-dependent protein kinase. J. Biol. Chem. **276:** 17625–17628.
10. HARRIS, M.B., H. JU, V.J. VENEMA, et al. 2001. Reciprocal phosphorylation and regulation of endothelial nitric oxide synthase in response to bradykinin stimulation. J. Biol. Chem. **276:** 16587–16591.
11. NAPOLI, C. & L.J. IGNARRO. 2001. Nitric oxide and atherosclerosis. Nitric Oxide **5:** 88–97.
12. RAIJ, L., J. NAGY, K. COFFEE, et al. 1993. Hypercholesterolemia promotes endothelial dysfunction in vitamin E- and selenium-deficient rats. Hypertension **22:** 56–61.
13. RUBINO, A. & G. BURNSTOCK. 1994. Recovery after dietary vitamin E supplementation of impaired endothelial function in vitamin E deficient rats. Br. J. Pharmacol. **112:** 515–518.
14. DAVIDGE, S.T., J. OJIMBA & M.K. MCLAUGHLIN. 1998. Vascular function in the vitamin E-deprived rat: an interaction between nitric oxide and superoxide anions. Hypertension **31:** 830–835.
15. KEANEY, J.F., JR, J.M. GAZIANO, A. XU, et al. 1993. Dietary antioxidants preserve endothelium-dependent vessel relaxation in cholesterol-fed rabbits. Proc. Natl. Acad. Sci. USA **90:** 11880–11884.
16. KEANEY, J.F., JR., J.M. GAZIANO, A. XU, et al. 1994. Low-dose alpha-tocopherol improves and high-dose alpha-tocopherol worsens endothelial vasodilator function in cholesterol-fed rabbits. J. Clin. Invest. **93:** 844–851.
17. STEWART-LEE, A.L., L.A. FORSTER, J. NOUROOZ-ZADEH, et al. 1994. Vitamin E protects against impairment of endothelium-mediated relaxations in cholesterol-fed rabbits. Arterioscler. Thromb. **14:** 494–499.
18. BOGER, R.H., S.M. BODE-BOGER, L. PHIVTHONG-NGAM, et al. 1998. Dietary L-arginine and alpha-tocopherol reduce vascular oxidative stress and preserve endothelial function in hypercholesterolemic rabbits via different mechanisms. Atherosclerosis **141:** 31–43.
19. RIBEIRO JORGE, P.A., L.C. NEYRA, R.M. OZAKI, et al. 1998. Improvement in the endothelium-dependent relaxation in hypercholesterolemic rabbits treated with vitamin E. Atherosclerosis **140:** 333–339.
20. TASINATO, A., D. BOSCOBOINIK, G.M. BARTOLI, et al. 1995. D-alpha-Tocopherol inhibition of vascular smooth muscle cell proliferation occurs at physiological concentrations, correlates with protein kinase C inhibition, and is independent of its antioxidant properties. Proc. Natl. Acad. Sci. USA **92:** 12190–12194.
21. MARTIN-NIZARD, F., A. BOULLIER, J.C. FRUCHART, et al. 1998. Alpha-Tocopherol but not beta-tocopherol inhibits thrombin-induced PKC activation and endothelin secretion in endothelial cells. J. Cardiovasc. Risk **5:** 339–345.
22. KEANEY, J.F., JR., Y. GUO, D CUNNINGHAM, et al. 1996. Vascular incorporation of alpha-tocopherol prevents endothelial dysfunction due to oxidized LDL by inhibiting protein kinase C stimulation. J. Clin. Invest. **98:** 386–394.
23. CHEN, X., R.M. TOUYZ, J.B. PARK, et al. 2001. Antioxidant effects of vitamins C and E are associated with altered activation of vascular NADPH oxidase and superoxide dismutase in stroke-prone SHR. Hypertension **38:** 606–611.
24. ÜLKER, S., P.P. MCKEOWN & U. BAYRAKTUTAN. 2003. Vitamins reverse endothelial dysfunction through regulation of eNOS and NAD(P)H oxidase activities. Hypertension **41:** 534–539.
25. SARABI, M., B. VESSBY, S. BASU, et al. 1999. Relationships between endothelium-dependent vasodilation, serum vitamin E and plasma isoprostane 8-iso-PGF(2alpha) levels in healthy subjects. J. Vasc. Res. **36:** 486–491.
26. KINLAY, S., J.C. FANG, H. HIKITA, et al. 1999. Plasma alpha-tocopherol and coronary endothelium-dependent vasodilator function. Circulation **100:** 219–221.
27. MCDOWELL, I.F., G.M. BRENNAN, J. MCENENY, et al. 1994. The effect of probucol and vitamin E treatment on the oxidation of low-density lipoprotein and forearm vascular responses in humans. Eur. J. Clin. Invest. **24:** 759–765.
28. GILLIGAN, D.M., M.N. SACK, V. GUETTA, et al. 1994. Effect of antioxidant vitamins on low-density lipoprotein oxidation and impaired endothelium-dependent vasodilation in patients with hypercholesterolemia. J. Am. Coll. Cardiol. **24:** 1611-1617.

29. MIETUS-SNYDER, M. & M.J. MALLOY. 1998. Endothelial dysfunction occurs in children with two genetic hyperlipidemias: improvement with antioxidant vitamin therapy. J. Pediatr. **133:** 35–40.
30. NEUNTEUFL, T., K. KOSTNER, R. KATZENSCHLAGER, *et al.* 1998. Additional benefit of vitamin E supplementation to simvastatin therapy on vasoreactivity of the brachial artery of hypercholesterolemic men. J. Am. Coll. Cardiol. **32:** 711–716.
31. HEITZER, T., S. YLA HERTTUALA, E. WILD, *et al.* 1999. Effect of vitamin E on endothelial vasodilator function in patients with hypercholesterolemia, chronic smoking or both. J. Am. Coll. Cardiol. **33:** 499–505.
32. CHOWIENCZYK, P.J., B.J. KNEALE, S.E. BRETT, *et al.* 1998. Lack of effect of vitamin E on L-arginine-responsive endothelial dysfunction in patients with mild hypercholesterolaemia and coronary artery disease. Clin. Sci. (London) **94:** 129–134.
33. GREEN, D., G. O'DRISCOLL, J.M. RANKIN, *et al.* 1998. Beneficial effect of vitamin E administration on nitric oxide function in subjects with hypercholesterolaemia. Clin. Sci. (London) **95:** 361–367.
34. ENGLER, M.M, M.B. ENGLER, M.J. MALLOY, *et al.* 2003. Antioxidant vitamins C and E improve endothelial function in children with hyperlipidemia: endothelial assessment of risk from lipids in youth (EARLY) trial. Circulation **108:** 1059–1063.
35. GAZIS, A., D.J. WHITE, S.R. PAGE, *et al.* 1999. Effect of oral vitamin E (alpha-tocopherol) supplementation on vascular endothelial function in type 2 diabetes mellitus. Diabet. Med. **16:** 304–311.
36. PINKNEY, J.H., L. DOWNS, M. HOPTON, *et al.* 1999. Endothelial dysfunction in type 1 diabetes mellitus: relationship with LDL oxidation and the effects of vitamin E. Diabet. Med. **16:** 993–999.
37. SKYRME-JONES, R.A., R.C. O'BRIEN, K.L. BERRY, *et al.* 2000. Vitamin E supplementation improves endothelial function in type I diabetes mellitus: a randomized, placebo-controlled study. J. Am. Coll. Cardiol. **36:** 94–102.
38. PAOLISSO, G., M.R. TAGLIAMONTE, M. BARBIERI, *et al.* 2000. Chronic vitamin E administration improves brachial reactivity and increases intracellular magnesium concentration in type II diabetic patients. J. Clin. Endocrinol. Metab. **85:** 109–115.
39. REGENSTEINER, J.G., S. POPYLISEN, T.A. BAUER, *et al.* 2003. Oral L-arginine and vitamins E and C improve endothelial function in women with type 2 diabetes. Vasc. Med. **8:** 169–175.
40. BECKMAN, J.A., A.B. GOLDFINE, M.B. GORDON, *et al.* 2003. Oral antioxidant therapy improves endothelial function in type 1 but not type 2 diabetes mellitus. Am. J. Physiol. Heart Circ. Physiol. **285:** H2392–H2398.
41. ELLIOTT, T.G., J.D. BARTH & G.B. MANCINI. 1995. Effects of vitamin E on endothelial function in men after myocardial infarction. Am. J. Cardiol. **76:** 1188–1190.
42. MOTOYAMA, T., H. KAWANO, K. KUGIYAMA, *et al.* 1998. Vitamin E administration improves impairment of endothelium-dependent vasodilation in patients with coronary spastic angina. J. Am. Coll. Cardiol. **32:** 1672–1679.
43. KINLAY, S., D. BEHRENDT, J.C. FANG, *et al.* 2004. Long-term effect of combined vitamins E and C on coronary and peripheral endothelial function. J. Am. Coll. Cardiol. **43:** 629–634.
44. GREEN, D., G. O'DRISCOLL, B. BLANKSBY, *et al.* 1995. Lack of effect of vitamin E administration on basal nitric oxide function in male smokers and non-smokers. Clin. Sci. (London) **89:** 343–348.
45. NEUNTEUFL, T., U. PRIGLINGER, S. HEHER, *et al.* 2000. Effects of vitamin E on chronic and acute endothelial dysfunction in smokers. J. Am. Coll. Cardiol. **35:** 277–283.
46. TOUSOULIS, D., C. ANTONIADES, C. TENTOLOURIS, *et al.* 2003. Effects of combined administration of vitamins C and E on reactive hyperemia and inflammatory process in chronic smokers. Atherosclerosis **170:** 261–267.
47. HELLER, R., F. MÜNSCHER-PAULIG, R. GRÄBNER, *et al.* 1999. L-Ascorbic acid potentiates nitric oxide synthesis in endothelial cells. J. Biol. Chem. **274:** 8254–8260.
48. HELLER, R., A. UNBEHAUN, B. SCHELLENBERG, *et al.* 2001. L-Ascorbic acid potentiates endothelial nitric oxide synthesis via a chemical stabilization of tetrahydrobiopterin. J. Biol. Chem. **276:** 40–47.

49. NEWAZ, M.A., N.N. NAWAL, C.H. ROHAIZAN, et al. 1999. alpha-Tocopherol increased nitric oxide synthase activity in blood vessels of spontaneously hypertensive rats. Am. J. Hypertens. **12:** 839–844.
50. FREEDMAN, J.E., L. LI, R. SAUTER, et al. 2000. alpha-Tocopherol and protein kinase C inhibition enhance platelet-derived nitric oxide release. FASEB J. **14:** 2377–2379.
51. LI, D., T. SALDEEN, F. ROMEO, et al. 2001. Different isoforms of tocopherols enhance nitric oxide synthase phosphorylation and inhibit human platelet aggregation and lipid peroxidation: implications in therapy with vitamin E. J. Cardiovasc. Pharmacol. Therapeut. **6:** 155–161.
52. HUANG, A., J.A. VITA, R.C. VENEMA, et al. 2000. Ascorbic acid enhances endothelial nitric-oxide synthase activity by increasing intracellular tetrahydrobiopterin. J. Biol. Chem. **275:** 17399–17406.
53. BAKER, T.A., S. MILSTIEN & Z.S. KATUSIC. 2001. Effect of vitamin C on the availability of tetrahydrobiopterin in human endothelial cells. J. Cardiovasc. Pharmacol. **37:** 333–338.
54. D'USCIO, L.V., S. MILSTIEN, D. RICHARDSON, et al. 2003. Long-term vitamin C treatment increases vascular tetrahydrobiopterin levels and nitric oxide synthase activity. Circ. Res. **92:** 88–95.
55. MAY, J.M., Z.-C. QU & S. MENDIRETTA. 1998. Protection and recycling of alpha-tocopherol in human erythrocytes by intracellular ascorbic acid. Arch. Biochem. Biophys. **349:** 281–289.
56. HELLER, R., M. HECKER, N. STAHMANN, et al. 2004. alpha-Tocopherol amplifies phosphorylation of endothelial nitric oxide synthase at serine 1177 and its short-chain derivative trolox stabilizes tetrahydrobiopterin. Free Radic. Biol. Med. **37:** 620–631.
57. RICCIARELLI, R., A. TASINATO, S. CLEMENT, et al. 1998. alpha-Tocopherol specifically inactivates cellular protein kinase C alpha by changing its phosphorylation state. Biochem. J. **334:** 243–249.
58. GHOSH, P.K., A. VASANJI, G. MURUGESAN, et al. 2002. Membrane microviscosity regulates endothelial cell motility. Nat. Cell Biol. **4:** 894–900.
59. DU, X.L., D. EDELSTEIN, S. DIMMELER, et al. 2001. Hyperglycemia inhibits endothelial nitric oxide synthase activity by posttranslational modification at the Akt site. J. Clin. Invest. **108:** 1341–1348.
60. MURATA, T., K. SATO, M. HORI, et al. 2002. Decreased endothelial nitric-oxide synthase (eNOS) activity resulting from abnormal interaction between eNOS and its regulatory proteins in hypoxia-induced pulmonary hypertension. J. Biol. Chem. **277:** 44085–44092.
61. HAMBRECHT, R., V. ADAMS, S. ERBS, et al. 2003. Regular physical activity improves endothelial function in patients with coronary artery disease by increasing phosphorylation of endothelial nitric oxide synthase. Circulation **107:** 3152–3158.

Vitamin E Mediates Cell Signaling and Regulation of Gene Expression

ANGELO AZZI, RENÉ GYSIN, PETRA KEMPNÁ, ADELINA MUNTEANU, YESIM NEGIS, LUIS VILLACORTA, THERESA VISARIUS, AND JEAN-MARC ZINGG

Institute of Biochemistry and Molecular Biology, University of Bern, Bern, Switzerland

ABSTRACT: α-Tocopherol modulates two major signal transduction pathways centered on protein kinase C and phosphatidylinositol 3-kinase. Changes in the activity of these key kinases are associated with changes in cell proliferation, platelet aggregation, and NADPH-oxidase activation. Several genes are also regulated by tocopherols partly because of the effects of tocopherol on these two kinases, but also independently of them. These genes can be divided in five groups: *Group 1*. Genes that are involved in the uptake and degradation of tocopherols: α-tocopherol transfer protein, cytochrome P450 (CYP3A), γ-glutamyl-cysteine synthetase heavy subunit, and glutathione-S-transferase. *Group 2*. Genes that are implicated with lipid uptake and atherosclerosis: CD36, SR-BI, and SR-AI/II. *Group 3*. Genes that are involved in the modulation of extracellular proteins: tropomyosin, collagen-α-1, MMP-1, MMP-19, and connective tissue growth factor. *Group 4*. Genes that are connected to adhesion and inflammation: E-selectin, ICAM-1 integrins, glycoprotein IIb, IL-2, IL-4, IL-1b, and transforming growth factor-β (TGF-β). *Group 5*. Genes implicated in cell signaling and cell cycle regulation: PPAR-γ, cyclin D1, cyclin E, Bcl2-L1, p27, CD95 (APO-1/Fas ligand), and 5a-steroid reductase type 1. The transcription of p27, Bcl2, α-tocopherol transfer protein, cytochrome P450 (CYP3A), γ-glutamyl-cysteine sythetase heavy subunit, tropomyosin, IL-2, and CTGF appears to be upregulated by one or more tocopherols. All the other listed genes are downregulated. Gene regulation by tocopherols has been associated with protein kinase C because of its deactivation by α-tocopherol and its contribution in the regulation of a number of transcription factors (NF-κB, AP1). A direct participation of the pregnane X receptor (PXR)/retinoid X receptor (RXR) has been also shown. The antioxidant-responsive element (ARE) and the TGF-β–responsive element (TGF-β-RE) appear in some cases to be implicated as well.

KEYWORDS: α-tocopherol (tocopherols, tocotrienols); vitamin E; cell regulation; gene expression; inhibition of cell proliferation; signal transduction; transcription factor; receptor

In 1982, Burton, Joyce, and Ingold published a letter in *Lancet* that claimed they had obtained the first proof that vitamin E is the major lipid-soluble, chain-breaking an-

Address for correspondence: Prof. Angelo Azzi, Institute of Biochemistry and Molecular Biology, University of Bern, Bühlstrasse 28, 3012 Bern, Switzerland. Voice: +41316314131; fax: +41316313737.
angelo.azzi@mci.unibe.ch

tioxidant in human blood plasma.[1] Just one year later, at a Ciba Foundation Symposium, Diplock proclaimed that the view that vitamin E functions in living systems primarily as a lipid antioxidant and free-radical scavenger had gained widespread acceptance. And it was concluded that as a result of a large recent increase in knowledge of the potentially damaging effects of certain oxygen metabolites, the role of vitamin E can now be placed in context as one factor in a complex protective system that includes superoxide dismutase, catalase, and peroxidases, including the selenoenzyme glutathione peroxidase.[2]

But not everything fit within this hypothesis. The same Diplock realized that α-tocopherol is capable of exerting a controlling influence upon the linoleyl and arachidonyl residues within membrane phospholipids, a capability that cannot be explained on the basis of the antioxidant function of the vitamin.[2] Also, other studies could not fit all results into the sole concept of an antioxidant action of α-tocopherol, such as its protection of erythrocytes from hemolysis induced by thermal injury. Bekiarova and associates conclude that two different mechanisms are responsible for the membrane-stabilizing effect of tocopherol, namely: 1) antiradical and 2) non-antioxidant, caused by interaction of tocopherol with phospholipid hydrolysis products by phospholipases A2 (free fatty acids and lysophospholipids).[3] Further data were not compatible with Ingold's postulate. For example, incompatible data were presented in a study on amiodarone and desethylamiodarone. In this study, which was conducted by Ruch and associates, it was suggested that prevention of hepatocyte toxicity by vitamin E was due to non-antioxidant effects.[4]

Despite these few examples, most articles have been restating, in different forms, and extended to all possible models, the assumption of Ingold's group. The PubMed request [vitamin E OR tocopherol] AND [antioxidant OR radical scavenger] gives today 24,370 results, showing an overwhelming conviction that vitamin E is the major lipid-soluble, chain-breaking antioxidant in human blood plasma as well as in membranes. In 1991, α-tocopherol was shown to act, in a non-antioxidant way, on protein kinase C,[5] thus influencing a series of events highly relevant to cellular functions. α-Tocopherol effects on protein kinase C have been documented since 1991 in more than 220 articles, and found to be the result of a specific dephosphorylation by the protein phosphatase PP2A.[6] A further word of caution about the antioxidant role of α-tocopherol came in 1994 from Lynch and associates. They observed that in plasma exposed to aqueous peroxyl radicals, lipid hydroperoxides and esterified F2-isoprostanes were formed simultaneously after endogenous ascorbate and ubiquinol-10 had been exhausted, despite the continued presence of urate, α-tocopherol, β-carotene, and lycopene, thus excluding a radical-scavenging role of tocopherol.[7]

The extremely large number of publications on the radical-scavenging properties of α-tocopherol has frequently confused the two elements of a scientific argument, the cause and the effect. The thesis has been very frequently embraced that because α-tocopherol has chemical radical-scavenging properties, shown by test-tube chemistry, all events modulated by α-tocopherol must be mediated by lipid-soluble free radicals. A non-allowed extension of the postulated unique lipid-soluble, chain-breaking antioxidant function of α-tocopherol not only has been that lipid-soluble, free radical reaction chains are interrupted by α-tocopherol, but also that α-tocopherol exerts a general antioxidant role (sometimes even indicated as redox function) at the level of all radicals, in water as well as in protein binding sites. A critical view against the notion of these degenerations has been recently published.[8]

Another unjustified syllogism frequently applied to α-tocopherol in cellular, tissue, or *in vivo* systems is the following: Radicals are produced in a system; in the presence of α-tocopherol, fewer radicals are present; α-tocopherol has scavenged the radicals. This interpretation would be analogous to the following: The sink is leaking water; after the intervention of the plumber, less water is visible on the floor; the plumber has dried up the floor. The latter event is quite possible, but a repair of the source of the leak must also be taken into consideration.

Analogously, it has been shown that α-tocopherol is able to block the production of radicals such as superoxide by inhibiting the NADPH oxidase.[9] The inhibition by α-tocopherol that has been shown to affect phospholipase A2,[10] cyclooxygenase,[11] and the stimulation of the synthesis of the γ–glutamylcysteine synthetase heavy subunit (γ-GCS HS)[12] may result in a coordinate diminution of radicals in a given system. The latter is not, however, due to the scavenging functions of tocopherol, but rather to specific effects not related to its antioxidant properties.

Logical, experimental, and evolutional criteria can be used to plead for a nonantioxidant function of α-tocopherol. If α-tocopherol acts as an antioxidant, other lipid-soluble, radical chain breaking molecules should act in the same way, especially if they are related molecules, such as other tocopherols and the tocotrienols. In several cases, it has been shown that α-tocopherol effects cannot be duplicated by any other molecule. If α-tocopherol performs its cell regulatory functions as a "radical scavenger,"[13,14] this implies that peroxy lipid radicals are entrusted in cell regulation. The difficulty of controlling the propagation of radical chain reactions makes such a mechanism unthinkable. However, if this were the case, all lipid-soluble radical scavengers would behave like cell regulators, but many investigations have demonstrated that there is no such behavior.[15]

The experimental reasoning comes from the recent data of Gohil and associates.[16] Deletion of the α-tocopherol transfer protein (α-TTP) gene in mice results in systemic deficiency of α-tocopherol and neurological dysfunction. mRNAs from brain cortex and liver of α-TTP gene–deficient mice[16] show regulation of a number of genes after 3 months of α-tocopherol deficiency. The classical antioxidant genes, superoxide dismutase, catalase, peroxidases, and heme oxygenase[17] were not upregulated, indicating that the absence of α-tocopherol did not cause oxidative stress. α-Tocopherol regulated a number of genes possibly involved in cell proliferation functions and neural signal transduction. A similar conclusion has been produced by the studies on rats deprived of α-tocopherol.[18]

Finally, we consider the evolutional criteria. α-TTP is specifically responsible for the uptake of α-tocopherol and is highly conserved in a number of species up to *Homo sapiens*. It is difficult to imagine how the specificity of α-tocopherol selection (α-TTP is not able to transport efficiently other tocopherols and tocotrienols[19]), realized through protein structural conservation, could have been kept if an equal evolutionary pressure was exerted by all other antioxidants. As discussed in the following text, α-tocopherol is entrusted with vital cellular functions, such as signal transduction regulation and gene expression, and it would be wasteful to expend it as a radical scavenger.[20] Rather, it would be important to give α-tocopherol, by means of alternative antioxidant defenses, such as catalase, peroxidases, superoxide dismutases, ascorbate, glutathione, uric acid, bilirubin, and α-lipoic acid, the same protection required by proteins, nucleic acids, and lipids. If these barriers are insufficient or if dietary intake of α-tocopherol is low, disease may result.

ENHANCEMENT OF THE EXPRESSION OF GENES IMPLICATED IN THE ABSORPTION AND METABOLISM OF α-TOCOPHEROL

α-TTP in the liver determines the plasma α-tocopherol level. The relative affinities for α-TTP are as follows: RRR-α-tocopherol, 100%; β-tocopherol, 38%; γ-tocopherol, 9%; δ-tocopherol, 2%; α-tocopherol acetate, 2%; α-tocopherol quinone, 2%; SRR-α-tocopherol, 11%; α-tocotrienol, 12%; trolox, 9%.[21] α-TTP in the liver is reduced by α-tocopherol deficiency, and α- and δ-tocopherol induce its expression, although the transcription factors involved have not yet been identified.[22] Two proteins, the cytochrome P450 enzymes CYP3A4 and CYP3A4, are involved in the metabolism of tocopherols in the liver. Tocopherols and tocotrienols enhance PXR-mediated expression of the endogenous CYP3A4 and CYP3A5 genes and therefore can modulate their own metabolism. These observations demonstrate that some forms of vitamin E can regulate gene activity via PXR.[23]

DOWNREGULATION OF GENES THAT ARE IMPLICATED WITH LIPID UPTAKE AND ATHEROSCLEROSIS

CD36 scavenger receptor (a receptor for oxidized low-density lipoprotein [LDL]), expressed in macrophages and human aortic smooth muscle cells, transports oxidized LDL into the cytosol. At physiological concentrations, α-tocopherol downregulates CD36 mRNA transcription and protein expression. Thus, the favorable action of α-tocopherol against atherosclerosis may be based, at least in part, on its lowering the uptake of oxidized lipoproteins, with resulting decrease of foam cell formation.[24,25] The scavenger receptor SR-A is affected also by α-tocopherol in a way similar to CD36.[26] The effect of α-tocopherol on scavenger receptor activity has been confirmed *in vivo*[27] α-Tocopherol-depleted rats show an increased expression of the scavenger receptor SR-B1[28] and CD36,[17] and CD36 gene deletion in apo-E null mice is associated with inhibition of plaque formation.[29] In cholesterol-fed rabbits, α-tocopherol is able to suppress a cholesterol-induced CD36 increase in aorta (Azzi and associates, unpublished results).

UPREGULATION OF GENES IMPLICATED IN THE MODULATION OF EXTRACELLULAR PROTEINS

α-Tocopherol treatment produces a time-dependent transient α-tropomyosin upregulation (mRNA, with a peak between 2 and 3 hr, and protein, with a peak at 5 hr). No effect is observed in cells treated with β-tocopherol.[30,31] In human skin fibroblasts, PKC-α protein expression increases during *in vivo* aging as a function of donor's age together with collagenase (MMP-1). α-Tocopherol is able to diminish collagenase gene transcription without altering the level of its natural inhibitor, tissue inhibitor of metalloproteinase (TIMP-1).[32] Long- and short-term supplementation with α-tocopherol to mice selectively decreases liver collagen mRNA by approximately 70%.[33] In primary cultures of quiescent stellate cells, inhibition of collagen α1(I) transactivation by α-tocopherol requires an "antioxidant"-responsive element (ARE) located at –0.22 kb of the 5′ region.[33,34] In humans, α-tocopherol prevents the fibrogenesis cascade in patients affected by chronic hepatitis and hepatic fibrogenesis.[34] The metalloproteinase MMP-19, the production of which can be upregulated by adhesion, is downregulated or even abrogated by α-tocopherol.[35]

With the use of gene array analysis, the expression of connective tissue growth factor (CTGF) gene is found to be 1.8-fold induced by α-tocopherol. The antioxidants β-tocopherol and N-acetylcysteine did not induce CTGF gene expression, suggesting a non-antioxidant mechanism for α-tocopherol action. Because CTGF promotes the synthesis of extracellular matrix, the normalization of CTGF gene expression by α-tocopherol may accelerate wound repair and tissue regeneration.[36]

DIMINUTION OF EXPRESSION OF INFLAMMATION-RELATED GENES

Integrin expression is reduced by α- but not β-tocopherol, negatively affecting monocyte adhesion, a main event in inflammation.[37] The decrease is specific for some integrins and for α-tocopherol, and it takes place at the transcriptional level (Visarius, unpublished results). α-Tocopherol significantly decreases adhesion of activated monocytes to endothelial cells by decreasing expression of CD11b and very late antigen-4 (VLA-4). In neutrophils, α-tocopherol significantly reduces platelet-activating factor (PAF)–induced CD11b/CD18 expression and IL-1-β-induced upregulation of intercellular adhesion molecule-1 (ICAM-1) and vascular cell adhesion molecule-1 (VCAM-1), respectively.[38] α-Tocopherol supplementation lowers the expression of plasminogen activator inhibitor-1 and P-selectin in type 2 diabetic patients.[39] Foreign body-type multinucleated giant cell formation is potently induced by α-tocopherol.[40] α-Tocopherol increases both cell-dividing and IL-2-producing capacity of naive T cells from old mice, with no effect on memory T cells[41]

The cytokine interleukin-1β (IL-1β) is found to be decreased by α-tocopherol. mRNA levels show that the inhibitory effect is exerted at the level of IL-1β gene expression.[42] Glycoprotein IIb, which functions as a specific receptor for platelet aggregation, shows downregulation by α-tocopherol of the 12-O-tetradecanoyl-13-phorbol acetate (TPA)–mediated glycoprotein IIb promoter activity. Reduction of glycoprotein IIb protein expression is consistent with the platelet aggregation inhibition produced by α-tocopherol.[43] α-Tocopherol has an inhibitory effect on LDL-induced production of adhesion molecules and adhesion of monocytes to endothelial cells, possibly via a direct regulatory effect on ICAM-1 expression.[44]

The experiments reported in the preceding text indicate that a number of genes involved in acute inflammation are downregulated by α-tocopherol.

REGULATION OF GENES INVOLVED IN CELL SIGNALING AND CELL CYCLE CONTROL

α-Tocopherol stimulates the synthesis of protein kinase C, but nothing is known about the molecular mechanism of this event.[30] In addition, α-tocopherol stimulates downregulation at the expression level of genes involved in the inhibition of apoptosis (defender against cell death 1 protein, Bcl2-L1) and the cell cycle (G1/S-specific cyclin D1).[45–48] The upregulation of the γ-glutamylcysteine synthetase catalytic subunit on the other side by increasing glutathione concentration stimulates telomerase activity and also slows down the cell cycle.[49] Tumors produced in animal by 7,12-dimethylbenz(a)anthracene (DMBA) develop significantly less after α-ocopherol supplementation and are characterized by a notably increased expression of p53.[38] Also, a reduced interaction of vitamin D receptor/retinoid X receptor complexes with putative α-tocopherol response elements has been suggested [45]

γ-Tocopherol inhibits human cancer cell cycle progression and cell proliferation by downregulating cyclins.[50] α-Tocopherol-treated prostate carcinoma cells (DU-145, a prostate cancer–derived cell line) show decreased progression into the S-phase. This effect is associated with reduced DNA synthesis and decreased levels of cyclin D1 and cyclin E.[50] These observation provide a theoretical basis for the putative chemopreventive effect of α-tocopherol.[51]

After partial hepatectomy, pretreatment with α-tocopherol induces a striking reduction of liver mass recovery and nuclear bromodeoxyuridine labeling, and it promotes a decreased expression of cyclin D1 and of the proliferating cell nuclear antigen. The latter could have a significant implication in the anti-tumorigenic effect ascribed to the treatment with α-tocopherol.[52]

PC-3 (a prostate cancer–derived cell line) proliferation is inhibited by α-tocopherol and γ-carboxyethyl hydroxychroman. Their effect is visible at 1 mM and reaches a maximum at approximately 10 mM with maximal inhibition values ranging between 70 and 82%.[51,53] High glucose inhibits the expression of Pax-3, a gene that is essential for neural tube closure; this effect is blocked by α-tocopherol. Impaired expression of essential developmental control genes could be the central mechanism by which neural tube defects occur during diabetic pregnancy.[54]

The peroxisome proliferator-activated receptor γ (PPAR-γ) is upregulated by α-tocopherol, and even more by γ-tocopherol. This behavior may have relevance not only to cancer prevention, but also to the management of inflammatory and cardiovascular disorders.[55]

In summary, the cell cycle–related proteins such as cyclin D, cyclin E1, P27, and P53 are affected by α- or by γ-tocopherol. Other genes, important in apoptosis inhibition (defender against cell death 1 protein, Bcl2-L1), are instead downregulated.

CONCLUSIONS

A number of genes are regulated by α-tocopherol and some by γ-tocopherol. A ligand-induced effect on specific proteins seems to be responsible for the α-tocopherol effects that appear to be unique and not imitated by structurally related antioxidant molecules.

Transcription factors or receptors apt to express α-tocopherol-dependent nuclear signaling have been intensively investigated, and a TRE (TPA-responsive element) has been found to be sensitive to tocopherol addition.[56] A deletion analysis of the promoter region of CTGF has indicated that a TGF-βRE is capable of activating, in the presence of α-tocopherol, the expression of the mRNA for CTGF (Villacorta and associates, unpublished results).

The search for a receptor has prompted the discovery of three tocopherol-associated proteins (TAP1, TAP2, and TAP3) that bind tocopherols as well as other hydrophobic ligands.[57–59] It has been suggested that tocopherol-associated protein-1

(TAP1) is a ligand-dependent transcriptional activator.[60] When a green fluorescent protein (GFP) fusion protein expression system was used, it was reported that TAP1 translocates from cytosol to nuclei in α-tocopherol-dependent fashion.[60] These data are apparently related to the construct. With the use of TAP-specific antibodies, no nuclear localization of TAP1 was observed (Kempná and Zingg, unpublished results). The claims that TAP activates the transcription of a reporter gene in an α-tocopherol-dependent manner[60] has so far not been confirmed.

α-Tocopherol activates the human pregnane X receptor-mediated gene expression in HepG2 cells. Tocopherols and tocotrienols enhance pregnane X receptor-mediated gene expression with different efficiency, whereas the tocopherol metabolic products do not.[61] The activation of genes, via the pregnane X receptor, is apparently restricted to those involved in the drug hydroxylation and elimination pathways (cytochromes P450 [CYP], such as CYP3A and some ABC transporters).[23,62] The role of TAPs and similar proteins may be that of conferring, through recognition, specificity to the action of the different tocopherols.

The large decrease in the expression of retinoic acid receptor-related orphan receptor-α mRNA in brains of α-tocopherol α-TTP-null mice may indicate that this receptor is involved in α-tocopherol molecular functions.[16]

Very recently it has been shown that α-tocopherylphosphate is able to produce cell signaling and gene expression more efficiently than tocopherols.[63] The question can be asked whether tocopherylphosphate is a "second messenger" responsible for some of the molecular action of α-tocopherol. Such a hypothesis is currently under experimental investigation.

ACKNOWLEDGMENTS

This study was made possible thanks to the support of the Swiss Science Foundation, the Swiss Krebsliga, and the Swiss Foundation for Nutrition Research in Switzerland.

REFERENCES

1. BURTON, G.W., A. JOYCE & K.U. INGOLD. 1982. First proof that vitamin E is major lipid-soluble, chain-breaking antioxidant in human blood plasma [letter]. Lancet **2:** 327.
2. DIPLOCK, A.T. 1983. The role of vitamin E in biological membranes. Ciba Found. Symp. **101:** 45–55.
3. BEKIAROVA, G.I., M.P. MARKOVA & V.G. KAGAN. 1989. alpha-Tocopherol protection of erythrocytes from hemolysis induced by thermal injury. Biull. Eksp. Biol. Med. **107:** 413–415.
4. RUCH, R.J. et al. 1991. Evaluation of amiodarone free radical toxicity in rat hepatocytes. Toxicol. Lett. **56:** 117–126.
5. BOSCOBOINIK, D. et al. 1991. Inhibition of cell proliferation by alpha-tocopherol: role of protein kinase C. J. Biol. Chem. **266:** 6188–6194.
6. RICCIARELLI, R. et al. 1998. alpha-Tocopherol specifically inactivates cellular protein kinase C alpha by changing its phosphorylation state. Biochem. J. **334:** 243–249.
7. LYNCH, S.M. et al. 1994. Formation of non-cyclooxygenase-derived prostanoids (F2-isoprostanes) in plasma and low-density lipoprotein exposed to oxidative stress in vitro. J. Clin. Invest. **93:** 998–1004.

8. AZZI, A., K.J. DAVIES & F. KELLY. 2004. Free radical biology: terminology and critical thinking. FEBS Lett. **558:** 3–6.
9. CACHIA, O. et al. 1998. alpha-Tocopherol inhibits the respiratory burst in human monocytes: attenuation of p47(phox) membrane translocation and phosphorylation. J. Biol. Chem. **273:** 32801–32805.
10. CHANDRA, V. et al. 2002. First structural evidence of a specific inhibition of phospholipase A2 by alpha-tocopherol (vitamin E) and its implications in inflammation: crystal structure of the complex formed between phospholipase A2 and alpha-tocopherol at 1.8 Å resolution. J. Mol. Biol **320:** 215–222.
11. JIANG, Q. et al. 2000. gamma-Tocopherol and its major metabolite, in contrast to alpha- tocopherol, inhibit cyclooxygenase activity in macrophages and epithelial cells. Proc. Natl. Acad. Sci. USA **97:** 11494–11499.
12. MARI, M. & A.I. CEDERBAUM. 2001. Induction of catalase, alpha, and microsomal glutathione S-transferase in CYP2E1 overexpressing HepG2 cells and protection against short-term oxidative stress. Hepatology **33:** 652–661.
13. MCCAY, P.B. et al. 1971. A function for alpha-tocopherol: stabilization of the microsomal membrane from radical attack during TPNH-dependent oxidations. Lipids **6:** 297–306.
14. URANO, S. & M. MATSUO. 1976. A radical scavenging reaction of alpha-tocopherol with methyl radical. Lipids **11:** 380–383.
15. RICCIARELLI, R., J.M. ZINGG & A. AZZI. 2001. Vitamin E 80th anniversary: a double life, not only fighting radicals. IUBMB Life **52:** 71–76.
16. GOHIL, K. et al. 2003. Gene expression profile of oxidant stress and neurodegeneration in transgenic mice deficient in alpha-tocopherol transfer protein. Free Radic. Biol. Med. **35:** 1343–1354.
17. TYRRELL, R.M. & S. BASU-MODAK. 1994. Transient enhancement of heme oxygenase 1 mRNA accumulation: a marker of oxidative stress to eukaryotic cells. Methods Enzymol. **234:** 224–235.
18. BARELLA, L. et al. 2004. Identification of hepatic molecular mechanisms of action of alpha-tocopherol using global gene expression profile analysis in rats. Biochim. Biophys. Acta **1689:** 66–74.
19. PANAGABKO, C. et al. 2003. Ligand specificity in the CRAL-TRIO protein family. Biochemistry **42:** 6467–6474.
20. AZZI, A. et al. 2002. Regulation of gene and protein expression by vitamin E. Free Radic. Res. **36:** 30–36.
21. HOSOMI, A. et al. 1997. Affinity for alpha-tocopherol transfer protein as a determinant of the biological activities of vitamin E analogs. FEBS Lett. **409:** 105–108.
22. FECHNER, H. et al. 1998. alpha- and delta-Tocopherol induce expression of hepatic alpha-tocopherol-transfer-protein mRNA. Biochem. J. **331**(part 2): 577–581.
23. LANDES, N. et al. 2002. Vitamin E activates hPXR-mediated gene expression in HEPG2 cells. Free Radic. Biol. Med. **33:** S189.
24. RICCIARELLI, R., J.M. ZINGG & A. AZZI. 2000. Vitamin E reduces the uptake of oxidized LDL by inhibiting CD36 scavenger receptor expression in cultured aortic smooth muscle cells. Circulation **102:** 82–87.
25. AZZI, A., R. RICCIARELLI & J.M. ZINGG. 2002. Non-antioxidant molecular functions of alpha-tocopherol (vitamin E). FEBS Lett. **519:** 8–10.
26. TEUPSER, D., J. THIERY & D. SEIDEL. 1999. alpha-Tocopherol downregulates scavenger receptor activity in macrophages. Atherosclerosis **144:** 109–115.
27. DEVARAJ, S., I. HUGOU & I. JIALAL. 2001. alpha-Tocopherol decreases CD36 expression in human monocyte-derived macrophages. J. Lipid Res. **42:** 521–527.
28. KOLLECK, I. et al. 1999. HDL is the major source of vitamin E for type II pneumocytes. Free Radic. Biol. Med. **27:** 882–890.
29. FEBBRAIO, M. et al. 2000. Targeted disruption of the class B scavenger receptor CD36 protects against atherosclerotic lesion development in mice. J. Clin. Invest. **105:** 1049–1056.
30. AZZI, A. et al. 1998. Molecular basis of alpha-tocopherol control of smooth muscle cell proliferation. Biofactors **7:** 3–14.

31. ARATRI, E. *et al.* 1999. Modulation of alpha-tropomyosin expression by alpha-tocopherol in rat vascular smooth muscle cells. FEBS Lett. **447:** 91–94.
32. RICCIARELLI, R. *et al.* 1999. Age-dependent increase of collagenase expression can be reduced by alpha-tocopherol via protein kinase C inhibition. Free Radic. Biol. Med. **27:** 729–737.
33. CHOJKIER, M. *et al.* 1998. Long- and short-term D-alpha-tocopherol supplementation inhibits liver collagen alpha1(I) gene expression. Am. J. Physiol. **275:** G1480–G1485.
34. HOUGLUM, K. *et al.* 1997. A pilot study of the effects of D-alpha-tocopherol on hepatic stellate cell activation in chronic hepatitis C. Gastroenterology **113:** 1069–1073.
35. MAUCH, S. *et al.* 2002. Matrix metalloproteinase-19 is expressed in myeloid cells in an adhesion-dependent manner and associates with the cell surface. J. Immunol. **168:** 1244–1251.
36. VILLACORTA, L. *et al.* 2003. alpha-Tocopherol induces expression of connective tissue growth factor and antagonizes tumor necrosis factor-alpha-mediated downregulation in human smooth muscle cells. Circ. Res. **92:** 104–110.
37. BREYER, I. & A. AZZI. 2001. Differential inhibition by alpha- and beta-tocopherol of human erythroleukemia cell adhesion: role of integrins. Free Radic. Biol. Med. **30:** 1381–1389.
38. YOSHIKAWA, T. *et al.* 1998. alpha-Tocopherol protects against expression of adhesion molecules on neutrophils and endothelial cells. Biofactors **7:** 15–19.
39. DEVARAJ, S., A.V. CHAN, JR. & I. JIALAL. 2002. alpha-Tocopherol supplementation decreases plasminogen activator inhibitor-1 and P-selectin levels in type 2 diabetic patients. Diabetes Care **25:** 524–529.
40. MCNALLY, A.K. & J.M. ANDERSON. 2003. Foreign body-type multinucleated giant cell formation is potently induced by alpha-tocopherol and prevented by the diacylglycerol kinase inhibitor R59022. Am. J. Pathol. **163:** 1147–1156.
41. ADOLFSSON, O., B.T. HUBER & S.N. MEYDANI. 2001. Vitamin E-enhanced IL-2 production in old mice: naive but not memory T cells show increased cell division cycling and IL-2-producing capacity. J. Immunol. **167:** 3809–3817.
42. AKESON, A.L. *et al.* 1991. Inhibition of IL-1 beta expression in THP-1 cells by probucol and tocopherol. Atherosclerosis **86:** 261–270.
43. CHANG, S.J., J.S. LIN & H.H. CHEN. 2000. alpha-Tocopherol downregulates the expression of GPIIb promoter in HEL cells. Free Radic. Biol. Med. **28:** 202–207.
44. MARTIN, A. *et al.* 1997. Vitamin E inhibits low-density lipoprotein-induced adhesion of monocytes to human aortic endothelial cells in vitro. Arterioscler. Thromb. Vasc. Biol. **17:** 429–436.
45. WU, C.G. *et al.* 1997. Correlation of repressed transcription of alpha-tocopherol transfer protein with serum alpha-tocopherol during hepatocarcinogenesis. Int. J. Cancer. **71:** 686–690.
46. FISCHER, A. *et al.* 2001. Effect of selenium and vitamin E deficiency on differential gene expression in rat liver. Biochem. Biophys. Res. Commun. **285:** 470–475.
47. WU, D. *et al.* 1998. Age-associated increase in PGE2 synthesis and COX activity in murine macrophages is reversed by vitamin E. Am. J. Physiol. **275:** C661–C668.
48. SCHWARTZ, J., G. SHKLAR & D. TRICKLER. 1993. p53 in the anticancer mechanism of vitamin E. Eur. J. Cancer B Oral. Oncol. **29B:** 313–318.
49. BORRAS, C. *et al.* 2004. Glutathione regulates telomerase activity in 3T3 fibroblasts. J. Biol. Chem. **279:** 34332–34335.
50. GYSIN, R., A. AZZI & T. VISARIUS. 2002. gamma-Tocopherol inhibits human cancer cell cycle progression and cell proliferation by down-regulation of cyclins. FASEB J. **16:** 1952–1954.
51. VENKATESWARAN, V., N.E. FLESHNER & L.H. KLOTZ. 2002. Modulation of cell proliferation and cell cycle regulators by vitamin E in human prostate carcinoma cell lines. J. Urol. **168:** 1578–1582.
52. TREJO-SOLIS, C. *et al.* 2003. Inhibitory effect of vitamin E administration on the progression of liver regeneration induced by partial hepatectomy in rats. Lab. Invest. **83:** 1669–1679.

53. GALLI, F. et al. 2004. The effect of alpha- and gamma-tocopherol and their carboxyethyl hydroxychroman metabolites on prostate cancer cell proliferation. Arch. Biochem. Biophys. **423:** 97–102.
54. CHANG, T.I. et al. 2003. Oxidant regulation of gene expression and neural tube development: insights gained from diabetic pregnancy on molecular causes of neural tube defects. Diabetologia **46:** 538–545.
55. CAMPBELL, S.E. et al. 2003. Gamma tocopherol upregulates peroxisome proliferator activated receptor (PPAR) gamma expression in SW 480 human colon cancer cell lines. BMC Cancer **3:** 25.
56. AZZI, A. et al. 1999. Vitamin E mediated response of smooth muscle cell to oxidant stress. Diabetes. Res. Clin. Pract. **45:** 191–198.
57. STOCKER, A. et al. 1999. Identification of a novel cytosolic tocopherol-binding protein: structure, specificity, and tissue distribution. IUBMB Life **48:** 49–55.
58. ZIMMER, S. et al. 2000. A novel human tocopherol-associated protein: cloning, in vitro expression, and characterization. J. Biol. Chem. **275:** 25672–25680.
59. KEMPNÁ, P. et al. 2003. Cloning of novel human SEC14p-like proteins: cellular localization, ligand binding and functional properties. Free Radic. Biol. Med. **34:** 1458–1472.
60. YAMAUCHI, J. et al. 2001. Tocopherol-associated protein is a ligand-dependent transcriptional activator. Biochem. Biophys. Res. Commun. **285:** 295–299.
61. BIRRINGER, M., D. DROGAN & R. BRIGELIUS-FLOHE. 2001. Tocopherols are metabolized in HepG2 cells by side chain omega-oxidation and consecutive beta-oxidation. Free Radic. Biol. Med. **31:** 226–232.
62. ORAM, J.F., A.M. VAUGHAN & R. STOCKER. 2001. ATP-binding cassette transporter A1 mediates cellular secretion of alpha-tocopherol. J. Biol. Chem. **276:** 39898–39902.
63. MUNTEANU, A. et al. 2004. Modulation of cell proliferation and gene expression by alpha-tocopheryl phosphates: relevance to atherosclerosis and inflammation. Biochem. Biophys. Res. Commun. **318:** 311–316.

Vitamin E and Gene Expression in Immune Cells

SUNG NIM HAN,[a] OSKAR ADOLFSSON,[a,d] CHEOL-KOO LEE,[b,e]
TOMAS A. PROLLA,[b] JOSE ORDOVAS,[c] AND SIMIN NIKBIN MEYDANI[a]

[a]*Nutritional Immunology Laboratory, Jean Mayer USDA Human Nutrition Research Center on Aging at Tufts University, Boston, Massachusetts 02111, USA*

[b]*Department of Genetics and Medical Genetics, University of Wisconsin, Madison, Wisconsin, USA*

[c]*Nutrition and Genomics Laboratory, Jean Mayer USDA Human Nutrition Research Center on Aging at Tufts University, Boston, Massachusetts, USA*

ABSTRACT: Aging is associated with dysregulation of immune cells, particularly T cells. Previous studies indicated that vitamin E improves T cell function, in part by a direct effect on T cells. We studied gene expression profile of T cells to better understand the underlying mechanisms of aging- and vitamin E–induced changes in T cell function. Young and old C57BL mice were fed diets containing 30 (control) or 500 (E) ppm of vitamin E for 4 weeks. T cells were purified from splenocytes by negative selection using magnetic beads (anti-Mac-1 and anti-MHC class II), then cultured with media or stimulated with anti-CD3 and anti-CD28. Gene expression profile was assessed using microarray analysis. Genes showing more than two-fold changes, $P < 0.05$ by ANOVA, and with at least one present call were selected. Aging had significant effects on genes involved in signal transduction, transcriptional regulation, and apoptosis pathways in T cells, while vitamin E had a significant effect on genes associated with the regulation of cell cycle.

KEYWORDS: vitamin E; gene expression; immune cells; aging

INTRODUCTION

Vitamin E is one of the nutrients that has been shown to have a significant impact on immune functions. Enhancement of immune functions by vitamin E is particularly pertinent for the aged because aging is associated with dysregulation of immune responses, which is believed to contribute to higher morbidity and mortality from infectious and neoplastic diseases. A reduced T cell function, as demonstrated by de-

---

Address for correspondence: Sung Nim Han, Ph.D., R.D., or Simin Nikbin Meydani, DVM, Ph.D., Nutritional Immunology Laboratory, Jean Mayer USDA Human Nutrition Research Center on Aging at Tufts University, 711 Washington Street, Boston, MA 02111. Voice: 617-556-3242 (Han) or 617-556-3129 (Meydani); fax: 617-556-3224.
 sungnim.han@tufts.edu or simin.meydani@tufts.edu
[d]Current address: Nestlé Research Center, Lausanne, Switzerland.
[e]Current address: Department of Biology, University of North Carolina, Chapel Hill, North Carolina, USA.

creased T cell proliferation and IL-2 production, and a shift toward greater proportions of antigen (Ag)-experienced memory T cells with fewer T cells of naïve phenotype[1] are some of the phenotypic and functional changes observed with aging in the immune system. Although several advances have been made in our understanding of changes in T cell response with aging, because activation of T cells involves simultaneous up- or downregulation of many different signaling pathways with complex interactions, it has been difficult to put together a comprehensive picture of molecular changes that lead to functional dysregulation of T cells.

Vitamin E has been consistently shown to enhance the immune functions in aged animals and humans. Vitamin E supplementation resulted in increased lymphocyte proliferation and IL-2 production, which was further shown to be due to an increase in the ability of naïve T cells from old mice to go through cell division cycles.[2] However, further studies are needed to elucidate the mechanisms by which vitamin E specifically enhances the functions of naïve T cells in the aged. Determining the global changes occurring in gene expression pattern of the immune cells with aging and vitamin E in T cells will help in identifying the pathways most profoundly affected with aging and vitamin E.

IMPACT OF AGING ON IMMUNE FUNCTIONS AND GENE EXPRESSION PROFILES OF IMMUNE CELLS

Among the immune cells, T cells are the main cells to show age-related changes. Aging is associated with reduced T cell function, as demonstrated by decreased T cell proliferation and IL-2 production.[1] One of the hallmarks of age-related changes is a shift toward greater proportions of antigen (Ag)-experienced memory T cells with fewer T cells of naïve phenotype. Naïve T cells have different response kinetics to Ag challenge than do memory T cells, with memory T cells responding faster and to a lower Ag dose than naïve T cells.[3] Recent evidence indicates that naïve T cells show an age-related functional decline in the earliest stages of activation induced by peptide/MHC complexes.[4] We showed that T cells from old mice go through lower activation-induced cell divisions, have fewer numbers of IL-2$^+$ cells, and produce less IL-2 per cell. These age-associated changes in T cells were only observed within the naïve T cell subpopulation.[2] Other researchers reported that IL-2 receptor expression is decreased in cells from elderly individuals,[5] and functional disruption of the CD28 gene transcriptional initiator is observed in senescent T cells.[6] The adverse effects of age is observed in various steps involved in the T cell activation pathway including tyrosine kinases such as ZAP-70, calcium/calmodulin-dependent protein kinases, and adaptor proteins.[7]

Thus far, only a limited number of studies have investigated the changes in gene expression profiles with aging in immune cells.[8–10] Mo et al.[8] stimulated purified CD4$^+$ T cells from young and old mice with anti-CD3 and anti-CD28 for 72 h and determined the gene expression profiles using Affymetrix microarray chips. They found significantly higher expression of CCR2, CCR5, and CXCR5 and lower expression of CCR7 in unstimulated CD4$^+$ T cells from old animals compared with those from the young. Distinct pattern of chemokine receptor expression is associated with polarization of Th1 and Th2 cells and a shift toward Th2 profile has been reported in T cells with aging.[11] However, Mo et al.[8] found that both Th1- and Th2-

associated chemokine receptors were increased in aged T cells. Visala Rao et al.[9] examined the heat-shock response (1 h at 42°C) of lymphocytes purified from two young and two old individuals using in-house microarray chips representing 4032 genes. The authors concluded that certain genes associated with signal transduction and mitochondrial respiration were upregulated while genes associated with heat-shock response and cell survival were downregulated in lymphocytes from old individuals after heat-shock treatment. We[10] investigated the effect of aging on purified T cells stimulated with anti-CD3 and anti-CD28 for 2 h on gene expression profiles. The results from our study suggest that aging is associated with increased susceptibility to apoptosis due to higher expression of Fas ligand and apoptotic Gadd45b and lower expression of antiapoptotic Bcl-2 in old T cells. Lower expression of Bcl-2 in the old T cells might be due to age-associated increase in oxidative stress. Reactive oxygen species have been shown to control the expression of Bcl-2, and treatment with synthetic antioxidants increased the expression of Bcl-2 in activated T cells.[12]

VITAMIN E AND IMMUNE FUNCTIONS

The beneficial effects of supplemental vitamin E on immune functions of the aged have been shown in animal studies and human clinical trials.[13,14] Vitamin E supplementation has been shown to increase delayed-type hypersensitivity response, in vitro T cell proliferation, and IL-2 production and to decrease macrophage production of the T cell–suppressive PGE_2.[13–15] In addition, the immunostimulatory effect of vitamin E is associated with increased resistance against infectious agents.[16]

Our previous study[2] demonstrated that vitamin E could enhance the functions of T cells from old mice directly, with preferential effect on naïve but not memory T cells. When young and old T cells supplemented with vitamin E were examined for their ability to go through activation-induced cell division over a 48-h period, vitamin E significantly increased the ability of naïve T cells from old mice to progress through one as well as two cell division cycles. This enhancing effect of vitamin E was not observed for memory T cells from old mice. Furthermore, by performing intracellular staining of IL-2, vitamin E supplementation increased IL-2 production by naïve T cells from old mice. Both the number of naïve $IL-2^+$ T cells from old mice and the staining intensity, an indication of the amount of IL-2 produced per cell, were increased by vitamin E.

IMPACT OF VITAMIN E ON GENE EXPRESSION OF IMMUNE CELLS

Vitamin E has been reported to have a significant impact on gene expression of cell cycle–related molecules in many different cell types including immune cells. Regulation of cell cycle and effect of vitamin E on cell-cycle regulatory machinery is depicted in FIGURE 1.

Aging is associated with decline of T cell proliferation. This has been partially attributed to the impairment of cell-cycle regulation. Dysregulation of cell cycles with aging has been reported to be due to a lower Cdk1 (Cdc2) activity as well as lower levels of cyclin B1 and Cdk1/cyclin B1 complex,[17] lower Cdk6 activity,[18] and decrease in cyclin D2 expression.[19] In our study, in which we looked at the gene ex-

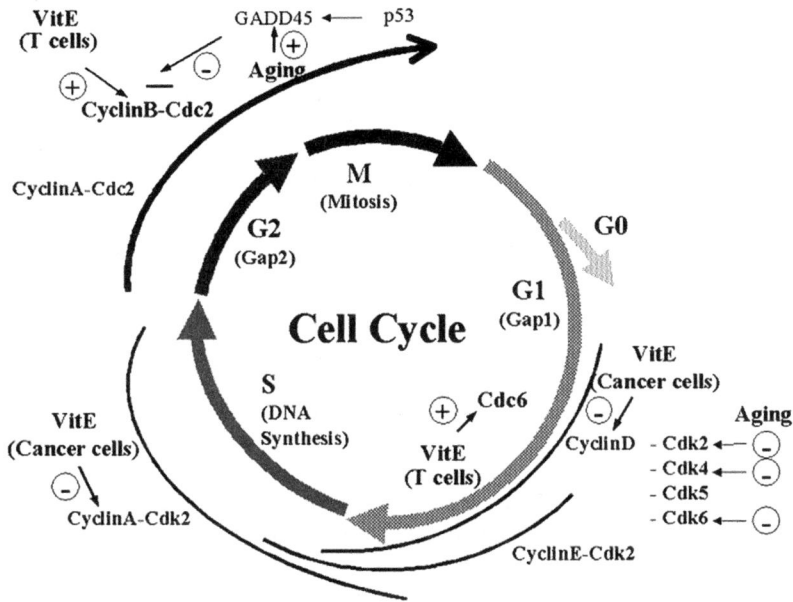

FIGURE 1. Effects of aging and vitamin E on cell-cycle regulation.

pression profiles of T cells from young and old mice, we observed that vitamin E supplementation in old mice increased the expression of cell cycle–related proteins, including cyclin B, Cdc2 (Cdk1), and Cdc6. Cyclin B and Cdc2 are important for entry of cells into M phase of the cell cycle, and Cdc6 is a key regulator in an early step of DNA replication.[17,20] In our previous study, vitamin E was shown to enhance the ability of naïve T cells from old mice to progress though cell cycle as determined by FACS analysis of CFSE-labeled cells following 48 h of anti-CD3 and anti-CD28 stimulation.[2] Thus, upregulation of the genes mentioned above by vitamin E might be the underlying mechanism through which vitamin E enhances the ability of naïve old T cells to go through the cell cycle.

Others have also reported vitamin E's effect on expressions and activities of cell-cycle regulatory proteins in different cell types. Fischer et al.[21] reported that deficiency of selenium and vitamin E resulted in a 3.1-fold decrease in expression of cyclin D1 in rat liver, which was 90% prevented by vitamin E. In cancer cells, vitamin E was suggested to inhibit cell growth by downregulating cell-cycle regulatory proteins.[22,23] Prostate cancer cells (LNCap cells) cultured in the presence of vitamin E succinate showed inhibition of growth and proliferation in a dose-dependent manner. Treatment with 20 μM of vitamin E succinate resulted in a decrease in protein expression of cyclin D1, cyclin D3, cdk2, cdk4, and cyclin E leading to cell-cycle blockage at the G1/S phase. In BT-20 breast cancer cells, vitamin E succinate inhibited the activity of cyclin A and decreased the level of cyclin A-cdk2 complex.[23] Differential effects of vitamin E on cell-cycle regulatory proteins in T cells and cancer cells are worth further investigation.

Vitamin E also seems to have a significant impact on expression of genes associated with Th1/Th2 balance. Previously, we observed an increase in IL-2–producing ability of the T cells and an enhancement of Th1 response with vitamin E supplementation.[2,16] In our gene expression study, vitamin E increased gene expressions of IL-2 and IL-1 receptor antagonist, and decreased the expression of IL-4, a major Th2 cytokine and stimulator of Th2 response. IL-1 receptor antagonist was reported to play a role in the upregulation of Th1 response.[24]

CONCLUSIONS

Vitamin E showed a significant impact on gene expression profiles of T cells in a few different categories of genes, including those involved in cell cycle and Th1/Th2 balance. Vitamin E increased expression of cyclin B2, Cdc2, and Cdc6 in old T cells, which might contribute to the increased ability of T cells from the old mice to progress through cell division and proliferate. This effect of vitamin E on cell-cycle regulation in T cells was in contrast to what has been observed in cancerous cells. Vitamin E also had a significant impact on expression of genes involved in Th1 response. The specific mechanisms through which vitamin E exerts its effect on expression of genes involved in regulation of Th1/Th2 balance and cell cycle needs further investigation. Such data would shed light on the implications of vitamin E supplementation on the risk and/or pathogenesis of several diseases.

REFERENCES

1. MILLER, R.A. 1996. The aging immune system: primer and prospectus. Science **273**: 70–74.
2. ADOLFSSON, O., B.T. HUBER & S.N. MEYDANI. 2001. Vitamin E-enhanced IL-2 production in old mice: naive but not memory T cells show increased cell division cycling and IL-2 -producing capacity. J. Immunol. **167**: 3809–3817.
3. ROGERS, P.R., C. DUBEY & S.L. SWAIN. 2000. Qualitative changes accompany memory T cell generation: faster, more effective responses at lower doses of antigen. J. Immunol. **164**: 2338–2346.
4. GARCIA, G.G. & R.A. MILLER. 2001. Single-cell analyses reveal two defects in peptide-specific activation of naive T cells from aged mice. J. Immunol. **166**: 3151–3157.
5. NAGEL, J.E., R.K. CHOPRA, F.J. CHREST, et al. 1988. Decreased proliferation, interleukin 2 synthesis, and interleukin 2 receptor expression are accompanied by decreased mRNA expression in phytohemagglutinin-stimulated cells from elderly donors. J. Clin. Invest. **81**:1096–1102.
6. VALLEJO, A.N., C.M. WEYAND & J.J. GORONZY. 2001. Functional disruption of the CD28 gene transcriptional initiator in senescent T cells. J. Biol. Chem. **276**: 2565–2570.
7. CHAKRAVARTI, B. 2001. T-cell signaling—effect of age. Exp. Gerontol. **37**: 33–39.
8. MO, R., J. CHEN, Y. HAN, et al. 2003. T cell chemokine receptor expression in aging. J. Immunol. **170**: 895–904.
9. VISALA RAO, D., G.M. BOYLE, P.G. PARSONS, et al. 2003. Influence of ageing, heat shock treatment and in vivo total antioxidant status on gene-expression profile and protein synthesis in human peripheral lymphocytes. Mech. Ageing Dev. **124**: 55–69.
10. HAN, S., O. ADOLFSSON, C. LEE, et al. 2003. Effect of age and vitamin E on gene expression profiles of T cells. FASEB J. **17**: A280.
11. GLOBERSON, A. & R.B. EFFROS. 2000. Ageing of lymphocytes and lymphocytes in the aged. Immunol. Today **21**: 515–521.

12. HILDEMAN, D.A., T. MITCHELL, J. KAPPLER & P. MARRACK. 2003. T cell apoptosis and reactive oxygen species. J. Clin. Invest. **111:** 575–581.
13. MEYDANI, S.N., M. MEYDANI, C.P. VERDON, et al. 1986. Vitamin E supplementation suppresses prostaglandin E_2 synthesis and enhances the immune response of aged mice. Mech. Ageing Dev. **34:** 191–201.
14. MEYDANI, S.N., M. MEYDANI, J.B. BLUMBERG, et al. 1997. Vitamin E supplementation and in vivo immune response in healthy subjects. JAMA **277:** 1380–1386.
15. WU, D., S.N. HAN & S.N. MEYDANI. 1996. Vitamin E supplementation inhibits macrophage cyclooxygenase activity of old mice. FASEB J. **10:** A191.
16. HAN, S.N., D. WU, W.K. HA, et al. 2000. Vitamin E supplementation increases T helper 1 cytokine production of old mice infected with influenza virus. Immunology **100:** 487–493.
17. QUADRI, R.A., A. ARBOGAST, M.A. PHELOUZAT, et al. 1998. Age-associated decline in cdk1 activity delays cell cycle progression of human T lymphocytes. J. Immunol. **161:** 5203–5209.
18. ARBOGAST, A., S. BOUTET, M.A. PHELOUZAT, et al. 1999. Failure of T lymphocytes from elderly humans to enter the cell cycle is associated with low Cdk6 activity and impaired phosphorylation of Rb protein. Cell. Immunol. **197:** 46–54.
19. HALE, T.J., B.C. RICHARDSON, L.I. SWEET, et al. 2002. Age-related changes in mature CD4+ T cells: cell cycle analysis. Cell. Immunol. **220:** 51–62.
20. PELIZON, C. 2003. Down to the origin: Cdc6 protein and the competence to replicate. Trends Cell Biol. **13:** 110–113.
21. FISCHER, A., J. PALLAUF, K. GOHIL, et al. 2001. Effect of selenium and vitamin E deficiency on differential gene expression in rat liver. Biochem. Biophys. Res. Commun. **285:** 470–475.
22. NI, J., M. CHEN, Y. ZHANG, et al. 2003. Vitamin E succinate inhibits human prostate cancer cell growth via modulating cell cycle regulatory machinery. Biochem. Biophys. Res. Commun. **300:** 357–363.
23. TURLEY, J.M., F.W. RUSCETTI, S.J. KIM, et al. 1997. Vitamin E succinate inhibits proliferation of BT-20 human breast cancer cells: increased binding of cyclin A negatively regulates E2F transactivation activity. Cancer Res. **57:** 2668–2675.
24. LIN, K.W., S.C. CHEN, F.H. CHANG, et al. 2002. The roles of interleukin-1 and interleukin-1 receptor antagonist in antigen-specific immune responses. J. Biomed. Sci. **9:**26–33.

Modulation of Hepatic Gene Expression by α-Tocopherol in Cultured Cells and *in Vivo*

GERALD RIMBACH,[a] ALEXANDRA FISCHER,[a] ELISABETH STOECKLIN,[b] AND LUCA BARELLA[b]

[a]*Institute of Human Nutrition and Food Science, Christian Albrechts University, D-24118 Kiel, Germany*

[b]*DSM Nutritional Products (registered as Roche Vitamins, Ltd.), CH-4002 Basel, Switzerland*

ABSTRACT: To obtain a comprehensive understanding of the molecular mechanisms of action of vitamin E (VE), global gene expression profiles using DNA arrays in rat liver and hepatocellular liver carcinoma cells (HepG2) were obtained. For the analysis of short-term (49 days) and long-term (290 days) VE deficiency, rats were fed semisynthetic diets either supplemented with or deficient in VE. In addition, HepG2 cells were treated with VE concentrations comparable to those that were achieved in the *in vivo* experiment. Differential gene expression in rat liver and that in HepG2 cells were measured by DNA arrays comprising up to 7,000 genes. Dietary VE deficiency over a 7-week period did not induce any significant changes in the expression profile among the genes evaluated. However, long-term VE deficiency upregulated coagulation factor IX (FIX), 5-α-steroid reductase type 1, and CD36 mRNA levels. Furthermore, VE deficiency resulted in a significant downregulation of hepatic γ-glutamyl-cysteinyl synthetase, the rate-limiting enzyme of glutathione synthesis. According to the rat experiment, VE supplementation changed coagulation factor IX and CD36 expression in HepG2 cells; thus, *in vivo* data could be partly confirmed with the *in vitro* model. Overall, the current studies reveal that dietary VE has important long-term effects on liver gene expression with potential downstream effects on extrahepatic tissues.

KEYWORDS: vitamin E; gene expression; liver; rat; HepG2

INTRODUCTION

It has been shown that cellular oxidant/antioxidant equilibrium is a key factor in determining redox-dependent gene expression. Recent advances in transcriptomics have led to the development of robust methods for the quantitative and comprehensive analyses of changes in mRNA level. These advances include gene chips. The po-

---

Address for correspondence: Prof. Gerald Rimbach, Institute of Human Nutrition and Food Science, Olshausenstrasse 40, D-24118 Kiel, Germany. Voice: +49-431-880-2583; fax: +49-431-880-2628.
rimbach@foodsci.uni-kiel.de

tential applications of transcriptomics in the field of vitamin E (VE) research are manifold. Gene chips can be used to analyze redox-dependent gene expression, thereby yielding more insights into the molecular functions of antioxidants. Furthermore, differences in the biopotency and bioavailability between different antioxidants (for example, RRR vs. all-rac tocopherol) may be detected by gene chip technology.

VE is the most important lipid-soluble antioxidant. Besides its well-established antioxidant activity, its cell signaling properties have been recently reported.[1] To obtain a comprehensive understanding of the molecular mechanisms of action of VE, global gene expression profiles in rat liver and hepatocellular liver cacrinoma cells (HepG2) were obtained. Our choice of tissue was reflected by the fact that the liver, as the central organ involved in endogenous VE metabolism, is highly susceptible to changes in dietary VE with potential downstream effects on extrahepatic tissues.

MATERIALS AND METHODS

Short-Term VE Deficiency

Two groups of eight male albino rats with an initial average live weight of 35 g were randomly assigned to semisynthetic diets that were based on torula yeast, corn starch, and tocopherol-stripped corn oil for 7 weeks. Control rats received diets supplemented with VE (75 mg/kg as RRR-α-tocopheryl acetate), whereas the VE animals were fed the basal diets.[2]

cDNA Array Hybridization

Total RNA was isolated from rat liver with the use of RNeasy Mini Kit (Qiagen, Hilden, Germany). Three samples within each group with the same diet treatment were pooled for preparing complex cDNA probes by simultaneous reverse transcription and radioactive labeling with ^{32}P. The primers used correspond to genes represented on the Atlas Rat cDNA Toxicology Array II (Clontech, Palo Alto, CA) comprising 465 genes. After hybridization at 68°C overnight, unbound and non-specifically bound probes were removed by high- and low-salt washes, and images of specifically bound probes were obtained by phosphorimaging for 1 week to reveal the expression profiles.

Long-Term VE Deficiency

Two groups of 30 male albino rats with an initial average weight of 55 g were randomly assigned to either a VE-containing (60 mg/kg RRR-α-tocopheryl acetate) diet (VE^+) or to a VE-deficient diet (VE^-) for 290 days.[3]

Gene Chip Hybridization

Total RNA extraction, cRNA preparation, and Affymetrix gene chip (U34A) hybridization was conducted as described elsewhere.[3] A schematic representation of the analytical steps involved in the gene chip experiments is given in FIGURE 1. Differential expression profile analysis between the two treatment groups was per-

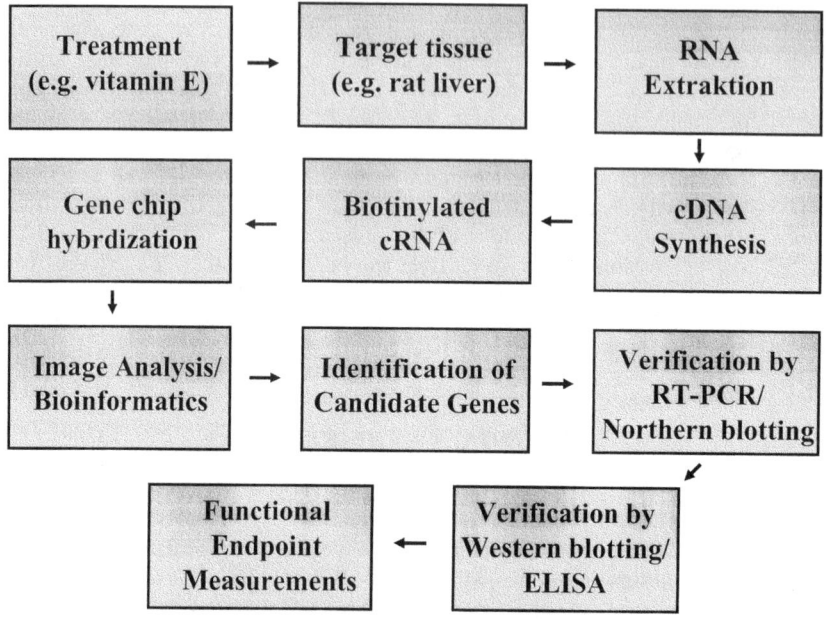

FIGURE 1. Major steps in the identification of VE-sensitive genes with the use of Affymetrix gene chip technology.

formed at four different time points (T1 = day 17 of feeding; T2 = day 91; T3 = day 191; T4 = day 269) over the 9-month study period. Data obtained during the different time points were compared, and only genes consistently upregulated or downregulated over a period of time greater than 170 days (three consecutive time points) were taken into consideration for further characterization.

Cell Culture Experiments Using HepG2 Cells

Human hepatocellular liver carcinoma cells (HepG2) were grown in Dulbecco's modified Eagle medium supplemented with 10% NU serum and antibiotics (100 U/mL of penicillin, 100 µg/mL of streptomycin) in a humidified atmosphere with 5% CO_2 at 37°C. Cells were passaged by trypsinization (1 × trypsin-EDTA solution) when 90% confluency was reached. The split ratio ranged from 1:4 to 1:16. Cells were seeded at a density of 50,000 cell/cm^2 in six-well tissue culture plates. Twenty-four hours after seeding, the culture medium was replaced by medium containing either 30 µM or 0 µM RRR-tocopheryl acetate. Cell were cultured for 7 days, and the cell culture medium was replaced every 24 hr. At day 7, cells were harvested in RLE buffer (Qiagen), and the RNA was isolated for Affymetrix gene experiments as mentioned earlier. For all experiments, VE was dissolved in ethanol so that the final ethanol concentration in the medium was ≤0.1% (v/v).

TABLE 1. Vitamin E–related changes in gene expression in liver of rats fed diets deficient or supplemented with vitamin E over 9 months

Affymetrix accession code	Change compared to –VE	Gene	Function
S65555_at	↑	Glutamyl cysteinyl synthetase	Glutathione synthesis
L38615_g_at	↑	GSH synthetase	Glutathione synthesis
S81448_s_at	↓	5 α–steroid reductase type 1	5 α–dihydrotesterone synthesis
M26247_at	↓	Factor IX	Blood coagulation
rc_AA925752_at	↓	CD 36	Scavenger receptor

NOTE: For a comprehensive analysis, genes with a differential change in expression greater than 0.25-fold or less than –0.25-fold (>25% increase or >25% decrease) combined with a significance level of P < 0.05 were selected. Differential expression profile analysis between the two treatment groups was performed at four different time points (T1 = day 17 of feeding; T2 = day 91; T3 = day 191; T4 = day 269). Data obtained during the different time points were compared, and only genes consistently upregulated or downregulated over a period of time exceeding 170 days (three consecutive time points) were taken into consideration for further characterization.

RESULTS

Rats fed diets supplemented with VE for 7 weeks had about 30-fold higher α-tocopherol liver concentrations as compared to non-supplemented control animals. Short-term VE deficiency did not induce any significant changes in the expression profile among the 465 genes evaluated as compared to the control animals. A difference in gene expression between groups was considered significant at a ratio threshold of two or more.

Out of the ~7,000 genes represented on the gene chip, only 14 annotations comprising 5 genes were consistently differentially expressed in response to VE in at least three consecutive time points. Long-term VE supplementation downregulated coagulation factor IX (FIX), 5-α-steroid reductase type 1 (5α-R1), and CD36 mRNA levels. Furthermore, dietary VE supplementation resulted in a significant upregulation of hepatic γ-glutamyl-cysteinyl synthetase (γ-GCS), the rate-limiting enzyme of glutathione synthesis and glutathione synthetase (TABLE 1).

In the *in vitro* experiments, HepG2 cells were supplemented with 30 μM RRR-tocopheryl acetate. When rats were fed VE-supplemented diets for 9 months, an average plasma VE concentration of 27 ± 3 μM was measured by the end of the experimental trial. Thus, the VE concentrations used in the *in vitro* study are comparable to those achievable under *in vivo* conditions. Supplementing hepatocytes with VE for 7 days induced a downregulation of CD36 gene expression by 40% as compared to controls (FIG. 2). In VE-supplemented hepatocytes, FIX mRNA levels were 30% lower than in hepatocytes not supplemented with VE, but the data did not reach statistical significance. Expression levels of γ-GCS and glutathione synthetase were similar between VE-supplemented and VE-deficient hepatocytes. Contrary to the *in vivo* study, 5α-R1 was not expressed in HepG2 cells.

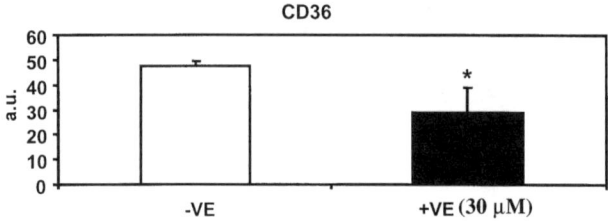

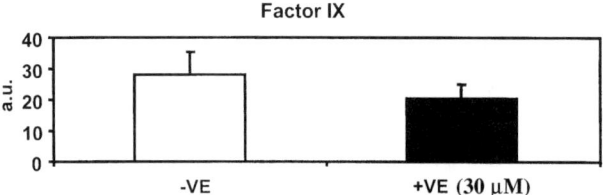

FIGURE 2. Effect of VE on mRNA levels of CD36 and FIX in HepG2 cells. Each value is a group mean ± SD ($n = 5$). An asterisk indicates a significant difference ($P < 0.05$).

DISCUSSION

Since the discovery of VE, studies have mainly focused on its antioxidant properties. In 1991, Angelo Azzi's group first described non-antioxidant, cell signaling functions of VE, demonstrating that α-tocopherol regulates protein kinase C activity in smooth muscle cells.[4] At the transcriptional level, α-tocopherol modulates the expression of the CD36 scavenger receptor in smooth muscle cells and monocyte-derived macrophages, the hepatic α-tocopherol transfer protein (α-TTP), as well as the expression of liver collagen α-1 collagenase and the α-tropomyosin gene.[5–9] Recently, a tocopherol-dependent transcription factor (tocopherol-associated protein, TAP) has been identified.[10] So far, most of the VE-sensitive genes have been discovered *in vitro*. Little is known about the effect of short- and long-term VE deficiency on differential gene expression *in vivo*.

Short-term VE deficiency over a period of time of 7 weeks did not induce any significant changes in expression profile among the genes evaluated.[2] However, when short-term VE deficiency was accompanied by selenium deficiency, alterations in the expression level of genes encoding for proteins involved in inflammation (multispecific organic anion exporter, SPI-3 serine protease inhibitor) and acute phase response (α-1 acid glycoprotein, metallothionein 1) were evident. In addition, a significant downregulation in the expression level of genes important in the inhibition of apoptosis (defender against cell death 1 protein, Bcl2-L1), cell cycle (G1/S-specific cyclin D1), and antioxidant defense (γ-glutamylcysteine synthetase catalytic

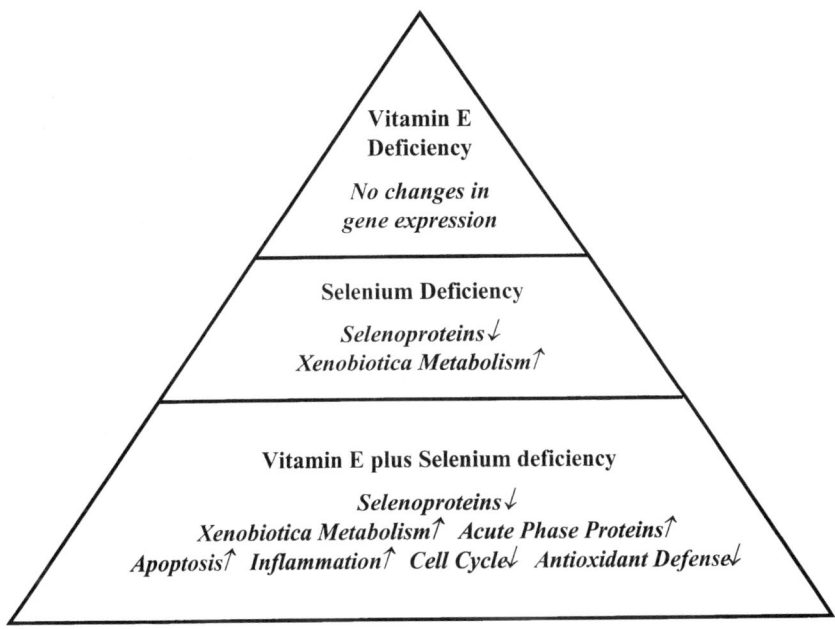

FIGURE 3. Effect of short-term (7-wk) dietary VE, selenium, and VE plus selenium deficiency on differential gene expression in rat liver. A difference in gene expression between groups was considered significant at a ratio threshold of two or more.

subunit) was demonstrated, as summarized in FIGURE 3. These data clearly underline the postulated synergism between Se and VE in their molecular functions as part of the so-called antioxidant network.

In the study mentioned earlier, changes in gene expression in response to VE were monitored at one time point and in pooled liver samples. Therefore, in the consecutive study, rats were followed for a period of 9 months at four individual time points, and animals were profiled individually.[3] Furthermore, changes in gene expression were tested for their ability to cause alterations in the corresponding biological endpoints. Dietary VE led to a significant upregulation of γ-GCS, the rate-limiting enzyme in GSH synthesis. Furthermore, VE induced a downregulation of FIX, 5α-R1, and CD36 mRNA levels. It is important that measurement of the corresponding biological endpoints, such as activated partial thromboplastin time, plasma dihydrotestosterone, and hepatic glutathione, substantiated the gene chip data that indicated dietary VE plays an important role in a range of metabolic processes within the liver.

Interstingly, CD36 and FIX mRNA levels in HepG2 were also downregulated in response to VE. Thus, current *in vivo* data were partly confirmed with the HepG2 *in vitro* model. However, other genes such γ-GCS, glutathione synthetase, and 5α-R1 responded differently in HepG2 cells in comparison to the *in vivo* situation in rats when VE-deficient and VE-supplemented diets were fed over 9 months. It might be that a longer VE supplementation in the cell culture experiment is necessary to induce similar changes in mRNA levels as observed in the *in vivo* experiment. In the current *in vitro* study, HepG2 cells were supplemented with VE for 7 days, whereas in most studies reported in the literature incubation periods of 24 hours have been chosen. It should be also taken into account that HepG2 cells, although they are from widely used and generally accepted transformed cell line, are of human origin, whereas the feeding study was conducted in rats. Furthermore, it would be interesting to test whether primary hepatocytes exhibit different patterns of gene expression as compared to HepG2 cells in response to VE supplementation.

Overall, the current *in vivo* and *in vitro* studies reveal that dietary VE has important long-term effects on liver gene expression with potential downstream effects on extrahepatic tissues and illustrates the application of genome-wide expression profiling in investigations of the biological action of essential dietary micronutrients.

REFERENCES

1. RIMBACH, G., A.M. MINIHANE, J. MAJEWICZ, *et al.* 2000. Regulation of cell signalling by vitamin E. Proc. Nutr. Soc. **61:** 415–425.
2. FISCHER, A., J. PALLAUF, K. GOHIL, *et al.* 2001. Effect of selenium and vitamin E deficiency on differential gene expression in rat liver. Biochem. Biophys. Res. Commun. **285:** 470–475.
3. BARELLA, L., P. MÜLLER, M. SCHLACHTER, *et al.* 2004. Identification of the hepatic molecular mechanism of action of alpha-tocopherol using global gene expression profile analysis in rats. Biochim. Biophys. Acta **1689**(1): 66–74.
4. BOSCOBOINIK, D., A. SZEWCZYK, C. HENSEY, *et al.* 1991. Inhibition of cell proliferation by alpha-tocopherol: role of protein kinase C. J. Biol. Chem. **266:** 6188–6194.
5. RICCIARELLI, R., J.M. ZINGG & A. AZZI. 2000. Vitamin E reduces the uptake of oxidized LDL by inhibiting CD36 scavenger receptor expression in cultured aortic smooth muscle cells. Circulation **102:** 82–87.
6. SHAW, H.M., & C. HUANG. 1998. Liver alpha-tocopherol transfer protein and its mRNA are differentially altered by dietary vitamin E deficiency and protein insufficiency in rats. J. Nutr. **128:** 2348-2354.
7. CHOJKIER, M., K. HOUGLUM, K.S. LEE & M. BUCK. 1998. Long- and short-term D-alpha-tocopherol supplementation inhibits liver collagen alpha1(I) gene expression. Am. J. Physiol. **275:** G1480–G1485.
8. RICCIARELLI, R., P. MARONI, N. OZER, *et al.* 1999. Age-dependent increase of collagenase expression can be reduced by alpha-tocopherol via protein kinase C inhibition. Free Radic. Biol. Med. **27:** 729–737.
9. ARATRI, E., S.E. SPYCHER, I. BREYER, *et al.* 1999. Modulation of alpha-tropomyosin expression by alpha-tocopherol in rat vascular smooth muscle cells. FEBS Lett. **447:** 91–94.
10. STOCKER, A., S. ZIMMER, *et al.* 1999. Identification of a novel cytosolic tocopherol-binding protein: structure, specificity, and tissue distribution. IUBMB Life **48:** 49–55.

α-Tocopherol Transfer Protein Deficiency in Mice Causes Multi-Organ Deregulation of Gene Networks and Behavioral Deficits with Age

KISHORCHANDRA GOHIL,[a] ROY GODZDANKER,[a] ERIN O'ROARK,[a] BETTINA C. SCHOCK,[b] RAMESH R. KAINI,[a] LESTER PACKER,[c] CARROLL E. CROSS,[a] AND MARET G. TRABER[d]

[a]*Center for Comparative Respiratory Biology and Medicine, Department of Internal Medicine, University of California, Davis, California 95616, USA*

[b]*Respiratory Research Group, Department of Medicine, Queen's University Belfast, UK*

[c]*Department of Molecular Pharmacology and Toxicology, University of Southern California, Los Angeles, California 90089-9121, USA*

[d]*Linus Pauling Institute, Department of Nutrition and Exercise Sciences, Oregon State University, Corvallis, Oregon 97331-6512, USA*

> ABSTRACT: Functions of α-tocopherol (α-T) *in vivo*, other than those for fertility in females, are intensely debated. The discovery of α-T deficiency in patients with ataxia (AVED) followed by the identification of mutations in the gene encoding α-tocopherol transfer protein (TTP) in AVED patients demonstrates an essential role of α-T and TTP for normal neurological function. α-T molecular targets that account for α-T–sensitive neurological dysfunction remain to be discovered. We have used high-density oligonucleotide arrays to search for putative α-T–sensitive genes in the CNS and other tissues in an *in vivo* model of α-T deficiency imposed at birth by the deletion of the TTP gene in mice. Repression of genes affecting synaptic function and myelination and induction of genes for neurodegeneration in the motor cortex of α-T–deficient mice were identified. The expression of retinoic acid–related orphan receptor alpha (ROR-α) was repressed in the cortex and adrenal glands of TTP-deficient mice. Deficiency of ROR-α causes ataxia in mice and may account for ataxia in AVED patients. These observations suggest that some of the actions of α-T are mediated by the transcription factor ROR-α. The behavior of young TTP-null mice was essentially normal, but older mice showed inactivity, ataxia, and memory dysfunction. mRNA profiles of old α-T–deficient cerebral cortices are compatible with repressed activity of oligodendrocytes and astrocytes. In conclusion, gene-expression profiling studies have identified novel α-T–modulated genes and cells in the CNS that may be causatively linked with delayed neurodegeneration and age-related decline in behavioral repertoires.

Address for correspondence: Kishorchandra Gohil, Center for Comparative Respiratory and Medicine, Department of Internal Medicine, University of California, Davis, CA 95616. Voice: 530-752-0674
kgohil@ucdavis.edu

KEYWORDS: vitamin E; gene expression; ROR-alpha; ataxia; transgenic; adrenal glands

INTRODUCTION

In 1922 Evans and Bishop reported "the existence of a hitherto unrecognized factor essential for reproduction."[1] The dietary factor, Factor X, was subsequently identified as a lipid-soluble factor present in lettuce, and later in wheat germ extracts, and was designated as vitamin E; its designation as tocopherol is derived from Greek (*tokos*, "childbirth" and *pherein*, "to bring forward"). There are eight distinct molecular entities that form the vitamin E family.[2] α-tocopherol (α-T) is the most biologically active member of the vitamin E family found in rodents and humans.

Physiological concentrations of α-T are primarily determined by the α-tocopherol tranfer protein (TTP) that preferentially binds α-T, compared to more abundant, naturally occurring isomers of vitamin E with similar antioxidant properties.[3] TTP is a member of the SEC14 family of proteins that bind and transfer specific lipids. For example, TTP binds α-T,[4–6] SEC14 binds phosphotidyl inositol,[7] retinaldehyde-binding protein binds retinaldehyde, and supernatant factor binds squalene.[8,9] The conservation of structural and functional properties of the members of the SEC14 family suggests that they play an important role in the assembly and functions of biological membranes and in secretory processes.

The precise mechanism of α-T's action in reproduction or its potential actions, other than its antioxidant function, in adults is unknown. α-T is required for growth and function of rat uterus and for maintaining normal plasma concentrations of luteinizing hormone.[10] α-T as a scavenger of reactive metabolites of oxygen in membranes may play an important role in its physiological function in fetal implantation[11] and for post-fetal life of mammals.[12–15] A need for α-T in post-natal humans remained controversial for decades because of the lack of a well-defined deficiency disease.[15] Discovery of vitamin E deficiency in patients with neurological diseases[16] in the past 20 years has rekindled the interest in the importance of α-T in humans. This group of patients showed mutations in the TTP gene, demonstrating an essential role of TTP in determining systemic concentrations of α-T, maintaining normal architecture of the nervous system and neurological functions. It is also noteworthy that mutations in the CRAL-TRIO domain, a motif that is conserved in TTP, may cause ataxia in humans and mice.[17]

Mice rendered deficient in TTP by genetic manipulation have a severe systemic deficiency of α-T[18] that is attributed to failure in the secretion of α-T from liver.[15] To emphasize this point, we will term these mice TTP-α-T–deficient. TTP-α-T–deficient mice show many features of age-related neurological diseases.[19] A common feature of these mice and human diseases associated with α-T deficiency is the delayed onset of ataxia, the most obvious disease phenotype. This may be attributed to a gradual loss of neurons and neuronal function caused by changes in the expression of the genome imposed by the deficiency of tocopherol transfer protein or α-tocopherol.

Collectively, the data from numerous *in vitro* and *in vivo* studies suggest that biological actions of α-T are mediated through diverse molecular mechanisms, including its non-antioxidant actions,[20] that may affect gene expression.[21–24] The hypothesis that the transcription of multiple genes is modulated by micronutrients and nutritional supplements has been tested using macro- and microarray tools.[24–26] The application of high-density oligonucleotide arrays showed that the systemic deficiency of α-T inflicted by the deletion of the TTP gene alters the transcriptional program of livers and brain.[22] Similarly chronic vitamin E deficiency in rats imposed by dietary vitamin E deficiency also alters the transcriptional program of livers.[21, 23]

In this report we further describe the effects of chronic vitamin E deficiency on genome-wide changes in mRNA expression profiles of adrenal glands, cerebral cortex, heart, liver, and spleen. The data show that vitamin E deficiency caused by TTP gene deletion in mice fed a diet with "adequate" levels of vitamin E alter the mRNA expression of multiple genes and gene families. A number of gene families in brain and adrenal glands were similarly repressed, suggesting an essential role of α-T in tissues derived from the neural crest. Gene-expression analysis of cerebral cortex identified repression of genes encoding synaptic synaptic and myelin proteins. A particularly noteworthy observation was the repression of mRNA encoding the transcription factor, retinoic acid receptor–related orphan receptor-alpha (ROR-α) in cerebral hemispheres[22] and in the adrenal glands. ROR-α deficiency causes severe ataxia in young mice[27] and may affect many other functions *in vivo*.[28] Behavioral analysis of TTP-α-T–deficient mice showed deficits in locomotion, anxiety and memory functions with age. These findings suggest that α-T plays a role in the expression of the transcription factor ROR-α and some of the genes regulated by the transcription factor that may affect behavioral phenotype with aging.

MATERIALS AND METHODS

Twenty female C57BL6J mice with a deletion in the *Ttpa* gene (TTP-deficient) and wild-type mice (WT) from our colony were used. Mice were housed in groups of four under conditions of constant temperature (18°C), light (6:00 AM to 6:00 PM), and access *ad libitum* to food (mouse chow, Purina Test Diet 5015, containing 35 IU of all-rac α-tocopheryl acetate/ kg diet) and water.

The colony of TTP-deficient mice in C57BL6 genetic background was obtained by back-crossing the original colony[18] of mixed (50% C57BL6J/ and 50% 129/Sv-Jae) mice heterozygous for the deletion TTP gene with C57BL6J WT mice. The offspring were genotyped using specific primers for *Ttpa* as previously described.[18] Additionally, the genotype of each animal was confirmed by Western blot analysis of liver TTP protein using an anti-TTP antiserum as previously described.[18] The concentrations of α-T in plasma, liver, and cortex were also determined[29] for confirmation of the predicted α-T status of the two groups of mice with distinct genotype.

Neurological Behavior Analysis

Behavioral analysis of learning and memory was performed in mice as described in Rodgers *et al.*[30] and Golub *et al.*[31]

The Morris Water Maze test was performed as described in Golub *et al.*[31] Sessions were run with a visible platform, with a hidden platform, and with no platform (probe trials). Anxiety levels were assessed with an elevated, plus-shaped maze consisting of two open arms and two closed arms equipped with rows of infrared photocells interfaced with a computer (Hamilton, Poway, CA). Mice were placed individually in the center of the maze and allowed free access to the arms for 10 min. They could spend their time either in a closed safe area (closed arms) or in an open area (open arms). Recorded beam brakes were used to calculate the time spent, the distance moved, and entries in the closed and open arms. Stride length was evaluated by first training mice to run down a narrow alley to an escape hole. The paws were then coated with ink, the alley was lined with white paper and a series of paw prints were collected for measurement of stride length (distance between paws in successive strides).

Statistical analysis: Behavioral data are expressed as mean ± SEM. The statistical significance of differences between groups was determined by ANOVA. $P<0.05$ was considered significant. Appropriate nonparametric tests were used when the data were not normally distributed.

RNA Extraction and Preparation of Biotin-Labeled RNA for GeneChip Analysis

These procedures were performed essentially as described previously.[22,32]

Data Analysis

Absolute mRNA expression (present or absent) and differential (TTP-deficient versus WT) mRNA expression analysis were obtained using the MAS 5.0 software. When the P value for detection signal was <0.039 (range of P value 0.0002 to 0.039) the expression of the mRNA was classified as present. All mRNAs with the P value for detection >0.039 were considered absent. The signal intensities for transcripts classified as present ranged from 5–7000 units.

To obtain the list of TTP-sensitive genes, the entire data set for each tissue from the two groups of mice was subjected to "batch analysis" that generated data with fold-change for each mRNA. The data that showed either an "increase" or a "decrease" of more than 2-fold and were present in at least one of the two samples in the pair were selected as TTP-sensitive genes. This conservative analysis excluded a large number of genes that were identified as significantly different between TTP-deficient and WT mice, but whose detection was of low confidence ($P>0.039$).

Validation of GeneChip Data.

We[32,33] and others[34,35] have shown that the changes in the expression of mRNAs selected by the conservative analysis of hybridization data as described above could be confirmed by independent analysis such as Northern blot, polymerase chain reaction (PCR), real-time PCR, and in some cases by immunoblot analysis of the encoded proteins.[32] In addition, the expression data and their interpretations were validated by comparison of the specificity of the expression levels of selected genes whose expression and the activities of the encoded proteins are known to be tissue-specific.[22] In addition, the expression of TTP mRNA, protein, and α-T concentrations was also measured.

RT-PCR: Five mg of total RNA from liver or adrenal gland was reverse-transcribed in the presence of oligo(dT)12–18 primer and SuperScriptRT (Invitrogen) according to manufacturer's protocol, except that α-^{32}P-dCTP was excluded from reaction mixture. TTP and β-actin mRNA expressions were determined in 5 mL of

1 in 100 and 1 in 1000 dilutions, respectively, of the cDNA solution from liver (in a final volume of 20 mL of PCR mix). TTP and β-actin mRNA expression in adrenal glands was determined in 1 in 10 and in 1 in 1000 dilutions, respectively, of cDNAs.

The oligonucleotide sequences (5' to 3') for the sets of primers are:

TTP(F), GATTTCGATCTGGA, TTP(R), CCACCTCCTGTACA and β-actin (F) CGAGAAGATGACCCAGATCATG, β-actin (R), AGTGATCTCCTTCTGCATC-CTG. The predicted and observed sizes of the amplified fragments were 280 and 630 bp, respectively. The PCR cycling conditions for 35 cycles were: 30 sec at 94°, 30 sec at 60°, and 60 sec at 72°. The amplified products were visualized with ethidium bromide after electrophoretic resolution in 2% agarose gel. The images were analyzed with NIH-Image software.

RESULTS AND DISCUSSION

Tissue-Specific Expression of Tocopherol Transfer Protein mRNA in Wild-Type and TTP-Deficient Mice: Validation of GeneChip Data and Interpretation

Analysis of liver TTP mRNA expression with GeneChips shows that TTP mRNA is highly expressed in wild-type mice and its expression is extremely low (14-fold) in livers from TTP-deficient mice (FIG. 1). TTP mRNA is moderately expressed in adrenal glands of wild-type mice but not in the TTP-deficient mice. TTP mRNA was very low in lungs of wild-type mice, but was undetectable in hearts and spleens.

Using RT-PCR, we found that the expected 270-bp fragment of TTP-mRNA was clearly detectable in livers of wild-type mice, but was expressed at very low levels in the TTP-deficient mice (FIG. 2). There was a ~17-fold difference in the intensities of the band from the wild-type and deficient mice, a similar value to that obtained by GeneChip assay. RT-PCR also showed low expression of TTP-mRNA in adrenal glands of wild-type mice. There was a ~7-fold difference between livers and adrenals in the expression of TTP-mRNA; this ratio is also in good agreement with the data obtained by the GeneChip assay (compare FIGS. 1 and 2).

FIGURE 3A shows that the TTP-deficient mice also showed a very low expression of TTP in liver. Concentrations of α-tocopherol in plasma and cerebral cortex were much lower in TTP-deficient mice than those detected in livers and brains of wild-type mice (FIG. 3B).

Tissue-Specific Effects of TTP and Vitamin E Deficiency

"Differentially" expressed, TTP-α-T–sensitive genes were determined by comparative analysis of the gene-expression profiles from five tissues obtained from wild-type mice and TTP-deficient mice (FIG. 4). All the tissues examined were sensitive to the deletion of the TTP gene and the resulting vitamin E deficiency. There does not appear to be any direct correlation between the expression of the TTP gene and the changes in gene-expression profile, but rather to differences in α-tocopherol concentrations. For example, TTP-mRNA expression in liver is about 6-fold higher that that in adrenal glands (FIGS. 1 and 2); however, adrenal gland shows ~2000 TTP-α-T–sensitive genes compared to liver, which shows only 50 differentially ex-

α-tocopherol transfer protein mRNA expression by GeneChip Assay

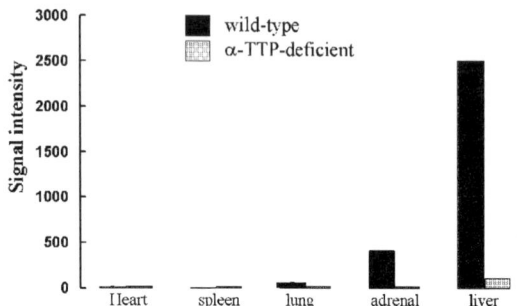

FIGURE 1. Expression of TTP mRNA in different tissues of the wild-type and the TTP-deficient mice. The data show that the GeneChip assay reliably measures the expression of TTP-mRNA as shown by low to undetable expression of the gene in liver and adrenal glands in TTP-null mice.

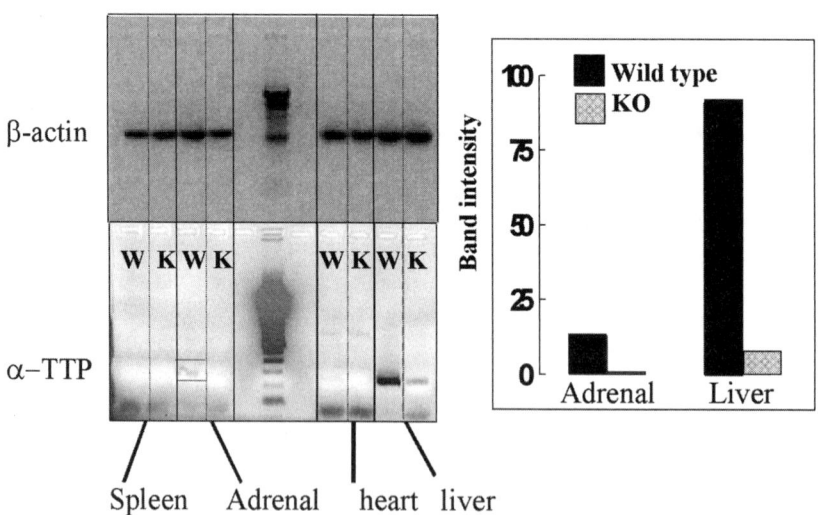

FIGURE 2. Confirmation of GeneChip data by RT-PCR. Total RNA from the various tissues was reverse-transcribed and then subjected to PCR in the presence of specific primers for either TTP mRNA or beta-actin mRNA. cDNAs for TTP assay were diluted 1 in 100 and those for beta-actin were diluted 1 in 1000. Beta actin expression (*upper left panel*) was similar in all the tissues, but TTP (*lower left panel*) was expressed only in livers and adrenal glands of wild-type (W), but not TTP-null (K) mice. The bar chart shows densitometric analysis of the scanned image for TTP expression in liver and adrenals.

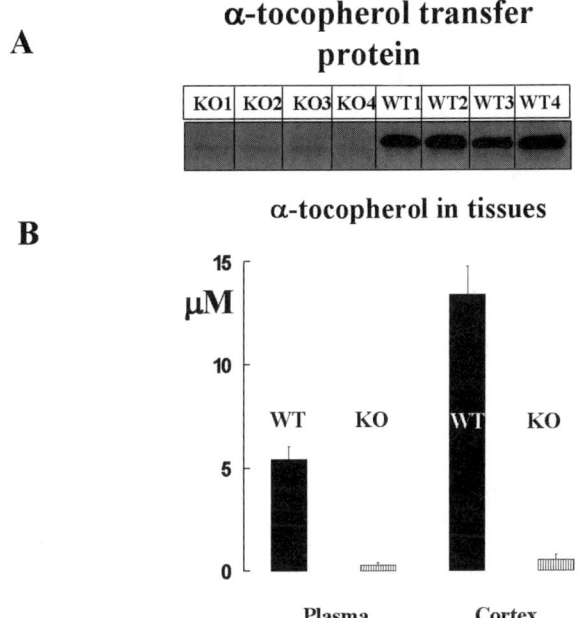

FIGURE 3. TTP gene deletion causes loss of hepatic tocopherol transfer protein (**A**) and depletion of α-tocopherol from plasma and cerebral cortex of mice fed diet with normal levels of vitamin E (**B**). KO = TTP-deficient mice; WT = wild-type mice.

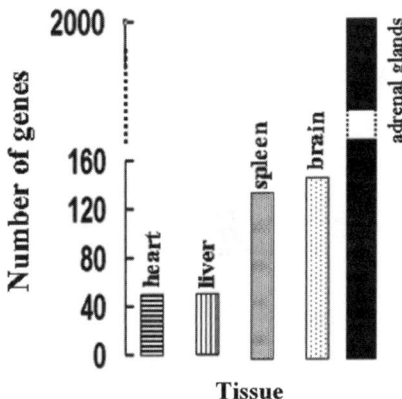

FIGURE 4. TTP gene deletion and the resulting depletion of tissue α-tocopherol cause tissue-specific changes in gene expression. About 10,000 genes were detected in the tissues of wild-type (WT) and TTP-deficient mice (KO). Differential analysis of WT and KO profiles generated the TTP-α-T-deficient list of genes (described in the MATERIALS AND METHODS section). The figure shows numbers of genes in each tissue that are sensitive to the absence of TTP and α-T.

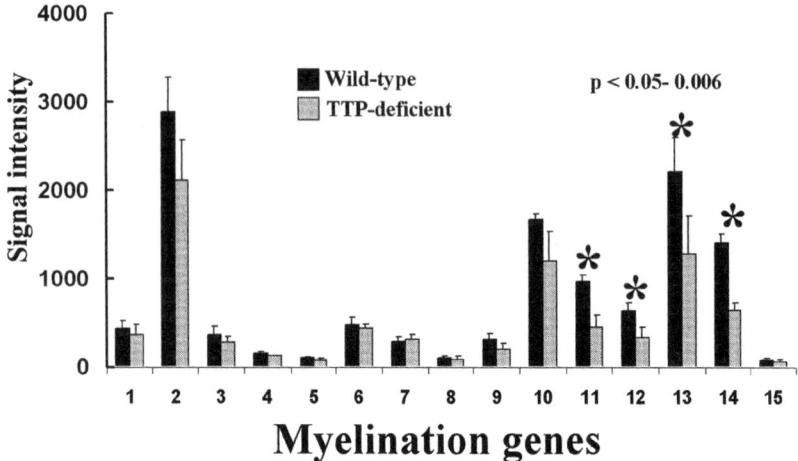

FIGURE 5. α-Tocopherol is required for the normal expression of selected genes for myelination. TTP gene deletion represses the expression of selected genes for myelination. GeneChip data from cerebral cortex of wild-type ($n = 3$) and TTP-deficient ($n = 3$) mice were searched for genes encoding myelin proteins. The expression of 15 genes were detectable by the GeneChip assay and, of these, 4 mRNAs were significantly ($P<0.05$) repressed in the cerebral cortex of TTP-deficient mice. These genes encoded myelin-associated oligodendrocyte-specific protein (MOSP) and proteolipid protein (PLP); 11 and 12 are two distinct probe sets for MOSP and 13 and 14 are two distinct probe sets for PLP.

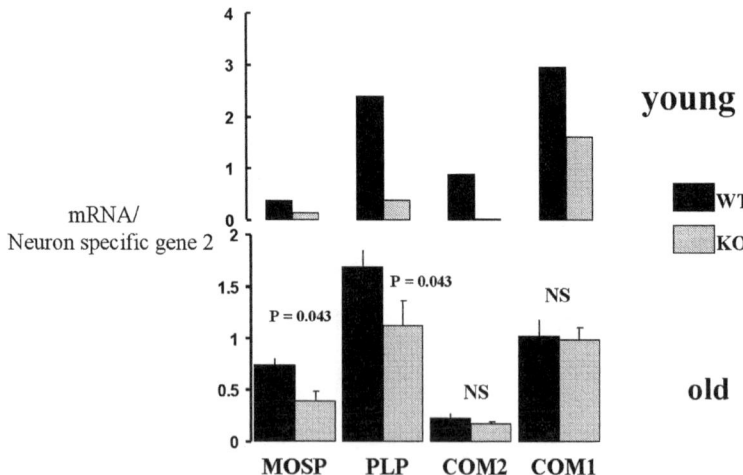

FIGURE 6. Synaptic degeneration and demyelination in vitamin E–deficient cortex: differential effects of age on the markers of myelination and synapse in wild-type and TTP-deficient mice. In younger mice, TTP deficiency resulted in lowered expression of the selected markers. In older mice, only the markers of myelination were repressed in the TTP-deficient mice. MOSP = myelin-associated oligodendrocyte-specific protein; PLP = proteolipid protein; COM1 = complexin 1; COM2 = complexin 2.

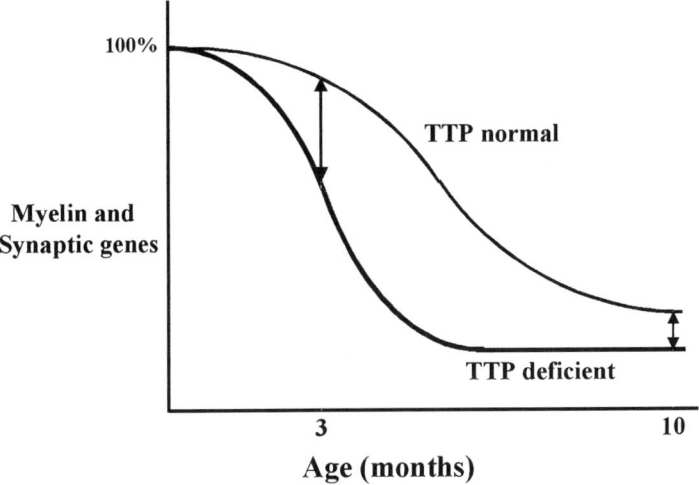

FIGURE 7. Hypothetical explanation for smaller differences in synaptic markers between older and younger wild-type and TTP-deficient mice. The TTP-deficient mice lose their synapses early at a faster rate and reach a plateau. The process is much slower in wild-type mice that reach this plateau as they age. This hypothesis may explain the lack of difference in synaptic markers shown in FIGURE 6.

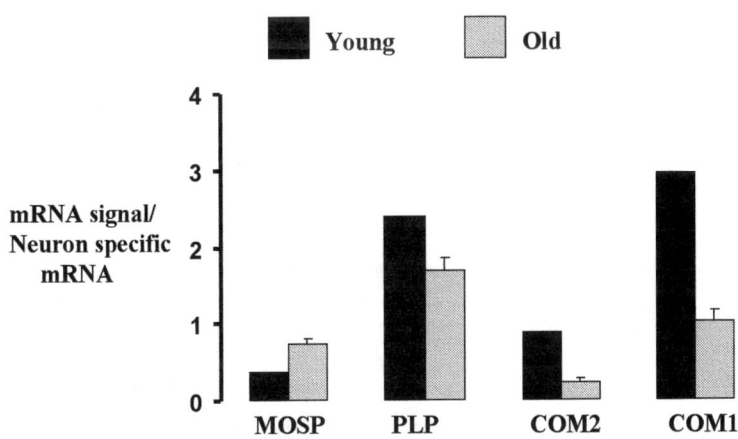

FIGURE 8. Aging represses mRNAs encoding selected myelin and synaptic proteins in TTP-NORMAL mice. Gene-expression profiles of young and old wild-type mice were "mined" for the expression of the four genes. The data were normalized per the signal intensity of neuron-specific mRNA. The data show that both the genes associated with synaptic functions were repressed in older mice. MOSP = myelin-associated oligodendrocyte-specific protein; PLP = proteolipid protein; COM1 = complexin 1; COM2 = complexin 2.

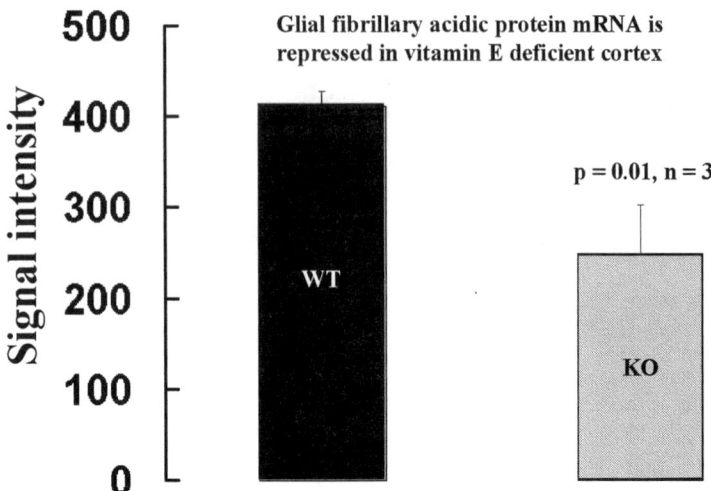

FIGURE 9. Is α-tocopherol required for the expression of astrocyte functions? The expression of glial fibrillary acidic protein mRNA, a marker for astrocyte function, was repressed in mice TTP-α-T deficiency.

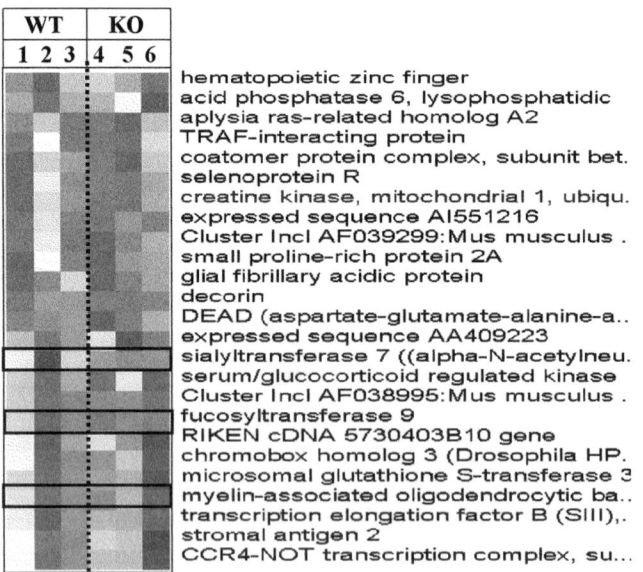

FIGURE 10. α-Tocopherol regulated genes in 10-month-old cerebral cortex. D-chip analysis of mRNA expression data of cerebral cortex from wild-type ($n = 3$) and TTP-deficient mice ($n = 3$) demonstrated 25 genes that were significantly affected by TTP-α-T deficiency. WT = wild-type; KO = TTP-deficient.

pressed genes. Both liver and heart showed similar sensitivities whereas spleens and brains were more sensitive to the TTP and α-T deficiencies.

Suppression of Myelination and Synaptic Markers

We have previously shown that gene-expression profiles of young cerebral corticees indicated inhibition of myelination and synaptogenesis in TTP-aT–deficient mice.[22] Therefore, the gene-expression profiles of older mice were searched for the expression of mRNAs encoding myelination genes. Four myelination genes were decreased 30–50% ($P<.05$) in TTP-α-T–deficient cortex (FIG. 5). The selective decrease in the oligodendrocyte-specific mRNAs encoding myelin-associated oligodendrocyte basic protein and proteolipid protein suggests that TTP-α-T is essential for the functions of oligodendrocyte, the primary cell type for elaborating myelin. However, two genes that encode synaptic proteins, complexins 1 and 2, did not show any difference between the two genotypes (FIG. 6, lower panel). This was particularly surprising because younger mice showed remarkable repression of the two genes in TTP-α-T–deficient mice when compared to age-matched wild-type mice. One possible explanation for this observation is that there is an age-dependent loss of synaptic function in the wild-type mice (FIG. 7). The TTP-deficient mice may lose their synapses early and hence this might account for the large difference between the younger wild-type and TTP-deficient mice (FIG. 7). This difference is minimal in the older mice because wild-type mice continue to lose their synapses with age. This hypothesis is supported by the observation that older compared with younger wild-type mice have lower expression of complexin 1 and 2 mRNAs (FIG. 8). In addition, the expression of glial cell–specific gene encoding glial fibrillary acidic protein was significantly ($P<0.01$) repressed by about 40% in TTP-aT–deficient mice (FIG. 9). Glial cells play an important role in the survival and functions of neurons.[36,37]

The entire data set of mRNA expression profiles from cortex ($n = 3$) of wild-type and TTP-α-T–deficient mice was analyzed with model-based hierarchical cluster analysis[38] to obtain a list of TTP-α-T–sensitive genes (FIG. 10). For example the repression of gene-encoding glial fibrillary acidic protein was detected by the two different analytical methods and supports our hypothesis that TTP-aT is required for normal functioning of glial cells. Similarly, repression of genes encoding myelin-associated basic protein, fucosyltransferase 9 and sialyltransferase 7, suggests an essential role of vitamin E for oligodendrocyte functions.

α-Tocopherol is Required for the Expression of Retinoic Acid–Related Orphan Receptor-α (ROR-α)

Our previous studies in young mice showed that TTP-α-T deficiency resulted in a 13-fold decrease in the expression of ROR-α mRNA in cerebral cortex[22] (FIG. 11). Expression of ROR-a protein in cerebral cortex by immunoblot analysis demonstrated that TTP-α-T–deficient mice had a significant 60% decrease in ROR-α protein expression ($P<0.04$) (FIG. 12). Further, the expression of ROR-α mRNA and mRNAs of other members of this nuclear receptor family were also repressed in adrenal glands by TTP-α-T deficiency (FIG. 11).

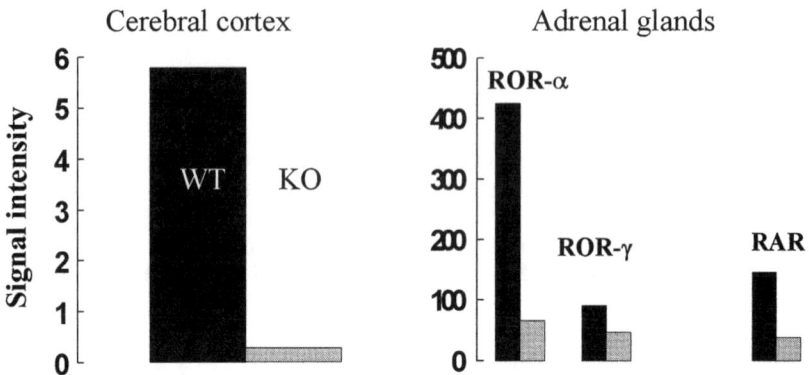

FIGURE 11. α-Tocopherol is required for ROR-α mRNA expression. ROR-α mRNA expression is higher in adrenal glands compared to cerebral cortex of wild-type mice. TTP-α-T deficiency results in the repression of ROR-α mRNA. Additionally, ROR-γ and retinoic acid receptor (RAR) mRNA expression is much lower than that of ROR-α in the adrenal glands and their expression is also repressed by TTP-α-T deficiency. The data were obtained from gene profiles of pooled samples ($n = 3$) of each genotype.

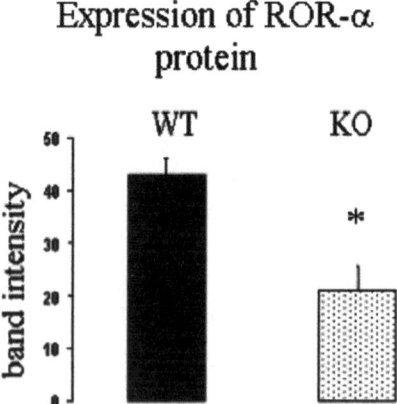

FIGURE 12. Expression of retinoic acid–related orphan receptor alpha (ROR-α) protein is repressed in the cortex of TTP-deficient (KO) mice compared to that in the wild-type (WT) mice. The data show band intensities (mean ± SD, $n = 3$) identified by rabbit anti-ROR-α antiserum.

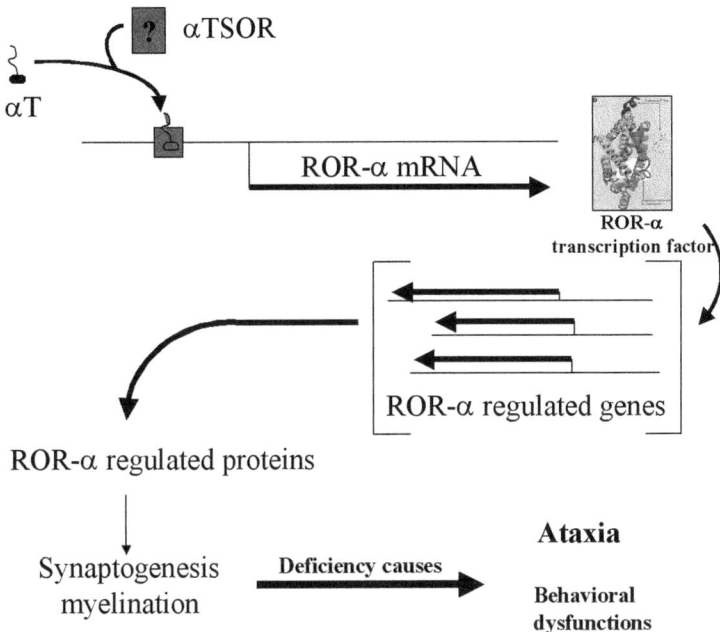

FIGURE 13. Hypothesis from gene-expression data. TTP-α-T deficiency represses mRNA and protein for ROR-α, a transcription factor that regulates the expression of multiple genes. The hypothesis predicts that some of the genes encoding myelin and synaptic proteins are driven by ROR-α. Therefore low expression of ROR-α in chronic vitamin E deficiency may account for some of the neurologic deficits such as ataxia.

These data suggest that α-tocopherol regulates the expression of ROR-α mRNA. Since ROR-α is a transcription factor, we suggest that some of the genes differentially expressed and driven by ROR-α are dependent on aT concentrations (FIG. 13). This hypothesis may account for previously described neurological abnormalities caused by chronic deficiency of vitamin E.[39,40] It is also noteworthy that *staggerer* mice have a mutation in the ROR-α gene[41] and transgenic mice with a deletion in ROR-α also show staggerer phenotype.[27] These observations suggest that the onset of ataxia reported in these TTP-deficient mice[19] is delayed because ROR-α is only partially repressed.

The effects of TTP-α-T deficiency on ataxia, anxiety, and memory function were also assessed. TTP-deficient mice develop ataxia with age (FIG. 14). Our data confirm the observations of Yokoto *et al.*,[19] who have independently generated TTP-deficient mice and shown abrogation of electrophysiological activity in the cortex and manifestation of ataxia with age. Although ataxia can be reliably measured, the cellular and molecular basis of ataxia is multi-factorial. Ataxia can be caused by mitochondrial dysfunction[42,43] abnormal glucose metabolism,[44] and severe deficiency of vitamin E.[45,46] In some ataxias the neuroanatomical substrates reside in the cerebellum. Severe ataxia in ROR-a–deficient mice is attributed to failure in the develop-

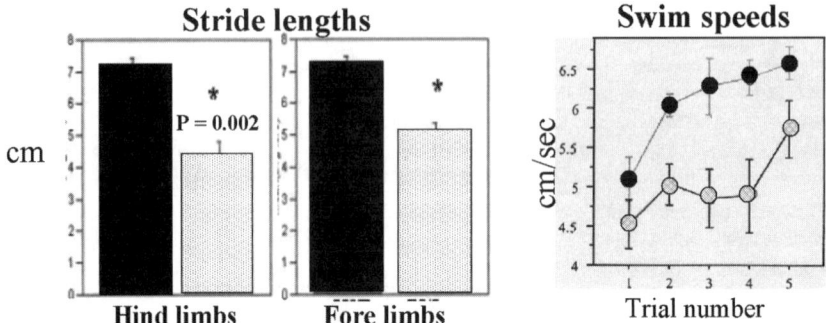

FIGURE 14. Ataxia in older TTP-deficient mice. Young (3-month-old) TTP-deficient mice were not significantly different from wild-type mice (data not shown). However, older (10–12 months) TTP-α-T–deficient mice showed significant ataxia. The older TTP-α-T–deficient mice also showed slower swim speeds, a possible indication of cerebellar dysfunction, peripheral neuropathy, and muscle weakness.

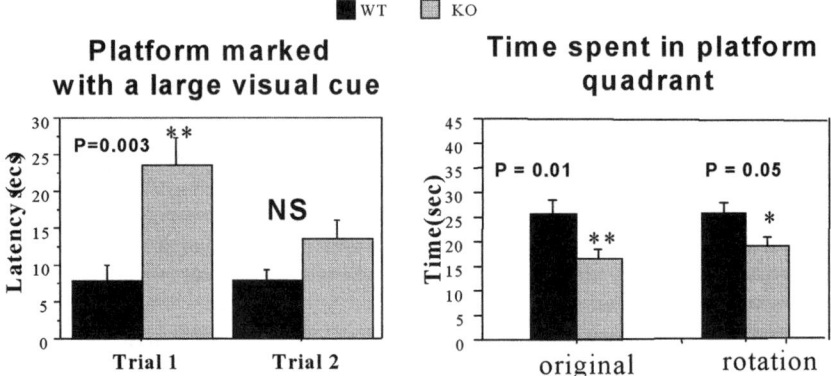

FIGURE 15. Performance in Morris Water Maze: TTP-α-T–deficient mice showed significantly longer latency in locating the escape platform, but were able to learn its location after the first trial (*left*). Some evidence of impaired memory was suggested by the data (*right*) that show that the TTP-deficient mice spent less time in the quadrant that previously contained the escape platform.

ment of Purkinje cells in the cerebellum and, as a result, loss of granule cells.[47] Delayed ataxia in TTP-deficient mice with repressed expression of ROR-α suggests a possible causative link between deficiency of cellular α-tocopherol, ROR-α, myelination and synaptic genes (FIG. 13), and neuropathy. Additional suggestion of cerebellar dysfunction in TTP-deficient mice was indicated by slower swim speeds of the TTP-deficient mice during the Morris Maze challenge (FIG. 14). The data from the Morris Maze test also suggest deficiency in hippocampal function; TTP-deficient mice were less successful in recalling the quadrant with the hidden escape platform (FIG., left panel). However, the mice were able to learn the location of the visible platform after one trial (FIG. 15, right panel).

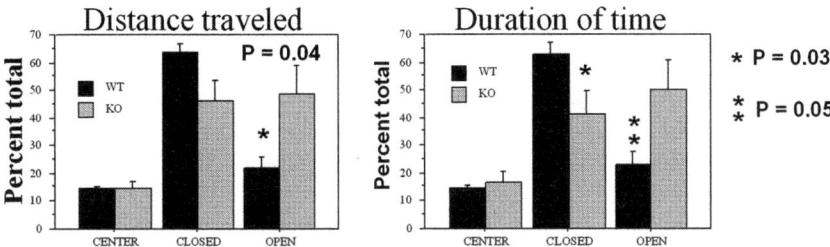

FIGURE 16. Performance in Elevated Plus Maze: TTP-α-T–deficient mice displayed lower levels of anxiety than the wild-type mice. The data show that the TTP-null mice traveled longer distances and spent more time in the open arm. Both are indications of less fear and anxiety than in the wild-type mice.

There was a suggestion of age-dependent changes in the anxiety behavior of TTP-deficient mice. We have previously shown that young (3 months) TTP-deficient mice displayed increased anxiety.[22] In this study 9–12-month-old mice showed decreased anxiety as shown by significantly ($P < 0.04$) increased time spent and distance traveled in the open arms of the elevated plus maze (FIG. 16).

SUMMARY AND CONCLUSIONS

Analysis of mRNA-expression profiles of cerebral cortex, heart, liver, lungs, and spleen of C57BL6 mice identified tissue-specific expression of a large number of genes, including those encoding tocopherol transfer protein (TTP). TTP mRNA was most abundant in the liver, moderately expressed in adrenal glands and was very low or undetectable in cerebral cortex, lungs, heart, and spleen. As expected, the expression of TTP mRNA was very low or undetectable in liver and adrenal glands of transgenic mice lacking TTP. The latter observations provide strong support for the validity of GeneChip analysis. Differential gene-expression analysis of wild-type and TTP-deficient mice identified the adrenal gland to be the most sensitive organ (~2000 genes) and liver and heart to be the least sensitive (~50 genes) to the deletion of TTP gene. TTP gene deletion causes early and chronic deficiency of α-tocopherol concentration in all tissues despite normal dietary concentration of vitamin E. Therefore differential gene-expression profiles of tissues such as cerebral cortex that lack TTP may primarily be attributed to the effects of α-tocopherol. The data showed repression of genes encoding myelin and synaptic proteins in cerebral cortex and those encoding synaptic proteins in adrenal glands. The data also suggest that the activities of oligodendrocytes and glial cells are affected by the deletion of the TTP gene, most probably due to depletion of cellular α-tocopherol. A particularly remarkable outcome of the gene-expression analysis was the observation that TTP-α-tocopherol regulates the tissue-specific expression of ROR-α gene. We postulate that some of the effects of α-tocopherol on gene expression are likely to be mediated by the transcription factor, ROR-α, a member of nuclear receptor superfamily.

ACKNOWLEDGMENTS

This research was supported by NIH Grants ES11528-02 and ES05707, and an unrestricted gift to the Regents of the University of California by BASF Human Nutrition and Scientific Affairs. Behavioral analyses were performed by the Murine Behavioral Assessment Laboratory of University of California, Davis.

REFERENCES

1. EVANS, H.M. & B.K. BISHOP. 1922. On the existence of a hitherto unrecognized dictatory factor essential for reproduction. Science **56:** 650–651.
2. BLATT, D.H., S.W. LEONARD & M.G. TRABER. 2001. Vitamin E kinetics and the function of tocopherol regulatory proteins. Nutrition **17:** 799–805.
3. BRIGELIUS-FLOHE, R. & M.G. TRABER. 1999. Vitamin E: function and metabolism. FASEB J. **13:** 1145–1155.
4. SATO, Y., H. ARAI, A. MIYATA, et al. 1993. Primary structure of alpha-tocopherol transfer protein from rat liver: homology with cellular retinaldehyde-binding protein. J. Biol. Chem. **268:** 17705–17710.
5. ARITA. M., Y. SATO, A. MIYATA, et al. 1995. Human alpha-tocopherol transfer protein: cDNA cloning, expression and chromosomal localization. Biochem. J. **306:** 437–443.
6. ZIMMER, S, A. STOCKER, M.N. SARBOLOUKI, et al. 2000. A novel human tocopherol-associated protein: cloning, in vitro expression, and characterization. J. Biol. Chem. **275:** 25672–25680.
7. SHA, B., S.E. PHILLIPS, V.A. BANKAITIS & M. LUO. 1998. Crystal structure of the *Saccharomyces cerevisiae* phosphatidylinositol- transfer protein. Nature **391:** 506–510.
8. SHIBATA, N., M. ARITA, Y. MISAKI, et al. 2001. Supernatant protein factor, which stimulates the conversion of squalene to lanosterol, is a cytosolic squalene transfer protein and enhances cholesterol biosynthesis. Proc. Natl. Acad. Sci. USA **98:** 2244–2249.
9. SINGH, D.K., V. MOKASHI, C.L. & T.D. PORTER. 2003. Phosphorylation of supernatant protein factor enhances its ability to stimulate microsomal squalene monooxygenase. J. Biol. Chem. **278:** 5646–5651.
10. DAS, P. & M. CHOWDHURY. 1999. Vitamin E-deficiency induced changes in ovary and uterus. Mol. Cell. Biochem. **198:** 151–156.
11. JISHAGE, K., M. ARITA, K. IGARASHI, et al. 2001. Alpha-tocopherol transfer protein is important for the normal development of placental labyrinthine trophoblasts in mice. J. Biol. Chem. **276:** 1669–1672.
12. TAPPEL, A.L. 1980. Vitamin E and selenium protection from in vivo lipid peroxidation. Ann. N.Y. Acad. Sci. **355:** 18–31.
13. TAPPEL, A.L. & C.J. DILLARD. 1981. In vivo lipid peroxidation: measurement via exhaled pentane and protection by vitamin E. Fed. Proc. **40:** 174–178.
14. BRIGELIUS-FLOHE, R. & M.G. TRABER. 1999. Vitamin E: function and metabolism. FASEB J. **13:** 1145–1155.
15. TRABER, M.G. & H. ARAI. 1999. Molecular mechanisms of vitamin E transport. Annu. Rev. Nutr. **19:** 343–355.
16. YOKOTA, T., T. SHIOJIRI. T. GOTODA, et al. 1997. Friedreich-like ataxia with retinitis pigmentosa caused by the His101Gln mutation of the alpha-tocopherol transfer protein gene. Ann. Neurol. **41:** 826–832.
17. BOMAR, J.M., P.J. BENKE, E.L. SLATTERY, et al. 2003. Mutations in a novel gene encoding a CRAL-TRIO domain cause human Cayman ataxia and ataxia/dystonia in the jittery mouse. Nat. Genet. **35:** 264–269.
18. TERASAWA, Y., Z. LADHA, S.W. LEONARD, et al. 2000. Increased atherosclerosis in hyperlipidemic mice deficient in alpha-tocopherol transfer protein and vitamin E. Proc. Natl. Acad. Sci. USA **97:** 13830–13834.

19. YOKOTA, T., K. IGARASHI, T. UCHIHARA, et al. 2001. Delayed-onset ataxia in mice lacking alpha-tocopherol transfer protein: model for neuronal degeneration caused by chronic oxidatiat stress. Proc. Natl. Acad. Sci. USA **98:** 15185–15190.
20. AZZI, A. 2004. The role of alpha-tocopherol in preventing disease. Eur. J. Nutr. (Suppl 1) **43:** I18–I25.
21. FISCHER, A., J. PALLAUF, K. GOHIL, et al. 2001. Effect of selenium and vitamin E deficiency on differential gene expression in rat liver. Biochem. Biophys. Res. Commun. **285:** 470–475.
22. GOHIL, K., B.C. SCHOCK, A.A. CHAKRABORTY, et al. 2003. Gene expression profile of oxidant stress and neurodegeneration in transgenic mice deficient in alpha-tocopherol transfer protein. Free Radic. Biol. Med. **35:** 1343–1354.
23. BARELLA, L., P.Y. MULLER & M. SCHLACHTER, et al. 2004. Identification of hepatic molecular mechanisms of action of alpha-tocopherol using global gene expression profile analysis in rats. Biochim. Biophys. Acta **1689:** 66–74.
24. GOHIL, K. & A.A. CHAKRABORTY. 2004. Applications of microarray and bioinformatics tools to dissect molecular responses of the central nervous system to antioxidant micronutrients. Nutrition **20:** 50–55.
25. GOHIL, K., S. ROY, L. PACKER & C.K. SEN. 1999. Antioxidant regulation of gene expression: analysis of differentially expressed mRNAs. Methods Enzymol. **300:** 402–410.
26. GOHIL, K. & L. PACKER. 2002. Global gene expression analysis identifies cell and tissue specific actions of Ginkgo biloba extract, EGb 761. Cell Mol. Biol. (Noisy-le-grand) **48:** 625–631.
27. STEINMAYR, M., E. ANDRE, F. CONQUET, et al. 1998. Staggerer phenotype in retinoid-related orphan receptor alpha-deficient mice. Proc. Natl. Acad. Sci. USA **95:** 3960–3965.
28. JETTEN, A.M. & E. UEDA. 2002. Retinoid-related orphan receptors (RORs): roles in cell survival, differentiation and disease. Cell Death Differ. **9:** 1167–1171.
29. LEONARD, S.W., Y. TERASAWA, R.V. FARESE, JR. & M.G. TRABER. 2002. Incorporation of deuterated RRR- or all-rac-alpha-tocopherol in plasma and tissues of alpha-tocopherol transfer protein–null mice. Am. J. Clin. Nutr. **75:** 555–560.
30. RODGERS, R.J., N.J. JOHNSON, J.C. COLE, et al. 1996. Plus-maze retest profile in mice: importance of initial stages of trial 1 and response to post-trial cholinergic receptor blockade. Pharmacol. Biochem. Behav. **54:** 41–50.
31. GOLUB, M.S., S.L. GERMANN & K.C. LLOYD. 2004. Behavioral characteristics of a nervous system-specific erbB4 knock-out mouse. Behav. Brain Res. **153:** 159–170.
32. GOHIL, K., R.K. MOY, S. FARZIN, et al. 2000. mRNA expression profile of a human cancer cell line in response to Ginkgo biloba extract: induction of antioxidant response and the Golgi system. Free Radic. Res. **33:** 831–849.
33. WATANABE, C.M., S. WOLFFRAM, P. ADER, et al. 2001. The in vivo neuromodulatory effects of the herbal medicine ginkgo biloba. Proc. Natl. Acad. Sci. USA **98:** 6577–6580.
34. LOCKHART, D.J., H. DONG, M.C. BYRNE, et al. 1996. Expression monitoring by hybridization to high-density oligonucleotide arrays. Nat. Biotechnol. **14:** 1675–1680.
35. THIBAULT, C., C. LAI, N. WILKE, et al. 2000. Expression profiling of neural cells reveals specific patterns of ethanol-responsiat gene expression. Mol. Pharmacol. **58:** 1593–600.
36. EMSLEY, J.G., P. ARLOTTA & J.D. MACKLIS. 2004. Star-cross'd neurons: astroglial effects on neural repair in the adult mammalian CNS. Trends Neurosci. **27:** 238-240.
37. PRIVAT A. 2003. Astrocytes as support for axonal regeneration in the central nervous system of mammals. **43:** 91–93.
38. LI, C. & W.H. WONG. 2001. Model-based analysis of oligonucleotide arrays: expression index computation and outlier detection. Proc. Natl. Acad. Sci. USA **98:** 31-36.
39. TOWFIGHI, J. 1981. Effects of chronic vitamin E deficiency on the nervous system of the rat. Acta Neuropathol. (Berl.) **54:** 261–267.
40. SOUTHAM, E., P.K. THOMAS, R.H. KING, et al. 1991. Experimental vitamin E deficiency in rats: morphological and functional evidence of abnormal axonal transport secondary to free radical damage. Brain 114: 915–936.

41. HAMILTON, B.A., W.N. FRANKEL, A.W. KERREBROCK, *et al.* 1996. Disruption of the nuclear hormone receptor ROR alpha in staggerer mice. Nature **379:** 736–739.
42. LARSSON, N.G. & P. RUSTIN. 2001. Animal models for respiratory chain disease. Trends Mol. Med. **7:** 578–581.
43. KAPLAN J. 2002. Spinocerebellar ataxias due to mitochondrial defects. Neurochem. Int. **40:** 553–557.
44. RISTOW, M. 2004. Neurodegenerative disorders associated with diabetes mellitus. J. Mol. Med. **82:** 510–529.
45. TRABER M.G. & H. SIES. 1996. Vitamin E in humans: demand and delivery. Annu. Rev. Nutr. **16:** 321–347.
46. ASLAM, A., S.A. MISBAH, K. TALBOT & H. CHAPEL. 2004. Vitamin E deficiency induced neurological disease in common variable immunodeficiency: two cases and a review of the literature of vitamin E deficiency. Clin. Immunol. **112:** 24–29.
47. SONMEZ, E. & K. HERRUP. 1984. Role of staggerer gene in determining cell number in cerebellar cortex. II. Granule cell death and persistence of the external granule cell layer in young mouse chimeras. Brain Res. **314:** 271–283.

Tocotrienol

The Natural Vitamin E to Defend the Nervous System?

CHANDAN K. SEN, SAVITA KHANNA, AND SASHWATI ROY

Laboratory of Molecular Medicine, Department of Surgery, Davis Heart & Lung Research Institute and The Ohio State University Medical Center, Columbus, Ohio 43210 USA

ABSTRACT: Vitamin E is essential for normal neurological function. It is the major lipid-soluble, chain-breaking antioxidant in the body, protecting the integrity of membranes by inhibiting lipid peroxidation. Mostly on the basis of symptoms of primary vitamin E deficiency, it has been demonstrated that vitamin E has a central role in maintaining neurological structure and function. Orally supplemented vitamin E reaches the cerebrospinal fluid and brain. Vitamin E is a generic term for all tocopherols and their derivatives having the biological activity of RRR-α-tocopherol, the naturally occurring stereoisomer compounds with vitamin E activity. In nature, eight substances have been found to have vitamin E activity: α-, β-, γ- and δ-tocopherol; and α-, β-, γ- and δ-tocotrienol. Often, the term vitamin E is synonymously used with α-tocopherol. Tocotrienols, formerly known as ζ, ε, or η-tocopherols, are similar to tocopherols except that they have an isoprenoid tail with three unsaturation points instead of a saturated phytyl tail. Although tocopherols are predominantly found in corn, soybean, and olive oils, tocotrienols are particularly rich in palm, rice bran, and barley oils. Tocotrienols possess powerful antioxidant, anticancer, and cholesterol-lowering properties. Recently, we have observed that α-tocotrienol is multi-fold more potent than α-tocopherol in protecting HT4 and primary neuronal cells against toxicity induced by glutamate as well as by a number of other toxins. At nanomolar concentration, tocotrienol, but not tocopherol, completely protected neurons by an antioxidant-independent mechanism. Our current work identifies two major targets of tocotrienol in the neuron: c-Src kinase and 12-lipoxygenase. Dietary supplementation studies have established that tocotrienol, fed orally, does reach the brain. The current findings point towards tocotrienol as a potent neuroprotective form of natural vitamin E.

KEYWORDS: nutrient; glutamate; neurotoxicity; antioxidant; neuroprotection

Vitamin E is essential for normal neurological function.[1,2] The nervous system is vulnerable to the damaging effects of highly reactive free radicals for several reasons. The brain contains high amounts of polyunsaturated (20:4 and 22:6) fatty acids

Address for correspondence: Dr. Chandan K. Sen, 512 Davis Heart & Lung Research Institute, 473 West 12th Avenue, The Ohio State University Medical Center, Columbus, Ohio 43210. Voice: 614-247-7786; fax: 614-247-7818.
sen-1@medctr.osu.edu

that are susceptible to lipid peroxidation, receives a large percentage of oxygen, and is relatively deficient in certain antioxidant enzymes. In addition, specific regions of the brain have high iron concentrations. Thus, antioxidant defenses are critically important to protect the brain and neural tissues from oxidative damage.[3] Indeed, numerous pathophysiological conditions have been associated with increased levels of oxidative stress indices.[4-6]

Neuroprotection by antioxidants has therefore drawn much interest. The majority of the available research on the role of antioxidant nutrients in neurological function and disease has focused on vitamin E. Vitamin E is the major lipid-soluble, chain-breaking antioxidant in the body, protecting the integrity of membranes by inhibiting lipid peroxidation. Mostly on the basis of symptoms of primary vitamin E deficiency, it has been demonstrated that vitamin E has a central role in maintaining neurological structure and function.[2] Orally supplemented vitamin E reaches the cerebrospinal fluid and brain.[7] One of the most extensively studied aspects of vitamin E is its antioxidant property. Most of the vitamin E–sensitive neurological disorders are associated with elevated levels of oxidative damage markers. This has led to a popular hypothesis stating that the neuroprotective effects of vitamin E are wholly mediated by its antioxidant property.[8]

THE VITAMIN E FAMILY: TOCOPHEROLS AND TOCOTRIENOLS

Vitamin E is a generic term for all tocopherols and their derivatives having the biological activity of RRR-α-tocopherol, the naturally occurring stereoisomer compounds with vitamin E activity.[9,10] In nature, eight substances have been found to have vitamin E activity: α-, β-, γ- and δ-tocopherol and α-, β-, γ- and δ-tocotrienol (FIG. 1). Often, the term vitamin E is synonymously used with α-tocopherol. Although d-α-tocopherol (RRR-α-tocopherol) has the highest bioavailability and is the standard against which all the others must be compared, it is only one out of eight natural forms of vitamin E. Tocotrienols, formerly known as ζ, ε or η-tocopherols (FIG. 1), are similar to tocopherols except that they have an isoprenoid tail with three unsaturated points instead of a saturated phytyl tail (FIG. 1). Although tocopherols are predominantly found in corn, soybean, and olive oils, tocotrienols are particularly rich in palm, rice bran, and barley oils.[9,10]

Interestingly, tocotrienols possess powerful antioxidant, anticancer, and cholesterol-lowering properties (TABLE 1). Some studies have confirmed that tocotrienol activity as an antioxidant, anticancer, and cholesterol-reducing substance to be stronger than tocopherols. Tocotrienols are thought to have more potent antioxidant properties than α-tocopherol.[43,52] The unsaturated side-chain of tocotrienol allows for more efficient penetration into tissues, such as the brain and liver, that have saturated fatty layers.[36] Experimental research examining the antioxidant, free-radical scavenging effects of tocopherol and tocotrienols revealed that tocotrienols appear superior because of their better distribution in the fatty layers of the cell membrane.[36] Although tocotrienols have shown better beneficial effects than α-tocopherol in a limited number of situations, as indicated in the foregoing text, little is known about the exact mechanism of action. Among the pathophysiological situations cited above, only one mechanism of action that accounts for the hypocholesterolemic property of tocotrienol has been characterized. Micromolar amounts of

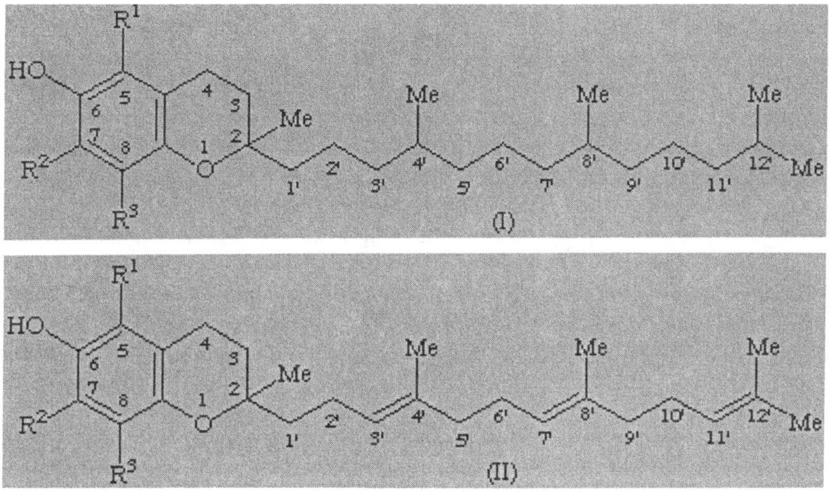

FIGURE 1. Vitamin E: variations and nomenclature. The term tocopherol(s) is a generic descriptor for all monomethyltocols, dimethyltocols, and trimethyltocols. Thus, this term is *not* synonymous with the term vitamin E. Compound I (R1 = R2 = R3 = Me), known as α-tocopherol, is designated α-tocopherol or 5,7,8-trimethyltocol; compound I (R1 = R3 = Me; R2 = H), known as β-tocopherol, is designated, β-tocopherol or 5,8-dimethyltocol; compound I (R1 = H; R2 = R3 = Me), known as γ-tocopherol, is designated γ-tocopherol or 7,8-dimethyltocol; compound I (R1 = R2 = H; R3 = Me), known as δ-tocopherol, is designated δ-tocopherol or 8-methyltocol; compound II (R1 = R2 = R3 = H), 2-methyl-2-(4,8,12-trimethyltrideca-3,7,11-trienyl)chroman-6-ol, is designated tocotrienol; compound II (R1 = R2 = R3 = Me), formerly known as ζ1 or ζ2-tocopherol, is designated 5,7,8-trimethyltocotrienol or α-tocotrienol. The name tocochromanol-3 has also been used; compound II (R1 = R3 = Me; R2 =), formerly known as ε-tocopherol, is designated 5,8-dimethyltocotrienol or β-tocotrienol; compound II (R1 = H; R2 = R3 = Me), formerly known as η-tocopherol, is designated 7,8-dimethyltocotrienol or γ-tocotrienol. The name plastochromanol-3 has also been used; compound II (R1 = R2 = H; R3 = Me) is designated 8-methyltocotrienol or δ-tocotrienol.[120]

tocotrienol have been shown to suppress the activity of HMG-CoA reductase, the hepatic enzyme responsible for cholesterol synthesis.[33,40]

GLUTAMATE-INDUCED TOXICITY: GENERAL MECHANISMS

Mammalian cells possess an Na^+-independent anionic amino acid transport system, designated as x_c^-, highly specific for cystine and glutamate.[53] This system imports cystine into cells in exchange for glutamate. Cystine taken up by the cell via system x_c^- is rapidly reduced to cysteine, which is incorporated into proteins and glutathione.[54] Because cysteine is a rate-limiting precursor for glutathione synthesis, the intracellular level of glutathione is regulated by the system x_c^- activity.[55] Impaired cellular cystine uptake in human immunodeficiency virus–infected (HIV^+) patients because of high plasma glutamate level has been suggested to be a causative factor of low leukocyte reduced glutathione (GSH) level in these patients.[56,57]

TABLE 1. Biological properties of tocotrienol (1986–2000)

Biological Action	Year of Study	Description/Reference
Neuroprotective	2000	*Mouse*; protects against glutamate-induced neuronal death by suppressing inducible pp60 c-Src kinase activation[11]
Antiaging/antioxidant	2000	*C. elegans*; α-tocopherol acetate did not work[12]
Hypocholesterolemic, antioxidant, and antitumor	2000	*Chicken*; the number and position of methyl substituents in tocotrienols affect their hypocholesterolemic, antioxidant, and antitumor properties; tocotrienol better than α-tocopherol[13]
Antiproliferative and apoptotic	2000	*Mouse*; preneoplastic and neoplastic mammary epithelial cells: α- and γ-tocopherol had no effect on cell proliferation[14]
Modulating normal mammary gland growth, function, and remodeling	2000	*Mouse*; mammary epithelial cells more easily or preferentially took up tocotrienols as compared to tocopherols[15]
Anti-cancer (breast)	1999	*Human*; naturally occurring tocotrienols and RRR-delta-tocopherol are effective apoptotic inducers for human breast cancer cells[16]
ApoB level reduction in hypercholesterolemic subjects	1999	*Human*; in HepG2 cells it (not tocopherol) stimulates apoB degradation, possibly as the result of decreased apoB translocation into the endoplasmic reticulum lumen[17]
Lowering blood pressure; antioxidant	1999	*SHR*; supplement of γ-tocotrienol may prevent increased blood pressure, reduce lipid peroxides in plasma and blood vessels, and enhance total antioxidant status[18]
Anti-cancer	1999	*Human*; apoptosis and cell-cycle arrest in human and murine tumor cells are initiated by isoprenoids[19]
Serum lipoproteins; platelet function	1999	*Human*; in men at risk for cardiovascular disease tocotrienol supplements had no marked favorable effects[20]
Serum triglycerides	1999	*Rat;* lower in tocotrienol fed; higher IgM productivity of spleen lymphocytes and IgA, IgG, and higher IgM productivity of mesenteric lymph node lymphocytes[21]
Immune function	1999	*Rats*; feeding affects proliferation and function of spleen and mesenetric lymph node lymphocytes[22]
Anti-cancer	1998	*Human*; inhibits the growth of human breast cancer cells irrespective of estrogen receptor status[23]
Transfer protein	1997	α-tocopherol transfer protein binds α-tocotrienol with 11% efficiency compared to a-tocopherol[24]
Anti-cancer	1997	*Human*; inhibited proliferation of estrogen receptor-negative MDA-MB-435 and -positive MCF-7 breast cancer cells[25] *Mouse*; isoprenoids suppress the growth of murine B16 melanomas *in vitro* and *in vivo*[26]

TABLE 1. (*continued*) **Biological properties of tocotrienol (1986–2000)**

Biological Action	Year of Study	Description/Reference
Lymphatic transport	1996	*Rat*; preferential absorption of alpha-tocotrienol compared to gamma- and delta-tocotrienols and alpha-tocopherol[27]
Antioxidant	1995	*Human*; controls the course of carotid atherosclerosis[28]
Hypocholesterolemic	1995	*Human*; lowered plasma cholesterol level in hypercholesterolemic subjects [29]
Anti-cancer	1995	*Human*; tocotrienol, not tocopherol, suppresses growth of a human breast cancer cell line in culture[30]
Antioxidant	1995	*Rat*; Protects brain against oxidative damage[31]
Hypocholesterolemic	1995	Isoprenoid-mediated suppression of mevalonate synthesis depletes tumor tissues of two intermediate products, farnesyl pyrophosphate and geranylgeranyl pyrophosphate, which are incorporated post-translationally into growth control-associated proteins[32]
Hypocholesterolemic	1994	*HepG2;* the farnesyl side chain and the methyl/hydroxy substitution pattern of gamma-tocotrienol responsible for HMG CoA reductase suppression[33]
Anti-cancer	1994	*Human;* suppresses activation of Epstein-Barr virus early antigen expression in PMA-activated lymphoblastoid Raji cells[34]
Hypocholesterolemic and antioxidant	1993	*Rat;* spares plasma tocopherol[35]
Antioxidant	1993	*In vitro;* tocotrienol is better than tocopherol; tocotrienol is located closer to the cell membrane surface[36]
Antioxidant	1993	*Human;* dietary tocotrienols become incorporated into circulating human lipoproteins where they react with peroxyl radicals as efficiently as the corresponding tocopherol isomers [7]
Anti-cancer	1993	*Rat*; tocotrienol. chemopreventive in hepatic tumor model[38]
Hypocholesterolemic	1993	Regulates cholesterol production in mammalian cells by post-transcriptional suppression of 3-hydroxy-3-methylglutaryl-coenzyme A reductase[39]
Hypocholesterolemic	1992	*In vitro*; posttranscriptional suppression of HMG-CoA reductase by a process distinct from other known inhibitors of cholesterol biosynthesis[40]
Anti-hypertensive	1992	*Rat*; depressed (better than α-tocopherol) age-related increase in the systolic blood pressure of spontaneously hypertensive rats[41]
Antioxidant regeneration	1992	*In vitro*; facilitates antioxidant recycling[42]
Antioxidant (lipid-phase)	1991	*In vitro*; better than α-tocopherol[43]

TABLE 1. (*continued*) Biological properties of tocotrienol (1986–2000)

Biological Action	Year of Study	Description/Reference
Hypocholesterolemic	1991	*Human*; lowered serum cholesterol in hypercholesterolemics[44]; lowered both serum total cholesterol (TC) and low-densitylipoprotein cholesterol[45] *Pigs;* reduced plasma cholesterol, apolipoprotein B, thromboxane B2, and platelet factor 4 in pigs with inherited hyperlipidemias [6]
Anti-cancer	1991	*Rat*; tocotrienol. chemopreventive in hepatic tumor model[47]
Anti-cancer	1991	*Rat*; tocotrienol, but not tocopherol, was chemopreventive in mammary tumor model [8]
Anti-cancer	1989	*Rat*; tocotrienol-rich palm oil prevented chemicallyinduced mammary tumorigenesis[49]
Anti-cancer	1989	*Mouse*; intraperitoneally injected tocotrienol prevented transplanted tumors[50]
Anti-cholesterol	1986	*Chicken*; three double bonds in the isoprenoid chain essential for the inhibition of cholesterogenesis; tocopherols do not share this property[51]

NOTE: SHR: spontaneously hypertensive rats; HMG CoA reductase: 3-hydroxy-3-methylglutaryl coenzyme A reductase.

Our initial interest was focused on the rescue of human lymphocytes from glutamate-induced oxidative damage, loss of thiols, and death.[58,59] We observed that several antioxidants are effective in preventing glutamate-induced lymphocyte toxicity.[54,58–60] Glutamate toxicity is a major contributor to pathological cell death within the nervous system and appears to be mediated by reactive oxygen species (ROS).[61] There are two forms of glutamate toxicity: receptor-initiated excitotoxicity[62] and non-receptor-mediated, glutamate-induced toxicity.[63] One model used to study oxidative stress–related neuronal death is to inhibit cystine uptake by exposing cells to high levels of glutamate.[64] The induction of oxidative stress by glutamate in this model has been demonstrated to be a primary cytotoxic mechanism in C6 glial cells,[65,66] PC-12 neuronal cells,[67,68] immature cortical neurons cells,[64] and oligodendroglial cells.[69] We were therefore led to investigate the role of oxidants and antioxidants in glutamate-induced death of cells of the nervous system.

Our first study in this direction was with C6 glial cells, where we noted that 0.1–1 mM lipoic acid or *N*-acetyl-L-cysteine was able to protect C6 glial cells against glutamate-induced death. This effect of these thiol antioxidants was mediated by their ability to increase cellular GSH levels.[66] Glutamate challenge to C6 cells was with associated increased accumulation of [ROS]i. Because the glutamate-induced cell death process was antioxidant-inhabitable and oxidant-associated, we sought to characterize the cellular events that are regulated by oxidants and antioxidants during the course of glutamate-induced death. HT neuronal cells, lacking a functional excitotoxic pathway, are commonly used to characterize the oxidative stress component of cell death.[63,70–81]

In HT4 cells,[82] we observed that glutamate challenge resulted in elevated $[ROS]_i$ and depleted $[GSH]_i$ and that the death process was inhibited in cells pretreated with several chemical classes of antioxidants.[83] We observed that compared to water-soluble antioxidants, lipophilic antioxidants were clearly more effective in preventing glutamate-induced death.[83] Our focus was therefore turned on the vitamin E family.[11] A comparison of the efficiency of α-tocopherol with α-tocotrienol to protect HT4 cells challenged with glutamate showed that tocotrienol was clearly more potent than tocopherol on a matched concentration basis.[11] The neuroprotective property of tocotrienol was clearly observed at a concentration of 50 nmol/L, and complete protection was achieved with 100 nmol/L even when tocotrienol was treated 2–3 hours after glutamate challenge. At these concentrations, tocopherol clearly failed to protect. After supplementation to humans, the level of α-tocotrienol in the plasma has been estimated to be 0.98 ± 0.8 mM.[84,85] Therefore, the neuroprotective effects of tocotrienol that we were observing corresponded to 1/10th of the concentration found in the plasma of supplemented humans. The observation that nanomolar concentrations of tocotrienol had neuroprotective properties was of outstanding interest. Particularly so because our observation constituted the first evidence that an antioxidant vitamin could have such potent cell regulatory properties at nanomolar concentrations. Later studies in our laboratory confirmed that the neuroprotective properties of nanomolar concentrations of tocotrienol were also applicable to primary fetal rat cortical neurons challenged with HCA or glutamate or even buthionine-S-R-sulfoximine.[86] Nanomolar concentrations of tocotrienol failed to protect against chemically generated peroxyl radicals. Micromolar concentration of tocotrienol was required for such protection.[11,86]

We were thus led to the conclusion that at nanomolar concentration, tocotrienol functions by an antioxidant-independent mechanism. Further study of the molecular processes suggested that nanomolar concentrations of tocotrienol potently regulate key signaling pathways involved in neuronal death. These findings constitute the first evidence establishing that trace amounts of tocotrienol may have potent signal transduction regulatory properties.[11]

MOLECULAR CHECKPOINTS IN NEURONAL CELL DEATH: OPPORTUNITIES FOR TOCOTRIENOL REGULATION

Executioners of cellular death in the nervous system are of diverse nature and are known to recruit a multitude of signaling pathways. It is not within the scope of this section to discuss such complexities. We undertake to focus on those specific mediators of neuronal death that have been identified by us to be tocotrienol sensitive in neuronal cells.[11,86]

pp60 c-Src

Our results indicate that inhibition of inducible pp60 c-Src kinase and extracellular signal responsive kinase activation represent a key mechanism by which nanomolar concentrations of tocotrienol protects glutamate-challenged HT4 cells.[11] In neurons and astrocytes, pp60 c-Src is present at levels 15–20 times higher than those found in fibroblasts. The specific activity of the c-Src protein from neuronal cultures is 6- to 12-times higher than that from the astrocyte cultures, suggesting a key function of this protein in neurons.[87] Src family kinases are able to induce caspase-independent cytoplasmic events leading to cell death.[88] We noted that glutamate-induced death of HT4 neurons is not sensitive to caspase inhibitors.

Extracellular Signal Responsive Kinase

The extracellular signal responsive kinase (ERK) subfamily of mitogen-activated protein kinases (MAPKs) has been implicated in the regulation of cell growth and differentiation.[89] The role of ERK in neuronal degeneration is less clear and may depend upon the specific neuronal cell type. ERK activation is typically associated with cell survival, proliferation, and differentiation, given the activation by mitogens and some cell survival factors.[90–92] However, activation of ERK contributes to neuronal cell death in certain *in vitro* models of neurotoxicity.[93–96]

Recently we[11] and others[80] have demonstrated that sustained activation of ERK plays a central role in mediating glutamate-induced death of murine hippocampal HT cells. Consistent with these findings supporting the role of ERK in neuronal cell death, inhibition of MEK-1/2, the upstream activators of ERK, afforded some degree of protection against apoptosis generated by nerve growth factor withdrawal of differentiated PC12 cells.[97] MEK-1 inhibition also protects against neuron cell damage induced by focal cerebral ischemia in rats.[98]

Activation of ERK involves a two-step protein kinase cascade lying upstream from ERK, in which the Raf family are the MAP kinase kinase and the MEK1/MEK2 isoforms are the MAP kinases. The linear sequence of Raf MEK ERK constitutes a major component of the ERK cascade. Growth factor-regulated–receptor protein tyrosine kinases and G protein–coupled receptors represent two major modulators of inducible ERK function.[99] More recently, Src family tyrosine kinases have been identified to possess inducible ERK regulatory function.[100–103] Whether glutamate-induced activation of c-Src in HT4 cells directly or indirectly regulates ERK induction remains to be determined.

The Eicosanoid Pathway

Lowered $[GSH]_i$ and elevated lipid peroxidation represents one of the early cellular events after glutamate challenge. Reduced glutathione is a key survival factor in cells of the nervous system, and lowered $[GSH]_i$ is one of the early markers of neurotoxicity induced by a variety of agonists.[104,105] With the use of immature cortical neurons and HT cells, it has been shown that a decrease in $[GSH]_i$ triggers the activation of neuronal 12-lipoxygenase (12-LOX), which leads to the production of peroxides, the influx of Ca^{2+}, and ultimately to cell death.[72]

We have noted that in neuronal cells, a decrease in $[GSH]_i$ is not lethal *per se*, but that it may serve as a signal to activate mechanisms that signal for death.[86] Our observations bring to light that strategies to inhibit 12-LOX are able to rescue neuronal cells from glutamate-induced death. Given that Src kinase activity is also known to regulate inducible lipoxygenase activity,[106] it is difficult to delineate the relative contribution of lowered [GSH]i and activated Src in activating lipoxygenase in glutamate-treated cells. Of importance, metabolites of the lipoxygenase pathway are known to be able to activate ERK. Hydroxyeicosatetraenoic acid (HETE), a lipoxygenase metabolite of arachidonic acid (AA), leads to activation of Erk via the Raf-1/MEK signal transduction pathway.[107] More recently, 12(S)-hydroxyeicosatetraenoic acid (12(S)-HETE), a 12-LOX metabolite of AA, has been specifically shown to be responsible for ERK1/2 induction.[108]

Although our studies indicate that 12-LOX may play a central role in glutamate-induced death of HT4 cells, the source of substrate (that is, AA for 12-LOX) remains unidentified. AA can be produced from phospholipids by the actions of PL (phospholipase) A2, PLC, or PLD. Cleavage of phosphatidylcholine by PC-PLC yields diacylglycerol, which can give further rise to AA through the action of diacylglycerol lipase. Diacylglycerol, subject to negative regulation by vitamin E,[109] can signal for the activation of protein kinase C (PKC), and PKC modulates glutamate toxicity. Various neuropathological conditions appear to be associated with the activation of phospholipases, which release lipid metabolites that either are directly toxic to neurons or act as second messengers.[110,111] Phosphatidylcholine constitutes the majority of phospholipid in brain tissues, and it has been shown that PC-PLC inhibitor blocks glutamate toxicity in neuronal cells by uncoupling cystine uptake from glutamate inhibition, allowing the maintenance of glutathione synthesis and cell viability.[73] Exposure of synaptosomal membranes to phospholipases A2, C, and D results in their depolarization and an increase of the negative surface potential. In the case of phospholipases A2 and C, these changes are associated with a decrease of the microviscosity of the membrane lipid bilayer. Vitamin E has been shown to stabilize synaptosomal membranes against the damaging action of the phospholipases. This stabilization is caused by reconstitution of the transmembrane potential and an increase of microviscosity of the phospholipase-treated membranes.[112]

DIETARY TOCOTRIENOL IN THE BRAIN

The concern that dietary tocotrienol may not reach the brain[113] has substantially dampened general interest to investigate the neuroprotective properties of tocotrienol. In this context, it is important to note that tocotrienols are relatively unstable and may not be retained well when added to the laboratory chow. We have found that gavaging of tocotrienol suspended in vitamin E–deficient corn oil represents an effective approach of delivery of the vitamin to laboratory rodents. In our first study that looked at the tissue availability of tocotrienol, we fed rats a tocotrienol-rich fraction (TRF; 1.23 mmol α-tocotrienol and 0.94 mmol α-tocopherol per g weight) isolated from palm oil[15,23,30,114–116] provided by the Carotech Sdn Bhd of Malaysia. Eight-day pregnant rats were fed daily (intragastrically) with 1 g/kg body weight of TRF suspended in vitamin E–stripped corn oil for nine days. On day 17 of pregnancy, rats were killed and tissues collected from the mother and fetus. Vitamin E content in the whole brain was measured with the use of a 12-channel CouloArray high-performance liquid chromatography-ultraviolet (HPLC-UV) electrochemical system.[117] We observed that TRF feeding increased α-tocopherol and α-tocotrienol content in the maternal brain by 0.1-fold and 5-fold, respectively. Dietary TRF increased fetal brain α-tocotrienol content more than 20-fold. These results provide the first evidence that dietary tocotrienol does reach the brain. Subsequent studies with lower doses of tocotrienol (5 mg/kg body weight; Tocomin, Carotech, Malaysia) over a longer period of time support observations of our first study that dietary tocotrienol is clearly available to the brain.

VITAMIN E–SENSITIVE GENES IN THE BRAIN

We have determined that lowering vitamin E in the diet of pregnant mothers results in marked vitamin E deficiency in the fetal tissues. Using this system as a model, we sought to identify vitamin E–sensitive genes in the developing fetal brain.[118] The transcriptomes of developing fetal brains from E-sufficient and E-deficient groups were compared with the use of the U34A rat genome high-density oligonucleotide GeneChip array. This array analyzed approximately 7,000 full-length sequences and approximately 1,000 EST clusters. With the use of raw data from all replicates available from both groups, a total of six pair-wise comparisons were generated. The average (six pair-wise comparisons) fold-changes of all the genes that were differentially expressed were calculated.

Our results indicated that a majority of genes remained unchanged in response to dietary vitamin E deficiency. A total of 645 (7.3%) genes were upregulated in the E-sufficient compared to the E-deficient group. Of these candidates, the expression of 416 genes increased by a magnitude of 2-fold or more. On the other hand, 152 (1.7%) of the genes were downregulated with 74 of them lowered by 2-fold or more. With the use of the t-test analysis, a total 144 genes were observed to have changed significantly in the E-deficient group compared to the E-sufficient group. Next, genes for those in which the concordance exceeded 50% in pair-wise comparisons were selected, especially if the gene was detected with redundant probe sets. With the use of this approach to data analysis, a total of 19 probe sets were found to be upregulated and 34 repressed in the E-sufficient group compared to the E-deficient group.

Among the upregulated genes, two probe sets targeting hemeoxygenase-3 (HO-3) were increased by 3.9- and 3.1-fold, respectively. In contrast, the expression of maspin, glyceraldehyde-3-phosphate dehydrogenase (GAPDH), apolipoprotein B (apoB), and G protein beta1 subunit (rGb1) genes was highly (3- to 5-fold) repressed. HO-3 was one of the few E-sensitive genes upregulated in fetal brains. HO isozymes, HO-1, HO-2, and HO-3, are heat shock protein 32 protein cognates with a known function of catalyzing the isomer-specific oxidation of the heme molecule, including that of NO synthase. HO-1 is highly inducible, whereas HO-2 and HO-3 are constitutively expressed. These proteins play a central role in cellular defense mechanisms. HO activity is responsible for the production of equimolar amounts of CO, biliverdin, and free Fe. Recent findings with the HO suggest that these proteins may serve as an intracellular "sink" for NO.

LINE1 was identified to be another E-sensitive transcript. The long interspersed elements 1 (LINE-1) or L1 family of interspersed repeats accounts for at least 10% of the mammalian genome. Like other interspersed repeat DNA families in genomes of other organisms, L1 is dispersed and amplified throughout the genome by a series of duplicative transposition events. Because of the high copy number of L1 sequences in the genome, L1 is abundantly represented in the RNA population of most cells. However, most of the transcripts that contain L1 are the result of fortuitous transcription and are not intermediates in L1 retrotransposition. This high background of L1-

containing transcripts, many of which are truncated and rearranged, makes it difficult to distinguish the transcript encoded by an active L1 element(s).

ApoB mRNA was one of top candidates that were lower in the E-sufficient group compared to the E-deficient fetal brain. ApoB plays a central role in lipoprotein metabolism and exists in two isoforms in plasma, apoB-100 and apoB-48. High levels of apoB and LDL cholesterol have been associated with an increased risk for coronary heart disease. An earlier study has shown that administration of TRF (100 mg/day) decreases serum apoB. Tocopherol has been shown to inhibit PKC activity in cells.[119] PKC-regulated chloride channel was one of the genes suppressed in the E-sufficient fetal brain.[118]

SIGNIFICANCE

The critical significance of vitamin E in neurological health and disease was recognized several decades ago. Since then, vitamin E research has developed in a highly asymmetric fashion, with emphasis on α-tocopherol in particular, and with the least studied natural vitamin E being the tocotrienols. Tocotrienols are naturally occurring and are routinely consumed by humans with no documented adverse effects. Our work builds on the striking observation showing that trace amounts of tocotrienol possess potent neuroprotective properties. The observation is indeed "striking" because, as a general trend, nutrients are required at high micromolar or millimolar levels to influence biological responses. The neuroprotective ability of 100 nM (1/10th of the concentration achieved in the plasma of humans receiving supplement) tocotrienol may be viewed as the most potent of all properties of vitamin E characterized so far. Thus, a new frontier defining the molecular basis of vitamin E action is unfolding.

ACKNOWLEDGMENT

This study was supported by NIH-NINDS R01NS42617 (to C.K.S.).

REFERENCES

1. MULLER, D.P. & M.A. GOSS-SAMPSON. 1989. Role of vitamin E in neural tissue. Ann. N.Y. Acad. Sci. **570:** 146–155.
2. MULLER, D.P. & M.A. GOSS-SAMPSON. 1990. Neurochemical, neurophysiological, and neuropathological studies in vitamin E deficiency. Crit. Rev. Neurobiol. **5:** 239–263.
3. FLOYD, R.A. 1999. Antioxidants, oxidative stress, and degenerative neurological disorders. Proc. Soc. Exp. Biol. Med. **222:** 236–245.
4. REITER, R.J. 1995. Oxidative processes and antioxidative defense mechanisms in the aging brain. FASEB J. **9:** 526–533.
5. SCHULZ, J.B., et al. 2000. Glutathione, oxidative stress and neurodegeneration. Eur. J. Biochem. **267:** 4904–4911.
6. ZHANG, Y., V.L. DAWSON & T.M. DAWSON. 2000. Oxidative stress and genetics in the pathogenesis of Parkinson's disease. Neurobiol. Dis. **7:** 240–250.
7. VATASSERY, G.T., S. FAHN & M.A. KUSKOWSKI. 1998. alpha-Tocopherol in CSF of subjects taking high-dose vitamin E in the DATATOP study: Parkinson Study Group. Neurology **50:** 1900–1902.

8. VATASSERY, G.T. 1998. Vitamin E and other endogenous antioxidants in the central nervous system. Geriatrics **53**(Suppl. 1): S25–S27.
9. TRABER, M.G. & H. SIES. 1996. Vitamin E in humans: demand and delivery. Annu. Rev. Nutr. **16:** 321–347.
10. TRABER, M.G. & L. PACKER. 1995. Vitamin E: beyond antioxidant function. Am. J. Clin. Nutr. **62:** 1501S–1509S.
11. SEN, C.K. *et al.* 2000. Molecular basis of vitamin E action: tocotrienol potently inhibits glutamate-induced pp60(c-Src) kinase activation and death of HT4 neuronal cells. J. Biol. Chem. **275:** 13049–13055.
12. ADACHI, H. & N. ISHII. 2000. Effects of tocotrienols on lifespan and protein carbonylation in *Caenorhabditis elegans*. J. Gerontol. Ser. A Biol. Sci. Med. Sci. **55:** B280–B285.
13. QURESHI, A.A. *et al.* 2000. Isolation and identification of novel tocotrienols from rice bran with hypocholesterolemic, antioxidant, and antitumor properties. J. Agric. Food Chem. **48:** 3130–3140.
14. MCINTYRE, B.S. *et al.* 2000. Antiproliferative and apoptotic effects of tocopherols and tocotrienols on preneoplastic and neoplastic mouse mammary epithelial cells. Proc. Soc. Exp. Biol. Med. **224:** 292–301.
15. MCINTYRE, B.S. *et al.* 2000. Antiproliferative and apoptotic effects of tocopherols and tocotrienols on normal mouse mammary epithelial cells. Lipids **35:** 171–180.
16. YU, W. *et al.* 1999. Induction of apoptosis in human breast cancer cells by tocopherols and tocotrienols. Nutr. Cancer **33:** 26–32.
17. THERIAULT, A. *et al.* 1999. Effects of gamma-tocotrienol on ApoB synthesis, degradation, and secretion in HepG2 cells. Arterioscler, Thromb. Vasc. Biol. **19:** 704–712.
18. NEWAZ, M.A. & N.N. NAWAL. 1999. Effect of gamma-tocotrienol on blood pressure, lipid peroxidation and total antioxidant status in spontaneously hypertensive rats (SHR). Clin. Exp. Hypert. (New York) **21:** 1297–1313.
19. MO, H. & C.E. ELSON. 1999. Apoptosis and cell-cycle arrest in human and murine tumor cells are initiated by isoprenoids. J. Nutr. **129:** 804–813.
20. MENSINK, R.P. *et al.* 1999. A vitamin E concentrate rich in tocotrienols had no effect on serum lipids, lipoproteins, or platelet function in men with mildly elevated serum lipid concentrations. Am. J. Clin. Nutr. **69:** 213–219.
21. KAKU, S. *et al.* 1999. Effect of dietary antioxidants on serum lipid contents and immunoglobulin productivity of lymphocytes in Sprague–Dawley rats. Biosci. Biotechnol. Biochem. **63:** 575–576.
22. GU, J.Y. *et al.* 1999. Dietary effect of tocopherols and tocotrienols on the immune function of spleen and mesenteric lymph node lymphocytes in Brown Norway rats. Biosci. Biotechnol. Biochem. **63:** 1697–1702.
23. NESARETNAM, K. *et al.* 1998. Tocotrienols inhibit the growth of human breast cancer cells irrespective of estrogen receptor status. Lipids **33:** 461–469.
24. HOSOMI, A. *et al.* 1997. Affinity for alpha-tocopherol transfer protein as a determinant of the biological activities of vitamin E analogs. FEBS Lett. **409:** 105–108.
25. GUTHRIE, N. *et al.* 1997. Inhibition of proliferation of estrogen receptor-negative MDA-MB-435 and -positive MCF-7 human breast cancer cells by palm oil tocotrienols and tamoxifen, alone and in combination. J. Nutr. **127:** 544S–548S.
26. HE, L. *et al.* 1997. Isoprenoids suppress the growth of murine B16 melanomas in vitro and in vivo. J. Nutr. **127:** 668–674.
27. IKEDA, I. *et al.* 1996. Lymphatic transport of alpha-, gamma- and delta-tocotrienols and alpha-tocopherol in rats. Int. J. Vit. Nutr. Res. **66:** 217–221.
28. TOMEO, A.C. *et al.* 1995. Antioxidant effects of tocotrienols in patients with hyperlipidemia and carotid stenosis. Lipids **30:** 1179–1183.
29. QURESHI, A.A. *et al.* 1995. Response of hypercholesterolemic subjects to administration of tocotrienols. Lipids **30:** 1171–1177.
30. NESARETNAM, K. *et al.* 1995. Effect of tocotrienols on the growth of a human breast cancer cell line in culture. Lipids **30:** 1139–1143.
31. KAMAT, J.P. & T.P. DEVASAGAYAM. 1995. Tocotrienols from palm oil as potent inhibitors of lipid peroxidation and protein oxidation in rat brain mitochondria. Neurosci. Lett. **195:** 179–182.

32. ELSON, C.E. & A.A. QURESHI. 1995. Coupling the cholesterol- and tumor-suppressive actions of palm oil to the impact of its minor constituents on 3-hydroxy-3-methylglutaryl coenzyme A reductase activity. Prostag. Leukotr. Essent. Fatty Acids **52:** 205–207.
33. PEARCE, B.C. et al. 1994. Inhibitors of cholesterol biosynthesis. 2. Hypocholesterolemic and antioxidant activities of benzopyran and tetrahydronaphthalene analogues of the tocotrienols. J. Med. Chem. **37:** 526–541.
34. GOH, S.H. et al. 1994. Inhibition of tumour promotion by various palm-oil tocotrienols. Int. J. Cancer **57:** 529–531.
35. WATKINS, T. et al. 1993. gamma-Tocotrienol as a hypocholesterolemic and antioxidant agent in rats fed atherogenic diets. Lipids **28:** 1113–1118.
36. SUZUKI, Y.J. et al. 1993. Structural and dynamic membrane properties of alpha-tocopherol and alpha-tocotrienol: implication to the molecular mechanism of their antioxidant potency. Biochemistry **32:** 10692–10699.
37. SUARNA, C. et al. 1993. Comparative antioxidant activity of tocotrienols and other natural lipid-soluble antioxidants in a homogeneous system, and in rat and human lipoproteins. Biochim. Biophys. Acta **1166:** 163–170.
38. RAHMAT, A. et al. 1993. Long-term administration of tocotrienols and tumor-marker enzyme activities during hepatocarcinogenesis in rats. Nutrition **9:** 229–232.
39. PARKER, R.A. et al. 1993. Tocotrienols regulate cholesterol production in mammalian cells by post-transcriptional suppression of 3-hydroxy-3-methylglutaryl-coenzyme A reductase. J. Biol. Chem. **268:** 11230–11238.
40. PEARCE, B.C. et al. 1992. Hypocholesterolemic activity of synthetic and natural tocotrienols. J. Med. Chem. **35:** 3595–3606.
41. KOBA, K. et al. 1992. Effects of alpha-tocopherol and tocotrienols on blood pressure and linoleic acid metabolism in the spontaneously hypertensive rat (SHR). Biosci. Biotechnol. Biochem. **56:** 1420–1423.
42. KAGAN, V.E. et al. 1992. Recycling of vitamin E in human low density lipoproteins. J. Lipid Res. **33:** 385–397.
43. SERBINOVA, E. et al. 1991. Free radical recycling and intramembrane mobility in the antioxidant properties of alpha-tocopherol and alpha-tocotrienol. Free Radic. Biol. Med. **10:** 263–275.
44. QURESHI, A.A. et al. 1991. Lowering of serum cholesterol in hypercholesterolemic humans by tocotrienols (palmvitee). Am. J. Clin. Nutr. **53:** 1021S–1026S.
45. TAN, D.T. et al. 1991. Effect of a palm-oil-vitamin E concentrate on the serum and lipoprotein lipids in humans. Am. J. Clin. Nutr. **53:** 1027S–1030S.
46. QURESHI, A.A. et al. 1991. Dietary tocotrienols reduce concentrations of plasma cholesterol, apolipoprotein B, thromboxane B2, and platelet factor 4 in pigs with inherited hyperlipidemias. Am. J. Clin. Nutr. **53:** 1042S–1046S.
47. NGAH, W.Z. et al. 1991. Effect of tocotrienols on hepatocarcinogenesis induced by 2-acetylaminofluorene in rats. Am. J. Clin. Nutr. **53:** 1076S–1081S.
48. GOULD, M.N. et al. 1991. A comparison of tocopherol and tocotrienol for the chemoprevention of chemically induced rat mammary tumors. Am. J. Clin. Nutr. **53:** 1068S–1070S.
49. SUNDRAM, K. et al. 1989. Effect of dietary palm oils on mammary carcinogenesis in female rats induced by 7,12-dimethylbenz(a)anthracene. Cancer Res. **49:** 1447–1451.
50. KOMIYAMA, K. et al. 1989. Studies on the biological activity of tocotrienols. Chem. Pharmaceut. Bull. **37:** 1369–1371.
51. QURESHI, A.A. et al. 1986. The structure of an inhibitor of cholesterol biosynthesis isolated from barley. J. Biol. Chem. **261:** 10544–10550.
52. SERBINOVA, E.A. & L. PACKER. 1994. Antioxidant properties of alpha-tocopherol and alpha-tocotrienol. Methods Enzymol. **234:** 354–366.
53. BANNAI, S. et al. 1984. Amino acid transport systems [letter]. Nature **311:** 308.
54. SEN, C.K. 1997. Nutritional biochemistry of cellular glutathione. J. Nutr. Biochem. **8:** 660–672.
55. SATO, H. et al. 1998. Induction of cystine transport via system x-c and maintenance of intracellular glutathione levels in pancreatic acinar and islet cell lines. Biochim. Biophys. Acta **1414:** 85–94.

56. DROGE, W., H.P. ECK & S. MIHM. 1992. HIV-induced cysteine deficiency and T-cell dysfunction: a rationale for treatment with N-acetylcysteine. Immunol. Today **13:** 211–214.
57. DROGE, W. et al. 1994. Functions of glutathione and glutathione disulfide in immunology and immunopathology. FASEB J. **8:** 1131–1138.
58. SEN, C.K. et al. 1997. Regulation of cellular thiols in human lymphocytes by alpha-lipoic acid: a flow cytometric analysis. Free Radic. Biol. Med. **22:** 1241–1257.
59. HAN, D. et al. 1997. Lipoic acid increases de novo synthesis of cellular glutathione by improving cystine utilization. Biofactors **6:** 321–338.
60. SEN, C.K., S. ROY & L. PACKER. 1998. Oxidants and antioxidants in glutamate induced cytotoxicity. In Biological Oxidants and Antioxidants: Molecular Mechanisms and Health Effects. L. Packer & A.S. Ong, Eds.: 5–13. AOCS Press. Champaign, IL.
61. COYLE, J.T. & P. PUTTFARCKEN. 1993. Oxidative stress, glutamate, and neurodegenerative disorders. Science **262:** 689–695.
62. CHOI, D.W. 1990. Methods for antagonizing glutamate neurotoxicity. Cerebrovasc. Brain Metab. Rev. **2:** 105–147.
63. TAN, S. et al. 1998. The regulation of reactive oxygen species production during programmed cell death. J. Cell Biol. **141:** 1423–1432.
64. MURPHY, T.H., R.L. SCHNAAR & J.T. COYLE. 1990. Immature cortical neurons are uniquely sensitive to glutamate toxicity by inhibition of cystine uptake. FASEB J. **4:** 1624–1633.
65. KATO, S. et al. 1992. A mechanism for glutamate toxicity in the C6 glioma cells involving inhibition of cystine uptake leading to glutathione depletion. Neuroscience **48:** 903–914.
66. HAN, D. et al. 1997. Protection against glutamate-induced cytotoxicity in C6 glial cells by thiol antioxidants. Am. J. Physiol. **273:** R1771–R1778.
67. PEREIRA, C.M. & C.R. OLIVEIRA. 1997. Glutamate toxicity on a PC12 cell line involves glutathione (GSH) depletion and oxidative stress. Free Radic. Biol. Med. **23:** 637–647.
68. FROISSARD, P., H. MONROCQ & D. DUVAL. 1997. Role of glutathione metabolism in the glutamate-induced programmed cell death of neuronal-like PC12 cells. Eur. J. Pharmacol. **326:** 93–99.
69. OKA, A. et al. 1993. Vulnerability of oligodendroglia to glutamate: pharmacology, mechanisms, and prevention. J. Neurosci. **13:** 1441–1453.
70. SCHUBERT, D., H. KIMURA & P. MAHER. 1992. Growth factors and vitamin E modify neuronal glutamate toxicity. Proc. Natl. Acad. Sci. USA **89:** 8264–8267.
71. LI, Y., P. MAHER & D. SCHUBERT. 1997. Requirement for cGMP in nerve cell death caused by glutathione depletion. J. Cell. Biol. **139:** 1317–1324.
72. LI, Y., P. MAHER & D. SCHUBERT. 1997. A role for 12-lipoxygenase in nerve cell death caused by glutathione depletion. Neuron **19:** 453–463.
73. LI, Y., P. MAHER & D. SCHUBERT. 1998. Phosphatidylcholine-specific phospholipase C regulates glutamate-induced nerve cell death. Proc. Natl. Acad. Sci. USA **95:** 7748–7753.
74. SAGARA, Y. et al. 1998. Cellular mechanisms of resistance to chronic oxidative stress. Free Radic. Biol. Med. **24:** 1375–1389.
75. MAHER, P. & D. SCHUBERT. 2000. Signaling by reactive oxygen species in the nervous system. Cell. Mol. Life Sci. **57:** 1287–1305.
76. POST, A., F. HOLSBOER & C. BEHL. 1998. Induction of NF-kappaB activity during haloperidol-induced oxidative toxicity in clonal hippocampal cells: suppression of NF-kappaB and neuroprotection by antioxidants. J. Neurosci. **18:** 8236–8246.
77. BEHL, C. 1998. Effects of glucocorticoids on oxidative stress-induced hippocampal cell death: implications for the pathogenesis of Alzheimer's disease. Exp. Gerontol. **33:** 689–696.
78. SATOH, T. et al. 2000. Neuroprotection by MAPK/ERK kinase inhibition with U0126 against oxidative stress in a mouse neuronal cell line and rat primary cultured cortical neurons. Neurosci. Lett. **288:** 163–166.
79. VEDDER, H. et al. 2000. Characterization of the neuroprotective effects of estrogens on hydrogen peroxide-induced cell death in hippocampal HT22 cells: time and dose dependency. Exp. Clin. Endocrinol. Diabetes **108:** 120–127.

80. STANCIU, M. et al. 2000. Persistent activation of ERK contributes to glutamate-induced oxidative toxicity in a neuronal cell line and primary cortical neuron cultures. J. Biol. Chem. **275:** 12200–12206.
81. XIAO, N. et al. 1999. Geldanamycin provides posttreatment protection against glutamate-induced oxidative toxicity in a mouse hippocampal cell line. J. Neurochem. **72:** 95–101.
82. MORIMOTO, B.H. & D.E. KOSHLAND, JR. 1990. Excitatory amino acid uptake and N-methyl-D-aspartate-mediated secretion in a neural cell line. Proc. Natl. Acad. Sci. USA **87:** 3518–3521.
83. TIROSH, O. et al. 1999. Neuroprotective effects of alpha-lipoic acid and its positively charged amide analogue. Free Radic. Biol. Med. **26:** 1418–1426.
84. O'BYRNE, D. et al. 1999. Supplementation with alpha-tocotrienyl acetate enhances LDL oxidative resistance without lowering serum cholesterol in hypercholesterolemic humans. FASEB J. **13:** A536.
85. O'BYRNE, D. et al. 2000. Studies of LDL oxidation following alpha-, gamma-, or delta-tocotrienyl acetate supplementation of hypercholesterolemic humans. Free Radic. Biol. Med. **29:** 834–845.
86. KHANNA, S. et al. 2003. Molecular basis of vitamin E action: tocotrienol modulates 12-lipoxygenase, a key mediator of glutamate-induced neurodegeneration. J. Biol. Chem. Epub Aug 13.
87. BRUGGE, J.S. et al. 1985. Neurones express high levels of a structurally modified, activated form of pp60c-src. Nature **316:** 554–557.
88. LAVOIE, J.N. et al. 2000. Adenovirus E4 open reading frame 4-induced apoptosis involves dysregulation of Src family kinases. J. Cell Biol. **150:** 1037–1056.
89. IMPEY, S., K. OBRIETAN & D. R. STORM. 1999. Making new connections: role of ERK/MAP kinase signaling in neuronal plasticity. Neuron **23:** 11–14.
90. XIA, Z. et al. 1995. Opposing effects of ERK and JNK-p38 MAP kinases on apoptosis. Science **270:** 1326–1331.
91. SEGAL, R.A & M.E. GREENBERG. 1996. Intracellular signaling pathways activated by neurotrophic factors. Annu. Rev. Neurosci **19:** 463–489.
92. BOULTON, T.G. et al. 1991. ERKs: a family of protein-serine/threonine kinases that are activated and tyrosine phosphorylated in response to insulin and NGF. Cell **65:** 663–675.
93. CREEDON, D.J., E.M. JOHNSON & J.C. LAWRENCE. 1996. Mitogen-activated protein kinase-independent pathways mediate the effects of nerve growth factor and cAMP on neuronal survival. J. Biol. Chem. **271:** 20713–20718.
94. MURRAY, B. et al. 1998. Inhibition of the p44/42 MAP kinase pathway protects hippocampal neurons in a cell-culture model of seizure activity. Proc. Natl. Acad. Sci. USA **95:** 11975–11980.
95. RUNDEN, E. et al. 1998. Regional selective neuronal degeneration after protein phosphatase inhibition in hippocampal slice cultures: evidence for a MAP kinase-dependent mechanism. J. Neurosci. **18:** 7296–7305.
96. BHAT, N.R. & P. ZHANG. 1999. Hydrogen peroxide activation of multiple mitogen-activated protein kinases in an oligodendrocyte cell line: role of extracellular signal-regulated kinase in hydrogen peroxide-induced cell death. J. Neurochem. **72:** 112–119.
97. KUMMER, J.L., P.K. RAO & K.A. HEIDENREICH. 1997. Apoptosis induced by withdrawal of trophic factors is mediated by p38 mitogen-activated protein kinase. J. Biol. Chem. **272:** 20490–20494.
98. ALESSANDRINI, A. et al. 1999. MEK1 protein kinase inhibition protects against damage resulting from focal cerebral ischemia. Proc. Natl. Acad. Sci. USA **96:** 12866–12869.
99. SUGDEN, P.H. & A. CLERK. 1997. Regulation of the ERK subgroup of MAP kinase cascades through G protein-coupled receptors. Cell. Signal. **9:** 337–351.
100. AIKAWA, R. et al. 1997. Oxidative stress activates extracellular signal-regulated kinases through Src and Ras in cultured cardiac myocytes of neonatal rats. J. Clin. Invest. **100:** 1813–1821.
101. BENARD, O., Z. NAOR & R. SEGER. 2001. Role of dynamin, Src and Ras in the protein kinase C-mediated activation of ERK by gonadotropin-releasing hormone. J. Biol. Chem. **276:** 4554–4563.

102. DAULHAC, L. et al. 1999. Src-family tyrosine kinases in activation of ERK-1 and p85/ p110-phosphatidylinositol 3-kinase by G/CCKB receptors. J. Biol. Chem. **274:** 20657–20663.
103. MIGLIACCIO, A. et al. 1998. Activation of the Src/p21ras/Erk pathway by progesterone receptor via cross-talk with estrogen receptor. EMBO J. **17:** 2008–2018.
104. DRINGEN, R., J.M. GUTTERER & J. HIRRLINGER. 2000. Glutathione metabolism in brain metabolic interaction between astrocytes and neurons in the defense against reactive oxygen species. Eur. J. Biochem. **267:** 4912–4916.
105. BAINS, J.S. & C.A. SHAW. 1997. Neurodegenerative disorders in humans: the role of glutathione in oxidative stress-mediated neuronal death. Brain Res. Brain Res. Rev. **25:** 335–358.
106. LEPLEY, R.A., D.T. MUSKARDIN & F.A. FITZPATRICK. 1996. Tyrosine kinase activity modulates catalysis and translocation of cellular 5-lipoxygenase. J. Biol. Chem. **271:** 6179–6184.
107. CAPODICI, C. et al. 1998. Integrin-dependent homotypic adhesion of neutrophils: arachidonic acid activates Raf-1/Mek/Erk via a 5-lipoxygenase- dependent pathway. J. Clin. Invest. **102:** 165–175.
108. SZEKERES, C.K. et al. 2000. Eicosanoid activation of extracellular signal-regulated kinase1/2 in human epidermoid carcinoma cells. J. Biol. Chem. **275:** 38831–38841.
109. TRAN, K., P.R. PROULX & A.C. CHAN. 1994. Vitamin E suppresses diacylglycerol (DAG) level in thrombin-stimulated endothelial cells through an increase of DAG kinase activity. Biochim. Biophys. Acta **1212:** 193–202.
110. STEPHENSON, D.T. et al. 1996. Cytosolic phospholipase A2 (cPLA2) immunoreactivity is elevated in Alzheimer's disease brain. Neurobiol. Dis. **3:** 51–63.
111. KANFER, J.N. et al. 1996. Phospholipid metabolism in Alzheimer's disease and in a human cholinergic cell. J. Lipid Med. Cell Signal. **14:** 361–363.
112. ERIN, A.N. et al. 1986. Stabilization of synaptic membranes by alpha-tocopherol against the damaging action of phospholipases: possible mechanism of biological action of vitamin E. Brain Res. **398:** 85–90.
113. PODDA, M. et al. 1996. Simultaneous determination of tissue tocopherols, tocotrienols, ubiquinols, and ubiquinones. J. Lipid Res. **37:** 893–901.
114. THIELE, J.J. et al. 1997. Ozone depletes tocopherols and tocotrienols topically applied to murine skin. FEBS Lett. **401:** 167–170.
115. WEBER, C. et al. 1997. Efficacy of topically applied tocopherols and tocotrienols in protection of murine skin from oxidative damage induced by UV irradiation. Free Radic. Biol. Med. **22:** 761–769.
116. NESARETNAM, K. et al. 1993. Influence of palm oil or its tocotrienol-rich fraction on the lipid peroxidation potential of rat liver mitochondria and microsomes. Biochem. Mol. Biol. Int. **30:** 159–167.
117. ROY, S. et al. 2002. Simultaneous detection of tocopherols and tocotrienols in biological samples using HPLC-coulometric electrode array. Methods Enzymol. **352:** 326–332.
118. ROY, S. et al. 2002. Vitamin E sensitive genes in the developing rat fetal brain: a high-density oligonucleotide microarray analysis. FEBS Lett. **530:** 17–23.
119. RICCIARELLI, R. et al. 1998. alpha-Tocopherol specifically inactivates cellular protein kinase C alpha by changing its phosphorylation state. Biochem. J. **334:** 243–249.
120. LIEBECQ, C. 1992. Biochemical Nomenclature and Related Documents. IUPAC-IUBMB Joint Commission on Biochemical Nomenclature and Nomenclature Commission of IUBMB347.

Tocotrienol-Rich Fraction from Palm Oil and Gene Expression in Human Breast Cancer Cells

KALANITHI NESARETNAM,[a] ROBERTO AMBRA,[b]
KANGA RANI SELVADURAY,[a] AMMU RADHAKRISHNAN,[c]
RAFFAELLA CANALI,[b] AND FABIO VIRGILI[b]

[a]*Malaysian Palm Oil Board, 6 Persiaran Institusi, Bandar Baru Bangi, 4300 Selangor, Malaysia*

[b]*National Institute for Food and Nutrition Research, Rome, Italy*

[c]*International Medical University, Kuala Lumpur, Malaysia*

ABSTRACT: Vitamin E is important not only for its cellular antioxidant and lipid-lowering properties, but also as an antiproliferating agent. It has also been shown to contribute to immunoregulation, antibody production, and resistance to implanted tumors. It has recently been shown that tocotrienols are the components of vitamin E responsible for growth inhibition in human breast cancer cells *in vitro* as well as *in vivo* through estrogen-independent mechanisms. Although tocotrienols act on cell proliferation in a dose-dependent manner and can induce programmed cell death, no specific gene regulation has yet been identified. In order to investigate the molecular basis of the effect of a tocotrienol-rich fraction (TRF) from palm oil, we performed a cDNA array analysis of cancer-related gene expression in estrogen-dependent (MCF-7) and estrogen-independent (MDA-MB-231) human breast cancer cells. The human breast cancer cells were incubated with or without 8 μg/mL of tocotrienols for 72 h. RNA was subsequently extracted and subjected to reverse transcription before being hybridized onto cancer arrays. Tocotrienol supplementation modulated significantly 46 out of 1200 genes in MDA-MB-231 cells. In MCF-7 cells, tocotrienol administration was associated with a lower number of affected genes. Interestingly, only three were affected in a similar fashion in both cell lines: c-myc binding protein MM-1, 23-kDa highly basic protein, and interferon-inducible protein 9-27 (IFITM-1). These proteins are most likely involved in the cell cycle and can exert inhibitory effects on cell growth and differentiation of the tumor cell lines. These data suggest that tocotrienols are able to affect cell homeostasis, possibly independent of their antioxidant activity.

KEYWORDS: vitamin E; tocopherols; tocotrienols; human breast cancer cells; gene expression

INTRODUCTION

The pathogenesis of many diseases can involve free radical–mediated lipid peroxidation of biological membranes. Vitamin E compounds are recognized as important antioxidants that regulate peroxidation reactions and function by quenching free radicals or reacting with their products.[1,2] Uncontrolled production of free radicals are associated with damage to cell structures and functions. Epidemiological studies indicate that vitamin E, alone or in combination with other antioxidants are associated with a decreased incidence of various disorders such as atherosclerosis and certain forms of cancer,[3] including breast cancer.[4] Vitamin E is a generic term that refers to an entire class of compounds that are further divided into two subgroups called tocopherols and tocotrienols. Just as there are several forms of tocopherol (α, β, γ, and δ), there are also α-, β-, γ-, and δ-tocotrienols. Tocopherols are commonly found in high concentrations in vegetable oils, animal fats, grains, vegetables, and fruits,[5] whereas tocotrienols are relatively rare and found in appreciable levels only in a few specific vegetable fats such as palm oil and rice bran oil.[6] Previous studies have demonstrated that dietary intake of palm oil, in contrast to other high-fat diets, suppressed carcinogen-induced mammary tumorigenesis in experimental animals.[7–9] Similarly, dietary supplementation with TRF has also been shown to inhibit mammary tumorigenesis.[10] However, if tocotrienols are removed from palm oil, protective effects of high palm oil diets against mammary tumorigenesis were no longer observed.[10]

Recent work has shown that tocotrienols can exert direct inhibitory effects on cell growth in human breast cancer cell lines *in vitro*[11–15] and that inhibitory effects occurred irrespective of estrogen receptor status of the cells.[12] The inhibitory effect on cell growth was more pronounced with γ- and δ-tocotrienols.[12,13] The mechanism of action is unknown, with previous data suggesting that action does not reside in antagonism of estrogen action or in alterations to growth-inhibitory insulin-like growth factor binding proteins in MCF-7 cells.[12] α-Tocopherol itself has no inhibitory action on breast cancer cell growth,[11–13] but work with α-tocopheryl succinate has shown growth-inhibitory effects.[16,17] Suggested mechanisms of action range from adenylate cyclase/AMP protein pathways,[18,19] to actions on protein kinase C,[20] to induction of apoptosis through transforming growth factor beta[16,17,21] through AP1/Jun[22,23] or through Fas signaling.[24]

The exact reason why tocotrienols display greater anticancer activity than tocopherols is still under investigation. Tocopherols and tocotrienols have the same basic structure, characterized by a long phytyl chain attached at the 1 position of a chromanol ring structure. However, tocopherols have a saturated phytyl chain while tocotrienols have an unsaturated phytyl chain. It is possible that the level of saturation may be critical in determining the antiproliferative activity of tocopherols and tocotrienols.

Changes in the rates of cell proliferation and death play an important role in initiation and progression of chronic disease and utilize constitutive and signaling pathways. To further understand the molecular basis of some of these effects, we performed a cDNA array analysis of cancer-related gene expression in estrogen-dependent (MCF-7) and estrogen-independent (MDA-MB-231) human breast cancer cells supplemented with tocotrienols.

MATERIALS AND METHODS)

Isolation of Tocotrienol-Rich Fraction

The tocotrienol-rich fraction (TRF) was obtained from Golden Hope Plantation (Malaysia). Extraction of TRF from palm oil has been described by Sundram and Gapor.[25] In brief: palm oil fatty acid distillate was converted into methyl esters by esterification. The methyl esters were then removed by distillation, leaving a vitamin E concentrate. This was further concentrated by crystallization and passed through an ion-exchange column to give 60–70% pure vitamin E. Further purification was achieved by washing and then drying the concentrate followed by a second molecular distillation stage. The final purity of the vitamin E preparation, TRF, was 95–99%.

Culture of Stock Cells

MCF-7 human breast cancer cells were kindly provided by Dr. K. Osborne at passage number 390.[26] Stock cells were grown as monolayer cultures in Dulbecco's modified Eagle's medium (DMEM) supplemented with 5% fetal calf serum (FCS, Gibco, BRL Life Technologies Incorporated, Grand Island, NY), 10^{-8} M estradiol, in a humidified atmosphere of 5% carbon dioxide in 95% air at 37°C. Cells were subcultured at weekly intervals by suspension with 0.06% trypsin/0.02% EDTA (pH 7.3). MDA-MB-231 human breast cancer cells were obtained from the American Tissue Culture Collection (Manassas, VA). The cells were maintained in monolayer culture in DMEM supplemented with 10% FCS. Cells were synchronized for cell cycle prior to start of experiments.

RNA Isolation and Purification

Cells were plated onto 75-cm^2 plastic tissue culture flasks in 16-mL aliquots of phenol red–free RPMI 1640 medium with 5% Dextran charcoal-coated fetal calf serum (DCFCS). After 24 h, the medium was changed to phenol red–free RPMI 1640 medium containing 5% DCFCS with or without 10^{-8} M estradiol or 8 µg/mL TRF for 72 h. Estradiol was dissolved in ethanol and TRF in dimethyl sulfoxide. Control cultures contained the same volume of dimethyl sulfoxide or ethanol vehicle alone.

Total RNA was extracted from cells using the Trizol solution (Life Technologies) according to manufacturer's instructions with some minor modifications. Tissues and cells were homogenized in Trizol solution and incubated for 15 min at room temperature. After the addition of 20% volume of chloroform, homogenates were vortexed for 2 min and centrifuged at $12,000 \times g$ for 20 min at 4°C. The resulting inorganic phase was subjected to three extractions with acid-phenol:chloroform:isoamyl-alcohol (125:24:1, AMBION) and one extraction with chloroform. RNA was precipitated overnight at 4°C with 0.75 volumes of 7.5 M LiCl and then centrifuged at $12,000 \times g$ for 10 min at 4°C. The pellet was resuspended in 400 mL distilled water, reprecipitated with 40 mL 3 M Na-acetate (pH 5.2) and 1 mL ethanol and washed with 70% ethanol. RNA integrity was checked by denaturing gel electrophoresis. Before labeling, total RNA was treated with 25 units of DNase I to remove any contaminating DNA.

cDNA Labeling and Atlas™ Cancer Array Membrane Hybridization, Exposure and Analysis

Atlas™ Human Cancer cDNA Expression Arrays (Cat. #7851-1) were purchased from Clontech Laboratories Inc. Array membranes contained 10 ng of each gene-specific cDNA from 1176 known genes and 9 housekeeping genes (see <http://www.clontech.com> for the complete list of genes). Poly A+ RNA enrichment, cDNA Probe Synthesis and purification were performed using the Atlas Pure RNA Labeling system (Clontech) following the manufacturer's instructions, starting from 50 mg total RNA and using [α-32P]dATP (NEN). Membrane arrays were hybridized for 18 h at 68°C into rolling bottles with 5 mL ExpressHyb hybridization solution (Clontech) containing the denatured probes (10 × 106 cpm) and 5 mg Cot-1 DNA. Membranes were then washed in bottles for 2 h at 68°C in 2 × SSC, 1% SDS with three changes of solutions, and for 30 min at 68°C in 0.1 × SSC, 0.5% SDS. Finally, membranes were rinsed in 2 × SSC at room temperature and exposed to X-ray films (Kodak Biomax or Amersham MP) at −70° for 1 to 6 days. Films were acquired with a scanner for transparencies and images analyzed with the AtlasImage software (Version 2.01, Clontech). Software analysis results were confirmed by eye-inspection of hybridization signals to ensure reliability. Since tocotrienols were found to modulate the expression of one of the housekeeping genes included in the array (see RESULTS), a global gene-normalization method was preferred. In such a method, the normalization coefficient is calculated using the average value of all genes in the array, instead of the expression of housekeeping genes.

Reproducibility and Precision Limits

Previous studies addressing the application of cDNA array indicated that the coefficient of variation for differential gene expression in cultured cells is 10–15%.[27] Studies on the reproducibility and variability of array results indicate that a two-fold or greater difference in the expression of a particular gene is to be considered a real difference in transcript abundance.[28,29] A difference in gene expression between the TRF-treated samples and controls was therefore considered significant, at a ratio of two folds or more and if both readings had a signal intensity above 2500 units. Data discussed herein were confirmed by Northern hybridization technique (see below).

Northern Hybridization

Total RNA (10 mg) separated through electrophoresis in 1.2% agarose gels were blotted onto Genescreen-N nylon membranes (Dupont) and hybridized according to the manufacturer's instructions. Gene transcripts of MIC-1, CD74/Ii, IFITM-1, and 23-kDa HBP were detected using [α-^{32}P]dATP (NEN) random-primed (Boehringer) DNA ampliclones obtained by PCR using sequence-specific primers (see TABLE 1 for sequences). Normalization of gene expression was achieved by hybridization of the same membranes with a labeled PCR fragment of the GAPDH gene. The Scion Image® software was used for quantification of the transcripts' relative abundance.

TABLE 1. Nucleotide sequences (from 5′ to 3′) of primers used for the preparation of probes in Northern hybridizations

	Forward	Reverse
MIC1	CGC GCA ACG GGG ACC ACT	TGA GCA CCA TGG GAT TGT AGC
CD74/Ii	ACC TCA TCC CAT GAG ACC TG	TCC AAA ACA TTG GCT CTT CC
IFITM-1	TGC ACA AGG AGG AAC ATG AG	TGA ATC CAA TGG TCA TGA GG
23-kDa HBP	GGA CCG TCT CAA GGT GTT TG	GTG GGT CTT GAG GAC CTC TG
GAPDH	TGA AGG TCG GAG TCA ACG GAT TTG G	CAT GTG GGC CAT GAG GTC CAC CAC

RESULTS

Effect of TRF Supplementation on Gene Expression in Cultured MCF-7 and MDA-MB-231 Human Breast Cancer Cells

In order to analyze the molecular basis of the response to TRF in the breast cancer cell lines, the differential expression of 1176 genes was investigated by cDNA array analysis. We report here that the supplementation with TRF from palm oil was able to significantly modulate 46 of 277 genes displaying a reliable signal intensity in MDA-MB-231 cells (22 upregulated and 24 genes downregulated) (TABLE 2). A lower number of genes were affected in the MCF-7 cells (21 of the 268 detectable genes) where 3 genes were upregulated and 18 genes were downregulated. The complete list of significant changes in gene expression after supplementation with tocotrienols in both cultured cell lines is presented in TABLE 2. They have been classified into 14 functional groups according to the putative function of the encoded protein, although data discussed hereafter focus on a selected subsample of genes involved in cell cycle control and immune response.

Only three significantly modulated genes were shared by the two cell lines, namely, the c-myc binding protein MM-1, the 23-kDa highly basic protein (23-kDa HBP), and the interferon-inducible protein 9-27 (IFITM-1). Such results suggest a complex response of tumor cells; also that different pathways are likely to be involved in the previously observed growth inhibition by tocotrienols in MCF-7 and MDA-MB-231 cells.[12,13] However, these three genes were regulated in the same way in both cell lines: IFITM-1 was downregulated whereas c-myc binding protein MM-1 and 23-kDa HBP were upregulated. Moreover, an analysis of gene effects including those that do not reach the two-fold threshold (see METHODS) shows that the most significant changes detected in one cell line are likely induced in the other (FIG. 1).

The largest functional group of genes modulated in our system is that coding for extracellular cell signaling proteins: of the 46 genes displaying significant differential expression in MDA-MB-231 cells, 12 genes code for such proteins. In particular, 5 genes were found upregulated and 7 downregulated. Within this group, only one gene was detected as significantly modulated in MCF-7 cells, the insulin-like growth factor binding protein 4 precursor (IGFBP4) gene (TABLE 2). IGFB family members regulate and modify the insulin-like growth factor 1 actions.[30] The finding that TRF treatment is associated with a significant reduction of IGFB4 gene expression in MCF-7 cells could indicate that proliferation-inhibitory properties of TRF could rely on their effect on IGFB4. Similarly, growth inhibition of MCF-7 cells by antiestro-

TABLE 2. Changes in gene expression in the two cell lines (MCF-7 and MDA-MB-231 cells) treated with TRF versus control

	Genbank	MDA-MB-231	MCF-7
Cell cycle			
Growth inhibitory factor; metallothionein-III (MT-III)	D13365; M93311	+0.51	−1.09
G2/mitotic-specific cyclin B1 (CCNB1)	M25753	low	−1.32
Cell division protein kinase 5 (CDK5); tau protein kinase II catalytic subunit (TPKII catalytic subunit); PSSALRE protein kinase	X66364	−1.06	−0.51
Cyclin-dependent kinase 4 inhibitor D (CDKN2D); p19-INK4D	U40343; U20498	−1.06	low
Extracellular signal–regulated kinase 3 (ERK3); MAP kinase 3 (MAPK3; p97-MAPK); PRKM5	X80692	low	−1.15
Cyclin-dependent kinase inhibitor 1 (CDKN1A); melanoma differentiation–associated protein 6; CDK-interacting protein 1 (CIP1); WAF1	U09579; L25610	−0.34	−1.36
CDC25B; CDC25HU2; M-phase inducer phosphatase 2	M81934; S78187	low	−1.43
23-kDa highly basic protein; 60S ribosomal protein L13A (RPL13A)	X56932	+1.22	+1.49
Oncogenes and tumor suppressors			
IFITM-1 (interferon-inducible protein 9–27)	J04164	−1.74	−1.29
c-*myc* binding protein MM-1	D89667	+1.48	+1.01
Myelodysplasia/myeloid leukemia factor 2 (MLF2)	U57342	+1.05	−0.22
Nucleoside diphosphate kinase A (NDKA); tumor metastatic process–associated protein; metastasis inhibition factor NM23 (NM23-H1)	X17620	+1.49	+0.06
B-myb	X13293	low	−1.22
Cullin homologue 2 (CUL2)	U83410	−1.25	low
Active breakpoint cluster region–related protein	U01147	−1.32	+0.01
Apoptosis-associated proteins and DNA binding and damage signaling/repair proteins			
Growth arrest & DNA-damage–inducible protein 153 (GADD153); DNA-damage–inducible transcript 3 (DDIT3); CHOP	S40706; S62138	+1.57	+0.16
Damage-specific DNA binding protein p48 subunit (DDBB P48); implicated in xeroderma pigmentosum group E (DDB2)	U18300	low	−1.25
High-mobility group protein (HMG-I)	M23619	+1.23	−0.09
Nuclear protein	X83703	+1.76	low

TABLE 2. (*continued*) Changes in gene expression in the two cell lines (MCF-7 and MDA-MB-231 cells) treated with TRF versus control

	Genbank	MDA-MB-231	MCF-7
Immune system proteins			
HLA-DR antigen–associated invariant subunit (CD74/Ii ANTIGEN)	X00497	−1.32	low
FC-epsilon-receptor gamma subunit	M33195	−1.60	low
Lymphoid-restricted membrane protein	U10485	−1.09	low
Macrophage inhibitory cytokine 1 (MIC1)	AF019770	+3.05	+0.14
Extracellular cell signaling and cell receptors			
Neurotrophin-3 precursor (NT-3); neurotrophic factor (HDNF); nerve growth factor 2 (NGF-2)	X53655; M37763	−1.09	+0.21
Glial cell line–derived neurotropic factor precursor (GDNF)	L19063	−1.36	low
Secretogranin I precursor (SGI); chromogranin B	Y00064	−1.15	low
Glia-activating factor precursor (GAF); fibroblast growth factor 9 (FGF9); HBGF9	D14838	+1.02	low
Vascular endothelial growth factor precursor (VEGF); vascular permeability factor (VPF)	M32977; M27281	+1.21	+0.08
Heparin-binding growth factor 2 precursor (HBGF2); prostatropin; basic fibroblast growth factor (BFGF; FGFB; FGF2)	M27968	−1.29	low
CYR61 protein (cysteine-rich, angiogenic inducer, 61)	AF031385	+1.38	low
Jagged 1 (HJ1)	AF028593	−1.03	low
Wnt-5A	L20861	+1.26	low
DNAX activation protein 12	AF019562	−1.43	low
Cytokine receptor class II CRF2-4 precursor	Z17227	−1.22	low
Insulin-like growth factor binding protein 4 precursor (IGF-binding protein 4; IGFBP4; IBP4)	M62403	low	−1.15
Intracellular transducers/effectors/modulators			
B-cell receptor-associated protein (hBAP)	U72511	+1.21	+0.31
SH3-binding protein 2	AF000936	+1.40	low
Serine/threonine protein kinase KRS2	U60207	+1.88	low
Protein phosphatase with EF-hands-2 long form (PPEF2)	AF023456	−1.15	low
Tyrosine kinase receptor tie-1 precursor	X60957; S89716	low	−1.06
Transcription activators/repressors			
E2F-3	Y10479	−1.18	low
Retinoic acid receptor alpha 1 (RAR-alpha 1; RARA) + PML-RAR protein	X06538; X06614 + M73779	low	−1.40

TABLE 2. (*continued*) Changes in gene expression in the two cell lines (MCF-7 and MDA-MB-231 cells) treated with TRF versus control

	Genbank	MDA-MB-231	MCF-7
Early growth response protein 1 (hEGR1); transcription factor ETR103; KROX24; zinc finger protein 225; AT225	X52541; M62829	−0.04	**+1.15**
Stress response proteins			
(2′–5′)Oligoadenylate synthetase 1 [(2–5′)oligo(A) synthetase 1; 2–5A synthetase 1]	M11810	low	**−1.47**
(2′–5′)Oligoadenylate synthetase 2 [(2–5′)oligo(A) synthetase 2; 2–5A synthetase 2]	M87434	low	**−1.60**
Glutathione synthetase (GSH synthetase; GSH-S); glutathione synthase	U34683	**−1.06**	−0.23
Glutathione-S-transferase (GST) homologue	U90313	**+1.44**	−0.22
Translation proteins			
Ribosomal protein S21 (RPS21)	L04483	**+1.06**	+0.52
Elongation factor 1 alpha (EF1 alpha)	M27364	**+1.80**	+0.82
Protein turnover			
Cathepsin D precursor (CTSD)	M11233	−0.34	**−1.00**
Placental protein 11 precursor (PP11)	M32402	**+1.41**	low
Leukocyte elastase inhibitor (LEI); monocyte/neutrophil elastase inhibitor) (EI)	M93056	**−1.00**	+0.92
Matrix metalloproteinase 14 precursor (MMP14); membrane-type matrix metalloproteinase 1 (MT-MMP1); MMP-X1	D26512; X83535	**−1.15**	low
Matrix metalloproteinase 16 precursor (MMP16); membrane-type matrix metalloproteinase 3 (MT-MMP3); MMP-X2	D50477	**−1.06**	low
Metabolism			
Fatty acid synthase	S80437	−0.12	**−1.60**
DR-nm23	U29656	**+1.26**	+0.31
Cell adhesion proteins			
Thrombospondin 2 precursor (THBS2; TSP2)	L12350	**−1.06**	−0.76
Integrin alpha 7B precursor (IGA7B)	X74295	**−1.51**	−0.12
Desmocollin 3A/3B precursor (DSC3) + desmocollin 4 (DSC4)	X83929 + D17427	**−1.12**	low
Membrane channels and transporters			
ADP/ATP carrier protein	J02683	**+2.62**	+0.55
Trafficking and extracellular matrix proteins			
Vitronectin precursor (VTN); serum spreading factor; S-protein	X03168	−0.56	**−1.12**

TABLE 2. (*continued*) Changes in gene expression in the two cell lines (MCF-7 and MDA-MB-231 cells) treated with TRF versus control

	Genbank	MDA-MB-231	MCF-7
Interferon-regulated resistance GTP-binding protein MXA (IFI-78K); interferon-induced protein P78	M33882	−0.23	**−2.74**
Importin beta 1 subunit; karyopherin beta 1 subunit; importin 90; nuclear factor p97	L38951	**+1.30**	low
Type I cytoskeletal 10 keratin; cytokeratin 10 (K10)	M19156	low	**−1.00**

NOTE: Values are expressed as the $\log_2$ of the ratio between treated versus control. The $\log_2$ is used to make the changes symmetric and closer to a normal distribution. Effects on gene expression considered significant are > +1.00 (equal to a twofold increase) and < −1.00 (equal to a twofold decrease) are indicated in boldface. Low = signal too low for calculation.

gens is associated with reduced levels of IGFB4 in the conditioned medium.[31] On the other hand, in this cell line we also found that within the group of genes encoding for cell cycle regulators, five genes were found to be downregulated after supplementation with TRF (TABLE 2).

Four immune-related genes were found modulated in MDA-MB-231 cells: the MHC class 11–associated invariant chain (CD74/Ii), the FC ε-receptor γ subunit and the lymphoid-restricted membrane protein were downregulated and the macrophage inhibitory cytokine 1 (MIC-1) was strongly upregulated.

Northern Hybridization

RNA extracted from MCF-7 and MDA-MB-231 cells treated with TRF were subjected to Northern hybridization to confirm data obtained by means of cDNA array analysis. Northern blot analysis was performed on a selected number of genes (i.e., MIC-1, CD74, IFITM-1, 23-kDa HBP, and GAPDH). Their hybridization signals together with the quantification obtained after the normalization to the expression of GAPDH is shown in FIGURE 2. IFITM-1 was confirmed to be two-fold downregulated in both cell lines. MIC-1 and CD74 genes showed a five-fold upregulation and two-fold downregulation, respectively, in MDA cells. Finally, the upregulation of 23-kDa HBP by tocotrienols in the two cell lines, which was considered significant in the array analysis (see TABLE 2), was also detected, though by a lesser extent (just below the threshold limit of twofold), by Northern hybridization.

DISCUSSION

Recent indications have shown that vitamin E (both tocopherols and tocotrienols) has anti-tumor activity in several experimental systems. However, it has been reported that the anti-tumor activity of vitamin E may be independent of its antioxidant activity.[3] On the other hand, it is thought that vitamin E exerts its anti-tumor activity by modulating a number of intracellular signaling pathways involved in mitogenesis[32,33] and apoptosis.[32,34,35] This study reports the effect of the adminis-

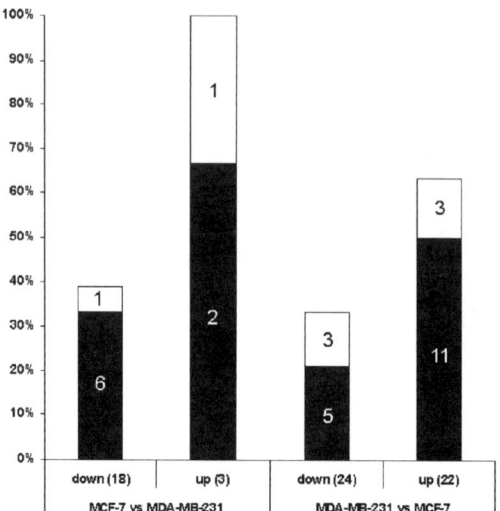

FIGURE 1. Comparison between gene changes induced by TRF in MCF-7 (18 down- + 3 upregulated genes) versus MDA-MB-231 (24 down- + 22 upregulated genes). TRF modulatory effects in the two cell lines were in the same (*black*) or opposite (*white*) directions. Data indicate that most of the changes in the two cell lines are common. Genes showed in the figure also include those displaying a lower than twofold modulatory change.

tration of TRF, a standardized tocotrienol-rich extract from palm oil, on gene expression, by means of a macroarray analysis, in the human breast cancer cell lines MCF-7 and MDA-MB-231.

Results obtained demonstrate that different complex molecular effects are induced by TRF from palm oil in the two breast cancer cell lines used. First, a different number of genes were affected, for example, 46 in MDA-MB-231 cells and 21 in MCF-7 cells. Moreover, although significant modulation of gene expression was found as a whole in 64 different genes (reported in TABLE 2), only three genes were affected in the same direction in the two cell lines, namely, the c-myc binding protein MM-1, the 23-kDa highly basic protein (23-kDa HBP), and the interferon-inducible protein 9-27 (IFITM-1). Such results suggest a complex response of tumor cells and also that growth inhibition by tocotrienols previously reported in MCF-7 and MDA-MB-231 cells,[12,13] is the result of the differential modulation of regulatory pathways in the two cell lines. Accordingly, it has recently been suggested that the induction of apoptosis in breast cancer cell lines *in vitro* relies on cell type–specific and multiple apoptotic mechanisms.[36] In fact, death induced by a polyamine analogue was associated with the modulation of Bcl-2 and Bax protein levels and with the phosphorylation of c-Jun in MDA-MB-465 and MDA-MB-231 cells, but not in MCF-7 cells.[36]

In spite of the evidence that different pathways are modulated by TRF in the two cell lines, if we consider genes that were not significantly affected according to our criteria, it is possible to remark that similarities in cell response exist. These are sum-

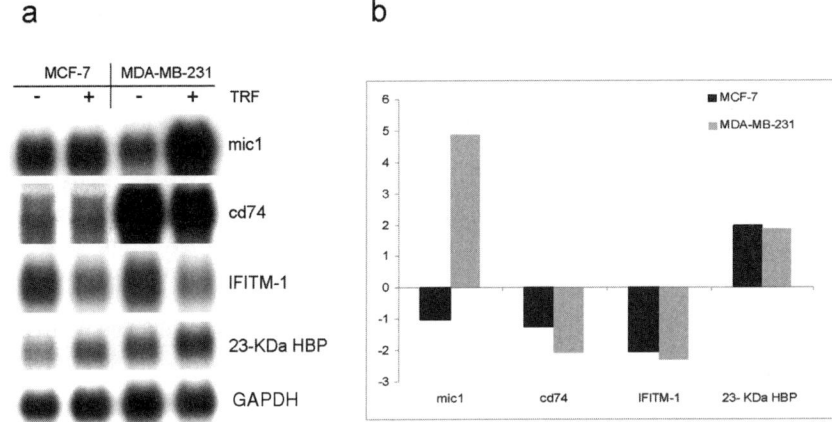

FIGURE 2. Northern analyses of TRF effects on expression of *mic1, cd74, IFITM-1, and 23-kDa HBP* in the two cell lines. Fold changes in gene expression calculated using the Scion software and normalized by hybridization signals of the GAPDH gene.

marized in FIGURE 1, showing that most of the significant changes in one cell line are present also in the other, even though changes are not "significant." These similarities suggest that some common pathways might exist in the way the two cancer cell lines respond to TRF.

We observed the upregulation both in MCF-and MDA-MB-231 cells of the 23-kDa HBP gene (ribosomal protein L13a). 23-kDa HBP is a housekeeping gene that has recently been described by Jesnowski *et al.*[37] as a reliable standard for gene expression analysis, at least in the pancreas and prostate. According to previously reported data on tocotrienols' ability to arrest MCF-7 and MDA-MB-231 cell growth,[12,13] our results are in agreement with the role suggested by Chen and Ioannou[38] of the coded protein as a proliferation checkpoint able to induce G2/M arrest of cell growth.

The interferon-induced protein 1 (IFITM-1) is a membrane protein that has been isolated by differential screening on the basis of its α- and γ-interferon inducibility in tumor cell lines. It has been shown to be a component of a multimeric complex involved in the transduction of antiproliferative and adhesion signals.[39] The inhibition of IFITM-1 by TRF in MCF-7 and MDA cells indicates a possible role of these genes in the modulation of cell growth by tocotrienols. Interferons are also known to exert their inhibitory effect on cell growth by acting at many levels, such as directly affecting the function of proteins (c-myc and Rb) involved in cell cycle.[40] Among these regulatory proteins, cyclins play an important role in cell cycle control by acting through the formation of enzymatic complexes with different cyclin- dependent kinases. Cyclin b1 was found to be overexpressed in various human breast cancer cell lines and tumor tissues.[41] The finding that the expression of cyclin b1 is downregulated by tocotrienols in MCF-7 and MDA-MB-231 cells is consistent with our previous results on the ability of these compounds to inhibit growth of tumor cell both *in vitro* and *in vivo*.[12]

The MHC class II–associated invariant chain (CD74/Ii) has been reported to play a central role in the biological function of the MHC class Ii molecules.[42] This invariant chain plays a critical role in the presentation of processed peptides to the CD4+ T lymphocytes by influencing the expression and peptide loading of the MHC class II molecules.[43] Several tumor cells overexpress CD74/Ii and are thought to escape activated cytotoxic T lymphocytes by evading detection by the host immune response. Treatment of animals with a specific monoclonal antibody against this protein induces selective apoptosis of neoplastic cells.[44] Our array analysis showed that the expression of CD74/Ii was significantly reduced by tocotrienols in the MDA-MB-231 cells. The findings were confirmed by Northern blot hybridization that demonstrated reduced expression of the gene by tocotrienols also in MCF-7 cells (FIG. 2). These results suggest that tocotrienols may operate their anti-tumor effect by inhibiting the ability of the tumor cells to escape from host immune system by either decreasing or inhibiting the expression of CD74/Ii in tumor cells.

The macroarray analysis identified changes in the expression of the gene encoding for the macrophage-inhibitory cytokine-1 (MIC-1), a member of the transforming growth factor-β (TGF-β) superfamily.[45] MIC-1 is not expressed in monocyte/macrophage undifferentiated resting cells but is progressively upregulated upon differentiation of these cells by a number of activation agents. It has been suggested that MIC-1 could be an autocrine inhibitor of macrophage activation.[46,47] We found a strong upregulation of the gene in MDA-MB-231 breast cancer cells (see FIG. 2). The expression of MIC-1 by nonmacrophage cells suggests an exocrine mechanism of regulating macrophage activation. The different activation of MIC1 by tocotrienols in the two cells lines suggests that tocotrienols could interfere with the transduction pathway of estrogen at some defined stage as a mediator of cellular stress signaling. cDNA array analyses identified two other TRF-sensitive genes coding for immune system proteins: the IgG receptor Fc large subunit p51 precursor (FcRN, neonatal Fc receptor) and the glycoprotein CD59. FcRn is a major histocompatibility complex class I–related receptor that plays a role both in the passive delivery of immunoglobulin from mother to the fetus during the colostrum formation and in the regulation of serum IgG transport to tissues.[48] CD59 is a potent complement inhibitor protein. It has been reported that CD59 binding to the membrane is able to inhibit the formation of the membrane attack complex (MAC) on the surface of tumor cells, thus inhibiting the direct cytolytic activity of the MAC against tumor cells.[49] Even though more studies are warranted to understand the role of these immune-related genes, it seems that TRF is able to modulate the immune signaling in our breast cancer model.

In conclusion, our study shows that TRF from palm oil selectively alters the expression of broad functional group of genes. Of interest is their ability to modulate immune modulatory genes as well as genes involved in cell cycle. This could be due to the induction of protein expression involved in cell growth inhibition such as the interferon-induced protein-1 (IFITM-1). Tocotrienols may also exert their anti-tumor effects by inhibiting the ability of the breast tumor cells to escape from host immune system through a decrease/inhibition of CD74/Ii expression in tumor cells. An alternative, parallel activity would involve the increase of host immune cells as a response to the invading tumor cells.

Even though more studies are warranted to understand the role of some of these proteins, it clearly appears that TRF supplementation is able to modulate gene expression in a fashion that is evidently independent from the antioxidant activity in our *in vitro* human breast cancer cell growth-inhibitory effects previously reported in both cell lines.[12]

REFERENCES

1. PACKER, L. & S. LANDVIK. 1989. Vitamin E: introduction to biochemistry and health benefits. Ann. N.Y. Acad. Sci. **570:** 1–6.
2. BURTON, G.W. & K.U. INGOLD. 1989. Vitamin E as an *in vitro* and *in vivo* antioxidant. Ann. N.Y. Acad. Sci. **570:** 7–22.
3. PACKER, L. 1991. Protective role of vitamin E in biological systems. Am. J. Clin. Nutr. **53:** 1050S–1055S.
4. KIMMICK, G.G., R.A. BELL & R.M. BOSTICK. 1997. Vitamin E and breast cancer: a review. Nutr. Cancer **27:** 109–117.
5. COMBS, G.F. 1992. The Vitamins: Fundamental Aspects in Nutrition and Health. Academic Press. San Diego, CA.
6. ONG, A.S.H. 1992. Natural sources of tocotrienols. *In* Vitamin E in Health and Disease. L. Packer & J. Fuchs, Eds.: 3–8. Marcel Dekker. New York.
7. SYLVESTER, P.W. *et al.* 1986. Comparative effects of different animal and vegetable fats fed before and during carcinogen administration on mammary tumorigenesis, sexual maturation, and endocrine function in rats. Cancer Res. **46:** 757–762.
8. GOULD, M.N. *et al.* 1991. A comparison of tocopherol and tocotrienol for the chemoprevention of chemically induced rat mammary tumors. Am. J. Clin. Nutr. **53:** 1068S–1070S.
9. KRITCHEVSKY, D., M.M. WEBER & D.M. KLURFELD. 1992. Influence of different fats on chemically-induced mammary tumours in rats. Nutr. Res. **12:** 879–892.
10. NESARETNAM, K. *et al.* 1992. The effect of vitamin E tocotrienols from palm oil on chemically induced mammary tumourigenesis in female rats. Nutr. Res. **12:** 879–892.
11. NESARETNAM, K. *et al.* 1995. Effect of tocotrienols on the growth of a human breast cancer cell line in culture. Lipids **30:** 1139–1143.
12. NESARETNAM, K. *et al.* 1998. Tocotrienols inhibit the growth of human breast cancer cells irrespective of estrogen receptor status. Lipids **33:** 461–469.
13. NESARETNAM, K., S. DORASAMY & P.D. DARBRE. 2000. Tocotrienols inhibit growth of ZR-75-1 breast cancer cells. Int. J. Food Sci. Nutr. **51:** S95–103.
14. CAROLL, K.K. *et al.* 1995. Anti-cancer properties of tocotrienols from palm oil. A.S.H. Ong, E. Niki & L. Packer, Eds.: 117–121. *In* Nutrition, Lipids, Health and Disease. AOCS Press. Champaign, IL.
15. GUTHRIE, N. *et al.* 1997. Inhibition of proliferation of estrogen receptor-negative MDA-MB-435 and -positive MCF-7 human breast cancer cells by palm oil tocotrienols and tamoxifen, alone and in combination. J. Nutr. **127:** 544S–548S.
16. CHARPENTIER, A. *et al.* 1993. RRR-alpha-tocopheryl succinate inhibits proliferation and enhances secretion of transforming growth factor-beta (TGF-beta) by human breast cancer cells. Nutr. Cancer **19:** 225–239.
17. DJURIC, Z. *et al.* 1997. Growth inhibition of MCF-7 and MCF-10A human breast cells by alpha-tocopheryl hemisuccinate, cholesteryl hemisuccinate and their ether analogs. Cancer Lett. **111:** 133–139.
18. SAHU, S.N., J. EDWARDS-PRASAD & K.N. PRASAD. 1988. Effect of alpha tocopheryl succinate on adenylate cyclase activity in murine neuroblastoma cells in culture. J. Am. Coll. Nutr. **7:** 285–293.
19. TORELLI, S., F. MASOUDI & K.N. PRASAD. 1988. Effect of alpha tocopheryl succinate on cyclic AMP-dependent protein kinase activity in murine B-16 melanoma cells in culture. Cancer Lett. **39:** 129–136.
20. CHATELAIN, E. *et al.* 1993. Inhibition of smooth muscle cell proliferation and protein kinase C activity by tocopherols and tocotrienols. Biochim. Biophys. Acta **1176:** 83–89.
21. YU, W. *et al.* 1999. Induction of apoptosis in human breast cancer cells by tocopherols and tocotrienols. Nutr. Cancer **33:** 26–32.

22. ZHAO, B. *et al.* 1997. Involvement of activator protein-1 (AP-1) in induction of apoptosis by vitamin E succinate in human breast cancer cells. Mol. Carcinogenesis **19**: 180–190.
23. YU, W. *et al.* 1997. Evidence for role of transforming growth factor-beta in RRR-alpha-tocopheryl succinate-induced apoptosis of human MDA-MB-435 breast cancer cells. Nutr. Cancer **27**: 267–278.
24. TURLEY, J.M. *et al.* 1997. Vitamin E succinate induces Fas-mediated apoptosis in estrogen receptor-negative human breast cancer cells. Cancer Res. **57**: 881–890.
25. SUNDRAM, K. & A. GAPOR. 1992. Vitamin E from palm oil: its extraction and nutritional properties. Lipid Technol. **4**: 137–141.
26. OSBORNE, C.K., K. HOBBS & J.M. TRENT. 1987. Biological differences among MCF-7 human breast cancer cell lines from different laboratories. Breast Cancer Res. Treat. **9**: 111–121.
27. YUE, H. *et al.* 2001. An evaluation of the performance of cDNA microarrays for detecting changes in global mRNA expression. Nucleic Acids Res. [online] **29**: E41–9.
28. FISCHER, A. *et al.* 2001. Effect of selenium and vitamin E deficiency on differential gene expression in rat liver. Biochem. Biophys. Res. Commun. **285**: 470–475.
29. HELLMANN, G.M., W.R. FIELDS & D.J. DOOLITTLE. 2001. Gene expression profiling of cultured human bronchial epithelial and lung carcinoma cells. Toxicol. Sci. **61**: 154–163.
30. JONES, J.I. & D.R. CLEMMONS. 1995. Insulin-like growth factors and their binding proteins: biological actions. Endocr. Rev. **16**: 3–34.
31. PRATT, S.E. & M.N. POLLAK. 1994. Insulin-like growth factor binding protein 3 (IGF-BP3) inhibits estrogen-stimulated breast cancer cell proliferation. Biochem. Biophys. Res. Commun. **198**: 292–297.
32. SCHWENKE, D.C. *et al.* 2002. Alpha-tocopherol protects against diet induced atherosclerosis in New Zealand white rabbits. J. Lipid Res. **43**: 1927–1938.
33. RICCIARELLI, R., J.M. ZINGG & A. AZZI. 2001. Vitamin E: protective role of a Janus molecule. FASEB J. **15**: 2314–2325.
34. KLINE, K., W. YU & B.G. SANDERS. 2001. Vitamin E: mechanisms of action as tumor cell growth inhibitors. J. Nutr. **131**: 161S–163S.
35. MCINTYRE, B.S. *et al.* 2000. Antiproliferative and apoptotic effects of tocopherols and tocotrienols on preneoplastic and neoplastic mouse mammary epithelial cells. Proc. Soc. Exp. Biol. Med. **224**: 292–301.
36. HUANG, Y. *et al.* 2003. A novel polyamine analog inhibits growth and induces apoptosis in human breast cancer cells. Clin. Cancer Res. **9**: 2769–2777.
37. JESNOWSKI, R. *et al.* 2002. Ribosomal highly basic 23-kDa protein as a reliable standard for gene expression analysis. Pancreatology **2**: 421–424.
38. CHEN, F.W. & Y.A. IOANNOU. 1999. Ribosomal proteins in cell proliferation and apoptosis. Int. Rev. Immunol. **18**: 429–448.
39. DEBLANDRE, G.A. *et al.* 1995. Expression cloning of an interferon-inducible 17-kDa membrane protein implicated in the control of cell growth. J. Biol. Chem. **270**: 23860–23866.
40. GUTTERMAN, J.U. 1994. Cytokine therapeutics: lessons from interferon alpha. Proc. Natt. Acad. Sci. USA **91**: 1198–1205.
41. YU, M., Q. ZHAN & O.J. FINN. 2002. Immune recognition of cyclin B1 as a tumor antigen is a result of its overexpression in human tumors that is caused by non-functional p53. Mol. Immunol. **38**: 981–987.
42. EYNON, E.E., C. SCHLAX & J. PIETERS. 1999. A secreted form of the major histocompatibility complex class II-associated invariant chain inhibiting T cell activation. J. Biol. Chem. **274**: 26266–26271.
43. TOPILSKI, I. *et al.* 2002. Preferential Th1 immune response in invariant chain-deficient mice. J. Immunol. **168**: 1610–1617.
44. VIDOVIC, D. & J.I. TORAL. 1998. Selective apoptosis of neoplastic cells by the HLA-DR-specific monoclonal antibody. Cancer Lett. **128**: 127–135.
45. BAUSKIN, A.R. *et al.* 2000. The propeptide of macrophage inhibitory cytokine (MIC-1), a TGF-beta superfamily member, acts as a quality control determinant for correctly folded MIC-1. EMBO J. **19**: 2212–2220.

46. FAIRLIE, W.D. et al. 2001. The propeptide of the transforming growth factor-beta superfamily member, macrophage inhibitory cytokine-1 (MIC-1), is a multifunctional domain that can facilitate protein folding and secretion. J. Biol. Chem. **276:** 16911–16918.
47. FAIRLIE, W.D. et al. 1999. MIC-1 is a novel TGF-beta superfamily cytokine associated with macrophage activation. J. Leukocyte Biol. **65:** 2–5.
48. GHETIE, V. & E.S. WARD. 2000. Multiple roles for the major histocompatibility complex class I- related receptor FcRn. Annu. Rev. Immunol. **18:** 739–766.
49. DURRANT, L.G. & I. SPENDLOVE. 2001. Immunization against tumor cell surface complement-regulatory proteins. Curr. Opin. Invest. Drugs **2:** 959–966.

Vitamin E and the Oxidative Stress of Exercise

M.J. JACKSON, M. KHASSAF, A. VASILAKI, F. McARDLE, AND A. McARDLE

School of Clinical Sciences, University of Liverpool, Liverpool, L69 3GA, U.K.

ABSTRACT: There is clear evidence that contracting skeletal muscle generates a complex set of reactive oxygen and nitrogen species and that the pattern and magnitude of this generation is influenced by the type and frequency of the muscle contraction protocol. The functions of these species in exercising organisms are still unclear although data have been presented indicating that they play a role in contraction-induced muscle damage and/or in signaling adaptive responses to contractions. Vitamin E has been claimed to exert a regulatory effect on the actions of contraction-induced oxidants for a considerable time, although evidence for any specific role in this area is lacking. A review of studies in this area suggests that vitamin E supplements are unlikely to reliably reduce the severity of contraction-induced muscle damage but, in contrast, appear capable of modulating redox-regulated adaptive responses to contractions. Full evaluation of the roles of oxidants and antioxidants such as vitamin E in responses of muscle to contractions should enable the manipulation of these processes with potential beneficial effects on maintenance of optimal muscle function.

KEYWORDS: vitamin E; reactive oxygen species; oxidative stress; nitric oxide; skeletal muscle; contraction; muscle damage; heat-shock protein; stress response

GENERATION OF REACTIVE OXYGEN SPECIES DURING EXERCISE

Reactive oxygen species (ROS) are generated as part of normal metabolism in mammalian cells. A great deal of data has now been presented showing that unaccustomed or demanding exercise leads to oxidation of lipids, DNA, and protein in a variety of body tissues in man and animals.[1] Relatively little data have been presented from studies attempting to delineate the major tissue sources of the increased oxidant detected during whole-body exercise. Exercise can increase oxygen utilization 200-fold above resting levels in active muscle fibers,[2] and it has been suggested that superoxide production increases with this large increase in oxygen flux through muscle mitochondria during exercise.[3] Data from our laboratory and others also indicates that skeletal muscle cells release superoxide[4] and generate hydroxyl radicals[5,6] in the extracellular fluid during contraction. Skeletal muscle also contains nitric oxide (NO) synthases and releases NO to the extracellular fluid during contractile activity.[7] Skeletal muscle is therefore one of the tissues that contributes to

Address for correspondence: Professor M.J. Jackson, School of Clinical Sciences, University of Liverpool, Liverpool, L69 3GA, U.K. Voice: +441517064072; fax: +441517065802.
mjj@liv.ac.uk

the oxidative stress of exercise and is arguably the major source of ROS generation at those times.[4]

Exercise-Induced Muscle Damage

A number of the earliest studies in this area examined the possibility that the ROS generated during exercise might contribute to the damage that sometimes occurs to muscle following unaccustomed or excessive exercise. Overall skeletal muscle is remarkably resistant to exercise-induced muscle damage although exposure to some specific types of muscle contractions greatly increases the tendency to cause muscle damage. Of particular importance is whether the muscle shortens during the contraction (concentric activity), remains at the same length (isometric activity), or increases in length (lengthening contractions or pliometric contractions that are commonly, but incorrectly, referred to as eccentric contractions). In both humans and rodents, the muscles are injured to a greater extent when exercise involves predominantly lengthening contractions rather than isometric or concentric activity.[8,9] This occurs mainly in activities such as running downhill.

Adaptations to Exercise

Skeletal muscle is a very adaptable tissue that can remodel and adapt rapidly following exposure to different types or degrees of contractile activity. Evidence from both animal and human studies indicate that many cell types specifically adapt to increased exposure to oxidants to reduce the risk of damage to the tissue.[4,10–12] An acute bout of exercise increases the activities of SOD, glutathione peroxidase, glutathione reductase, and catalase in skeletal muscle of rats.[13] Longer-term exercise training also appears to increase the activity of several antioxidant enzymes, such as SOD and CAT[14] or glutathione peroxidase[13] in muscle, although these are not consistent findings.[15] In humans, exercise training has been reported to increase skeletal muscle SOD activities[16,17] and the activities of various protective enzymes in blood.[18]

In addition to adaptive changes in protective enzymes, oxidative and other stresses to cells are also known to induce increased production of stress or heat-shock proteins (HSPs). These proteins are an important component of the cellular protective response.[19] This occurs in blood cells, such as lymphocytes,[11] and recent data also indicate that an increase in muscle HSP content occurs following exercise in rats[20] and mice.[4] HSPs act as molecular chaperones facilitating the correct folding of newly synthesized cellular proteins and translocation to cellular compartments.[21] Studies in a variety of tissues indicate that prior stimulation of the synthesis of HSPs protects tissues against a variety of (normally damaging) stresses, such as ischemic-reperfusion injury or intracellular calcium overload.[6,22,23]

Few data have been presented on the expression of HSPs in human skeletal muscle. Liu et al.[24] reported an increase in the HSP70 content of *vastus lateralis* muscle after 1–4 weeks of rowing training whereas Puntschart and co-workers[25] found the HSP70 mRNA to be increased in muscle following exercise with no increase in HSP70 protein content. We have previously demonstrated that muscle HSP60 and HSP70 contents were increased following a single episode of cycle ergometry.[26]

We have previously speculated that the exercise-induced increase in muscle HSP content was stimulated by an increased production of oxidants during muscle contractile activity.[4,26] Studies in mice demonstrated that a demanding period of nondamaging isometric contractions resulted in an increased production of a range of ROS and a transient and reversible oxidation of the protein thiols in muscle,[4,6] and we hypothesize that this increased oxidation results in increased HSP production via activation of the heat-shock transcription factor HSF-1.[4] There is increasing awareness that ROS may play a role in many cell types to stimulate changes in gene expression by modulation of the activity of various signaling molecules and transcription factors.[27] Of particular interest is the role of oxidants in stimulating activation of NFκB.[28] Currently, the effect of antioxidant supplementation on these pathways is incompletely understood.[27]

Effects of Vitamin E on Skeletal Muscle

Some of the first studies of exercise-induced ROS generation used vitamin E depletion or supplementation as tools to investigate the effects of ROS on physiological and pathological processes.[3,29,30] In this current paper, we concentrate on current understanding of the effects of vitamin E in two key processes that may be modulated by ROS: exercise-induced muscle damage and adaptive responses to exercise.

Vitamin E and Exercise-Induced Muscle Damage

An increase in oral intake of the so-called nutritional antioxidants has been proposed to be beneficial in reducing oxidant damage to tissues,[31] including skeletal muscle.[3,32] Many early studies examined the possibility that the vitamin E content muscle could influence the extent of muscle damage in a variety of different models (e.g., see Refs. 3, 30, and 33) with varying levels of efficacy. Several studies examined the effect of vitamin E supplementation on markers of oxidation in tissues,[34–36] but examination of the potential effects of supplemental antioxidants against contraction-induced muscle damage have been relatively unrewarding despite early high expectations.[32] In lengthening contraction-induced damage to muscle, there is evidence that ROS generated by invading phagocytic cells and neutrophils leads to oxidation of muscle tissue that contributes to the damage that occurs several days after the initial insult.[37] In addition, Zerba et al.[38] demonstrated that this secondary injury was almost completely blocked by prior treatment of animals with polyethylene glycol-tagged superoxide dismutase (PEG-SOD), supporting a role for extracellular superoxide in this process.

Multiple studies of the potential protective effects of vitamin E supplementation in models of lengthening contraction-induced muscle damage have been contradictory. Meydani et al.[39] reported that subjects who took vitamin E supplements and subsequently ran downhill on a treadmill had a decreased serum creatine kinase (CK) activity at 5 days post-exercise in comparison with a control non-supplemented group, while Jakeman and Maxwell[40] found no effect of oral vitamin E supplementation against force deficit or elevated serum CK activities after box-stepping. Similarly in rodents, animals given vitamin E supplements showed no difference in muscle force deficit or elevated serum CK activities compared to control non-supplemented animals following downhill running.[41] In more recent studies, Petersen et al.[42] also

TABLE 1. Differential effects of vitamin E supplements on serum CK activities and histologic evidence of muscle damage[a]

	Non-exercised control animals	Exercised vehicle-treated rats	Exercised vitamin E–treated rats
% of damaged fibers at 3 days post-contraction protocol	0	32 ± 5	29 ± 3
Serum CK activity at 1 day post-contraction protocol (U/L)	52 ± 5	170 ± 40[b]	65 ± 30
Serum CK activity at 3 days post-contraction protocol (U/L)	52 ± 5	120 ± 35[b]	60 ± 10

[a]Data derived from Van der Meulen et al.[43]
[b]Significantly different from non-exercised animals and exercised, vitamin E–treated control rats.

saw no protective effect of prior vitamin E supplementation against markers of muscle damage following downhill running in human subjects.

In an attempt to clarify any potential role for vitamin E in protecting skeletal muscle against lengthening contraction-induced damage, we examined a well-characterized model of lengthening contractions in rodents in which a single discrete muscle (in this case the *extensor digitorum longus*, EDL) is damaged in a highly reproducible manner.[43] These data provided evidence that vitamin E supplements may have differential effects on individual measures of damage to muscle. Animals subjected to a protocol of 225 lengthening contractions had a force deficit of 64 ± 7% at 3 days post-exercise and morphological damage to 38 ± 5% of the EDL fibers on histological examination. This was associated with a significant elevation of the serum CK activity at 3 h and 3 days post-exercise. Prior vitamin E supplementation of the rats had no effect on the loss of force generation by the EDL or on the percentage of damaged fibers, but surprisingly prevented the rise in circulating CK activity (TABLE 1) and pyruvate kinase activities[43] that occurred post-exercise.

This apparent selective effect of vitamin E on the release of cytosolic enzymes from the damaged muscle is consistant with *in vitro* data suggesting that vitamin E can stabilize muscle membranes by interaction with phospholipids[33] and may provide an explanation for at least some of the apparently discrepant data in this area. Measurements of the serum activities of CK and other cytosolic enzymes are frequently used as readily accessible measures of muscle damage in exercise studies.

Vitamin E and Adaptive Changes in Muscle Gene Expression after Contractile Activity

We have previously described a model system in which exercise of untrained subjects leads to an increased expression of a number of cytoprotective proteins and HSPs in human muscle, and we speculated that this process involves activation of muscle gene expression through exercise-induced oxidative stress.[26] We have examined the effect of supplementary vitamin C on the responses of human lymphocytes and skeletal muscle to exogenous and endogenous oxidants.[17] These studies demonstrated that supplementary vitamin C caused an attenuation of adaptive responses to oxidants, and we concluded that this was due to an increased baseline expression of systems that are protective against oxidative stress (including SOD, catalase, and HSPs) following supplementation. An alternative explanation would be that an elevation in the tissue content of antioxidants could quench the change in ROS during exercise and thus abolish the subsequent activation of transcription. We have also examined the effect of supplementation with either vitamin E or β-carotene on the stress response of muscle to exercise. We hypothesized that these lipid-soluble antioxidants would reduce the responses of skeletal muscle to the oxidative stress of contractile activity.

The study was undertaken with 22 healthy, untrained male volunteers. All were non-smokers and not taking any routine medication or vitamin supplements and none participated in regular sport or exercise training. Their heights, masses, and ages were 1.71 ± 0.01 m, 68.6 ± 1.5 kg, and 23.3 ± 1.1 years (mean ± SEM), respectively. The protocol was approved by the Research Ethical Committee of the Liverpool Research Ethics Committee, and all subjects gave informed written consent. Subjects were randomized to receive either 400 mg RRR-α-tocopherol/day (Roche, Basel, Switzerland) in the form of two 200-mg tablets, or 15 mg β-carotene/day (Boots, Nottingham, UK) or no supplements for 8 weeks. Two days prior to beginning the supplement, subjects gave a blood sample and muscle biopsy and undertook an exercise protocol followed by a second muscle biopsy two days later. Eight weeks later, the blood and muscle sampling and the exercise test were repeated. Eight volunteers took the α-tocopherol supplement, nine volunteers took the β-carotene, and five had no supplement.

Each subject exercised at a cadence of 70 rpm, using a single leg, on a friction–loaded cycle ergometer (Monark 864, Sweden) that was modified specifically for this purpose.[26] Prior to randomization, an incremental work test was performed to determine peak oxygen uptake, during which the workload was increased by 35 watts every 4 min to volitional exhaustion. Expired air was monitored continuously during exercise using an on-line gas analysis system. Because the subjects were unaccustomed to this exercise protocol, a second incremental work test was performed within a week of the first test to assess the reliability of the measurements. During the experimental protocols, the subjects each cycled at 70% VO_2 peak for 45 min using the contralateral leg to that used for the preliminary incremental tests.

Blood samples and muscle biopsies from *vastus lateralis* muscle of the exercised leg were taken at 2 days prior to the exercise protocol. Two days following the exercise, further muscle biopsies were obtained. Biopsies were taken under local anesthesia using a Bergstrom-type needle (6.5-mm diameter). Samples (approximately 100 mg) were obtained and immediately frozen in liquid nitrogen and stored at 70°C until analyzed. HSPs in the muscle tissue were analyzed as previously.[17]

Subjects showed a rise in circulating levels of vitamin E or β-carotene following these levels of supplementation as anticipated from previous studies.[44] Eight weeks of supplementation with vitamin E at a dose of 400 mg/day were found to increase the mean serum vitamin E concentration from 14.0 ± 1.5 mg/mL at baseline to 19.0 ± 1.0 mg/mL with supplementation ($P < 0.01$). Eight weeks of supplementation with β-carotene increased plasma levels from 1.0 ± 0.3 μg/mL to 2.3 ± 0.5 μg/mL ($P < 0.05$).

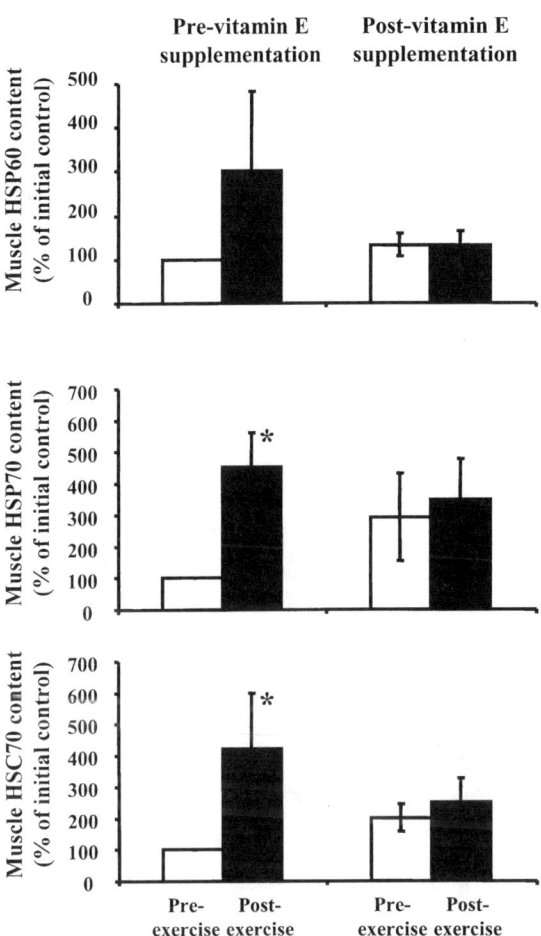

FIGURE 1. Relative content of HSP60 (FIG. 1A), HSP70 (FIG. 1B), and HSC70 (FIG. 1C) in the *vastus lateralis* muscles of a group of volunteer subjects prior to, and at two days following, 45 min of exercise on a cycle ergometer. The effect of supplementation for 8 weeks with 400 mg vitamin E/day is also shown. Data are presented as mean ± SEM and as a percentage of the initial HSP content prior to either exercise or supplementation. *Values significantly different from pre-stimulation, non-supplemented values.

The effect of the vitamin E supplementation on muscle HSP60, HSP70, and HSC70 content prior to, and at 2 days following, exercise is shown in FIGURE 1, and the equivalent data from the β-carotene–supplemented subjects is shown in FIGURE 2. Prior to supplementation, the exercise protocol significantly increased HSP70 and HSC70 contents of muscle, but this exercise effect was not seen following 8 weeks of either vitamin E or β-carotene supplements.

The mechanisms activating transcription of HSPs in muscle following contractile activity are unclear. In previous studies in mice, we have shown that increased ex-

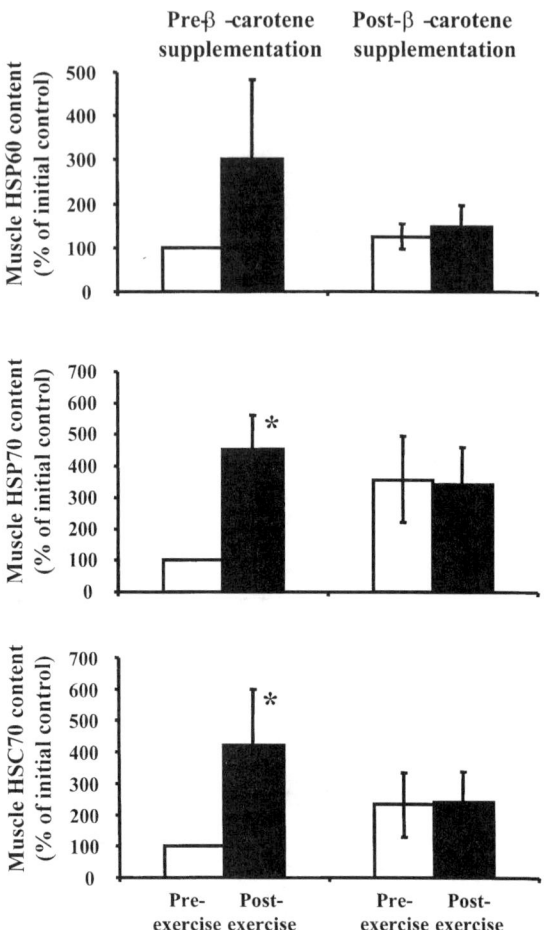

FIGURE 2. Relative content of HSP60 (FIG. 2A), HSP70 (FIG. 2B), and HSC70 (FIG. 2C) in the *vastus lateralis* muscles of a group of volunteer subjects prior to, and at two days following, 45 min of exercise on a cycle ergometer. The effect of supplementation for 8 weeks with 15 mg β-carotene/day is also shown. Data are presented as mean ± SEM and as a percentage of the initial HSP content prior to either exercise or supplementation. *Values significantly different from pre-stimulation, non-supplemented values.

pression of HSPs following contractile activity is associated with an increase in oxidant generation by skeletal muscle and a transient oxidation of protein thiols.[4] Oxidation of protein thiols has been shown to be part of a signaling process leading to induction of HSPs in other cell types,[45] and we have hypothesized that increased skeletal muscle HSP expression post-exercise is initiated by increased oxidant generation during contractile activity.[4,26]

Vitamin E and β-carotene supplementation had similar effects on the expression of HSPs in skeletal muscle. Both supplements effectively abolished any adaptive response in HSP70 and HSC70 that followed exercise in the non-supplemented group, but tended to increase the baseline content of the HSPs. The implication of these data is that activation of HSP transcription involves formation of lipid-soluble free radical species that are scavenged by vitamin E or β-carotene. Potential candidate radicals would include alkyl or alkoxy species, and there is previous evidence that such species are generated and released from skeletal muscle during exercise or ischemia and reperfusion and that they are relatively long-lived and detectable in the circulation of animals and man.[46] HSF1, the transcription factor involved in activation of HSP transcription is redox sensitive,[27] and these data support the possibility that activation of this transcription factor may be inhibited by vitamin E or β-carotene.

We have previously reported that supplementation with vitamin C also leads to an attenuation of the increase in skeletal muscle HSP70 content following contractile activity in humans.[17] In those studies, we also observed that vitamin C supplementation suppressed the HSP response of lymphocytes to hydrogen peroxide challenge.[17] We have not observed similar effects of vitamin E or β-carotene, suggesting that lipid soluble antioxidants do not play a role in this process (data not shown in detail). In the vitamin C supplementation studies, a significant increase in the baseline muscle content of HSP70 was also seen following vitamin C supplementation. It was proposed that this reduced adaptive response may be due to an increase in overall cellular protection against oxidants because vitamin C additionally induced an increase in the expression of other potential protective systems against oxidative stress with lymphocytes having an increased baseline activity of SOD and catalase enzymes and an elevated HSP60 content. Similar mechanisms cannot be invoked for the effects of vitamin E or β-carotene reported here because these supplements had no effect on lymphocyte or muscle catalase or SOD activities (data not shown in detail).

Since both vitamin E and β-carotene supplements appear to reduce HSP expression following exercise, it is relevant to consider whether this will have beneficial effects on muscle. There is increasing interest in the potential role of heat-shock proteins in maintenance of cell integrity in skeletal muscle. Data from studies with cardiac and other tissues demonstrates that these proteins have significant cytoprotective effects against a variety of damaging processes, and experimental animal studies indicate that these proteins can provide cytoprotective effects against contraction-induced damage and other stresses to skeletal muscle.[4,6,23] It can be argued that suppression of the expression of these proteins following stress to skeletal muscle will not be beneficial to skeletal muscle viability over the longer term. The validity of this hypothesis will be evaluated by further studies on the importance of post-exercise HSP expression in the recovery and adaptation of skeletal muscle following contractile activity and will help define whether antioxidant supplements are likely to be beneficial in this area.

CONCLUSIONS

After 25 years of study, it is clear that vitamin E (and potentially other lipid-soluble antioxidants) can influence responses of muscle tissue to contractile activity. Initial optimistic studies indicating protective effects of vitamin E supplements against exercise-induced muscle damage have not been substantiated, but redox-regulation of gene expression appears to play a role in adaptive responses to exercise, and vitamin E can influence these processes. Optimization of the activity of vitamin E in these actions is an important goal for future research in this area.

ACKNOWLEDGMENTS

We would like to acknowledge the generous financial support of the U.K. Ministry of Agriculture, Fisheries and Food and the Wellcome Trust. The late Professor Anthony Diplock, Dr. Robert Child, Dr. Christian Esanu, and Professor David Brodie have all provided advice concerning this work. Mr. Chris Price provided technical assistance for parts of the studies.

REFERENCES

1. REZNICK, A.Z., L. PACKER, C.K. SEN, et al. 1998. Oxidative Stress in Skeletal Muscle. Birkhauser. Basel.
2. KEUL, J., E. DOLL & D. KOPPLER. 1972. Oxidative Energy Supply. Karger. Basel.
3. DAVIES, K.J.A., A.T. QUINTANILLA, G.A. BROOKS & L. PACKER. 1982. Free radicals and tissue damage produced by exercise. Biochem. Biophys. Res. Commun. **107:** 1198–1205.
4. MCARDLE, A., D. PATTWELL, A. VASILAKI, et al. 2001. Contractile activity-induced oxidative stress: cellular origin and adaptive responses. Am. J. Physiol. Cell Physiol. **280:** C621–C627.
5. O'NEILL, C.A., C.L. STEBBINS, S. BONIGUT, et al. 1996. Production of hydroxyl radicals in contracting skeletal muscle of cats. J. Appl. Physiol. **81:** 1197–1206.
6. MCARDLE, A., J. VAN DER MEULEN, G.L. CLOSE, et al. 2004. Role of mitochondrial superoxide dismutase in contraction-induced generation of reactive oxygen species in skeletal muscle extracellular space. Am. J. Physiol. Cell Physiol. **286:** C1152–C1158.
7. BALON, T.W. & J.L. NADLER. 1994. Nitric oxide release is present from incubated skeletal muscle preparations. J. Appl. Physiol. **77:** 2519–2521.
8. ARMSTRONG, R.B., R.W. OGILVIE & J.A. SCHWANE. 1983. Eccentric exercise-induced injury to rat skeletal muscle. J. Appl. Physiol. **54:** 80–93.
9. NEWHAM, D.J., G. MCPHAIL, K.R. MILLS & R.H. EDWARDS. 1983. Ultrastructural changes after concentric and eccentric contractions of human muscle. J. Neurol. Sci. **61:** 109–122.
10. NIWA, Y., O. IIZAWA, K. ISHIMOTO, et al. 1993. Age-dependent basal level and induction capacity of copper-zinc and manganese superoxide dismutase and other scavenging enzyme activities in leukocytes from young and elderly adults. Am. J. Pathol. **143:** 312–320.
11. MARINI, M., F. FRABETTI, D. MUSIANI & C. FRANCESCHI. 1996. Oxygen radicals induce stress proteins and tolerance to oxidative stress in human lymphocytes. Int. J. Radiat. Biol. **70:** 337–350.
12. JONES, S.A., F. MCARDLE, C.I.A. JACK & M.J. JACKSON. 1999. Effect of antioxidant supplementation on the adaptive responses of human skin fibroblasts to UV-induced oxidative stress. Redox Rep. **4:** 291–299.
13. JI, L.L. 1993. Antioxidant enzyme response to exercise and ageing. Med. Sci. Sports Exercise **25:** 225–231.
14. HIGUCHI, M., L.J. CARTIER, M. CHEN & J.O. HOLLOSZY. 1985. Superoxide dismutase and catalse in skeletal muscle: adaptive response to exercise. J. Gerontol. **40:** 281–286.
15. ALESSIO, H.M. & A.H. GOLDFARB. 1988. Lipid peroxidation and scavenger enzymes during exercise: adaptation to training. J. Appl. Physiol. **64:** 1333–1336.
16. JENKINS, R.R., R. FRIEDLAND & H. HOWALD. 1984. The relationship of oxygen uptake to superoxide dismutase and catalase activity in human skeletal muscle. Int. J. Sports Med. **5:** 11–14.

17. KHASSAF, M., A. MCARDLE, C. ESANU, et al. 2003. Effect of vitamin C supplements on antioxidant defence and stress proteins in human lymphocytes and skeletal muscle. J. Physiol. **549:** 645–652.
18. ROBERTSON, J.D., R.G. MAUGHAN, G,G. DUTHIE & P.C. MORRICE. 1991. Increased blood antioxidant systems of runners in response to training load. Clin. Sci. **80:** 611–618.
19. SMOLKA, M.B., C.C. ZOPPI, A.A. ALVES, et al. 2000. HSP72 as a complementary protection against oxidative stress induced by exercise in the soleus muscle of rats. Am. J. Physiol. Regul. Integr. Comp. Physiol. **279:** R1539–R1545.
20. SALO, D.C., C.M. DONOVAN & K.J.A. DAVIES. 1992. HSP70 and other possible heat shock or oxidative proteins are induced in skeletal muscle, heart and liver during exercise. Free Radical Biol. Med. **11:** 239–246.
21. FIEGE, U., R.I. MORIMOTO, I. YAHARA & B.S. POLLA. 1996. Stress-Inducible Cellular Responses. Birkhauser Verlag. Basel.
22. MARBER, M.S., R. MESTRIL, S.H. CHI, et al. 1995. Overexpression of the rat inducible 70-kD heat stress protein in a transgenic mouse increases the resistance of the heart to ischemic injury.J. Clin. Invest. **95:** 1446–1456.
23. MAGLARA, A.A., A. VASILAKI, M.J. JACKSON & A. MCARDLE. 2003. Damage to developing mouse skeletal muscle myotubes in culture: protective effect of heat shock proteins. J. Physiol. **548:** 837–846.
24. LIU, Y., S. MAYR, A. OPITZ-GRESS, et al. 1999. Human skeletal muscle HSP70 response to training in highly trained rowers. J. Appl. Physiol. **86:** 101–104.
25. PUNTSCHART, A., M. VOGT, H.R. WIDMER, et al. 1996. Hsp70 expression in human skeletal muscle after exercise. Acta Physiol. Scand.**157:** 411–417.
26. KHASSAF, M., R.B. CHILD, A. MCARDLE, et al. 2001. Time course of responses of human skeletal muscle to exercise-induced oxidative stress. J. Appl. Physiol. **90:** 1031–1036.
27. JACKSON, M.J., S. PAPA, J. BOLANOS, et al. 2002. Antioxidants, reactive oxygen and nitrogen species, gene induction and mitochondrial function. Mol. Aspects Med. **23:** 209–285.
28. HOLLANDER, J., R. FIEBIG, M. GORE, et al. 2001. Superoxide dismutase gene expression is activated by a single bout of exercise in rat skeletal muscle. Pflugers Arch. **442:** 426–4234.
29. DILLARD, C.J., R.E. LITOV, W.M. SAVIN, et al. 1978. Effects of exercise, vitamin E, and ozone on pulmonary function and lipid peroxidation. J. Appl.Physiol. **45:** 927–932.
30. JACKSON, M.J., D.A. JONES & R.H.T. EDWARDS. 1983. Vitamin E and skeletal muscle. Ciba Found. Symp. **101:** 224–239.
31. GEY, K.F. 1993. Prospects for the prevention of free radical disease, regarding cancer and cardiovascular diseases. In Free Radicals in Medicine. K.H. Cheeseman & T.F. Slater, Eds. Br. Med. Bull. **49:** 679–699.
32. BENDICH, A. 1991. Exercise and free radicals: effects of antioxidant vitamins. In Advances in Nutrition and Top Sport. F. Brouns, Ed.: 59–78. Karger. Basel.
33. PHOENIX, J., R.H. EDWARDS & M.J. JACKSON. 1991. The effect of vitamin E analogues and long hydrocarbon chain compounds on calcium-induced muscle damage. A novel role for alpha-tocopherol? Biochim. Biophys. Acta **1097:** 212–218.
34. KANTER, M.M., L.A. NOLTE & J.O. HOLLOSZY. 1993. Effects of an antioxidant vitamin mixture on lipid peroxidation at rest and postexercise. J. Appl. Physiol. **74:** 965–969.
35. GOLDFARB, A.H., M.K. MCINTOSH, B.T. BOYER & J. FATOUROS. 1994. Vitamin E effects on indexes of lipid peroxidation in muscle from DHEA-treated and exercised rats. J. Appl. Physiol. **76:** 1630–1635.
36. KUMAR, C.T., V.K. REDDY, M. PRASAD, et al. 1992. Dietary supplementation of vitamin E protects heart tissue from exercise-induced oxidant stress. Mol. Cell. Biochem. **111:** 109–115.
37. MCARDLE, A., J.H. VAN DER MEULEN, M. CATAPANO, et al. 1999. Free radical activity following contraction-induced injury to the extensor digitorum longus muscles of rats. Free Radical Biol. Med. **26:** 1085–1091.
38. ZERBA, E., T.E. KOMOROWSKI & J.A. FAULKNER. 1990. Free radical injury to skeletal muscles of young, adult, and old mice. Am. J. Physiol. **258:** C429–C435.

39. MEYDANI, M., W.J. EVANS, G. HANDELMAN, et al. 1993. Protective effect of vitamin E on exercise-induced oxidative damage in young and older adults. Am. J. Physiol. **264:** R992–R998.
40. JAKEMAN, P. & S. MAXWELL. 1993. Effect of antioxidant vitamin supplementation on muscle function after eccentric exercise. Eur. J. Appl. Physiol. Occup. Physiol. **67:** 426–430.
41. WARREN, J.A., R.R. JENKINS, L. PACKER, et al. 1992. Elevated muscle vitamin E does not attenuate eccentric exercise-induced muscle injury. J. Appl. Physiol. **72:** 2168–2175.
42. PETERSEN, E.W., K. OSTROWSKI, T. IBFELT, et al. 2001. Effect of vitamin supplementation on cytokine response and on muscle damage after strenuous exercise. Am. J. Physiol. Cell. Physiol. **280:** C1570–C1575.
43. VAN DER MEULEN, J.H., A. MCARDLE, M.J. JACKSON & J.A. FAULKNER. 1997. Contraction-induced injury to the extensor digitorum longus muscles of rats: the role of vitamin E. J. Appl. Physiol. **83:** 817–823.
44. MCARDLE, F., L.E. RHODES, R.A.G. PARSLEW, et al. 2004. Effects of oral vitamin E and β-carotene supplementation on UVR-induced oxidative stress in human skin. Am. J. Clin. Nutr. **80:** 1270–1275.
45. FREEMAN, M.L., M.J. BORELLI, K. SYED, et al. 1995. Characterisation of a signal generated by oxidation of protein thiols that activates the heat shock transcription factor. J. Cell. Physiol. **164:** 356–366.
46. PATTWELL, D., T. ASHTON, A. MCARDLE, et al. 2003. Ischemia and reperfusion of skeletal muscle lead to the appearance of a stable lipid free radical in the circulation. *Am. J. Physiol. Heart Circ. Physiol.* **284:** H2400–H2404.

Effect of Vitamin E on Gene Expression Changes in Diet-Related Carcinogenesis

JOSEPH LUNEC, EUGENE HALLIGAN, NALINI MISTRY, AND KATHERINE KARAKOULA

Genome Instability Group, University of Leicester, and the Department of Cancer & Molecular Medicine, Leicester, LE2 7LX, United Kingdom

ABSTRACT: Colorectal cancer (CRC) is responsible for the second highest associated mortality in Western Europe and the United States. Approximately 95% of CRC is sporadic and believed to involve environmental agents and chronic inflammation as causal elements. Several recent studies have suggested a link with diet, in particular, red meat, dietary fats, and low consumption of vegetables. Lipid peroxidation and arachidonic acid metabolism have specifically been implicated in genotoxicity, tumor initiation, and promotion. We have examined the global gene expression profiles (Affymetrix; HU133A) of differentiated vs. undifferentiated colonocytes (CRL-1807), with and without vitamin E supplementation, while undergoing a lipid peroxidative stress. Malondialdehyde and hydroxynonenal, generated by heating a mixture of linoleic and linolenic acid, caused DNA adduct formation identified by immunofluoresence. We also observed a decreased ability for vitamin E to upregulate detoxifying enzymes against free-radical peroxidation, with the exception of mitochondrial superoxide dismutase in undifferentiated cells. However, there was an increased ability in undifferentiated, rather than in differentiated, colonic cells to detect DNA damage, initiate cytostasis, and then effect subsequent DNA repair and apoptosis, in the presence of vitamin E. The expression profile implies less genotoxic stress is experienced in vitamin E–supplemented colonocytes, particularly undifferentiated cells, and points to a mechanism by which dietary supplementation may prevent genotoxic damage and subsequent carcinogenic events in the colon, by both antioxidant and non-antioxidant–related mechanisms.

KEYWORDS: colon cancer; vitamin E; microarray

INTRODUCTION

The risk of colorectal cancer (CRC) has been closely related to diet and lifestyle factors in many epidemiological, case control, and cohort studies.[1–3] Various studies have shown that risk is associated with an increased intake of dietary fat and a decreased intake of cereal grains and dietary fiber. Whereas analytical studies have associated risk with a decreased intake of vegetables and fruits, a sedentary lifestyle,

---

Address for correspondence: Professor Joe Lunec, Genome Instability Group, University of Leicester, Genome Instability Group, Department of Cancer & Molecular Medicine, Level 0, RKCSB, LRI, Leicester, LE2 7LX, U.K. Voice: 0116- 252-5890; fax: 0116-252-5887.
jl20@le.ac.uk

and obesity, a high intake of meat and sugar has also been implicated. However, large prospective cohort studies have failed to find a causal relationship between a high-fat diet and CRC. The inconsistencies in findings of dietary fat may relate to the fact that they are generally assessed in accordance with their quantity (total fat) or origin (animal or vegetable). There is now considerable epidemiological and experimental evidence to suggest a positive association between a high dietary intake of ω-6 polyunsaturated fatty acids (PUFAs), lauric and myristic acid, found in corn, safflower, and coconut oils, respectively, and increased risk of CRC,[4–6] whereas diets high in ω-3 PUFAs found in fish and olive oils have no enhancing effect on the incidence of CRC.[5,6] These dietary associations with CRC are characterized as typical of the Western diet and indeed countries such as Japan that are adopting a more Westernized diet are noting an increased colon cancer incidence.[7]

Nevertheless, despite these observations, the association between an increased dietary fat intake and CRC risk remains contentious, partly because of the lack of consensus on the mechanism of action of dietary fat in mammalian cells. Phospholipids of cell membranes contain significant amounts of PUFAs, which are highly susceptible to oxidation. Oxidation of the conjugated double bonds in PUFAs leads to a state of persistent oxidative stress that leads to generation of several reactive α,β-unsaturated aldehydes, which are potentially cytotoxic and are implicated in the pathophysiology of CRC.[8] The list of carbonyl compounds formed from the decomposition of lipid hydroperoxides is vast; for example, malondialdehyde (MDA); alkanals such as pentanal, hexanal, heptanal, octanal; alkenals such as 2-propenal (i.e., acrolein), 2-butenal (i.e. crotonaldehyde), 2-pentenal, 2-hexanal; ketones such as butanone, 2-pentanone, 2-octanone; 2,2-alkadienals such as heptadienal, nonadienal; 4,5-dihydroxydecanal; 4-hydroxy-2,5-nondienal; 5-hydroxy-octanol; various 4-hydroxy-2-alkenals such as 4-hydroxy-2-nonenal and 4-hydroxy-2-octenal.[9] Most of these compounds are generated via homolytic cleavage of carbon–carbon bonds in alkoxyl radicals.[10] Since many are not overtly toxic, or are only minor products of toxicological interest, research has focused on just a few compounds such as MDA, 4-hydroxy-2-nonenal (HNE), and various 2-alkenals. These have shown significant cytotoxicity and mutagenicity *in vitro*, following adduction with protein and DNA.[10] These DNA adducts possess strong miscoding potential *in vitro*,[11] and, of the DNA adducts formed by MDA, pyrimido(1,2α)purin-10(3H)one (M_1G) is readily detected in many human tissues. Other propano-adducts also originate from α,β–unsaturated aldehydes or enals such as acrolein (Acr), crotonaldehyde (Cro), glyoxal (Gly), and HNE. Adducts formed by HNE have also been detected in healthy human colon tissue.[12–13]

In this study, our aim was to observe any effects of vitamin E on aldehyde DNA adduct formation in colonocytes and combine this data with global gene expression analysis in order to establish novel mechanisms of protection afforded by vitamin E.

MATERIALS AND METHODS

Human Colon Epithelial Cell Culture

The human normal colon cell line CRL 1807 transformed with heat-sensitive SV40 virus (tsSV40) (American Tissue Culture Collection Repository, Rockville,

MD) was maintained in 25-cm^3 tissue culture flasks in Dulbecco's modified Eagle's medium supplemented with 10 % (v/v) fetal bovine serum, 50 µg/mL at 37°C in a humidified atmosphere containing 5% (v/v) CO_2.

Differentiation of CRL-1807 Colon Cells

CRL 1807 cells were seeded in to 75-cm^3 tissue culture flasks in Dulbecco's modified Eagle's medium supplemented with 10% fetal bovine serum, 50 µg/mL gentimycin, at 37°C in a humidified atmosphere of 5% CO_2. The cells were grown to approximately 75% confluency before the medium was replenished with fresh medium containing 20 mM retinoic acid and further incubated for three additional days. Three replicate determinations at each concentration were performed in each experiment.

Heat Oxidation of Linoleic/Linolenic Acid

In an open-top heat resistant tube, 1 mL of Me-linoleic acid and 1 mL Me-linolenic acid were mixed and heated to 180°C for 20 min in air. Following this incubation, the oils were allowed to cool to room temperature in air for 2 h. The oil mixture was stored at –20°C under an argon atmosphere until use.

Extraction of Heat-Oxidized Oil into Phosphate-Buffered Saline

Heat-oxidized oil (300 mL) was added to 2.7 mL phosphate-buffered saline (PBS) and vortexed for 2 min. Following this, the oil/PBS mixture was allowed to mix by rotation for 10 min. The oil/PBS mixture was then centrifuged at 1300 × g for 5 min, and the upper aqueous phase was removed and used immediately.

Exposure of Undifferentiated CRL-1807 Colon Cells to Heat-Oxidized Linoleic/Linolenic Acid

Conditioned medium was removed from undifferentiated CRL-1807 colon cells and replaced with fresh medium containing either 6 or 15 µL heat-oxidized oil/PBS (corresponding to 20 and 50 nM of MDA) extract, and was further incubated with cells for 24 h. Three replicate determinations at each concentration were performed in each experiment.

Preparation of CRL-1807 Cells for Fluorescence Microscopy

Following treatment with oil/PBS, conditioned medium was removed, and cells were washed twice with cold PBS. Cells were then fixed with 100% ice-cold ethanol for 5 min, following which excess ethanol was discarded and cells allowed to dry at room temperature. Immunoglobulin G purified antiserum 741, 200 µL/chamber (1:500 in PBS) were incubated for one hour at 37°C in a humidified atmosphere. Following two washes with PBS, a FITC-labeled anti-rabbit IgG antibody, 200 µL/chamber (1:100 in PBS), were added and incubated for a further hour as described above and protected from exposure to light. The slides were then washed twice with PBS before nuclear staining with 4,6-diamidino-2-phenylindole (DAPI), 200 µL/chamber (5 µg/ mL) for 5 min at room temperature. Following two washes with PBS, the chambers were removed and the cells were mounted using mounting medium consisting of glycerol in PBS with 0.1% sodium azide.

Imaging Software

Images were captured using a Hamamatsu 12-bit digital camera and FITC or DAPI filters on a 10-position filter wheel, which were controlled using Openlab 3.0 software (Improvision, University of Warwick Science Park, Coventry, UK). Additional software (advanced measurement and ratioing modules) allowed quantitative analysis of DNA damage as a ratio of the FITC/DAPI staining for each individual cell. In addition, the images were captured using an automated program such that the exposure and image capture parameters were unchanged for each reading.

Analysis for Aldehyde-DNA Adducts by Immunohistochemistry

Cells were allowed to reach room temperature (RT) for 30 min prior to analysis. They were then incubated for 30 min in a blocking solution of PBS, pH 7.2 containing 2% normal goat serum (NGS) at RT in a covered chamber. Following three PBS rinses, they were incubated with antiserum 741 at 1:500 dilution or monoclonal antibody M_1G at 1:500 dilution for two hours at RT in a covered chamber. Control cells were incubated with 2% NGS. Monoclonal antibody M_1G has been raised against malondialdehyde-deoxyguanosine adduct. The antibody was used at 1:500 dilution of 1.9 mg/mL stock and was a gift from L.J. Marnett. The cells were then washed three times with PBS and incubated with a biotinylated link antibody at 1:1000 dilution for one hour at RT in a covered chamber. For the detection of rabbit polyclonal primary antiserum and mouse monoclonal primary antibodies, biotinylated goat anti-rabbit immunoglobulins (DAKO E432), or biotinylated goat anti-mouse immunoglobulins (DAKO E433), were used, respectively. Control sections (without primary antibody) were treated with biotinylated goat anti-mouse immunoglobulins. Sections were washed three times with PBS. Incubation with FITC-labeled streptavidin (Vector Labs, SA-5001) at 1:100 dilution was for 30 min at RT in a covered chamber. All procedures from this point onward were carried out in the dark. Sections were rinsed three times with PBS and incubated with DAPI (1μg/ mL) for 5 min at RT. Sections were then rinsed three times with PBS and mounted using Vectashield fluorescence mounting medium.

Cells were viewed using a Zeiss Axioskop fluorescence microscope at ×20 magnification. Images were captured using a Hamamatsu 12-bit digital camera and FITC or DAPI filters on a 10-position filter wheel, which were controlled using Openlab 3.04 software (Improvision). Exposure time was set at 9 s.

Total RNA Extraction for Microarray Analysis

CRL-1807 cells were harvested and lysed in Tri reagent (Sigma Chemical Company, Pool, Dorset, UK) using repeated pipetting until no cell clumps were visible, and total RNA was isolated from each sample according to the manufacturer's instructions. The integrity of the total RNA from each replicate was established by formaldehyde gel electrophoresis (uniform RNA smear with intact 18 and 28S rRNA bands) before being pooled together for microarray analysis.

Hybridization and Staining for Microarray Analysis

In brief, a primer encoding the T7 RNA polymerase promoter linked to oligo dT24 was used to prime double-stranded cDNA synthesis from each total RNA sample using Superscript II reverse transcriptase (Invitrogen, Groningen, Holland). Each double-stranded cDNA sample was precipitated, then *in vitro* transcribed using T7 RNA polymerase (MEGAscript II T7, Ambion, Austin, TX), incorporating biotin-UTP and biotin-CTP (PerkinElmer Life Sciences Ltd, Cambridge, UK) into the resulting complementary RNA (cRNA). cRNA transcripts were fragmented at 95°C for 35 min in 30 mM magnesium acetate, 100 mM potassium acetate and 40 mM Tris-acetate to a mean size of ~50 to ~200 nucleotides, and hybridized to the HG-U95Av2 array for 16 h at 45°C. Arrays were washed, stained with streptavidin-R-phycoerythrin, and scanned at 3-mm resolution using an Agilent Gene Array Scanner.

Data Analysis

Scanned image files were visually inspected for hybridization anomalies (regions of intense/absent fluorescence) and analyzed following normalization with GeneChip™ 4.01 (Affymetrix) and dChip software.[14] The expression level (average difference) for each gene was determined by calculating the average of differences in intensity of fluorescence between perfect match and mismatch for each probe pair. MASS4.0 and dChip were used to filter and visualize genes whose fold change was ≥ 2.0 or ≤ -2.0 of baseline values and with absolute average difference intensity between baseline and experiment ≥ 50. Each sample corresponded to three separate and pooled total RNA preparations.

RESULTS AND DISCUSSION

The role of vitamin E, a potent lipid-soluble antioxidant, in the prevention of colon cancer is not clear. Harmful chemicals, such as lipid peroxides, in the diet and environment may be mutagenic to the colorectal epithelium and may promote colon cancer.[15,16] Food-derived lipid peroxides and reactive aldehydes are potent mutagens, and dietary antioxidants should prevent their formation; indeed, this appeared to be the case in our study (see FIGS. 1 and 2). We were able to detect a significant amelioration of the aldehyde adducts, identified by our antibodies, by preincubating cells for 24 h with vitamin E. This was the case for both antibodies but only with respect to undifferentiated colonocytes in each case. There was an apparent increase in DNA damage in vitamin E–treated differentiated cells, but this was probably due to a decrease in apoptosis. Vitamin E is a major lipid-soluble antioxidant and is widely known to prevent the propagation of lipid peroxides within membranes and by definition prevent the formation of toxic aldehydes such as MDA and HNE. It would be expected therefore that our experiment would show a protective effect against the heated oil–induced formation of the DNA adduct. It is well known that foods rich in polyunsaturated fatty acids are oxidized during the cooking process to produce mutagens such as lipid peroxides and MDA.[8] Furthermore, we know from the Iowa Women's Health Study, that a high intake of vitamin E is associated with a decreased incidence of colon cancer. In addition, we know that inflammatory bowel disease can also predispose to colon cancer. Inflammation can trigger the activation of leukocytes which results in the generation of various free-radical species such as nitric oxide and superoxide anion. Despite views to the contrary, it is possible to maintain a low-level, chronic flux of oxygen radicals and hydrogen peroxide in the colon that could diffuse into the colonic epithelial cells.[17] The latter process is also a potential source of endogenous lipid peroxides, which may be accelerated by the presence of unabsorbed iron in the large bowel.

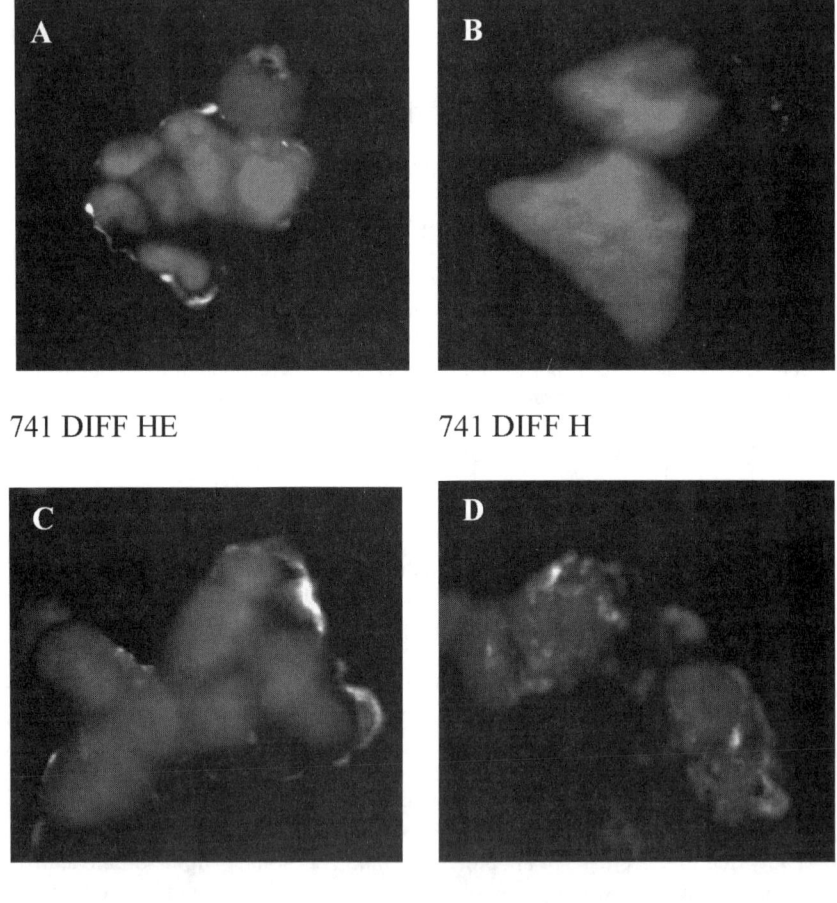

FIGURE 1. Immunocytochemical analysis of colon cells using antiserum 741. (**A** and **B**) Differentiated cells (CRL-1807) exposed to hot oil with and without vitamin E, respectively; (**C** and **D**) the corresponding undifferentiated cells exposed in exactly the same way. Antibody 741 was produced as a polyclonal antisera in rabbits and detected predominantly glyoxylated, HNE and acrolein DNA adducts.

One hundred eighteen genes were differentially expressed in the experiment. Some of the significant major gene groups included cell cycle; DNA damage and repair; cell signaling; and connective tissue–related genes. Their quantitative expression is summarized in TABLES 1–5. Cyclin D_1 is a nuclear protein whose expression is both necessary and rate-limiting for transit for G_1. The inhibition of cyclin D_1 expression by vitamin E in undifferentiated cells (TABLE 1) would suggest a lengthening of G_1. Cyclin D_1 is a target for chemoprevention in cancer, and its inhibition

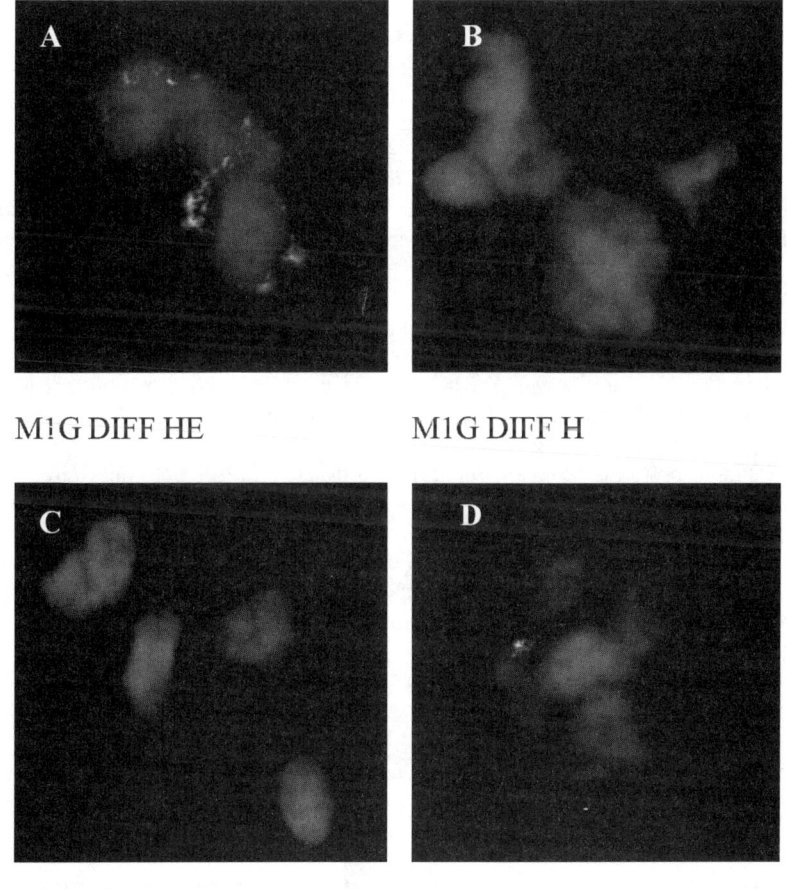

M1G DIFF HE M1G DIFF H

M1G UNDIFF HE UNDIFF H

FIGURE 2. Immunocytochemical analysis of colon cells using antiserum M1G. (**A** and **B**) Differentiated cells (CRL-1807) exposed to hot oil with and without vitamin E, respectively; (**C** and **D**) the corresponding undifferentiated cells treated in exactly the same way. This monoclonal antibody detects only MDA-DNA adducts.

would block cells from entering S phase. This result is consistent with the ability of vitamin E to promote the arrest of the cell cycle (see TABLE 2, Gadd 45α) and allow time for DNA repair. Gadd 45α plays an important role in maintaining genomic integrity. Gadd 45α–deficient cells have a slower rate of nucleotide excision repair and lack of G2/M arrest coupled with reduced DNA repair. It is induced under conditions of DNA damage because it primes the cell for arrest and DNA repair. It is clearly more active in differentiated compared to undifferentiated cells treated with vitamin E. This is consistent with the differential DNA damage exposed by our aldehyde-DNA antibodies.

p27 is repressed by mitogenic growth factors and induced by specific mitogenic signals. This gene is increased in vitamin-treated, undifferentiated cells relative to differentiated colonocytes. Furthermore, the relative increase in p21 in undifferentiated cells (−1.0 vs. −2.2) suggests that both cell types are protected from DNA damaging agents because p21 is required for regulation of DNA repair. This is most apparent in the undifferentiated cells. Again, this is entirely consistent with the corresponding effects of vitamin E on Gadd 45α expression.

Gadd 45α is highly expressed in undifferentiated cells whereas it is repressed in highly differentiated colonocytes under the influence of vitamin E. This is consistent with the extent of DNA damage induced in both cell types and the protection afforded by vitamin E (see FIGS. 1 and 2). E2F transcription factors are known to regulate the expression of genes involved in cell differentiation, development, proliferation, and apoptosis. P107 and p130 transcription factors are downstream effectors and when associated with E2F act as transcriptional repressors, whereas free E2F acts to activate transcription of genes.[18] The effects caused by incubating undifferentiated colonocytes with vitamin E appear to promote greater protection from the DNA damaging activity of the hot oil.

TABLE 3 shows the genes that are affected by vitamin E in both undifferentiated and differentiated cells in terms of cell signaling and DNA repair. From TABLES 1 and 2, we see that there is a relative upregulation in Gadd 45α and p21 in undifferentiated cells, apparently induced by the combined effects of vitamin E and hot oil. Both Gadd 45α and p21 act to coordinately arrest the growth of cells following DNA damage. In addition, Mdm2, which is also upregulated by p53, is markedly elevated in undifferentiated cells protected by vitamin E. Mdm2 protein is believed to have a role in regulating growth arrest by forming complexes with p53 and inhibiting its effects. In TABLE 3 it is clear that vitamin E has a profound effect on (stress-activated and growth-promoting) MAP kinase activity, suppressing it markedly compared to differentiated cells. This is a well-established effect of vitamin E. It is clear from the rest of the genes shown to be affected that vitamin E has a marked, upregulating effect on homologous recombination (RAD54), nucleotide excision repair, and transcription-coupled repair. However, vitamin E had little positive effect on mismatch repair (mut S or MSH2). It has previously been associated with colon cancer.[19] In TABLE 4 we see the general suppressive effect that vitamin E has on antioxidant enzymes with the exception of superoxide dismutase. However, metalothioneins are known to be protective against oxidative stress and are increased during the DNA damage response together with thrombospondin-1.[20] In TABLE 5 we see marked effects of vitamin E on tissue remodeling (wound healing) with relative upregulation of fibronectin, suppression of collagenase, and an elevation of tissue inhibitor of metalloproteinase (TIMP), particularly in undifferentiated cells.

TABLE 1. Cell cycle

				A^a			B^a
cyclin D1 (PRAD1: parathyroid adenomatosis 1)	M73554	1042.91 P	63.65 P	−16.39	1042.91 P	1449.77 P	1.39
cyclin D1 (PRAD1: parathyroid adenomatosis 1)	X59798	1488.49 P	91.86 P	−16.2	1488.49 P	2054.87 P	1.38
cyclin D1 (PRAD1: parathyroid adenomatosis 1)	M64349	387.24 P	97.44 P	−3.97	387.24 P	928.55 P	2.4
cyclin D3	M92287	546.3 P	240.66 P	−2.27	546.3 P	798.55 P	1.46
cyclin F	Z36714	286.19 P	131.77 P	−2.17	286.19 P	482.2 P	1.68
cyclin G2	U47414	58.2 P	196.44 P	3.38	52.2 P	25.96 P	−2.24
cyclin G2	U47414	157.5 P	330.64 P	2.1	157.5 P	46.57 P	−3.38
cyclin-dependent kinase inhibitor 3 (CDK2-associated)	L25876	320.31 P	737.7 P	2.3	320.31 P	480.96 P	1.5
cyclin-dependent kinase inhibitor 1B (p27, Kip1)	AL304854	207.58 P	360.97 P	1.74	207.58 P	99.31 P	−2.09
cyclin-dependent kinase inhibitor 1A (p21, Cip1)	U03106	2452.93 P	2322.43 P	−1.06	2452.93 P	1102.4 P	−2.23
cell division cycle 2-like 2	AL031282	213.48 P	87.56 P	−2.44	213.48 P	229.56 P	1.08

[a]Columns A and B represent fold change in some expression in vitamin E-treated undifferentiated and differentiated cells, respectively.

TABLE 2. DNA damage response[a]

				A			B
breast cancer 1, early onset	L7833	118.73 P	252.145 P	2.12	118.73 P	38.7 P	-3.07
Mdm2, transformed 3T3 cell double minute 2, p53 binding	U33202	51.54 P	396.45 P	7.69	51.54 P	44.49 A	-1.16
Mdm2, transformed 3T3 cell double minute 2, p53 binding	M92424	24.53 P	174.96 P	7.13	24.53 P	20.81 A	-1.18
growth arrest and DNA-damage–inducible, α	M60974	606.26 P	1606.88 P	2.65	606.26 P	193.31 P	-3.14
CHK1 checkpoint homologue (S. pombe)	AF016582	72.1 P	215.75 P	2.99	72.1 P	84.73 A	1.18
checkpoint suppressor 1	U68723	702.05 P	488.02 P	-1.44	702.05 P	320.55 P	-2.19
growth arrest-specific 6	L13720	1069.34 P	267.24 P	-4	1069.34 P	437.3 P	-2.45
programmed cell death 6	AF035606	628.22 P	258.63 P	-2.43	628.22 P	571.04 P	-1.1
PRKC, apoptosis, WT1, regulator	U63809	80.31 P	411.61 P	5.13	80.31 P	111.17 P	1.38
E2F transcription factor 4, p107/p130- binding	S75174	131.85 P	346.21 P	2.63	131.85 P	73.23 P	-1.8
E2F transcription factor 2	AL021154	243.23 P	1264.6 P	5.2	243.23 P	444.74 P	1.83

[a]Columns A and B represent fold change in some expression in vitamin E–treated undifferentiated and differentiated cells, respectively.

TABLE 3. Cell signaling/DNA repair[a]

				A			B
mitogen-activated protein kinase-activated protein kinase	U12779	1038.67 P	516.31 P	-2.01	1038.67 P	1123.21 P	1.08
mitogen-activated protein kinase kinase kinase	AB014587	177.6 P	65.82 P	-2.7	177.6 P	225.58 P	1.27
mitogen-activated protein kinase kinase 3	D87116	531.8 P	104.91 P	-5.07	531.8 P	924.59 P	1.74
mitogen-activated protein kinase-activated protein kinase	U09578	274.99 P	135.79 P	-2.03	274.99 P	459.59 P	1.67
TGFβ-inducible early growth response	S81439	58.68 P	194.61 P	3.32	58.68 P	104.55 P	1.78
RAD54-like (*S. cerevisiae*)	X97795	262.8 P	615.93 P	2.34	262.9 P	165.41 P	-1.59
excision repair cross-complementing rodent repair defic.	X52221	88.24 P	208.58 P	2.36	88.24 P	117.35 P	1.33
Cockayne syndrome 1 (classical)	U28413	114.4 P	312.16 P	2.73	114.4 P	86.76 P	-1.32
UV radiation resistance-associated gene	X99050	303.47 P	667.01 P	2.2	303.47 P	302.73 P	-1
MCM4 minichromosome maintenance deficient 4 (*S. cerevisiae*)	X74794	93.5 P	197.27 P	2.11	93.5 P	79.36 P	-1.18
mutS homologue 2, colon cancer, nonpolyposis type 1	U02911	302.96 P	127.96 P	-2.37	302.96 P	299.38 P	-1.01
mutS homologue 2, colon cancer, nonpolyposis type 1	U03911	200.25 P	89.06 P	-2.25	200.25	115.18 P	-1.74
5′ nucleotidase (CD73)	X55740	1011.72 P	138.31 P	-7.31	1011.72 P	713.17 P	-1.42
Fanconi anemia, complementation group G	AC004472	686.85 P	244.33 P	-2.81	686.85 P	811.4 P	1.18
nucleotide binding protein	U13919	246.27 P	115.98 P	-2.12	246.27 P	327.44 P	1.33
PMS1 postmeiotic seregation increased 1 (*S. cerevisiae*)	U13695	253.36 P	171.71 P	-1.48	253.36 P	103.26 P	-2.45
damage-specific DNA dinding protein 2 (48kD)	U18300	388.47 P	273.1 P	-1.32	388.47 P	145.72 P	-2.67
topoisomerase (DNA) 1 alpha (170kD)	J04088	360.39 P	613.59 P	1.7	360.39 P	360.39 P	-2.22

[a]Columns A and B represent fold change in some expression in vitamin E–treated undifferentiated and differentiated cells, respectively.

TABLE 4. Antioxidants[a]

				A			B
metallothionein 1L	AA224832	179.99 P	406.98 P	2.26	179.99 P	263.23 P	1.46
metallothionein 2A	AI547258	191.83 P	87.83 P	-2.18	191.83 P	231.52 P	1.21
NADH dehydrogenase (ubiquinone) 1 α subcomple.	L04490	113.5 P	85.67 P	-1.32	113.5 P	231.19 P	2.04
NADH dehydrogenase (ubiquinone) Fe-S protein 6 (13k)	AI360249	413.6 P	200.55 P	-2.06	413.6 P	746.13 P	1.8
NADH dehydrogenase (ubiquinone) Fe-S protein 8 (23k)	AF038406	1012.89 P	490.56 P	-2.06	1012.89 P	1115.01 P	1.1
superoxide dismutase 2, mitochondrial	X07834	88.65 P	229.5 P	2.59	88.65 P	159.89 P	1.8
glutathione-S-transferase-like; glutathione transferase c	U90313	1911.21 P	700.51 P	-2.73	1911.21 P	2057.48 P	1.08
thrombospondin 1	X14787	21.4 P	130.5 P	6.1	21.4 P	30.6 A	1.43
glutaredoxin (thioltransferase)	X76648	398.75 P	156.23 P	-2.55	398.75 P	308.9 P	-1.29
quinone oxidoreductase homolog	AF010309	279.75 P	60.83 P	-4.6	279.75 P	94.99 P	-2.95

[a]Columns A and B represent fold change in some expression in vitamin E-treated undifferentiated and differentiated cells, respectively.

TABLE 5. Connective tissue/proteases[a]

			A			B
fibronectin 1	M10905	797.18 P	1003.11 P	1.26	797.18	253.11 P	−3.15
fibronectin 1	M10905	587.14 P	713.65 P	1.22	587.14 P	219.51 P	−2.67
collagen, type X, α1 (Schmid metaphyseal chondr.)	X60382	31.31 P	195.51 P	6.24	31.31 P	52.22 P	1.67
collagen, type XIII, α1	M59217	152.84 P	17.15 P	−8.91	152.84	80.62 P	−1.9
collagen, type V, α2	Y14690	926.24 P	2816.2 P	3.04	926.24 P	638.33 P	−1.45
collagen, type VIII, α1	X57527	687.9 P	305.88 P	−2.25	687.9 P	290.98 P	−2.36
collagen, type XIII, α1	M33653	357.86 P	24.95 A	−14.34	357.86 P	127.08 P	−2.82
collagen, type XV, α1	L25286	181.86 P	106.45 P	−1.71	181.86 P	23.45 P	−7.76
matrix metalloproteinase 1 (interstitial collagenase)	M13509	676.33 P	116.6 P	−5.8	676.33 P	1530.45 P	2.26
cathepsin K (pycnodysostosis)	X82153	219.31 P	92.09 P	−2.38	219.31 P	52.29 P	−4.19
tissue inhibitor of metalloproteinase 3 (Sorsby fundus d.)	U14394	159.67 P	323.78 P	2.03	159.67 P	98.4 P	−1.62
tissue inhibitor of metalloproteinase 3 (Sorsby fundus d.)	U14394	214.42 P	559.8 P	2.61	214.42 P	142.44 P	−1.51
chondroitin sulfate proteoglycan 4 (melaoma-associated)	X96753	463.01 P	87.18 P	−5.31	463.01 P	512.2 P	1.11

[a]Columns A and B represent fold change in some expression in vitamin E–treated undifferentiated and differentiated cells, respectively.

The colonic mucosa is composed of crypts lined with epithelial cells, all of which are at varying degrees of proliferation and differentiation. Precursor or stem cells lining the base of the crypt are undifferentiated and have a large proliferative capacity and migrate towards the luminal surface.[21–23] These migrating cells undergo numerous divisions before acquiring the fundamental functional abilities of a typical differentiated colonocyte.[24] This ordered growth program of colonic epithelial cells breaks down during colonic tumorgenesis.[25] In 1974, Lipkin proposed a multi-step model of colon carcinogenesis in which colonic epithelial cells do not repress DNA synthesis during migration along the crypt axis and may consequently aid the development of additional abnormal properties enabling them to be retained in the mucosa and produce adenomatous lesions. Lipid peroxides, generated during the cooking of oils or generated endogenously by inflammatory activity, may represent a continuous stress, which causes genotoxicity, particularly in undifferentiated cells. The overall suggestion is that undifferentiated cells in the crypt may be more vulnerable to the consequences of DNA damage.[26]

In this study, we have utilized Affymetrix high-density oligonucleotide U133A arrays, with probe sets complimentary to more than 26,000 human genes, to monitor levels of mRNA expression. We have evaluated the relative efficacy of vitamin E in both undifferentiated and differentiated CRL-1807 cells in protecting against the lipid peroxides and aldehydes present in heated oils. This experiment was designed specifically to test the theory that the undifferentiated cells of the crypt may be a particular focus of lipid peroxide–mediated DNA damage and early carcinogenesis.[27] Hence, the addition of vitamin E would arguably protect cells that were most vulnerable. The gene expression profile of differentiated versus undifferentiated colonocytes, with the added vitamin E protection, observed in this experiment, points to an almost equal ability to protect the genome from damaging detoxifying enzymes against free-radical peroxidation; an increased ability to detect and subsequently repair DNA damage; and an enhanced ability in undifferentiated cells to effect cytostasis, subsequent DNA repair, and apoptosis. This indicates that undifferentiated cells such as those lining the crypt may indeed be more vulnerable to the effects of DNA damage and that, in the presence of vitamin E, protection is complex and due not only to antioxidant action.

REFERENCES

1. POTTER, J.D. *et al.* 1993. Colon cancer: a review of the epidemiology. Epidemiol. Rev. **15:** 499–545.
2. HOWE, G.R. *et al.* 1992. Dietary intake of fiber and decreased risk of cancers of the colon and rectum: evidence from the combined analysis of 13 case-control studies. J. Natl. Cancer Inst. **84:** 1887–1896.
3. HOWE, G.R. *et al.* 1997. The relationship between dietary fat intake and risk of colorectal cancer: evidence from the combined analysis of 13 case-control studies. Cancer Causes Control **8:** 215–228.
4. POTTER, J.D. 1995. Risk factors for colon neoplasia: epidemiology and biology. Eur. J. Cancer **31A:**1033–1038.
5. REDDY, B.S., C. BURILL & J. RIGOTTY. 1991. Effects of diets high in ω-3 and ω-6 fatty acids on initiation and postination stages of colon carcinogenesis. Cancer Res. **51:** 487–491.
6. DESCHNER, E.E. *et al.* 1990. The effects of dietary omega-3 fatty acids (fish oil) on azomethanol-induced focal areas of dysplasia and colon tumor incidence. Cancer **66:** 2350–2356.

7. WILLETT, WC. 2001. Diet and cancer: one view at the start of the millennium. Cancer Epidemiol. Biomarkers Prev. **10:** 3–8.
8. VACCA, C.E., J. WILHELM & M. HARMS-RINGDAHL. 1988. Interaction of lipid peroxidation products with DNA: a review. Mutat. Res. **195:**137–149.
9. ESTERBAUER, H. *et al.* 1982. Separation and characterization of the aldehydic products of lipid peroxidation stimulated by ADP-Fe2+ in rat liver microsomes. Biochem. J. **208:** 129–140.
10. ESTERBAUER, H., R.J. SCHAUR & H. ZOLLNER. 1991. Chemistry and biochemistry of 4-hydroxynonenal, malondialdehyde and aldehydes. Free Radical Biol. Med. **11:** 81–128.
11. MARNETT, L.J. & A.L. WILCOX. 1995. The chemistry of lipid alkoxyl radicals and their role in metal amplified lipid peroxidation. Biochem. Soc. Symp. **61:** 65–72.
12. SCHAEFERHENRICH, A. *et al.* 2003. Human adenoma cells are highly susceptible to the genotoxic action of 4-hydroxy-2-nonenal. Mutat. Res. **526:** 19–32.
13. BACH, S.P., A.G. RENEHAN & C.S. POTTEN. 2000. Stem cells: the intestinal stem cell as a paradigm. Carcinogenesis **21:** 469–476.
14. LI, C. & W.H. WONG. 2001. Model based analysis of oligonucleotide arrays: expression index computation and outlier detection. Proc. Natl. Acad. Sci. **91:** 31–38.
15. BARTSCH, H., J. NAIR & R.W. OWEN. 1999. Dietary polyunsaturated fatty acids and cancers of the breast and colorectum: emerging evidence for their role as risk modifiers. Carcinogenesis **20:** 2209–2218.
16. BABBS, C.F. 1980. Hypothesis paper: free radicals and the etiology of colon cancer. Free Radical Biol. Med. **8:** 191–200.
17. ERHARDT, G. *et al.* 1997. A diet rich in fat and poor in dietary fibre increases the *in vitro* formation of reactive oxygen species in human feces. J. Nutr. **127:** 106–109.
18. MULLER, H. *et al.* 2001. E2Fs regulate the expression of genes involved in differentiation, development, proliferation, and apoptosis. Genes Dev. **15:** 267–285.
19. FISHEL, R. *et al.* 1993. The human mutator gene homolog MSH2 and its association with hereditary nonpolyposis colon cancer. Cell **75:** 1027–1038.
20. JASANI, B. *et al.* 1998. Clonal overexpression of metallothionein is induced by somatic mutation in morphologically normal colonic mucosa. J. Pathol. **184:** 144–147.
21. LIPKIN, M. 1974. Proliferative changes in the colon. Am. J. Dig. Dis. **19:**1029–1032.
22. HALL, P.A. & F.M. WATT. 1989. Functional-characterization of a stem-cell population from cultured human keratinocytes [abstract]. J. Pathol. **157:** A172.
23. HONG, M.Y. *et al.* 1997. Relationship among colonocyte proliferation, differentiation, and apoptosis as a function of diet and carcinogen. Nutr. Cancer **28:** 20–29.
24. LAMPRECT, S. A. & M. LIPKIN. 2002. Migrating colonic crypt epithelial cells: primary targets for transformation. Carcinogenesis **23:** 1777–1780.
25. POTTEN, C.S *et al.* 1992. A possible explanation for the differential cancer incidence in the intestine, based on distribution of the cytotoxic effects of carcinogens in the murine large-bowel. Carcinogenesis **13:** 2305–2312.
26. KANAZAWA, A. *et al.* 2002. Dietary lipid peroxidation products and DNA damage in colon carcinogenesis. Eur. J. Lipid Sci. Technol. **13:** 439–447.

Oral Supplementation with *All-Rac-* and *RRR*-α-Tocopherol Increases Vitamin E Levels in Human Sebum after a Latency Period of 14–21 Days

SWARNA EKANAYAKE-MUDIYANSELAGE,[a,b] KLAUS KRAEMER,[c] AND JENS J. THIELE[a]

[a]*Department of Dermatology, Northwestern University Medical School, Chicago, Illinois, USA*

[b]*Department of Dermatology, Friedrich Schiller University, Jena, Germany*

[c]*BASF, Ludwigshafen, Germany*

ABSTRACT: In human skin, highest α-tocopherol levels are found in facial sebum. We hypothesized that the bioavailability of vitamin E in human skin is, at least in part, dependent on sebaceous gland secretion. To test this, 24 volunteers were subjected to a randomized daily supplementation with either 400 mg *RRR*-α-tocopheryl acetate (*RRR*-α-toc) or 400 mg *all-rac*-α-tocopheryl acetate (*all-rac*-α-toc) for 14 days. Fasting blood samples, facial sebum samples, and lower-arm skin-surface lipids (SSL) were taken at time-points between 0–21 days. Samples were analyzed by HPLC for α-tocopherol and squalene concentrations. Increased serum α-tocopherol levels were detectable as early as 12 h after supplementation of *RRR*-α-toc or *all-rac*-α-toc and peaked on day 7. No significant changes were observed in lower-arm SSL. Remarkably, while unchanged until day 14, α-tocopherol sebum levels were increased on day 21 in both the *RRR*-α-toc and the *all-rac*-α-toc group by 87% and 92%, respectively. With respect to dietary supplementation of vitamin E and its bioavailability in human skin, these results suggest that (1) sebaceous gland secretion is a relevant delivery mechanism; (2) the bioavailabilities of *RRR*-α-toc and the *all-rac*-α-toc are similar; and (3) significant accumulation requires a daily supplementation period of at least 2–3 weeks.

KEYWORDS: antioxidants; sebum; vitamin E; tocopherol; sebaceous gland

ABBREVIATIONS: SC, stratum corneum; SSL, skin-surface lipids; SQ, squalene; UV, ultraviolet; ECD, electrochemical detection; RRR-α-toc, RRR-α-tocopheryl acetate; all-rac-α-toc, all-rac-α-tocopheryl acetate; BHT, butylated hydroxytoluene; HPLC, high-pressure liquid chromatography.

Address for correspondence: Jens J. Thiele, M.D., Ward Building 9-321, Department of Dermatology, Northwestern University, 303 East Chicago Avenue, Chicago, IL 60611. Voice and fax: 312-503-4843

j-thiele@northwestern.edu

INTRODUCTION

Vitamin E, an essential lipophilic nutrient, is a key component of all biological membranes and is provided to the human organism by dietary intake.[1] α-Tocopherol, the major biologically active vitamin E homologue, is generally regarded as the most important lipid-soluble antioxidant in human tissues.[2] While numerous studies have demonstrated penetration and beneficial effects of topically applied vitamin E, little is known on the cutaneous bioavailability of dietary vitamin E and its various homologues. Werninghaus et al. found unchanged tocopherol levels in full-skin thickness biopsies taken from buttocks of human volunteers after supplementation with 400 IU (approximately 295 mg) of oral vitamin E.[3] Subsequent studies have indicated that upper epidermal layers are particularly susceptible to vitamin E depletion and oxidative stress induced by environmental factors, such as solar UV exposure.[4,5] It was concluded that α-tocopherol may play a crucial role not only for protecting lipid bilayers in viable cell membranes, but also in the stratum corneum (SC).[6] As the outermost layer of human skin, the SC functions as a biophysical penetration barrier of the human body. In skin regions rich in sebaceous glands, such as in facial skin, the outer SC layers contain high amounts of skin-surface lipids (SSL), which are derived from both epidermal lipids and as well as from lipids synthesized by sebaceous glands ("sebum").[7,8] The secretion of sebum is controlled by hormonal factors that regulate the proliferation, differentiation, and maturation of sebaceous cells.[9] While the upper SC layers of human skin generally contain very low amounts of vitamin E, its concentrations in human facial skin were found to be elevated in the outermost SC layers.[10] Consequently, it was demonstrated that human sebum contains the highest amounts of α-tocopherol detected in human skin and accounts for the high levels of vitamin E found in the outermost SC layers and SSL of facial skin. On the basis of the good correlation found between physiological levels of α-tocopherol and the sebum marker lipid squalene (SQ) in human sebum, it was suggested that the role of vitamin E is to maintain low levels of SQ oxidation products in skin surface lipids.[11,12] Adverse effects known to result from skin exposure to SQ peroxides[13,14] may be prevented by physiological antioxidants such as vitamin E.[15]

On the basis of these findings, we postulated that sebaceous gland secretion is a major pathway of vitamin E delivery to human skin and accounts for the high levels of α-tocopherol found in facial SSL by re-penetration of the upper SC.[10] Indeed, a recent study confirmed that orally supplemented deuterium-labeled α-tocopherol was recovered in SSL extractions of forehead skin of four human volunteers.[16] However, since SSL are derived from both epidermal and sebaceous lipids,[8] the role of sebaceous glands and sebum in dietary vitamin E delivery still remains to be elucidated. The goal of the present study was (1) to evaluate whether daily oral intake of 400 mg tocopheryl acetate results in increased levels of α-tocopherol in sebum; (2) to investigate the accumulation of α-tocopherol in sebum as well as in SSL from skin with poor density of sebaceous glands; and (3) to compare the sebaceous bioavailability of *RRR*-α-tocopheryl acetate and *all-rac*-α-tocopheryl acetate over a period of up to 3 weeks.

MATERIAL AND METHODS

Chemicals

All chemicals and solvents were of highest analytical or HPLC grade, unless specified otherwise. HPLC-grade ethanol and methanol were from Roth GmbH, Karlsruhe, Germany. α-Tocopherol used for standard curve calibration was from Merck, Darmstadt, Germany, lithium perchlorate from ABC Chemie, Germany. SQ, SDS, BHT and EDTA were all from Sigma–Aldrich, Steinheim, Germany.

Volunteers

Approval for this human subject study was granted by the ethical commission of the Friedrich Schiller University, Jena. Written, informed consent was obtained from all individuals entering the study. Twenty-four healthy volunteers (12 females, 12 males; average age: 29.5 ± 8.8 years; Fitzpatrick skin types: II: 11, III: 13) entered this study and 23 participants completed the entire study (one drop-out at day 2 due to repeated hypotensive episodes during venipuncture). Exclusion criteria were: history of dermatologic disorders, current medical problems or systemic medication, oral or topical antioxidant supplementation, smoking, exclusive vegetarian diet, pregnancy, and exposure to intense solar or artificial UV-exposure/ tanning salons in the 3 months preceding the start of the study. Participants were asked not to apply any creams and ointments to the skin or to take any oral or topical antioxidant supplementation 14 days prior to and during the entire study. Over the same period, test subjects were provided with vitamin E–free skin care products (Palmolive Sensitive® fluid soap for sensitive skin [Colgate Palmolive, Piscataway, NJ]; Penaten No Tears® Baby Shampoo [Johnson & Johnson, Duesseldorf, Germany] and instructed not to use other products. The study was performed in the winter months of February and March 2003 to ensure the lowest possible environmental UV-exposure levels.

Experimental Protocol

A randomized, single-blinded study design was applied. All volunteers were randomly assigned to either *RRR*-α-tocopheryl acetate ("*RRR*-α-toc"; natural source of vitamin E, $n = 12$) or *all-rac*-α-tocopheryl acetate ("*all-rac*-α-toc"; synthetic source of vitamin E, $n = 12$) supplementation group. Both supplements were administered as single doses of 400 mg, given once daily in form of soft gelatin capsules (provided by BASF, Ludwigshafen, Germany) for 14 consecutive days. Participants were instructed to take the vitamin E capsules in the morning along with a standardized candy bar meal (Mars Mini®, Masterfoods, Verden, Germany). Fasting blood samples, sebum samples from foreheads, and skin-surface lipid samples from volar forearms skin were taken at $t = 0h$, 12h, 1d, 2d, 3d, 7d, 14d, and 21d after starting the oral supplementation. In order to avoid contamination, investigators wore powder-free latex gloves that were routinely changed after each individual sampling procedure.

Blood Samples

Blood samples (9 mL) were collected after overnight fasting prior to the volunteers' first meal by venipuncture using sterile monovettes (S-Monovette, Sarstedt,

Nuermbrecht, Germany). Plasma and serum were separated by centrifugation (10 min at 4°C) and the serum was immediately stored at −80°C.

Serum Analysis

Serum amounts of 20 μL were transferred into 15-mL test tubes (Cellstar, Greiner-Bio-one, Frickenhausen, Germany) on ice, and 500 μL EDTA (1 mM in PBS) and 50 μL BHT (10 mg/mL ethanol, 4°C) were added and vortexed. 250 μL 0.1M SDS was added, vortexed for 1 min at room temperature, and then mixed with 1 mL ethanol and vortexed for 1 min at 4°C. Thereafter, 2 mL hexane was added and the whole sample vigorously vortexed for 5 minutes, and then centrifuged at 4°C. 1 mL of the hexane phase was then transferred into a 1.5-mL Eppendorf tube and evaporated using a SpeedVac system (Thermo-Electron, Karlsruhe, Germany). The residue was resolved in 100 μL ethanol, vortexed for 1 min, centrifuged for 3 min at 4°C, and 10 μL was directly injected into the HPLC system.

Sebum Collection

Sebum samples were collected from the foreheads of each volunteer using Sebutapes® (Cuderm, Dallas, Texas) as previously described.[17] In brief: forehead skin was cleaned prior to sample acquisition using a sterile gauze ball (Gazin®, Lohmann & Rauscher International GmbH, Rengsdorf, Germany) that was soaked in 1 mL 70% (v/v) ethanol. Black borders of the Sebutapes were removed prior to application. Each tape was individually weighed before and after sebum collection to calculate the amount of sebum collected. For each time point given, four Sebutapes were applied onto the forehead skin for 60 minutes. Overall, the average amount of sebum collected per Sebutape in this study was 0.89 mg ± 0.33 mg ($n = 736$; means ± SD). Immediately after collection and weighing, sebum-enriched tapes were stored in Eppendorf tubes at −80°C until further analysis.

Sebum Lipid Extraction

Each sebum-enriched Sebutape was extracted in 975 μL HPLC-grade ethanol and 25 μL BHT (10 mg/mL ethanol) by vortexing for 1 minute in 1.5-mL Eppendorf tubes. Thereafter, tapes were removed and the remainder centrifuged at 4000 rpm and 4°C for 10 min (5415R, Eppendorf, Hamburg, Germany). The supernatant was transferred into another Eppendorf tube and immediately subjected to HPLC analysis.

Skin-Surface Lipid Extraction and Analysis

SSL extractions were performed at each given time point in two volar forearm sites (duplicate sampling for each time point). A round glass cup of 2.9 cm inner diameter was placed in the center of one forearm and 1 mL HPLC-grade ethanol was pipetted into the cup. The ethanol-covered skin area was gently rubbed using a glas rod in a standardized pattern for 1 minute. Subsequently, ethanol extracts were removed using a pipette, transferred into a 1.5-mL Eppendorf tube and centrifuged at 4000 rpm and 4°C for 10 min to remove SC squames and debris. Supernatants of each sample were taken, and vortexed with 25 μL BHT (10 mg/mL HPLC-grade ethanol). 100 μL of each collected sample was used for HPLC analysis.

HPLC Analysis of α-Tocopherol and SQ in Human Sebum, Skin-Surface Lipids, and Serum

High-performance liquid chromatography (HPLC) was performed using a Gynkotek HPLC system (Dionex-Softron GmbH, Germering, Germany) as described.[17] The HPLC system included an auto sampler (Gina 50), pump (M480G), degasser, UV/Vis-detector (UVD 340S, all from Gynkotek/Dionex-Softron), and an electrochemical detector (ECD) (ANTEC, Leyden, the Netherlands). All samples were analyzed at room temperature (20–22°C) using a Luna 5μ C18(2) column (250 × 4.6 mm, Phenomenex®, Hösbach, Germany). The mobile phase consisted of HPLC-grade ethanol and methanol (1:1, v/v) and 20 mM lithium perchlorate. The flow rate was 1.4 mL/min. Control standards of SQ and α-tocopherol standards were prepared from commercially available pure SQ and α-tocopherol. SQ standards were detected by UV-detection at 210 nm and α-tocopherol by in-line electrochemical detection (ECD) operating with an oxidation potential of 500 mV at a scale of 0.02 × 100 nA/V. Peak integration and quantitation were performed by Gynkotek Software 5.6 (Dionex-Softron GmbH, Germering, Germany).

Statistical Analysis

Statistical analysis was carried out using repeated measures paired one-way ANOVA (Sofware Graph Pad Instat®, Graph Pad Software, Inc., San Diego, USA). All data are given as means ± standard error of the means.

RESULTS

Serum Levels of Vitamin E

Baseline serum concentrations of α-tocopherol taken prior to the supplementation period were 21.4 ± 1.12 μmol/L in the *RRR*-α-toc group, and 21.0±0.93 μmol/L in the *all-rac*-α-toc group, respectively (means ± SEM; FIG. 1). Serum α-tocopherol levels were significantly increased as early as 12h after the first supplementation of *RRR*-α-toc or *all-rac*-α-toc and peaked on day 7 with an average increase of 76% and 73%, respectively (FIG. 1). One week after the last supplementation (day 21), α-tocopherol levels were decreased in both groups (*RRR*-α-toc group: 22.8 ±1.23 μmol/L; *all-rac*-α-toc-group: 24.6 ±2.01 μmol/L). No significant differences were observed between the two groups during the entire investigation period (FIG. 1).

SQ Levels in Sebum

Baseline levels of SQ in facial sebum were equally distributed over the study groups and remained unchanged during the entire observation period (FIG. 2). Specifically, baseline SQ concentrations were 96.2±5.4 μmol/mg sebum in the *RRR*-α-toc group and 99.2 ± 6.42 μmol/mg sebum in the *all-rac*-α-toc group. No significant differences were observed between the two groups.

SQ and α-Tocopherol Levels in Skin-Surface Lipids (SSL)

As was found in sebum, SQ levels in SSL remained unchanged during the entire study (data not shown). Average baseline α-tocopherol levels ranged from 1.9 ±

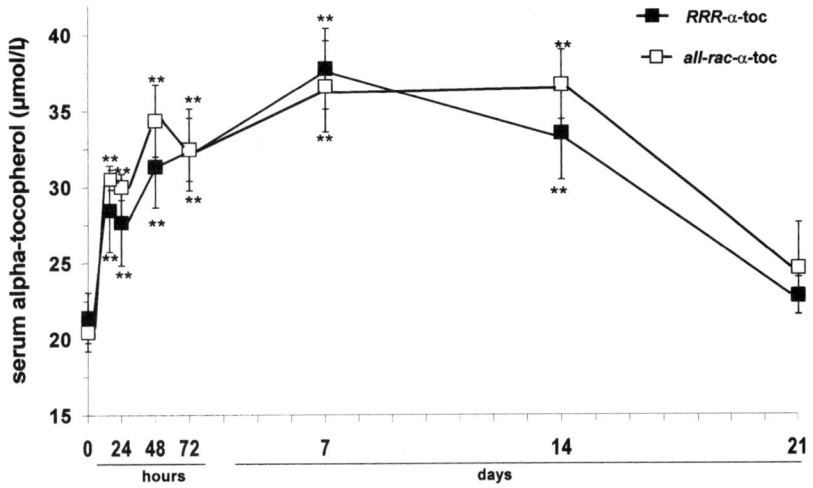

FIGURE 1. Serum α-tocopherol kinetics upon supplementation with both natural and synthetic vitamin E. All blood samples (except for the 12-h time-point) were taken after overnight fasting. α-Tocopherol was analyzed by HPLC. *RRR*-α-tocopheryl acetate supplementation group ("*RRR*-α-toc"): $n = 12$; *all-rac*-α-tocopheryl acetate supplementation group ("*all-rac*-α-toc"): $n = 11$; **$P<0.01$ vs. baseline.

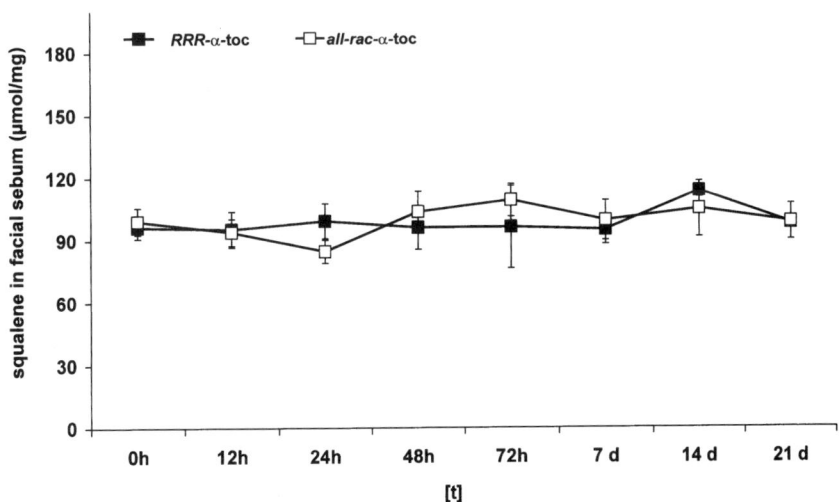

FIGURE 2. Sebum squalene levels remain constant during the investigation period. Sebum was obtained from the foreheads of volunteers using Sebutapes®, extracted and analyzed for squalene levels by HPLC. *RRR*-α-tocopheryl acetate supplementation group ("*RRR*-α-toc"): $n = 12$; *all-rac*-α-tocopheryl acetate supplementation group ("*all-rac*-α-toc"): $n = 11$.

0.47 to 3.8±0.82 pmol/nmol/cm^2 and exhibited high inter-individual variations. Notably, neither supplementation with *RRR*-α-toc nor with *all-rac*-α-toc resulted in significant changes of α-tocopherol levels in SSL during the observation period of 21 days.

α-Tocopherol Levels in Facial Sebum

Sebum secretion rates and, thus, the absolute amounts of sebum collected per one-hour collecting time intervals exhibited significant inter-individual variance. Therefore, α-tocopherol levels measured in human sebum were normalized using the simultaneously detected sebum marker lipid SQ, which was continuously secreted at constant levels during the entire observation time (FIG. 2). Baseline levels of sebaceous α-tocopherol were similar in both groups (*RRR*-α-toc: 1.3 ± 0.16 pmol/μmol SQ; *all-rac*-α-toc: 1.1 ± 0.09 pmol/μmol SQ). At day 21, significantly increased absolute α-tocopherol levels were detected in both supplementation groups (*RRR*-α-toc: 2.4±0.37pmol/μmol SQ; *all-rac*-α-toc: 2.2±0.27; both $P<0.01$). To better reflect the individual changes, relative increases of α-tocopherol levels from baseline levels were calculated for each subject (FIG. 3). Again, significant increases were detected on day 21 in both supplementation groups: α-tocopherol levels in the *RRR*-α-toc and the *all-rac*-α-toc group were increased by 87% and 92%, respectively (both $P<0.01$; FIG. 3). Similarly, when α-tocopherol levels were not normalized by co-extracted

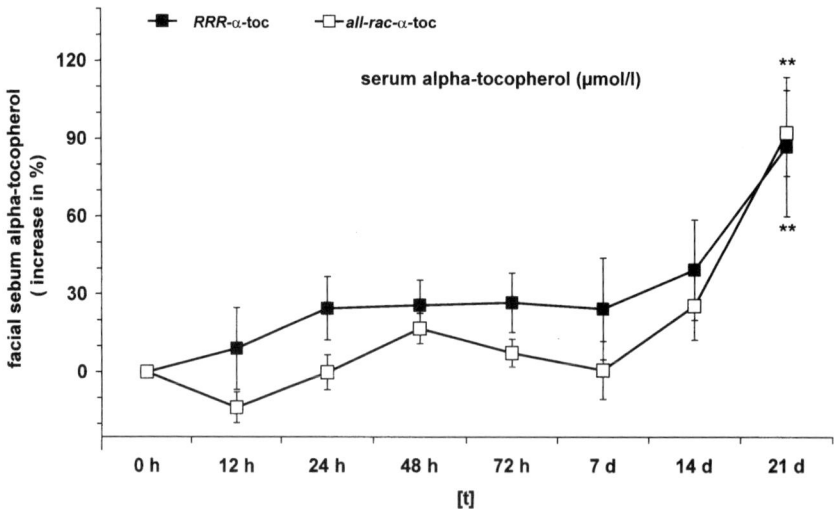

FIGURE 3. Sebum α-tocopherol levels increase between 2–3 weeks after starting dietary vitamin E supplementation. Sebum was obtained from the foreheads of volunteers by Sebutapes®, extracted and analyzed for α-tocopherol concentrations by HPLC. α-Tocopherol levels in sebum were normalized using co-extracted sqalene concentrations. Changes are expressed as percent increase from baseline levels on day 0. *RRR*-α-tocopheryl acetate supplementation group ("RRR-α-toc"): $n = 12$; *all-rac*-α-tocopheryl acetate supplementation group ("*all-rac*-α-toc"): $n = 11$; **$P<0.01$ vs. baseline.

SQ, but by the sebum amounts collected (mg), highest levels were detected in both groups on day 21: α-tocopherol levels in the RRR-α-toc and the all-rac-α-toc group were increased by 74% and 90%, respectively (both $P<0.01$).

DISCUSSION

With respect to dietary supplementation of vitamin E and its bioavailability in human skin, these results suggest that (1) sebaceous gland secretion is a major mechanism leading to site-specific differences; (2) the bioavailability of RRR-α-toc and the all-rac-α-toc is similar; and (3) possible protective effects require a daily pre-supplementation period of at least 2–3 weeks.

Baseline α-tocopherol serum levels detected in this study were in accordance with published data.[18,19] It was previously shown that plasma α-tocopherol concentrations in normal subjects can only be raised up to 2–3-fold, regardless of the duration, amount, or frequency of vitamin E supplementation.[20] The liver, expressing the hepatic α-tocopherol transfer protein (α-TTP), plays a central role in maintaining plasma vitamin E concentrations and in discriminating between the different homologues and stereoisomers of vitamin E.[2,20] In the present study, no significant differences were found for serum concentration in response to RRR-α-tocopheryl acetate (RRR-α-toc) or all-rac-α-tocopheryl acetate (all-rac-α-toc) during 14 days of daily supplementation with 400 mg and 7 days after cessation of supplementation. While the bioavailability of vitamin E and its homologues has been studied intensively in human blood plasma and serum,[21] little is known on its response in human skin.[22]

Human sebum is generated in sebaceous glands, where many of its constituting lipids, such as SQ, are formed. Its major components are triglycerides (40–60%), wax ester (19–26%), and SQ (11–15%), an unsaturated lipid that is considered a sebum-specific marker lipid.[8,23–26] Previously, we have demonstrated that human sebum contains high levels of α-tocopherol, which is secreted onto the skin surface, repenetrates the upper SC, and thus contributes to SSL.[10] Sebaceous glands are considered to be able to synthesize all components of sebum lipids[27,28] except for lipid-soluble vitamins. Sebaceous glands, particularly the large ones found in facial skin, are richly supplied with blood vessels.[29] Therefore, one might conclude that sebaceous vitamin E is taken up from the blood circulation. A few $in\ vivo$ studies have demonstrated an influence of specific dietary factors on the production of sebum lipids.[30,31] However, the transport and delivery of oral vitamin E to human skin is still little investigated. A recent study by Passi and co-workers provided good evidence for a significant deposition of vitamin E in SSL and lower SC layers using topical application. However, the complex study design employing antioxidant mixtures but not single antioxidants, the combination of topical and dietary antioxidants but not dietary antioxidants alone, as well as the low amounts of vitamin E in the oral supplement (25 mg RRR-α-tocopheryl acetate) did not allow conclusive interpretations with respect to the uptake of oral α-tocopherol by sebaceous glands.[32] There is evidence that orally administered lipophilic antifungal agents, such as ketoconazole, itraconazole, and terbinafine, accumulate in human sebum.[33] Terbinafine is delivered to the SC through sebum and only to a minor extent by direct diffusion through the dermal–epidermal junction.[34] Since lipophilic drugs, such as terbinafine, have been recovered in human sebum within the first 48 hours, similar kinetics were ex-

time [days]	0	0.5	1	2	3	4	5	6	7	8	9	10	11	12	13	14	15	16	17	18	19	20	21
Vitamin E supplementation	x		x	x	x	x	x	x	x	x	x	x	x	x		x		x		x			
Venipuncture	x[1]	x	x	x	x				x							x							x
Sebum collection	x[1]	x	x	x	x				x							x							x
SSL collection	x[1]	x	x	x	x				x							x							x

FIGURE 4. Study sampling scheme. Post-application time (days) for individual sampling procedures: α–tocopherol supplementation (*RRR* or *all-rac* α-tocopherol); venipuncture (blood); sebum collection from forehead; SSL collection from lower arm. Superscript ([1]) = sampling immediately prior to first supplementation.

pected for vitamin E. Accordingly, the study design included a number of early sebum and SSL sampling time-points (FIG. 4). Hence, the late increase of sebaceous vitamin E levels between 2 and 3 weeks after initiation of the oral supplementation (FIG. 3) was rather unexpected. Interestingly, our data on sebum confirm the finding that steady-state levels in tissues lag behind steady-state plasma vitamin E concentrations following *RRR*- or *all-rac*-α-toc supplementation, which are reached after 5 half-lives or 10–15 days.[35] Moreover, our results are supported by recent work by Vaule and co-workers, who measured the recovery of orally administered deuterium-labeled tocopherol in SSL of four human subjects: labeled α-tocopherol was undetectable in SSL for approximately 1 week and then reached highest recovery on day 19, more than 10 days after cessation of supplementation.[16] While changes in the SSL composition may reflect both delivery via dermal–epidermal or sebaceous gland routes, the results of the present study demonstrate that dietary α-tocopherol is delivered to the skin surface via sebum secretion. In contrast, SSL in anatomical locations with a low density of sebaceous glands, such as the lower volar arm, were not significantly enriched with α-tocopherol. However, one should not rule out the possibility of alternate pathways of vitamin E delivery to human skin. Dietary vitamin E is likely to also reach basal keratinocytes through diffusion from the well-perfused papillary dermis. Considering the epidermal turnover time of approximately 4 weeks, it may take a longer observation period than the 3 weeks in the present study until vitamin E increases are detectable in the SC/SSL of skin areas exhibiting low sebum levels. Post-divisional lipid cell movement studies revealed that the renewal rate of average-sized sebaceous lobules in humans takes from 21 to 25 days.[36,37] These sebocyte-specific turn-over times are in remarkable accordance with the kinetics of sebaceous vitamin E secretion detected in the present study and may well account for the observed 2–3-week delay of recovery. Interestingly, no significant differences were found between the *RRR*-α-toc and the *all-rac*-α-toc supplementation groups with respect to time course and concentration levels in plasma and sebum. These results suggest an equivalent bioavailabilty of both forms for human skin.

The herein-presented results demonstrate that dietary supplementation of 400 mg of vitamin E results in almost doubled levels of this important antioxidant in human sebum. To achieve this effect, a daily supplementation period of at least 2 weeks is required. In view of the recently identified susceptibility of sebaceous lipids to solar photo-oxidation, dietary vitamin E supplementation may help to protect human skin barrier lipids from environmental oxidative stress. Further studies investigating possible photo-protective effects of dietary vitamin E should consider choosing anatomical test sites exhibiting a different density and activity of sebaceous glands.

REFERENCES

1. STOCKER, A. & A. AZZI. 2000. Tocopherol-binding proteins: their function and physiological significance. Antiox. Redox Signal. **2:** 397–404.
2. TRABER, M.G. & H. SIES. 1996. Vitamin E in humans: demand and delivery. Annu. Rev. Nutr. **16:** 321–347.
3. WERNINGHAUS, K. et al. 1994. Evaluation of the photoprotective effect of oral vitamin E supplementation. Arch. Dermatol. **130:** 1257–1261.
4. THIELE, J.J., M. PODDA & L. PACKER. 1997. Tropospheric ozone: an emerging environmental stress to skin. Biol. Chem. **378:** 1299–1305.
5. THIELE, J.J., M.G. TRABER & L. PACKER. 1998. Depletion of human stratum corneum vitamin E: an early and sensitive in vivo marker of UV-induced photooxidation. J. Invest. Dermatol. **110:** 756–761.
6. THIELE, J.J. 2001. Oxidative targets in the stratum corneum: a new basis for antioxidative strategies. Skin Pharmacol. Appl. Skin Physiol. **14:** 87–91.
7. ELIAS, P.M. & K.R. FEINGOLD. 1992. Lipids and the epidermal water barrier: metabolism, regulation, and pathophysiology. Semin. Dermatol. **11:** 176–182.
8. DOWNING, D.T. et al. 1987. Skin lipids: an update. J. Invest. Dermatol. **88:** 2s–6s.
9. THODY, A. & S. SHUSTER. 1989. Control and function of sebaceous glands. Physiol. Rev. **69:** 383–416.
10. THIELE, J.J., S.U. WEBER & L. PACKER. 1999. Sebaceous gland secretion is a major physiological route of vitamin E delivery to skin. J. Invest. Dermatol. **113:** 1006–1010.
11. THIELE, J.J. et al. 2001. The antioxidant network of the stratum corneum. Curr. Probl. Dermatol. **29:** 26–42.
12. EKANAYAKE MUDIYANSELAGE, S. et al. 2003. Ultraviolet A induces generation of squalene monohydroperoxide isomers in human sebum and skin surface lipids *in vitro* and *in vivo*. J. Invest. Dermatol. **120:** 915–922.
13. CHIBA, K. et al. 2000. Comedogenicity of squalene monohydroperoxide in the skin after topical application. J. Toxicol. Sci. **25:** 77–83.
14. CHIBA, K. et al. 1999. Skin roughness and wrinkle formation induced by repeated application of squalene-monohydroperoxide to the hairless mouse. Exp. Dermatol. **8:** 471–479.
15. EKANAYAKE MUDIYANSELAGE, S., P. ELSNER & J.J. THIELE. 2003. SPT: a new sceening test for phototoxicity and photoprotection of topical formulation [abstract]. Arch. Dermatol. Res. **294:** 493.
16. VAULE, H., S.W. LEONARD & M.G. TRABER. 2004. Vitamin E delivery to human skin: studies using deuterated alpha-tocopherol measured by APCI LC-MS. Free Radic. Biol. Med. **36:** 456–463.
17. THIELE, J.J. & L. PACKER. 1999. Non-invasive measurement of alpha-tocopherol gradients in human stratum corneum by HPLC analysis of sequential tape strippings. Meth. Enzymol. **300:** 413–419.
18. TOMASCH, R., K.H. WAGNER & I. ELMADFA. 2001. Antioxidative power of plant oils in humans: the influence of alpha- and gamma-tocopherol. Ann. Nutr. Metab. **45:** 110–115.
19. DEVARAJ, S. et al. 1997. Dose-response comparison of RRR-alpha-tocopherol and all-racemic alpha-tocopherol on LDL oxidation. Arterioscler. Thromb. Vasc. Biol. **17:** 2273–2279.

20. TRABER, M.G. et al. 1998. Vitamin E dose response studies in humans using deuterated RRR-α-tocopherol. Am. J. Clin. Nutr. **68:** 847–853.
21. BRIGELIUS-FLOHE, R. et al. 2002. The European perspective on vitamin E: current knowledge and future research. Am. J. Clin. Nutr. **76:** 703–716.
22. THIELE, J.J., F. DREHER & L. PACKER. 2000. Antioxidant defense systems in skin. In Drugs vs. Cosmetics: Cosmeceuticals? P. Elsner & H.I. Maibach, Eds.: 145–188. Marcel Dekker. New York.
23. STEWART, M.E. & T.D. DOWNING. 1991. Chemistry and function of mammalian sebaceous lipids. In Skin Lipids, Vol. 24. P.M. Elias, Ed.: 263–301. Academic Press. San Diego.
24. KELLUM, R.E. 1967. Human sebaceous gland lipids. Arch. Dermatol. **85:** 218–220.
25. GREEN, S.C., M.E. STEWART & D.T. DOWNING. 1984. Variation in sebum fatty acid composition among adult humans. J. Invest. Dermatol. **83:** 114–117.
26. NICOLAIDES, N. 1974. Skin lipids: their biochemical uniqueness. Science **186:** 19–26.
27. CASSIDY, D.M. et al. 1986. Lipogenesis in isolated human sebaceous glands. FEBS Lett. 200: 173–176.
28. DOWNIE, M.M. & T. KEALEY. 1998. Lipogenesis in the human sebaceous gland: glycogen and glycerophosphate are substrates for the synthesis of sebum lipids. J. Invest. Dermatol. **111:** 199–205.
29. MONTAGNA, W. 1974. An introduction to sebaceous glands. J. Invest. Dermatol. **62:** 120–123.
30. DOGLIOTTI, M. et al. 1977. Nutritional influences of pellagra on sebum composition. Br. J. Dermatol. **97:** 25–28.
31. POCHI, P.E., D.T. DOWNING & J.S. STRAUSS. 1970. Sebaceous gland response in man to prolonged total caloric deprivation. J. Invest. Dermatol. **55:** 303–309.
32. PASSI, S. et al. 2003. The combined use of oral and topical lipophilic antioxidants increases their levels both in sebum and stratum corneum. Biofactors **18:** 289–297.
33. FAERGEMANN, J. et al. 1997. A double-blind comparison of levels of terbinafine and itraconazole in plasma, skin, sebum, hair and nails during and after oral medication. Acta Derm. Venereol. **77:** 74–76.
34. FAERGEMANN, J. et al. 1993. Levels of terbinafine in plasma, stratum corneum, dermis-epidermis (without stratum corneum), sebum, hair and nails during and after 250 mg terbinafine orally once per day for four weeks. Acta Derm. Venereol. **73:** 305–309.
35. HOPPE, P.P. & G. KRENNRICH. 2000. Bioavailability and potency of natural-source and all-racemic alpha-tocopherol in the human: a dispute. Eur. J. Nutr. **39:** 183–193.
36. PLEWIG, G. & E. CHRISTOPHERS. 1974. Renewal rate of human sebaceous glands. Acta Derm. Venereol. **54:** 177–182.
37. DOWNING, D.T. et al. 1975. Measurement of the time between synthesis and surface excretion of sebaceous lipids in sheep and man. J. Invest. Dermatol. **64:** 215–219.

Anti-inflammatory Effects of α-Tocopherol

UMA SINGH AND ISHWARLAL JIALAL

Laboratory for Atherosclerosis and Metabolic Research, University of California Davis Medical Center, Sacramento, California, 95817 USA

ABSTRACT: Cardiovascular disease (CVD) is the leading cause of morbidity and mortality in the western world. Its incidence has been increasing lately in the developing countries. Much evidence suggests a major role for inflammation in all phases of atherosclerosis. Cell adhesion molecules, cytokines, chemokines, and monocytes-macrophages as well as T lymphocytes play a pivotal role in atherogenesis. C-reactive protein (CRP), a downstream marker of inflammation, in addition to being a risk marker for CVD, could contribute to atherosclerosis. Dietary micronutrients with anti-inflammatory properties, specially α-tocopherol, may play an important role with regard to the prevention and treatment of CVD. α-Tocopherol has been shown to have anti-inflammatory effects both *in vitro* and *in vivo*. α-Tocopherol therapy, especially at high doses, has been shown to decrease release of pro-inflammatory cytokines (such as interleukin-1β, interleukin-6, and tumor necrosis factor-α) and the chemokine interleukin-8, and to decrease adhesion of monocytes to endothelium. In addition, α-tocopherol has been shown to decrease CRP levels in patients with CVD and having related risk factors for CVD (such as diabetes and smoking). Furthermore, pro-inflammatory cytokines and plasminogen activator inhibitor-1 (PAI-1) levels have also been shown to be decreased with α-tocopherol supplementation *in vivo*. In this review, our focus will be on anti-inflammatory effects of α-tocopherol reported in *in vivo* studies.

KEYWORDS: cardiovascular disease; C-reactive protein; inflammation; cytokines; α-tocopherol; monocytes

INFLAMMATION AND ATHEROSCLEROSIS

Much evidence supports a pivotal role for inflammation in all phases of atherosclerosis from the initiation of the fatty streak to the culmination in acute coronary syndromes (plaque rupture).[1,2] Various noxious insults, including hypertension, diabetes, smoking, dyslipidemia, and hyperhomocysteinemia, can result in endothelial cell dysfunction. Major cellular participants in atherosclerosis include monocytes, macrophages, active vascular endothelium, T lymphocytes, platelets, and smooth muscle cells.

Address for correspondence: Dr. Ishwarlal Jialal, Director, Laboratory for Atherosclerosis and Metabolic Research, University of California Davis Medical Center, 4635 Second Avenue, Res 1 Building, Room 3000, Sacramento, CA 95817.

ishwarlal.jialal@ucdmc.ucdavis.edu

Monocytes and macrophages are critical cells that are present at all stages of atherogenesis and that, when stimulated, can produce biologically active mediators that have a profound influence on the progression of atherosclerosis. Monocytes promote the peroxidation of lipids, such as low-density lipoproteins (LDLs) through the generation of reactive oxygen species. Monocytes and macrophages secrete several pro-inflammatory, pro-atherogenic cytokines, such as interleukin-1β (IL-1β) tumor necrosis factor-α (TNF-α), and interleukin-6 (IL-6), which have been shown to be present in the atherosclerotic lesion and are known to augment monocyte-endothelial adhesion. IL-1β has been shown to stimulate procoagulant activity, promote cholesterol esterification in macrophages, and stimulate smooth muscle proliferation via platelet-derived growth factor (PDGF). TNF-α has been shown to promote monocyte adhesion to endothelium and contribute to the necrotic core by promoting apoptosis of macrophages and smooth muscle cells.[3] Macrophages also release tissue factor, the major initiator of the blood coagulation cascade.[3]

Atherosclerosis is associated with impaired endothelial cell (EC) function, and these changes induce adhesion and transendothelial migration of monocytes.[3] Both IL-1β and TNF-α stimulate expression of adhesion molecules, such as vascular cell adhesion molecule-1 (VCAM-1), intercellular cell adhesion molecule-1 (ICAM-1), and E-selectin.[3] Chemotaxis and entry of monocytes into the subendothelial space are promoted by monocyte chemoattractant protein-1 (MCP-1), interleukin-8 (IL-8), and a newly reported chemokine, fractalkine. Several studies have shown a strong association between levels of soluble cell adhesion molecules (sCAMs), which are shed from activated cells such as endothelial cells, and coronary as well as carotid atherosclerosis.[4]

Many stimuli in response to inflammation, growth, and chemotactic factors from neighboring endothelial cells, monocytes, macrophages, and platelets induce smooth muscle cell (SMC) migration and subsequent proliferation, thereby resulting in the formation of the fibrous cap.[3] The earliest event after plaque fissure is the adhesion and aggregation of platelets, leading to thrombus formation. Increased platelet aggregation contributes to acute coronary syndrome such as myocardial infarction (MI). The inflammatory response of atherosclerosis is also mediated by specific subtypes of T lymphocytes at every stage. Thus, there is a complex interaction of a wide variety of cells, and their activation leads to release of hydrolytic enzymes, cytokines, chemokines, and growth factors that can result in further injury.

Several large population studies have indicated that biomarkers of inflammation predict an increased risk for cardiovascular disease (CVD).[1–3] The prototypic marker of inflammation is C-reactive protein (CRP), a member of the pentraxin family.[3,4] Its synthesis in the liver is triggered by various pro-inflammatory cytokines derived from numerous sources, including monocytes and macrophages and adipose tissue. The pro-inflammatory response includes an increased secretion of IL-1β and TNF-α, resulting in the release of the messenger cytokine, IL-6, from macrophages. IL-6, after engagement of its receptor on the liver, results in the secretion and release of CRP. Recent evidence points to the role of vascular cells, such as smooth muscle cells, in the production of CRP. CRP mRNA and protein have been shown to be expressed in the cells of the lesion at levels an order of magnitude higher than those observed in plasma.[5,6]

Many prospective studies from populations throughout the world have shown that elevated levels of CRP confer a greater risk of CVD.[3,7] In addition to indications that

CRP is a risk marker, a large body of evidence points to a pro-atherogenic role of CRP in vascular smooth muscle cells, monocytes-macrophages, and endothelial cells.[3,4] In monocytes, CRP induces the production of inflammatory cytokines and stimulates tissue factor expression and chemotaxis of monocytes.[3] A large body of evidence indicates that CRP also is pro-atherogenic in endothelial cells. CRP upregulates endothelin-1, PAI-1, and chemokines such as MCP-1 and IL-8, and it increases expression of cell adhesion molecules ICAM-1 and VCAM-1 as well as adhesion of monocytes to endothelial cells.[3] We and others have shown that CRP could result in endothelial dysfunction by downregulating synthesis, activity, and bioactivity of endothelial nitric oxide synthase (eNOS).[3] We recently showed that CRP decreases another potent vasodilator and inhibitor of platelet aggregation, prostacyclin release from aortic endothelial cells via nitration of prostacyclin synthase, which renders the enzyme inactive.[3] Thus, plasma CRP is considered to be a sensitive marker of systemic inflammation, and chronically high levels predict increased risk of future cardiovascular events (CVEs).[3,4] Data are beginning to emerge reporting inflammation (as manifested by an increase in CRP) in dialysis patients.[8] These findings also demonstrate a negative correlation between plasma CRP levels and plasma α-tocopherol levels, consistent with the hypothesis that inflammation depletes antioxidants. In a large cross-sectional study of dialysis patients, traditional risk factors such as hypertension and hypercholesterolemia have been found to have low predictive power, whereas markers of inflammation and malnutrition are highly correlated with cardiovascular morbidity.[9] Inflammation is a common feature of end-stage renal disease (ESRD), and it has been recognized that about 30 to 50% of predialysis, hemodialysis (HD), and peritoneal dialysis (PD) patients have serologic evidence of an activated inflammatory response.[10] Ward and McLeish[11] have reported that phagocytic cells that are "primed" in uremia may contribute to increased production of both reactive oxygen species as well as cytokines. An elevation of plasma CRP is one indication of a cytokine-driven (especially IL-6), acute-phase inflammatory response. The clinical significance of CRP in dialysis patients has been well documented in a series of recent studies in which an elevated CRP has been shown to be a strong predictor of adverse clinical outcomes and increased cardiovascular mortality.[12] Furthermore, inflammation is also involved in many of the abnormalities associated with the metabolic syndrome. A recent report by Ford[13] showed that in a representative sample of the U.S. population spanning 8,570 participants (>20 years old), those subjects with the metabolic syndrome were more likely to have elevated CRP levels than individuals without the syndrome. There seems to be a clear relationship between the number of metabolic disorders (dyslipidemia, upper body adiposity, insulin resistance, hypertension) and increasing high-sensitivity CRP (hsCRP) levels. In support of this, another study, reported by Ridker,[7] evaluated the potential interrelationships between CRP, the metabolic syndrome, and the incident cardiovascular events. CRP levels significantly increased with an increase in the number of components of the metabolic syndrome and correlated with an increase in the age-adjusted relative risk for future cardiovascular events. In fact, it has been reported that at all levels of severity of the metabolic syndrome, CRP added prognostic information with regard to subsequent risk of incident CVE. Furthermore, Type 2 diabetes appears to be a pro-inflammatory state, as evidenced by increased levels of pro-inflammatory cytokines and CRP levels.[14]

α-TOCOPHEROL

Given the central role played by inflammation in cardiovascular disease, antioxidants having anti-inflammatory effects, such as α-tocopherol, appear to be very important. The two major antioxidant forms of tocopherol, α- and γ-tocopherol, differ structurally only by a methyl group substitution at the five position. However, this additional methyl group allows α-tocopherol to be bound by the tocopherol transfer protein, and preferentially exported from hepatocytes and incorporated into lipoproteins, including LDLs.[15,16] α-Tocopherol is the principal and most potent lipid-soluble antioxidant in plasma and LDLs. *In vitro* studies demonstrate superior antioxidant properties of α-tocopherol in the prevention of LDL lipid peroxidation that are due to its lipid solubility and preferential incorporation into lipoproteins.[17]

In the Cambridge Heart Antioxidant Study (CHAOS),[18] patients received placebo or natural α-tocopherol (RRR-α-tocopherol) at a dose of either 400 or 800 IU/day. α-Tocopherol supplementation resulted in a significant increase in plasma α-tocopherol levels and a significant 47% reduction in the primary endpoint, defined as combined endpoint of cardiovascular death and non-fatal myocardial infarction. The Secondary Prevention with Antioxidants of Cardiovascular Disease in End-Stage Renal Disease (SPACE) study[19] was a double-blind, placebo-controlled, randomized, secondary prevention trial in hemodialysis patients. The primary endpoint was a composite variable consisting of myocardial infarction (fatal and non-fatal), ischemic stroke, peripheral vascular disease, and unstable angina. In addition to a significant increase in α-tocopherol levels, RRR-α-tocopherol (800 IU/day) significantly decreased the primary endpoint by 54%. However, no measure of biomarkers for inflammation has been reported in either of these studies.

We have tested the effect of RRR-α-tocopherol supplementation on monocyte function and inflammatory markers. Our group[20] has shown that supplementation with 1200 IU/day of α-tocopherol for 8 weeks significantly influenced monocyte function by decreasing lipid oxidation, decreasing release of superoxide (O_2^-) and hydrogen peroxide, decreasing release of the pro-atherogenic cytokine IL-1β, as well as decreasing monocyte-endothelial cell adhesion in 21 normal volunteers. Supplementation resulted in 2.5-fold increase in monocyte α-tocopherol levels. This supplementation led to a 90% inhibition of IL-1β and a 35% decrease in monocyte-endothelial cell adhesion, clearly documenting that supplementation with RRR-α-tocopherol is anti-inflammatory. In a further study[21] in Type 2 diabetic patients with and without macrovascular disease ($n = 25$ in both groups), we showed that diabetics monocytes secreted increased levels of superoxide and IL-1β and displayed greater adhesion to endothelial cells. α-Tocopherol supplementation (1200 IU/day for 3 months) resulted in a 2.5-fold increase in mononuclear cell α-tocopherol and significantly reduced O_{2-}, IL-1β, TNF-α, and monocyte adhesion to endothelial cells. In addition, α-tocopherol supplementation also resulted in a significant decrease in the levels of soluble cell adhesion molecules (ICAM, VCAM, and E-selectin). In a subsequent report,[22] we documented increased IL-6 release from monocytes and increased serum CRP levels in these diabetic patients. Both hsCRP and monocyte IL-6 were significantly decreased with α-tocopherol therapy.[22] This finding was also confirmed by another group.[23] They showed that RRR-α-tocopherol supplementation (800 IU/day, $n = 13$) in patients with Type 2 diabetes compared to placebo ($n = 12$) for a duration of 4 weeks resulted in a significant decrease in plasma CRP (49%,

TABLE 1. Summary of anti-inflammatory effects of α-tocopherol

- effective dose ≥600–800 RRR-α-tocopherol/day
- duration: ~ 1–3 months
- ↓ plasma hsCRP (in diabetic patients and smokers with acute coronary syndrome)
- ↓ pro-inflammatory cytokines (IL-β, IL-6 and TNF-α) from monocytes of Type 2 diabetic patients and control subjects
- ↓ cytokine production (IL-1β and TNF-α) from LPS-activated PBMCs
- ↓ soluble CAMs and PAI-1 levels in Type 2 diabetic patients

$P = .004$) as well. These findings were suggested to be relevant to strategies aimed at reducing risk of CVD in patients with diabetes.

Interestingly, van Tits and colleagues,[24] in a clinical trial of RRR-α-tocopherol administration (600 IU/day for 6 weeks) in primary hypertriglyceridemic ($n = 12$) and normolipidemic subjects ($n = 8$), measured the release of cytokines (TNF-α, IL-1β) and the chemokine IL-8 from peripheral blood mononuclear cells (PBMCs) before and after intervention. Following α-tocopherol supplementation, *in vitro* cytokine production and IL-8 in response to lipopolysaccharide (LPS) decreased significantly in both groups. Hence, it is suggested that α-tocopherol may influence the inflammatory response of immune cells infiltrating subendothelial spaces, and that its therapeutic implications become relevant in chronic inflammatory processes such as atherogenesis. This study confirms *in vitro* reports in the literature that *in vitro* α-tocopherol inhibited phorbol myristate acetate (PMA)-induced IL-1β expression in human monocyte leukemic cell line THP-1[25] as well as LPS-induced activation of rat Kupffer cells.[26]

Furthermore, Mol and colleagues[27] in diabetic patients and smokers examined the effect of all rac α-tocopherol supplementation (600 IU/day of all rac α-tocopherol for 4 weeks) on oxidative stress and inflammatory status, as reflected by circulating and LPS-stimulated levels of IL-1β and TNF-α and the levels of IL-1 receptor antagonist (IL-1RA) in whole blood. The lag time of oxidation after α-tocopherol supplementation increased in all three groups. Plasma thiobarbituric acid-reactive substances (TBARS) levels dropped significantly after α-tocopherol treatment in both diabetics and smokers, reaching values comparable to those in control subjects. However, total plasma oxysterols, which were significantly higher in smokers versus controls, were unaffected by α-tocopherol treatment. With respect to the inflammatory status, there were no differences in the levels of IL-1β and TNF-α, whereas there was an increased LPS-stimulated level of IL-1RA in both patients with diabetes and smokers versus controls. Increased levels of the cytokine IL-1RA have been observed in the acute phase of meningococcal disease and in rheumatoid arthritis[28,29] and is supposed to reflect an anti-inflammatory reaction. Thus, the results of IL-1RA levels in this study would indicate increased inflammation in patients with diabetes mellitus and smokers. This might be due to the increased oxidative stress to hyperglycemia and to toxic substances in cigarettes, but can also reflect an initiation of inflammation related to cardiovascular disease. Supplementation with all rac α-tocopherol decreased both TNF-α and corrected the increased IL-1RA response in smokers, but not in patients with diabetes mellitus. The form and dose of α-tocopherol could have influenced their findings because other groups, as reviewed above, have documented an anti-inflammatory effect with higher doses of RRR-α-tocopherol.

Recently, Murphy and colleagues[30] reported their findings aimed at elucidating effect of α-tocopherol supplementation (400 IU/day of RRR-α-tocopherol acetate for 6 months) in smokers in a randomized, double blind, placebo-controlled clinical trial of 110 patients with acute coronary syndrome. Patients with acute coronary syndrome were selected because this syndrome, in particular, is characterized by sustained inflammatory upregulation. In addition, as is clearly evident, the release of pro-inflammatory cytokines[31] and CRP is elevated in these patients. The endpoints selected were plasma α-tocopherol, CRP, IL-6, sICAM, sVCAM, sE-selectin, and sP-selectin. α-Tocopherol supplementation resulted in a significant increase in α-tocopherol levels with a concomitant and significant decrease in CRP levels in smokers only versus placebo. On the contrary, there was no effect on sCAMs as well as IL-6 levels. Importantly, this was the first report showing an association of α-tocopherol with a reduction in inflammatory markers in patients with acute coronary syndromes. This finding warrants a larger clinical trial assessing the impact of RRR-α-tocopherol on outcome in this patient population with a sustained elevation in inflammatory markers and a high short-term clinical event rate.

Smith and colleagues[32] reported on a small clinical trial of patients with endstage renal disease undergoing hemodialysis. This study assessed oxidative stress, measured as plasma concentrations of vitamin E metabolites such as α-carboxyethyl hydroxychromans (α-CEHC), γ-CEHC, α-tocopherol, γ-tocopherol, and F_2-isoprostane, and inflammatory biomarkers (TNF-α, IL-6, and CRP) in blood samples obtained from a group of patients ($n = 11$) before and after dialysis at two occasions prior to vitamin E supplementation and at 1 and 2 months of daily vitamin E supplementation (400 IU RRR-α-tocopherol). α-Tocopherol supplementation significantly increased plasma α-tocopherol concentrations and decreased γ-tocopherol concentrations. Both serum α- and γ-CEHC increased significantly. Plasma IL-6, CRP, TNF-α, and F_2-isoprostane concentrations were elevated throughout the study. However, the complex relationship between chronic inflammation and oxidative stress could not be mitigated by short-term α-tocopherol supplementation. We again suspect the negative outcome of this study is related to be the low dose of α-tocopherol used.

Another clinical trial, by Himmelfarb and colleagues,[10] enrolled 15 uremic patients undergoing dialysis. Five patients were supplemented with RRR-α-tocopherol (300 mg/day), and 10 received mixture of tocopherols (60% RRR-γ-tocopherol, 28% RRR-δ-tocopherol, and 18% RRR-α-tocopherol)for a duration of 14 days. The endpoints selected were serum CRP, IL-6, serum α- and γ-tocopherols, and α- and γ-CEHC as vitamin E metabolites. A potentially important observation in this study is that the administration of the γ-tocopherol-enriched preparation, but not the α-tocopherol preparation, significantly reduced CRP concentrations in hemodialysis patients. Although the authors did not observe a consistent reduction in CRP with α-tocopherol, an effect cannot be ruled out for α-tocopherol. Such a conclusion could not be supported because the study's sample size was too small ($n = 5$). Similarly, the observation of a slight increase in serum IL-6 levels after α-tocopherol administration is in contradistinction to other studies in diabetic patients and may also reflect the small sample size in this particular study. Because this study's small sample size limited its ability to assess inflammatory biomarkers, further studies with larger sample sizes will be required to more definitively address these important endpoints.

Finally, another clinical trial is being completed by our group testing the effect of RRR-α-tocopherol supplementation (1200 IU/day for 2 years) in patients with stable coronary artery disease. This trial is a randomized, placebo-controlled study. The various endpoints selected are biomarkers of oxidative stress as well as inflammation and carotid intimal-medial thickness. In the first 50 patients who have completed the study, RRR-α-tocopherol therapy compared to placebo resulted in a significant reduction in F_2-isoprostane and hsCRP levels.

The dose and form of α-tocopherol seem to be very important; that is, these factors could have an impact on the results. It seems a threshold dose of α-tocopherol, ≥600–800 IU/day, might be effective. Importantly, most of the reported anti-inflammatory effects of α-tocopherol seem to be due to RRR-α-tocopherol.[33] In this regard, we have shown that both 400 IU[34] and 800 IU[35] of all-rac-α-tocopherol, containing the eight isomers, failed to have any significant anti-inflammatory effects in normal subjects.

Although the inhibition of superoxide (O_2^-) appears to be via inhibition of protein kinase C (PKC),[36] α-tocopherol inhibits IL-1 release from activated human monocytes by inhibiting 5-lipoxygenase at the post-transcriptional levels.[37] Also, we have shown that α-tocopherol enrichment of monocytes inhibits subsequent adhesion to human endothelium via inhibition of counter-receptors macrophage adhesion molecule-1 (Mac-1/CD11b) and very-late antigen-4 (VLA-4) on the monocytes, possibly by inhibition of the transcription factor, nuclear factor-kappa B (NF-κB).[38]

CONCLUSION

Not only is α-tocopherol a potent antioxidant, as evidenced by decreased LDL oxidative susceptibility and F_2-isoprostanes, it also has pronounced anti-inflammatory effects as summarized in TABLE 1. For example, it is capable of decreasing monocyte pro-inflammatory activity, in terms of cytokine release, and decreasing plasma CRP. It is clear that RRR-α-tocopherol demonstrates a multifaceted effect promoting vascular homeostasis.

ACKNOWLEDGMENTS

This work was supported by the National Institutes of Health (grants NIH K24 AT00596 and RO1 AT 00005).

REFERENCES

1. ROSS, R. 1999. Atherosclerosis: an inflammatory disease. N. Engl. J. Med. **340:** 115–126.
2. LIBBY, P. 2002. Inflammation in atherosclerosis. Nature **420:** 868–874.
3. JIALAL, I. et al. 2004. C-reactive protein: risk marker or mediator in atherothrombosis? Hypertension **44:** 1–6.

4. JIALAL, I & S. DEVARAJ. 2001. Inflammation and atherosclerosis: the value of the high-sensitivity C-reactive protein assay as a risk marker. Am. J. Clin. Pathol. **116** (Suppl.): S108–S115.
5. KOBAYASHI, S. *et al.* 2003. Interaction of oxidative stress and inflammatory response in coronary plaque instability: important role of C-reactive protein. Arterioscler. Thromb. Vasc. Biol. **23**: 1398–1404.
6. YASOJIMA, K. *et al.* 2001. Generation of C-reactive protein and complement components in atherosclerotic plaques. Am. J. Pathol. **158**: 1039–1051.
7. RIDKER, P.M. 2003. Clinical application of C-reactive protein for cardiovascular disease detection and prevention. Circulation **168**: 363–369.
8. NGUYEN-KHOA, T. *et al.* 2001. Oxidative stress and haemodialysis: role of inflammation and duration of dialysis treatment. Nephrol. Dial. Transplant. **16**: 335–340.
9. HIMMELFARB, J. *et al.* 2002. The elephant in uremia: oxidant stress as a unifying concept of cardiovascular disease in uremia. Kidney Int. 2002. **62**: 1524–1538.
10. HIMMELFARB, J. *et al.* 2003. α- and γ-Tocopherol metabolism in healthy subjects and patients with end-stage renal disease. Kidney Int. **64**: 978–991.
11. WARD, R.A. & K.R. MCLEISH. 1995. Polymorphonuclear leukocyte oxidative burst is enhanced in patients with chronic renal insufficiency. J. Am. Soc. Nephrol. **5**: 1697–1702.
12. ARICI, M. & J. WALLS. 2001. End-stage renal disease, atherosclerosis, and cardiovascular mortality: is C-reactive protein the missing link? Kidney Int. **59**: 407–414.
13. FORD, E.S. 2003. The metabolic syndrome and C-reactive protein, fibrinogen, and leukocyte count: findings from the Third National Health and Nutrition Examination Survey. Atherosclerosis **168**: 351–358.
14. JIALAL, I. *et al.* 2002 . Oxidative stress, inflammation, and diabetic vasculopathies: the role of α-tocopherol therapy. Free Radic. Res. **36**:1331–1336.
15. STOCKER, A. & A. AZZI. 2000. Tocopherol-binding proteins: their function and physiological significance. Antioxid. Redox Signal. **2**: 397–404.
16. TRABER, M.G. & H. ARAI. 1999. Molecular mechanisms of vitamin E transport. Annu. Rev. Nutr. **19**: 343–355.
17. THOMAS, S.R. & R. STOCKER. 2000. Molecular action of vitamin E in lipoprotein oxidation: implications for atherosclerosis. Free Radic. Biol. Med. **28**: 1795–1805.
18. STEPHENS, N.G. *et al.* 1996. Randomized controlled trial of vitamin E in patients with coronary disease: Cambridge Heart Antioxidant Study (CHAOS). Lancet **347**: 781–786.
19. BOAZ, M. *et al.* 2000. Secondary prevention with antioxidants of cardiovascular disease in end-stage renal disease (SPACE): randomized placebo-controlled trial. Lancet **356**: 1213–1218.
20. DEVARAJ, S. *et al.* 1996. The effects of α-tocopherol supplementation on monocyte function: decreased lipid oxidation, interleukin-1β secretion, and monocyte adhesion to endothelium. J. Clin. Invest. **98**: 756–763.
21. DEVARAJ, S. & I. JIALAL. 2000. Low-density lipoprotein postsecretory modification, monocyte function, and circulating adhesion molecules in type 2 diabetic patients with and without macrovascular complications: the effect of α-tocopherol supplementation. Circulation **102**: 191–196.
22. DEVARAJ, S. & I. JIALAL. 2000. α-Tocopherol supplementation decreases serum C-reactive protein and monocyte interleukin-6 levels in normal volunteers and type 2 diabetic patients. Free Radic. Biol. Med. **29**: 790–792.
23. UPRITCHARD, J.E. *et al.* 2000. Effect of supplementation with tomato juice, vitamin E, and vitamin C on LDL oxidation and products of inflammatory activity in type 2 diabetes. Diabetes Care **23**: 733–738.
24. VAN TITS, L.J. *et al.* 2000. α-Tocopherol supplementation decreases production of superoxide and cytokines by leukocytes ex vivo in both normolipidemic and hypertriglyceridemic individuals. Am. J. Clin. Nutr. **71**: 458–464.
25. AKESON, A.L. *et al.* 1991. Inhibition of IL-1β expression in THP-1 cells by probucol and tocopherol. Atherosclerosis **86**: 261–270.
26. FOX, E.S. *et al.* 1997. *N*-Acetylcysteine and α-tocopherol reverse the inflammatory response in activated rat Kupffer cells. J. Immunol. **158**: 5418–5423.

27. MOL, M.J. *et al.* 1997. Plasma levels of lipid and cholesterol oxidation products and cytokines in diabetes mellitus and cigarette smoking: effects of vitamin E treatment. Atherosclerosis **129:** 169–176.
28. VAN DEUREN, M. *et al.* 1994. Differential expression of proinflammatory cytokines and their inhibitors during the course of meningococcal infections. J. Infect. Dis. **169:** 156–161.
29. BARRERA, P. *et al.* 1995. Effect of methotrexate alone or in combination with sulphasalazine on the production and circulating concentrations of cytokines and their antagonists: longitudinal evaluation in patients with rheumatoid arthritis. Br. J. Rheumatol. **34:** 747–755.
30. MURPHY, R.T. *et al.* 2004. Vitamin E modulation of C-reactive protein in smokers with acute coronary syndromes. Free Radic. Biol. Med. **36:** 959–965.
31. BRAUNWALD, E. 1998. Unstable angina: an etiological approach to management. Circulation **98:** 2219–2222.
32. SMITH, K.S. *et al.* 2003. Vitamin E supplementation increases circulating vitamin E metabolites tenfold in end-stage renal disease patients. Lipids **38:** 813–819.
33. JIALAL, I. & S. DEVARAJ. 2003. Antioxidants and atherosclerosis: don't throw out the baby with the bath water. Circulation **107:** 926–928.
34. KAUL, N. *et al.* 2001. Failure to demonstrate a major anti-inflammatory effect with α-tocopherol supplementation (400 IU/day) in normal subjects. Am. J. Cardiol. **87:** 1320–1323.
35. VEGA-LOPEZ, S. *et al.* 2004. Supplementation with omega3 polyunsaturated fatty acids and all-rac α-tocopherol alone and in combination failed to exert an anti-inflammatory effect in human volunteers. Metabolism **53:** 236–240.
36. AZZI, A. *et al.* 1998. Molecular basis of α-tocopherol control of smooth muscle cell proliferation. Biofactors **7:** 314.
37. DEVARAJ, S. & I. JIALAL. 1999. α-Tocopherol inhibits IL-β release by inhibition of 5-lipoxygenase. Arterioscler. Thromb. Vasc. Biol. **19:** 1125–1133.
38. ISLAM, K. *et al.* 1998. α-Tocopherol enrichment of monocytes decreases agonist-induced adhesion to human endothelial cells. Circulation **98:** 2255–2261.

Oxidative Stress and Antioxidant Treatment in Diabetes

JOSHUA A. SCOTT AND GEORGE L. KING

Research Division, Joslin Diabetes Center, Harvard Medical School, Boston, Massachusetts 02215, USA

ABSTRACT: The many studies on oxidative stress, antioxidant treatment, and diabetic complications have shown that oxidative stress is increased and may accelerate the development of complications through the metabolism of excessive glucose and free fatty acids in diabetic and insulin-resistant states. However, the contribution of oxidative stress to diabetic complications may be tissue-specific, especially for microvascular disease that occurs only in diabetic patients but not in individuals with insulin resistance without diabetes, even though both groups suffer from oxidative stress. Although antioxidant treatments can show benefits in animal models of diabetes, negative evidence from large clinical trials suggests that new and more powerful antioxidants need to be studied to demonstrate whether antioxidants can be effective in treating complications. Furthermore, it appears that oxidative stress is only one factor contributing to diabetic complications; thus, antioxidant treatment would most likely be more effective if it were coupled with other treatments for diabetic complications.

KEYWORDS: diabetic complications; oxidative stress; antioxidant treatment; vitamin E; PKC

Diabetes and insulin resistance can greatly increase the risk of cardiovascular disease in the many people displaying these increasingly prevalent disorders. Oxidative stress has also been postulated to be the main metabolic abnormality causing microvascular complications including retinopathy, nephropathy, and neuropathy as a result of hyperglycemia and diabetes.[1–4] Oxidative stress occurs when the amount of reactive oxygen species (ROS) exceeds the levels of neutralizing agents called antioxidants. The increase of oxidative stress in patients who have diabetes and poor glycemic control or insulin resistance is most likely a result of abnormal metabolism such as hyperglycemia, dyslipidemia, and elevated levels of free fatty acids (FFAs).[7–10] Although it has been shown that oxidant production is increased in vascular cells exposed to high glucose concentrations and in various cardiovascular tissues originating from diabetic and insulin-resistant states,[1–4] it is still relatively unknown how significant a role oxidative stress plays in the pathogenesis of diabetic microvascular and cardiovascular complications.[11] In this brief review, we will ex-

Address for correspondence: George L. King, M.D., Research Division, Joslin Diabetes Center, Harvard Medical School, One Joslin Place, Boston, MA 02215. Voice: 617-732-2660; fax: 617-732-2637.
george.king@joslin.harvard.edu

amine the increase in oxidative stress in diabetic and insulin-resistant states, the potential mechanisms of hyperglycemia-induced oxidant production, the vascular pathologies that may be associated with oxidative stress, and the effects of antioxidant treatment on treating diabetic complications in animals and clinical studies.

INDUCTION OF OXIDANTS BY DIABETIC OR INSULIN-RESISTANT STATES

There is a wealth of evidence showing that oxidant production is increased when microvascular or cardiovascular cells are exposed to hyperglycemia or elevated levels of FFAs.[12] Cultured vascular cells exposed to high concentrations of glucose and vascular tissues from animals and patients with diabetes have increased levels of oxidative stress markers such as gluco-oxidants, glycated compounds, oxidized low-density lipoprotein, superoxidants, and nitrotyrosine.[7,13–16] Likewise, diabetic animals and patients have been shown to have elevated levels of isoprostanes, 8-hydroxydeoxyguanosine, and lipid peroxides in the plasma or urine.[15–18] Despite the growing evidence that the production of oxidants is increased in diabetic and insulin-resistant states, it has not been clearly shown that oxidative stress is responsible for the microvascular or cardiovascular pathologies in diabetes and insulin resistance. A lack of clear and definitive evidence of tissue damage caused by oxidants could be due to the large reserve of antioxidants in both plasma and cells acting to diminish the effects of increased production of oxidants. This is corroborated by the findings that various antioxidants in plasma and cells have not been shown to be decreased consistently in the diabetic state.[19–22] For example, there are as many studies that have reported a decrease in plasma vitamin C or E levels as studies that have found no change in diabetic states.[19–24] However, it is also likely that antioxidant levels in the plasma are not reflective of the levels in the tissues. Nonetheless, ample evidence showing that oxidative stress markers are increased suggests that antioxidant defense in the tissues is not adequate to neutralize the oxidants produced by diabetes or insulin resistance.

PATHWAYS OF OXIDANT PRODUCTION

Increased oxidant production is a result of abnormal metabolism of glucose, FFAs, and other reactive metabolites in insulin-deficient and insulin-resistant states.[2,8–10] In hyperglycemia, increases of oxidants can arise from several processes. For example, gluco-oxidants and advanced glycated endproducts are created by non-enzymatic reactions thereby adding to the increased levels of oxidants.[24,25] These processes can also form oxidized low-density lipoprotein and nitrotyrosine both extracellularly and intracellularly. It has been suggested that the production of superoxide due to hyperglycemia can also be derived from glycolysis and mitochondrial oxidative phosphorylation.[7] Elevated intracellular glucose can alter the redox balance by increasing flux through the aldose reductase pathway, inhibition of the electron transport chain in the mitochondria, activation of oxidases, and alteration of NADPH/NADP ratios.[7,26–28] Furthermore, byproducts of these processes can cause activation of certain signaling cascades such as protein kinase C (PKC), which

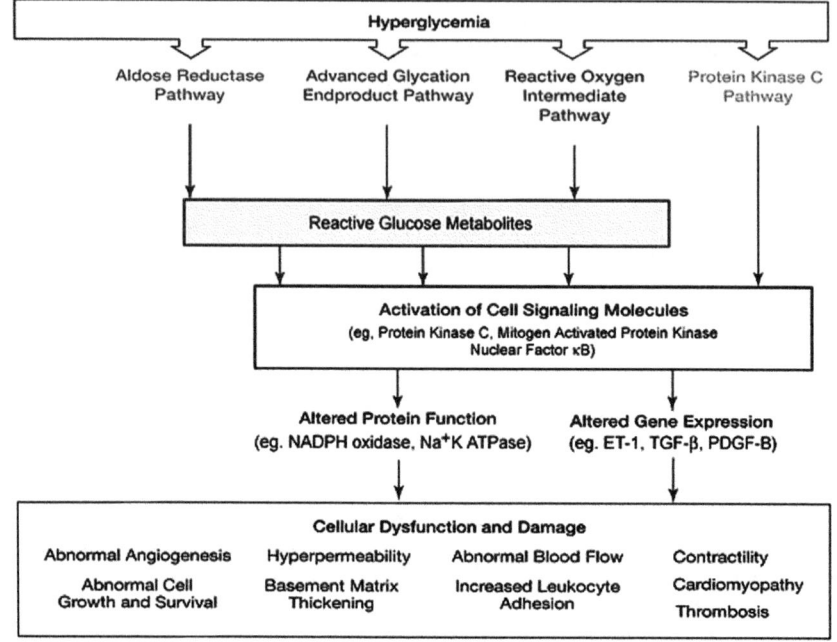

FIGURE 1. The toxins and signaling pathways contributing to hyperglycemias's adverse effects for complications.

can activate oxidases to increase superoxide production.[28] Thus, metabolism of high concentrations of glucose can activate NADPH oxidase in vascular cells independent of mitochondrial metabolism to increase oxidants.[28] For example, elevation of glucose can increase NADPH oxidase activity by activating or increasing the expression of the phox47 subunit of the enzyme in endothelial cells and monocytes by activation of PKC through the *de novo* synthesis of diacylglycerol (DAG).[28] In summary, oxidant production by hyperglycemia stems not just from a single dominant route but through multiple pathways that present several targets for therapeutic intervention (FIG. 1).

Elevated FFA levels, also a consequence of diabetes and insulin resistance, can increase oxidant production by β oxidative phosphorylation via mitochondrial metabolism.[8–10,28–30] It has been shown that malondialdehyde levels and NF-κB expression are increased in insulin-resistant states without hyperglycemia in vascular tissues as well as in muscle and adipose tissues.[10,31] Furthermore, it was demonstrated that glutathione levels in the plasma can be decreased by FFA infusion.[31] Therefore, increased oxidant production in diabetic and insulin-resistant states can originate from the metabolism of both glucose and FFAs through multiple pathways.

THE ROLE OF OXIDATIVE STRESS IN DIABETIC MICROVASCULAR AND CARDIOVASCULAR COMPLICATIONS

Clearly, there is ample evidence to support an increase of oxidative stress in diabetes and insulin resistance; however, it is far from proven that oxidative stress can cause the vascular abnormalities of diabetes. For cardiovascular disease, increases in oxidative stress have also been reported in aging and in non-diabetic patients.[32] Experimental findings indicate that increases in oxidative stress may be responsible for accelerating the risk of cardiovascular disease in diabetic or insulin-resistant states because of elevated levels of glucose or FFAs.[1,2] The sharing of common risk factors for cardiovascular disease amongst non-diabetic, insulin-resistant, and diabetic patients are reasonable because pathologies for cardiovascular disease amongst these three groups of patients are very similar, although the progression and severity of the pathologies are different. However, it is not clear at all whether oxidative stress is causing microvascular pathologies because microvascular pathologies are observed only in the diabetic state and are directly associated with hyperglycemia. In contrast, microvascular pathologies such as pericyte loss and mesangial expansion, which contribute to diabetic retinopathy and nephropathy, respectively, are not reported in the insulin-resistant state or aging populations even though they experience oxidative stress to a similar level as diabetes. Thus, an increase in oxidative stress induced by FFAs, lipids, or other processes are not adequate to cause microvascular pathologies of diabetes.[2,7,8,29] It is still possible that oxidative stress may accelerate the microvascular pathologies even though it is unlikely that microvessel pathologies of diabetes are initiated by oxidative stress. Lastly, the damage caused by oxidative stress is likely to be tissue specific because hyperglycemia appears to increase oxidant production in many cell types and tissues that do not manifest significant pathologies.

ANTIOXIDANTS AS THERAPEUTICS

Because oxidative stress may contribute to diabetic cardiovascular complications, it leaves the question as to whether antioxidants as therapeutics can prevent or delay the onset of complications in diabetic states. Many different types of antioxidants such as vitamin C, vitamin E, β-carotene, lipoic acids, and others have been studied in cultured vascular cells, in animal models of diabetes, and in diabetic patients.[22,33–41]

It has been reported that some antioxidants such as vitamins C and E, lipoic acid, antioxidative enzymes, taurine, acetylcysteine, and others prevented hyperglycemia-induced biological changes including cytokine expression, matrix synthesis, and cellular growth and turnover.[40–46] There is mounting evidence to support the notion that antioxidants such as those listed above can prevent, and even reverse, many early changes in the vascular and neurological tissues from diabetic animals. In the following, we will provide a brief review of the evidence available on the effects of antioxidant treatment to prevent or halt diabetic vascular complications.

Animal Studies

Similar to cell culture experiments, many antioxidant studies have used diabetic and insulin-resistant rodents. In the antioxidant studies that have used these rodents, antioxidants have been evaluated for their effectiveness in preventing or delaying the onset of vascular and neurological complications.[2,22,30,33,34,38,39,41,42,44,45] These studies have yielded mostly positive effects of antioxidant treatment on preventing or stopping the early changes of diabetic nephropathy, neuropathy, retinopathy, endothelial dysfunction, and surrogate markers of atherosclerosis.

Vitamins C and E and α-lipoic acid (a superoxide scavenger) are required to regenerate glutathione and oxidized vitamins C and E. Administered alone or in combination, they have been shown to be effective in ameliorating diabetic complications by demonstrating improvement of nerve conduction velocity and blood flow to the peripheral nerves, leukocyte adhesion in the retina, cataract formation, and mesangial expansion.[22,42,44–48] Surprisingly, α-lipoic acid alone has been reported to normalize other diabetic abnormalities besides oxidative stress, such as improving glycemic control, and may even prevent the onset of diabetes and insulin resistance.[49] Therefore, this leaves the question as to whether the effectiveness of α-lipoic acid in treating diabetic complications is due to antioxidative actions or an ability to mediate through another mechanism to improve glycemic control and preserve pancreatic islet function.[41] However, α-lipoic acid was not able to reverse several other vascular changes, such as the decrease in retinal blood flow corrected by high doses of vitamin E.[45] Although both α-lipoic acid and vitamin E are potent antioxidants, vitamin E was able to reverse many more neural and vascular changes of diabetes than was α-lipoic acid, indicating that vitamin E at high doses has a greater variety of effects than those typically associated with an antioxidant.

Many studies using a variety of diabetic animal models have characterized the effectiveness of vitamins C and E. When administered alone or in combination to diabetic animals, vitamins C and E normalized such parameters as levels of lipid peroxidation, isoprostanes, plasma malondialdehyde, and other cellular markers of oxidative stress such as NF-κB.[22,30,42,44–48,50] Furthermore, not only have vitamins C and E been shown to improve biochemical changes, they also have been shown to improve early functional markers of complications including diabetic retinopathy, nephropathy, and neuropathy. These vitamins can ameliorate or reverse cardiovascular abnormalities such as forearm blood flow, nerve conduction velocity, vascular permeability and contractility, endothelial dysfunction, and albuminuria.[44] Some studies have even reported that in diabetic animal models, late pathological changes in the retina and the peripheral nerves can be prevented by vitamins C and E.[33,46] In other studies, high doses of vitamin E normalized parameters of oxidative stress and inhibited vascular abnormalities caused by hyperglycemia-induced production of DAG and PKC activation in the retina and glomerulus.[46,48]

The mechanism by which vitamin E acts to prevent diabetic complications is still relatively unclear. However, doses of d-α-tocopherol at 50 μM or higher have been shown to decrease PKC activity by activating DAG kinase, thereby decreasing the levels of the DAG pool.[46] The action of d-α-tocopherol to reduce DAG levels and decrease glucose-induced PKC activation has been shown to occur not only in the retina, glomerulus, and macrophages of diabetic animals,[46,51] but also in cell types such as aortic smooth muscle cells in response to various growth factors, suggesting

TABLE 1. Results of clinical antioxidant trials for diabetic complications measuring hard endpoints

	No. of Patients	Treatment	Duration	End Point	Result
Gaede et al. (2001)	30	Vit. C (1250 mg) Vit. E (680 mg)	4 wk	Albuminuria	Decreased by 10% ($P = 0.04$)
SPACE Trial ERD (2001)	196	Vit. E (800 IU)	519 days	CV events	Decreased relative risk (0.46)
Chaos Trial (1999) DN and NDM	2002	Vit. E (400–800 IU)	510 days	Nonfatal MI	Decreased ($P = 0.0005$)
				CV death	No difference
HOPE Trial (2000)	3657	Vit. E (400 IU)	4 years	CV death, MI, stroke	No effect
Type 2				Neuropathy	No effect
SECURE (2001) DM and NDM	732	Vit. E (400 IU)	4.5 years	Intimal medial thickness	No effect

it may play a therapeutic role in preventing or delaying atherosclerosis in non-diabetic states.[50,52–54] Although these data generally suggest a positive effect for diabetic complications in animals without serious adverse side-effects of high- or low-dose antioxidant treatment, it has been shown to improve only early changes and potential surrogate markers of vascular or neurological complications. Besides the studies on early nonproliferative microvascular changes in the retina, very few studies have indicated that antioxidant treatment in animals will prevent or delay the onset of late pathologic changes of diabetic microvascular or cardiovascular diseases.[33]

Clinical Studies

In clinical studies, antioxidant treatments such as vitamins C and E and α-lipoic acid provided positive results to show that they can prevent or stop only early surrogate markers of diabetic retinopathy, nephropathy, neuropathy, and cardiovascular disease, in parallel with neutralizing oxidative markers in the plasma or circulatory monocytes. For example, studies have shown that α-lipoic acid improved symptoms of diabetic polyneuropathy and increased glucose transport in skeletal muscle cells.[38,41,55,56] Studies involving vitamins C and E, individually or in combination, been reported to improve early oxidative stress markers in the plasma, urine, and circulating cells, as well as endothelial dysfunction and microalbuminuria.[47,57,58] We have shown that retinal blood flow and renal hyperfiltration can be normalized with high doses of vitamin E (1800 IU/day) in type 1 diabetic patients in a placebo-controlled trial.[37] Although there is evidence that vitamin E can ameliorate early neuronal and vascular changes caused by oxidative stress, larger studies, such as the Heart Outcomes Prevention Study using a dose of 400 IU/day of vitamin E, d-α-tocopherol, did not show improvement of microvascular or cardiovascular damage in greater than 3,000 individuals who have had diabetes for several years.[59] However, smaller studies using a dose of 600 mg/day or higher of vitamin E, the Cambridge Heart Antioxidant Study and the Secondary Prevention with Antioxidants of Cardiovascular Disease in End-Stage Renal Disease (SPACE), provided suggestive evidence that vitamin E may improve cardiovascular function.[60,61] However, most large studies using vitamin E alone or in combination with other antioxidants have not yielded positive benefits for decreasing the development or progression of diabetic microvascular and cardiovascular pathologies or mortality (TABLE 1).

ACKNOWLEDGMENTS

This work was supported by a grant (DK53105) from the National Institutes of Health to G.L.K.

REFERENCES

1. DUCKWORTH, W.C. 2001. Hyperglycemia and cardiovascular disease. Curr. Atheroscler. Rep. **3:** 383–391.
2. GIUGLIANO, D., A. CERIELLO & G. PAOLISSO. 1996. Oxidative stress and diabetic vascular complications. Diabetes Care **19:** 257–267.
3. EGAN, B.M., E.L. GREENE & T.L. GOODFRIEND. 2001. Insulin resistance and cardiovascular disease. Am. J. Hypertens. **14:** 116S–125S.
4. GINSBERG, H.N. 2000. Insulin resistance and cardiovascular disease. J. Clin. Invest. **106:** 453–458.
5. KHAMAISI, M., O. KAVEL, M. ROSENSTOCK, et al. 2000. Effect of inhibition of glutathione synthesis on insulin action: in vivo and in vitro studies using buthionine sulfoximine. Biochem. J. **349:** 579–586.
6. MAECHLER, P., L. JORNOT & C.B. WOLLHEIM. 1999. Hydrogen peroxide alters mitochondrial activation and insulin secretion in pancreatic beta cells. J. Biol. Chem. **274:** 27905–27913.
7. BROWNLEE, M. 2001. Biochemistry and molecular cell biology of diabetic complications. Nature **414:** 813– 820.
8. EVANS, J.L., I.D. GOLDFINE, B.A. MADDUX & G.M. GRODSKY. 2003. Are oxidative stress-activated signaling pathways mediators of insulin resistance and beta-cell dysfunction? Diabetes **52:** 1–8.
9. BODEN, G. & G.I. SHULMAN. 2002. Free fatty acids in obesity and type 2 diabetes: defining their role in the development of insulin resistance and beta-cell dysfunction. Eur. J. Clin. Invest. **32**(Suppl. 3): 14–23.
10. ITANI, S.I., N.B. RUDERMAN, F. SCHMIEDER & G. BODEN. 2002. Lipid-induced insulin resistance in human muscle is associated with changes in diacylglycerol, protein kinase C, and IκB-α. Diabetes **51:** 2005–2011.
11. LONN, E., S. YUSUF, B. HOOGWERF, et al. 2002. Effects of vitamin E on cardiovascular and microvascular outcomes in high-risk patients with diabetes: results of the HOPE study and MICRO-HOPE substudy. Diabetes Care **25:** 1919–1927.
12. KING, G.L. & M. LOEKEN. 2004. Hyperglycemia-induced oxidative stress in diabetic complications. Histochem. Cell. Biol. July 15 [online].
13. KAWAMURA, M., J.W. HEINECKE & A. CHAIT. 1994. Pathophysiological concentrations of glucose promote oxidative modification of low-density lipoprotein by a superoxide-dependent pathway. J. Clin. Invest. **94:** 771–778.
14. ZOU, M.H., C. SHI & R.A. COHEN. 2002. Oxidation of the zinc-thiolate complex and uncoupling of endothelial nitric oxide synthase by peroxynitrite. J. Clin. Invest. **109:** 817–826.
15. SHINOMIYA, K., M. FUKUNAGA, H. KIYOMOTO, et al. 2002. A role of oxidative stress-generated eicosanoid in the progression of arteriosclerosis in type 2 diabetes mellitus model rats. Hypertens. Res. **25:** 91–98.

16. MEZZETTI, A., F. CIPOLLONE & F. CUCCURULLO. 2000. Oxidative stress and cardiovascular complications in diabetes: isoprostanes as new markers on an old paradigm. Cardiovasc. Res. **47:** 475–488.
17. KAKIMOTO, M., T. INOGUCHI, T. SONTA, et al. 2002. Accumulation of 8-hydroxy-2′-deoxyguanosine and mitochondrial DNA deletion in kidney of diabetic rats. Diabetes **51:** 1588–1595.
18. LEINONEN, J., T. LEHTIMAKI, S. TOYOKUNI, et al. 1997. New biomarker evidence of oxidative DNA damage in patients with non-insulin-dependent diabetes mellitus. FEBS Lett. **417:** 150-152.
19. RUIZ, C., A. ALEGRIA, R. BARBERA, et al. 1999. Lipid peroxidation and antioxidant enzyme activities in patients with type 1 diabetes mellitus. Scand. J. Clin. Lab. Invest. **59:** 99–105.
20. VESSBY, J., S. BASU, R. MOHSEN, et al. 2002. Oxidative stress and antioxidant status in type 1 diabetes mellitus. J. Intern. Med. **251:** 69–76.
21. MILLEN, A.E., M. GRUBER, R. KLEIN, et al. 2003. Relations of serum ascorbic acid and alpha-tocopherol to diabetic retinopathy in the Third National Health and Nutrition Examination Survey. Am. J. Epidemiol. **158:** 225–233.
22. BURSELL, S.E., A.C. CLERMONT, L.P. AIELLO, et al. 1999. High-dose vitamin E supplementation normalizes retinal blood flow and creatinine clearance in patients with type 1 diabetes. Diabetes Care **22:** 1245–1251.
23. CAMPOY, C., R.M. BAENA, E. BLANCA, et al. 2003. Effects of metabolic control on vitamin E nutritional status in children with type 1 diabetes mellitus. Clin. Nutr. **22:** 81–86.
24. WILL, J.C., E.S. FORD & B.A. BOWMAN. 1999. Serum vitamin C concentrations and diabetes: findings from the Third National Health and Nutrition Examination Survey, 1988–1994. Am. J. Clin. Nutr. **70:** 49–52.
25. BAYNES, J.W. & S.R. THORPE. 1999. Role of oxidative stress in diabetic complications: a new perspective on an old paradigm. Diabetes **48:** 1–9.
26. DUNLOP, M. 2000. Aldose reductase and the role of the polyol pathway in diabetic nephropathy. Kidney Int. Suppl. **77:** S3–S12.
27. KASHIWAGI, A., T. ASAHINA, M. IKEBUCHI, et al. 1994. Abnormal glutathione metabolism and increased cytotoxicity caused by H_2O_2 in human umbilical vein endothelial cells cultured in high glucose medium. Diabetologia **37:** 264–269.
28. INOGUCHI, T., P. LI, F. UMEDA, et al. 2000. High glucose level and free fatty acid stimulate reactive oxygen species production through protein kinase C-dependent activation of NAD(P)H oxidase in cultured vascular cells. Diabetes **49:** 1939–1945.
29. EVANS, J.L., I.D. GOLDFINE, B.A. MADDUX & G.M. GRODSKY. 2002. Oxidative stress and stress-activated signaling pathways: a unifying hypothesis of type 2 diabetes. Endocr. Rev. **23:** 599–622.
30. DOUILLET, C., M. BOST, M. ACCOMINOTTI, et al. 1998. Effect of selenium and vitamin E supplementation on lipid abnormalities in plasma, aorta, and adipose tissue of Zucker rats. Biol. Trace Elem. Res. **65:** 221–236.
31. PAOLISSO, G., A. GAMBARDELLA, M.R. TAGLIAMONTE, et al. 1996. Does free fatty acid infusion impair insulin action also through an increase in oxidative stress? J. Clin. Endocrinol. Metab. **81:** 4244–4248.
32. CECONI, C., A. BORASO, A. CARGNONI & R. FERRARI. 2003. Oxidative stress in cardiovascular disease: myth or fact? Arch. Biochem. Biophys. **420:** 217–221.
33. KOWLURU, R.A. & A. KENNEDY. 2001. Therapeutic potential of anti-oxidants and diabetic retinopathy. Expert Opin. Investig. Drugs **10:** 1665–1676.
34. DOI, K., F. SAWADA, G. TODA, et al. 2001. Alteration of antioxidants during the progression of heart disease in streptozotocin-induced diabetic rats. Free Radic. Res. **34:** 251–261.
35. HAAK, E., K.H. USADEL, K. KUSTERER, et al. 2000. Effects of alpha-lipoic acid on microcirculation in patients with peripheral diabetic neuropathy. Exp. Clin. Endocrinol. Diabetes **108:** 168–174.
36. LOEBSTEIN, R., D.C. LEHOTAY, X. LUO, et al. 1998. Diabetic nephropathy in hypertransfused patients with beta-thalassemia: the role of oxidative stress. Diabetes Care **21:** 1306–1309.

37. MOORADIAN, A.D. 2003. Cardiovascular disease in type 2 diabetes mellitus: current management guidelines. Arch. Intern. Med. **163:** 33–40.
38. PACKER, L., K. KRAEMER & G. RIMBACH. 2001. Molecular aspects of lipoic acid in the prevention of diabetes complications. Nutrition **17:** 888–895.
39. RUHE, R.C. & R.B. MCDONALD. 2001. Use of antioxidant nutrients in the prevention and treatment of type 2 diabetes. J. Am. Coll. Nutr. **20:** 363S–369S [discussion: 381S–383S].
40. MONTERO, A., K.A. MUNGER, R.Z. KHAN, et al. 2000. F(2)-isoprostanes mediate high glucose-induced TGF-beta synthesis and glomerular proteinuria in experimental type I diabetes. Kidney Int. **58:** 1963–1972.
41. GREENE, E.L., B.A. NELSON, K.A. ROBINSON & M.G. BUSE. 2001. Alpha-lipoic acid prevents the development of glucose-induced insulin resistance in 3T3-L1 adipocytes and accelerates the decline in immunoreactive insulin during cell incubation. Metabolism **50:** 1063–1069.
42. STUDER, R.K., P.A. CRAVEN & F.R. DERUBERTIS. 1997. Antioxidant inhibition of protein kinase C-signaled increases in transforming growth factor-beta in mesangial cells. Metabolism **46:** 918–925.
43. TRACHTMAN, H., S. FUTTERWEIT & R.S. BIENKOWSKI. 1993. Taurine prevents glucose-induced lipid peroxidation and increased collagen production in cultured rat mesangial cells. Biochem. Biophys. Res. Commun. **191:** 759–765.
44. CAMERON, N.E. & M.A. COTTER. 1999. Effects of antioxidants on nerve and vascular dysfunction in experimental diabetes. Diabetes Res. Clin. Pract. **45:** 137–146.
45. ABIKO, T., A. ABIKO, A.C. CLERMONT, et al. 2003. Characterization of retinal leukostasis and hemodynamics in insulin resistance and diabetes: role of oxidants and protein kinase-C activation. Diabetes **52:** 829–837.
46. KOYA, D., I.K. LEE, H. ISHII, et al. 1997. Prevention of glomerular dysfunction in diabetic rats by treatment with d-alpha-tocopherol. J. Am. Soc. Nephrol. **8:** 426–435.
47. GAEDE, P., H.E. POULSEN, H.H. PARVING & O. PEDERSEN. 2001. Double-blind, randomised study of the effect of combined treatment with vitamin C and E on albuminuria in type 2 diabetic patients. Diabet Med. **18:** 756–760.
48. KUNISAKI, M., S.E. BURSELL, A.C. CLERMONT, et al. 1995. Vitamin E prevents diabetes-induced abnormal retinal blood flow via the diacylglycerol-protein kinase C pathway. Am. J. Physiol. **269:** E239–E246.
49. PACKER, L., K. KRAEMER & G. RIMBACH. 2001. Molecular aspects of linoleic acid in the prevention of diabetes complications. Nutrition **17:** 888–895.
50. OZER, N.K. A. AZZI. 2000. Effect of vitamin E on the development of atherosclerosis. Toxicology **148:** 179–185.
51. SAKAMOTO, W., K. FUJIE, H. HANDA, et al. 1990. In vivo inhibition of superoxide production and protein kinase C activity in macrophages from vitamin E-treated rats. Int. J. Vitam. Nutr. Res. **60:** 338–342.
52. KEANEY, J.F., JR., D.I. SIMON & J.E. FREEDMAN. 1999. Vitamin E and vascular homeostasis: implications for atherosclerosis. FASEB J. **13:** 965–975.
53. SIRIKCI, O., N.K. OZER & A. AZZI. 1996. Dietary cholesterol-induced changes of protein kinase C and the effect of vitamin E in rabbit aortic smooth muscle cells. Atherosclerosis **126:** 253–263.
54. BOSCOBOINIK, D., A. SZEWCZYK & A. AZZI. 1991. Alpha-tocopherol (vitamin E) regulates vascular smooth muscle cell proliferation and protein kinase C activity. Arch. Biochem. Biophys. **286:** 264–269.
55. VAN DAM, P.S. 2002. Oxidative stress and diabetic neuropathy: pathophysiological mechanisms and treatment perspectives. Diabetes Metab. Res. Rev. **18:** 176–184.
56. KONRAD, D., R. SOMWAR, G. SWEENEY, et al. 2001. The antihyperglycemic drug alpha-lipoic acid stimulates glucose uptake via both GLUT4 translocation and GLUT4 activation: potential role of p38 mitogen-activated protein kinase in GLUT4 activation. Diabetes **50:** 1464–1471.
57. VENUGOPAL, S.K., S. DEVARAJ, T. YANG & I. JIALAL. 2002. Alpha-tocopherol decreases superoxide anion release in human monocytes under hyperglycemic conditions via inhibition of protein kinase C-alpha. Diabetes **51:** 3049–3054.

58. BECKMAN, J.A., A.B. GOLDFINE, M.B. GORDON & M.A. CREAGER. 2001. Ascorbate restores endothelium-dependent vasodilation impaired by acute hyperglycemia in humans. Circulation **103:** 1618–1623.
59. GERSTEIN, H.C., J. BOSCH, J. POGUE, *et al.* 1996. Rationale and design of a large study to evaluate the renal and cardiovascular effects of an ACE inhibitor and vitamin E in high-risk patients with diabetes. The MICRO-HOPE Study. Microalbuminuria, cardiovascular, and renal outcomes. Heart Outcomes Prevention Evaluation. Diabetes Care **19:** 1225–1228.
60. STEPHENS, N.G., A. PARSONS, P.M. SCHOFIELD, *et al.* Randomised controlled trial of vitamin E in patients with coronary disease: Cambridge Heart Antioxidant Study (CHAOS). Lancet **347:** 781–786.
61. BOAZ, M., S. SMETANA, T. WEINSTEIN, *et al.* 2000. Secondary prevention with antioxidants of cardiovascular disease in endstage renal disease (SPACE): randomised placebo-controlled trial. Lancet **356:** 1213–1218.+

Vitamin E and Respiratory Infection in the Elderly

SIMIN NIKBIN MEYDANI,[a,b] SUNG NIM HAN,[a] AND DAVIDSON H. HAMER[a,c]

[a]*Jean Mayer USDA Human Nutrition Research Center on Aging at Tufts University, Boston, Massachusetts 02111, USA*

[b]*Department of Pathology, Sackler Graduate School of Biomedical Sciences, Tufts University, Boston, Massachusetts, USA*

[c]*Center for International Health and Development, Boston University School of Public Health, Boston, Massachusetts, USA*

ABSTRACT: Respiratory infections are prevalent in the elderly, resulting in increased morbidity, mortality, and utilization of health care services. Contributing to the increased incidence of infection with age is the well-described decline in immune response, which has been correlated with patterns of illness in the elderly. For example, there are higher morbidity and mortality from cancer, pneumonia, and post-operative complications in those who have diminished, delayed-type hypersensitivity skin test responses. Nutritional status is an important determinant of immune function. We have shown in double-blind, placebo-controlled trials that vitamin E supplementation significantly improved immune response, including DTH and response to vaccines. Furthermore, subjects receiving vitamin E in the 6-month trial had a 30% lower incidence of infectious diseases. That study, however, was not powered to demonstrate statistical significance, and the infections were self-reported. To overcome these limitations, we conducted a double-blind, placebo-controlled trial to determine the effect of one-year supplementation with 200 IU/day vitamin E on the incidence and duration of respiratory infections in 617 elderly nursing home residents. The results of this clinical trial show that vitamin E supplementation significantly reduces the incidence rate of common colds and the number of subjects who acquire a cold among elderly nursing home residents. A nonsignificant reduction in the duration of colds was also observed. Because of the high rate and more severe morbidity associated with common colds in this age group, these findings have important implications for the well being of the elderly as well as for the economic burden associated with their care.

KEYWORDS: vitamin E supplementation; elderly; immune function; infectious diseases

Address for correspondence: Dr. Simin Nikbin Meydani, Nutritional Immunology Laboratory, Jean Mayer USDA Human Nutrition Research Center on Aging at Tufts University, 711 Washington Street, Boston, MA 02111. Voice: 617-556-3129; fax: 617-556-3224.
simin.meydani@tufts.edu

INTRODUCTION

Vitamin E is a potent chain-breaking antioxidant that protects membrane from free radical damage. Available evidence suggests that the beneficial effects of supplemental vitamin E are on immune function and related diseases. Vitamin E is perhaps one of the most studied nutrients in relation to its immunoregulatory effect. Results from animal and human studies indicate that vitamin E deficiency impairs both humoral and cell-mediated immune functions,[1,2] while supplementation with vitamin E above the recommended levels has been shown to enhance immune response and to be associated with increased resistance against several pathogens.[3,4]

A recommended dietary allowance (RDA) for vitamin E is currently set at 15 mg/day of α-tocopherol for adults (ages above 19),[5] increased from the 10 mg recommended in the 10th edition of the RDA book.[5] The average daily intake of vitamin E in the United States and other Western countries is estimated to be around 10 mg. Certain population groups, such as the elderly, are at greater risk for inadequate dietary intake of vitamin E.[6,7] Ryan et al.[6] reported that more than 40% of elderly (65 to 98 years) persons had intakes of vitamin E that were below two-thirds of the 1989 RDA.

This paper will summarize studies related to the role of vitamin E in modulating immune response and resistance to infectious diseases in humans.

VITAMIN E AND IMMUNE FUNCTION

The beneficial effect of dietary vitamin E supplementation above the recommended levels, especially in the aged, has been shown in animal studies and human clinical trials.[3,8,9]

Supplementation with vitamin E (800 mg per day) in the healthy elderly over 60 years old resulted in an increase in delayed-type hypersensitivity (DTH) response, *in vitro* T cell proliferation, and IL-2 production and a decrease in plasma lipid peroxide concentration and production of the T cell–suppressive PGE_2.[3] In a subsequent study, Meydani et al.[9] investigated the effect of 4½ months of vitamin E supplementation on *in vivo* indices of immune function in healthy elderly over 65 years old; 88 subjects were supplemented with placebo or 60, 200, and 800 mg of *dl*-α-tocopherol. All three vitamin E–supplemented groups showed a significant increase in DTH response compared with baseline. Subjects in the 200 mg/day group showed a significantly greater increase in median percentage change of DTH compared with those in the placebo group (65% vs. 17%, $P = 0.04$) and a significant increase in antibody titers to hepatitis B and tetanus vaccines. Lee and Wan[10] reported a significant increase in the proliferative response to phytohemagglutinin (PHA) or lipopolysaccharide (LPS) and a significant decrease in plasma malondialdehyde and urinary DNA adduct 8-hydroxy-2′-deoxyguanosine levels after short-term supplementation with vitamin E (400 IU *dl*-α-tocopherol/day for 28 days) in Chinese adults. De Waart et al.[11] observed no significant changes in mitogenic response to concavalin A (ConA) and PHA or levels of IgG and IgA against *Penicillium* after 3-month supplementation with vitamin E at 100 mg/day. The lower dose of vitamin E, as well as the use of previously frozen lymphocytes for determination of mitogenic response and evaluation of antibody levels without previous specific vaccination, may have contributed to the discrepancy observed between the results of De Waart et al.[11] and those of Meydani et al.[3,9] and Lee and Wan.[10] Pallast et al.[12] supplemented healthy elderly subjects (65–80 years old) with 50 or 100 mg/day of vitamin E for 6 months. Subjects in the vitamin E–supplemented group showed a significant increase in DTH (induration diameter and number of positive responses) compared with their own baseline values. Only the change in the number of positive DTH responses tended to be larger in the group supplemented with 100 mg than in the placebo group ($P = 0.06$). A significantly greater improvement in cumulative DTH score and the number of positive DTH responses was observed in a subgroup of subjects who received 100 mg vitamin E and had a low baseline DTH reactivity. There was no significant difference in PHA-stimulated IL-2 production between the vitamin E–treated groups relative to the placebo group.

Differences in results among human studies may reflect the differences in vitamin E status at baseline and supplementation dose, resulting in varied levels of changes in plasma vitamin E levels and methodology. Considering the results from the study by Meydani et al.[9] in which subjects in the upper tertile of serum vitamin E concentration (> 48.4 μmol/L) after supplementation had higher antibody response to hepatitis B as well as higher DTH responses than those in the lower tertile of serum vitamin E (19.9–34.7 μmol/L), the amount of increase in vitamin E levels achieved in the studies by others[11,12] might not have been adequate to observe a highly significant effect. It is also noteworthy that Lee and Wan[10] observed a significant increase in cell-mediated immune response with a 13.4 μmol/L increase in plasma vitamin E level, a level of increase comparable to those observed by De Waart et al.[11] and Pallast et al.[12] with 100-mg supplementation. A difference in baseline vitamin E status may explain the varied results observed in these latter studies, because subjects in the study by Lee and Wan[10] had significantly lower plasma vitamin E levels at baseline (14 μmol/L) compared with those in the studies by De Waart et al.[11] (33 μmol/L) and Pallast et al.[12] (31 μmol/L).

VITAMIN E AND INFECTIOUS DISEASES

The immunostimulatory effect of vitamin E has been shown to be associated with resistance to infections. Most of the animal studies that investigated the effect of vitamin E on infectious diseases reported a protective effect despite the variations in the dose and duration of the supplementation, infectious organisms involved, and route of administration as reviewed by Meydani, Fawzi, and Han.[13] Vitamin E supplementation in old mice resulted in significantly lower viral titer and preserved antioxidant nutrient status following influenza virus infection.[14] This protective effect of vitamin E against influenza infection seems to be partly due to enhancement of Th1 response, increased IL-2, and IFN-γ production.[15]

VITAMIN E AND RESPIRATORY INFECTIONS IN THE ELDERLY

Only a limited number of studies have investigated the effect of vitamin E on resistance against infections in humans. The subjects in these studies were mainly elderly. Infections, particularly respiratory infections (RIs), are common in the elderly, resulting in decreased daily activity, prolonged recovery times, increased health care service utilization, and more frequent complications, including death.[16–26]

It is predicted that 43% of all elderly persons will be admitted to a nursing home, with > 85% of them admitted to long-term (> 1 year) care facilities.[27] Infections occur more frequently in nursing home residents than among the independent-living elderly,[17–25,28] and RIs are a major cause of morbidity and mortality.[24,29,30]

Contributing to the increased incidence of infection with age is the well-described decline in immune response.[31] For example, there are higher morbidity and mortality from cancer, pneumonia, and postoperative complications in those who have diminished delayed-type hypersensitivity skin test responses.[32–34]

Nutritional status is an important determinant of immune function.[35,36] Nutritional supplementation has been shown to enhance older subjects' immune response.[37,38] In our earlier placebo-controlled, double-blind trials in elderly persons, vitamin E supplementation improved immune response, including DTH and response to vaccines.[9,39] In this study we also reported a nonsignificant ($P < 0.09$) 30% lower incidence of self-reported infections among the groups supplemented with vitamin E (60, 200, or 800 mg/day for 235 days) compared with the placebo group. Since infection was not the primary outcome, the study did not have enough power to detect significant differences in the incidence of infections. To overcome these limitations, we conducted a large double-blind, placebo-controlled trial to determine the effect of one-year supplementation with vitamin E on objectively recorded RIs in elderly nursing home residents.[40]

In this randomized, double-blind study, 617 people aged over 65 residing at 33 nursing homes in the Boston area who met the study's eligibility criteria received either a placebo or 200 IU of vitamin E (dl-α-tocopherol) daily for one year. All participants received a capsule containing half the RDA of essential vitamins and minerals. The main outcomes of the study were incidence of respiratory tract infections, number of persons and days with RI (upper and lower), and number of new antibiotic prescriptions for RIs among all randomized participants and those who completed the study.

Supplementation with vitamin E had no significant effect on the incidence or duration of all RIs taken together, or on upper or lower respiratory tract infections measured separately. However, fewer vitamin E–supplemented subjects acquired one or more RI (65% vs. 74%, RR = 0.87, CI = 0.73–0.99, $P = 0.035$), or upper respiratory infections (50% vs. 62%, RR = 0.81, CI = 0.65–0.96, $P = 0.015$). Further analysis on the foremost RI, the common cold, indicated that the vitamin E group had a lower incidence of common colds (0.66 vs. 0.83 per subject–year, RR = 0.80, CI = 0.64–1.00, $P = 0.046$), and fewer subjects in the vitamin E group acquired one or more common colds (46% vs. 57%, RR = 0.79, CI = 0.63–0.96, $P = 0.016$).[40] The vitamin E–treated group also had fewer days with common cold per person–year compared to the placebo group, but the difference did not reach statistical significance (22% less, $P = 0.11$).

In conclusion, the results of this clinical trial show that vitamin E supplementation significantly reduces the incidence rate of common colds and the number of subjects who acquire a cold among elderly nursing home residents. A nonsignificant reduction in the duration of colds was also observed. Because of the high rate and more severe morbidity associated with common colds in this age group, these findings have important implications for the well being of the elderly, as well as for the economic burden associated with their care.

Colds are common afflictions for all age groups, accounting for 30% of absenteeism in the United States.[41] Rhinoviruses and coronaviruses represent the majority of the documented causes of colds.[42–45] They exacerbate chronic obstructive pulmonary disease (COPD)[46] and are known to be associated with lower respiratory tract infections in the elderly.[45,47,48] For example, a prospective cohort study of community-based elderly found that rhinoviruses were associated with lower respiratory symptoms in nearly two-thirds of episodes: about one-fifth of patients were confined to bed, and 26% were unable to perform routine household activities.[48] Constitutional and lower respiratory tract symptoms and signs have been reported to be more common in the elderly compared to younger adults infected with cold viruses.[47] Nursing home populations may also be at risk for epidemic outbreaks of rhinovirus infections.[49] The common cold is generally less severe than influenza. However, its much higher incidence and its recognized morbidity in the elderly[45,47–50] make it an important public health problem in this age group.[51] This is particularly relevant because at present no clinically useful vaccine or antiviral therapy is available to combat colds.

The economic impact of non-influenza-related viral upper respiratory infections in general, and in the elderly in particular, has been overlooked. Fendrick et al.[51] showed that, because of their high attack rate, these diseases are responsible for an economic burdenthat approaches $40 billion annually. Thus, our finding that vitamin E supplementation reduces the common cold by 22% has significant implications for the elderly in reducing the burden of diseases and associated health care costs.

Previous studies on vitamin E and infection in the elderly have demonstrated mixed results. A retrospective study showed that subjects with plasma vitamin E levels above 16.7 mg/L had a significantly lower mean number of infections compared to those with plasma vitamin E levels below 12.2 mg/L (1.0 vs. 2.3, 95% CI for difference = 0.12–2.48).[52] Hemila et al.[53] evaluated the effect of long-term vitamin E and beta-carotene supplementation on the incidence of common cold episodes from a cohort of 21,796 male smokers from the Alpha-Tocopherol Beta-Carotene Cancer Prevention Study. Common-cold episodes were queried three times per year during a 4-year follow-up period. Vitamin E supplementation (50 mg) resulted in a slightly lower incidence of colds among subjects 65 years of age or older (RR = 0.95); this reduction was greatest among older city dwellers who smoked fewer than 15 cigarettes per day (RR = 0.72).

A recent double-blind trial of Dutch elderly[54] living in the community reported a rate ratio for all RIs among those receiving vitamin E as 1.12 (95% CI = 0.88–1.25), compared to those not receiving vitamin E. The Dutch study differed from that of Meydani et al.[40] in terms of the population and the way that respiratory infections were diagnosed. While our subjects were the institutionalized elderly, their incidence of respiratory infection was similar to that of the community-dwelling Dutch elderly.[54] Furthermore, we have previously shown that vitamin E is effective in improving the immune response in the community-dwelling elderly,[9,39] and although it did not have sufficient power to demonstrate statistical significance, one of these studies showed a 30% reduction of infection in the independently living elderly.[9]

In the Dutch study,[54] subjects self-reported their infections by telephone, and then the infections were confirmed by nurse visits. However, absence of infection in those not reporting was not confirmed, thus making the study results susceptible to reporting biases. In our study, the presence and type of RI, or absence, was documented by infectious-disease specialists on the basis of review of data gathered by trained research nurses during weekly subject interviews, review of medical records, and physical examination focused on respiratory infections using standardized case definitions.[28,47,55–57] Furthermore, our results indicate that vitamin E reduces upper respiratory infections, particularly common colds, with no effect on lower respiratory infections or seasonal allergies. Graat et al.[54] did not differentiate between types of infections or between respiratory infection and allergies, and thus might have overlooked any vitamin E effect on upper respiratory infections. In addition, in our study, adherence was checked by nursing-home medication records and by periodic plasma vitamin E measurements, whereas the Graat et al.[54] study measured plasma vitamin E levels only at baseline.

CONCLUSION

Several investigations have demonstrated that vitamin E significantly enhances immune functions in humans, especially in the elderly. Animal studies as well as recently completed clinical trials strongly suggest that this effect of vitamin E is associated with reduced risk of acquiring infections, particularly upper respiratory infections, in the elderly.

ACKNOWLEDGMENT

This work was supported by National Institute on Aging Grant No. 1R01-AG 13975, United States Department of Agriculture agreement 58-1950-9-001, and a grant for preparation of study capsules from Hoffmann-LaRoche Inc.

REFERENCES

1. GEBREMICHAEL, A., E.M. LEVY & L.M. CORWIN. 1984. Adherent cell requirement for the effect of vitamin E on in vitro antibody synthesis. J. Nutr. **114:**1297–1305.
2. KOWDLEY, K., S. MEYDANI, S. CORNWALL, et al. 1992. Vitamin E deficiency and impaired cellular immunity related to intestinal fat malabsorption. Gastroenterology **102:** 2139–2142.
3. MEYDANI, S.N., M.P. BARKLUND, S. LIU, et al. 1990. Vitamin E supplementation enhances cell-mediated immunity in healthy elderly subjects. Am. J. Clin. Nutr. **52:** 557–563.
4. HAN, S.N. & S.N. MEYDANI. 1999. Vitamin E and infectious diseases in the aged. Proc Nutr. Soc. **58:** 697–705.
5. FOOD AND NUTRITION BOARD. 2000. Vitamin E. Dietary Reference Intakes for Vitamin C, Vitamin E, Selenium, Carotenoids. :186–283. National Academy Press. Washington, DC.; NATIONAL RESEARCH COUNCIL. 1989. Vitamin E. Recommended Dietary Allowances.: 99–107. National Academy Press. Washington, DC.
6. RYAN, A.S., L.D. CRAIG & S.C. FINN. 1992. Nutrient intakes and dietary patterns of older Americans: a national study. J. Gerontol. **47:** M145–150.
7. PANEMANGALORE, M. & C.J. LEE. 1992. Evaluation of the indices of retinol and alpha-tocopherol status in free-living elderly. J. Gerontol. **47:** B98–B104.
8. MEYDANI, S.N., M. MEYDANI, C.P. VERDON, et al. 1986. Vitamin E supplementation suppresses prostaglandine E_2 synthesis and enhances the immune response of aged mice. Mech. Ageing Dev. **34:** 191–201.

9. MEYDANI, S.N., M. MEYDANI, J.B. BLUMBERG, et al. 1997. Vitamin E supplementation and in vivo immune response in healthy elderly subjects. A randomized controlled trial. JAMA **277:** 1380–1386.
10. LEE, C.-Y.J. & J.M.-F. WAN. 2000. Vitamin E supplementation improves cell-mediated immunity and oxidative stress of Asian men and women. J. Nutr. **130:** 2932–2937.
11. DE WAART, F., L. PORTENGEN, G. DOEKES, et al. 1997. Effect of 3 months vitamin E supplementation on indices of the cellular and humoral immune response in elderly subjects. Br. J. Nutr. **78:** 761–774.
12. PALLAST, E.G., E.G. SCHOUTEN, F.G. DE WAART, et al. 1999. Effect of 50- and 100-mg vitamin E supplements on cellular immune function in noninstitutionalized elderly persons. Am. J. Clin. Nutr. **69:**1273–1281.
13. MEYDANI, S.N., W.W. FAWZI & S.N. HAN. 2001. The effect of vitamin A deficiencies (E and A) and supplementation of infection and immune response. *In* Nutrition, Immunity, and infection in infants and children. R.M. Suskind & K. Tontisirin, Eds. Vol. 45: 213–241. Lippincott, Williams & Wilkins. Philadelphia.
14. HAYEK, M.G., S.F. TAYLOR, B.S. BENDER, et al. 1997. Vitamin E supplementation decreases lung virus titers in mice infected with influenza. J. Infect. Dis. **176:** 273–276.
15. HAN, S.N., D. WU, W.K. HA, et al. 2000. Vitamin E supplementation increases T helper 1 cytokine production of old mice infected with influenza virus. Immunology **100:** 487–493.
16. SCHNEIDER, E.L. 1983. Infectious diseases in the elderly. Ann. Intern. Med. **98:** 395–400.
17. GUGLIOTTI, R. 1987. The incidence of nosocomial infections in a skilled nursing facility. Conn. Med. **51:** 287–290.
18. ALVAREZ, S., C.G. SHELL, T.W. WOOLLEY, et al. 1988. Nosocomial Infections in long-term facilities. J. Gerontol. **43:** M9–M17.
19. GARIBALDI, R.A., S. BRODINE & S. MATSUMIYA. 1981. Infections among patients in nursing homes. N. Engl. J. Med. **305:** 731–735.
20. JACKSON, M.M., J. FIERE, E. BARRETT-CONNOR, et al. 1992. Intensive surveillance for infections in a three-year study of nursing home patients. Am. J. Epidemiol. **135:** 685–696.
21. NICOLLE, L.E., M. MCINTYRE, H. ZACHARIAS & J.A. MACDONELL. 1984. Twelve-month surveillance of infections in institutionalized elderly men. J. Am. Geriatr. Soc. **32:** 513–519.
22. FARBER, B.F., C. BRENNEN, A.J. PUNTERERI & J.P. BRODY. 1984. A prospective study of nosocomial infections in a chronic care facility. J. Am. Geriatr. Soc. **32:** 499–502.
23. PLEWA, M.C. 1990. Altered host response and special infections in the elderly. Emerg. Med. Clin. North Am. **8:** 193–206.
24. CROSSLEY, K.B. & P.K. PETERSON. 1996. Infections in the elderly. Clin. Infect. Dis. **22:** 209–215.
25. MEHR, D.R., B. FOXMAN & P. COLOMBO. 1992. Risk factors for mortality from lower respiratory infections in nursing home patients. J. Family Pract. **34:** 585–591.
26. HASLEY, P.B., F.L. BRANCATI, J. ROGERS, et al. 1993. Measuring functional change in community-acquired pneumonia. Med. Care **41:** 649–657.
27. GABREL, C.S. 2000. Characteristics of elderly nursing home current residents and discharges: data from the 1997 National Nursing Home Survey. Adv. Data **312:** 1–15.
28. RUBEN, F.L., S.R. DEARWATER, C.W. NORDEN, et al. 1995. Clinical infections in the non-institutionalized geriatric age group: methods utilized and incidence of infections. Am. J. Epidemiol. **141:**145–157.
29. MUDER, R.R. 1998. Pneumonia in residents of long-term care facilities: epidemiology, etiology, management, and prevention. Am. J. Med. **105:** 319–330.
30. MARSTON, B.J., J.F. PLOUFFE, T.M. FILE, JR., et al. 1997. Incidence of community-acquired pneumonia requiring hospitalization. Results of a population-based active surveillance study in Ohio. The Community-Based Pneumonia Incidence Study Group. Arch. Intern. Med. **157:** 1709–1718.
31. SISKIND, G.W. 1980. Immunological aspects of aging: an overview. *In* Biological Mechanism in Aging. R.T. Schimke, Ed.: 455–467. USDA, NIH. Washington, DC.

32. WAYNE, S.J., R.L. RHYNE, P.J. GARRY & J.S. GOODWIN. 1990. Cell-mediated immunity as a predictor of morbidity and mortality in the aged. J. Gerontol. Med. Sci. **45:** M45–48.
33. CHRISTOU, N.V., J. TELLADO-RODRIGUEZ, L. CHARTRAND, et al. 1989. Estimating mortality risk in preoperative patients using immunologic, nutritional, and acute-phase response. Ann. Surg. **210:** 69–77.
34. COHN, J.R., C.A. HOHL & C.E. BUCKLEY. 1983. The relationship between cutaneous cellular immune responsiveness and mortality in a nursing home population. J. Am. Geriatr. Soc. **31:** 808–809.
35. KEUSCH, G.T., C.S. WILSON & S.D. WAKSAL. 1983. Nutrition, host defenses, and the lymphoid system. Adv. Host Defense Mech. **2:** 275–306.
36. CHANDRA, R.K. 1990. Nutrition is an important determinant of immunity in old age. *In* Nutrition and Aging. D.M. Prinsley & H.H. Sandstead, Eds.: 321–334. Alan R. Liss, Inc. New York.
37. CHANDRA, R.K. 1992. Effect of vitamin and trace-element supplementation on immune responses and infection in elderly subjects. Lancet **340:** 1124–1127.
38. MEYDANI, S.N. & J.B. BLUMBERG. 1989. Nutrition and the immune function in the elderly. *In* Human Nutrition: A Comprehensive Treatise. H. Munro & A. Danforth, Eds. Vol. VII: 61–87. Plenum Press. New York.
39. MEYDANI, S.N., P.M. BARKLUND, S. LIU, et al. 1990. Effect of vitamin E supplementation on immune responsiveness of healthy elderly subjects. Am. J. Clin. Nutr. **52:** 557–563.
40. MEYDANI, S.N., L.S. LEKA, B.C. FINE, et al. 2004. Vitamin E and respiratory tract infections in elderly nursing home residents: a randomized controlled trial. JAMA **292:** 828–836.
41. MONTO, A.S. & B.M. ULLMAN. 1974. Acute respiratory illness in an American community. The Tecumseh study. JAMA **227:** 164–169.
42. ARRUDA, E., A. PITKARANTA, T.J. WITEK, et al. 1997. Frequency and natural history of rhinovirus infections in adults during autumn. J. Clin. Microbiol. **35:** 2864–2868.
43. TREANOR, J. & A. FALSEY. 1999. Respiratory viral infections in the elderly. Antiviral Res. **44:** 79–102.
44. MAKELA, M.J., T. PUHAKKA, O. RUUSKANEN, et al. 1998. Viruses and bacteria in the etiology of the common cold. J. Clin. Microbiol. **36:** 539–542.
45. NICHOLSON, K.G., J. KENT, V. HAMMERSLEY & E. CANCIO. 1997. Acute viral infections of upper respiratory tract in elderly people living in the community: comparative, prospective, population based study of disease burden. Br. Med. J. **315:** 1060–1064.
46. SEEMUNGAL, T., R. HARPER-OWEN, A. BHOWMIK, et al. 2001. Respiratory viruses, symptoms, and inflammatory markers in acute exacerbations and stable chronic obstructive pulmonary disease. Am. J. Respir. Crit. Care Med. **164:** 1618–1623.
47. FALSEY, A.R., R.M. MCCANN, W.J. HALL, et al. 1997. The "common cold" in frail older persons: impact of rhinovirus and coronavirus in a senior daycare center. J. Am. Geriatr. Soc. **45:** 706–711.
48. NICHOLSON, K.G., J. KENT, V. HAMMERSLEY & E. CANCIO. 1996. Risk factors for lower respiratory complications of rhinovirus infections in elderly people living in the community: prospective cohort study. Br. Med. J. **313:** 1119–1123.
49. WALD, T.G., P. SHULT, P. KRAUSE, et al. 1995. A rhinovirus outbreak among residents of a long-term care facility. Ann. Intern. Med. **123:** 588–593.
50. FALSEY, A.R., E.E. WALSH & F.G. HAYDEN. 2002. Rhinovirus and coronavirus infection-associated hospitalizations among older adults. J. Infect. Dis. **185:** 1338–1341.
51. FENDRICK, A.M., A.S. MONTO, B. NIGHTENGALE & M. SARNES. 2003. The economic burden of non-influenza-related viral respiratory tract infection in the United States. Arch. Intern. Med. **163:** 487–494.
52. CHAVANCE, M., B. HERBETH, C. FOURNIER, et al. 1989. Vitamin status, immunity and infections in an elderly population. Eur. J. Clin. Nutr. **43:** 827–835.
53. HEMILA, H., J. KAPRIO, D. ALBANES, et al. 2002. Vitamin C, vitamin E, and beta-carotene in relation to common cold incidence in male smokers. Epidemiology **13:** 32–37.

54. GRAAT, J.M., E.G. SCHOUTEN & F.J. KOK. 2002. Effect of daily vitamin E and multivitamin-mineral supplementation on acute respiratory tract infections in elderly persons. JAMA **288:** 715–721.
55. TYRRELL, D.A., S. COHEN & J.E. SCHLARB. 1993. Signs and symptoms in common colds. Epidemiol. Infect. **111:** 143–156.
56. DYKEWICZ, M.S., S. FINEMAN, D.P. SKONER, et al. 1998. Diagnosis and management of rhinitis: complete guidelines of the Joint Task Force on Practice Parameters in Allergy, Asthma and Immunology. American Academy of Allergy, Asthma, and Immunology. Ann. Allergy Asthma Immunol. **81:** 478–518.
57. MCGEER, A., B. CAMPBELL, T.G. EMORI, et al. 1991. Definition of infection for surveillance in long-term care facilities. Am. J. Infect. Control **19:** 1–7.

Tocopherols and the Treatment of Colon Cancer

WILLIAM L. STONE,[a] KOYAMANGALATH KRISHNAN,
[b]SHARON E. CAMPBELL,[b]MIN QUI,[a] SARAH G. WHALEY,[b]
AND HONGSONG YANG[b]

[a]*Department of Pediatrics, East Tennessee State University and James H. Quillen VA Medical Center, Johnson City, Tennessee 37614, USA*

[b]*Division of Hematology-Oncology, Department of Internal Medicine, East Tennessee State University and James H. Quillen VA Medical Center, Johnson City, Tennessee 37614 USA*

ABSTRACT: Colorectal cancer is the second most common cause of cancer deaths in the United States. Vitamin E (VE) and other antioxidants may help prevent colon cancer by decreasing the formation of mutagens arising from the free radical oxidation of fecal lipids or by "non-antioxidant" mechanisms. VE is not a single molecule, but refers to at least eight different molecules, that is, four tocopherols and four tocotrienols. *Methods:* Both animal models and human colon cancer cell lines were used to evaluate the chemopreventive potential of different forms of VE. Rats were fed diets deficient in tocopherols or supplemented with either α-tocopherol or γ-tocopherol. Half the rats in each of these groups received normal levels of dietary Fe and the other half Fe at eight times the normal level. In our cell experiments, we looked at the role of γ-tocopherol in upregulating peroxisome proliferator–activated receptor-γ (PPAR-γ) in the SW 480 human cell line. *Results:* Rats fed the diets supplemented with α-tocopherol had higher levels of VE in feces, colonocytes, plasma, and liver than did rats fed diets supplemented with γ-tocopherol. Dietary Fe levels did not influence tocopherol levels in plasma, liver, or feces. For colonocytes, high dietary Fe decreased tocopherol levels. Rats fed the γ-tocopherol-supplemented diets had lower levels of fecal lipid hydroperoxides than rats fed the α-tocopherol-supplemented diets. R*as-p21* levels were significantly lower in rats fed the γ-tocopherol-supplemented diets compared with rats fed the α-tocopherol-supplemented diets. High levels of dietary Fe were found to promote oxidative stress in feces and colonocytes. Our data with the SW480 cells suggest that both α- and γ-tocopherol upregulate PPAR-γ mRNA and protein expression. γ-tocopherol was, however, found to be a better enhancer of PPAR-γ expression than α-tocopherol at the concentrations tested.

KEYWORDS: vitamin E; tocopherols; colon cancer

Address for correspondence: William L. Stone, Ph.D., East Tennessee State University, James H. Quillen College of Medicine, Department of Pediatrics, Johnson City, TN 37614. Voice: 423-439-8762.
stone@etsu.edu

INTRODUCTION

Colorectal cancer is the second most common cause of cancer deaths in the United States and accounts for 10% of all cancer deaths <http://www.cdc.gov/nccdphp/burdenbook2002/02_colocancer.htm>. The risk of developing colorectal cancer dramatically increases with advancing age. There are, however, enormous country-to-country differences (40-fold) in the incidence of colon cancer throughout the world, suggesting that dietary factors could be critically important. Vitamin E (VE) and other antioxidants may help prevent colon cancer by decreasing the formation of mutagens arising from the free radical oxidation of fecal lipids or by "non-antioxidant" mechanisms. Conversely, dietary factors that contribute to the production of free radicals such as iron may contribute to colon cancer.[1,2] Most dietary iron is not absorbed and is concentrated in feces. Moreover, the respiratory activity of bacteria in feces produces superoxide radicals ($O^{\bullet-}_2$) that, in the presence of iron, can generate hydroxyl radicals by Fenton chemistry.

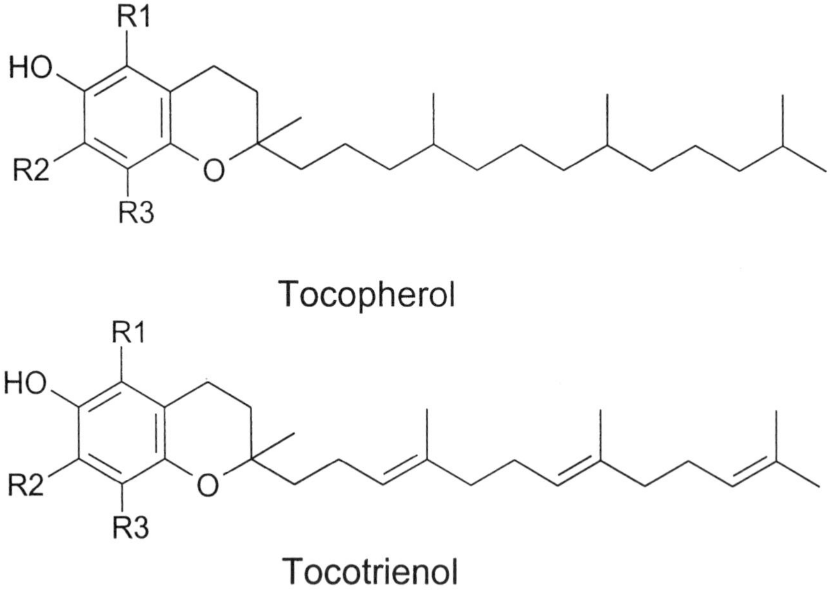

Tocopherol

Tocotrienol

TOCOPHEROLS AND TOCOTRIENOLS

	R1	R2	R3
α-T	CH$_3$	CH$_3$	CH$_3$
β-T	CH$_3$	H	CH$_3$
γ-T	H	CH$_3$	CH$_3$
δ-T	H	H	CH$_3$

FIGURE 1. Vitamin E is at least eight compounds.

Babbs[3] has observed that bacteria in the fecal mass adjacent to the mucosa can generate hydroxyl free radicals ($^{\bullet}$OH) at a rate corresponding to that produced by over 10,000 rads of gamma irradiation per day. Hydroxyl radicals are highly reactive and can react with the polyunsaturated fatty acids (PUFAs) in fecal lipids to initiate lipid peroxidation reactions leading to the formation of lipid hydroperoxides and reactive aldehydes (such as malondialdehyde and 4-hydroxynonenal). Malondialdehyde (MDA) is a well-characterized mutagen,[4] and evidence suggests that the reaction of MDA and deoxyguanosine forms a major adduct found in the DNA of human tissues.[5] The presence of vitamin E in feces should inhibit the process of lipid peroxidation and thereby reduce the formation of mutagenic peroxidation products.

VE is the major fat-soluble antioxidant, and it occurs naturally as eight compounds (FIG. 1). Four of these compounds have a tocol structure with a saturated C16 phytyl side-chain, and four have a tocotrienol structure with the phytyl side-chain having three double bonds. The number and position of the methyl groups determines the specific tocopherol (α-, β-, γ-, or δ-tocopherol) or tocotrienol compound (α-, β-, γ-, or δ-tocotrienol) as indicated in FIGURE 1. In the typical American diet, the levels of γ-tocopherol are about two to four times higher than the levels of α-tocopherol.[6] Nevertheless, plasma levels of α-tocopherol are about two to three times higher than γ-tocopherol levels. Most investigations studying the relationship between colon and cancer and VE have focused only on the α-tocopherol form of VE.[7,8] In this paper, we will review our *in vitro* and *in vivo* studies directed at evaluating the comparative chemopreventive properties of dietary RRR-γ-tocopherol and RRR-α-tocopherol in colon cancer.[7–10] Our experimental results reinforce the notion that γ-tocopherol should be considered in clinical studies relating tocopherol nutriture to colon cancer.

RESULTS AND DISCUSSION

In Vitro *Studies*

Comparative Cellular Uptake of α- and γ-Tocopherols

The protection of cellular DNA from free radical damage and subsequent chemical modification is likely to be very dependent upon intracellular VE levels rather than the levels in plasma. Surprisingly, there have been very few studies comparing the cellular uptakes of α- and γ-tocopherol. Tran and Chan[11] found a preferentially uptake (3-fold higher after 4 hr of incubation) of γ-tocopherol compared to α-tocopherol in cultured human umbilical endothelial cells. In contrast, Jiang and colleagues[12] found a similar incorporation of both α- and γ-tocopherol into RAW264.7 macrophages and only a slightly higher (30%) incorporation of γ-tocopherol (compared to α-tocopherol) in A549 endothelial cells.

Our results with RAW 264.7 macrophages (FIG. 2) showed a significantly greater uptake of γ-tocopherol compared to α-tocopherol with uptake being defined as the net difference between tocopherol transported into the cells and loss due to catabolism and/or *in vitro* oxidation.[13] When macrophages were incubated with α-tocopherol or γ-tocopherol individually, the macrophage level of α-tocopherol was just 10–20% of that of γ-tocopherol (FIG. 2A). In marked contrast, when macrophages

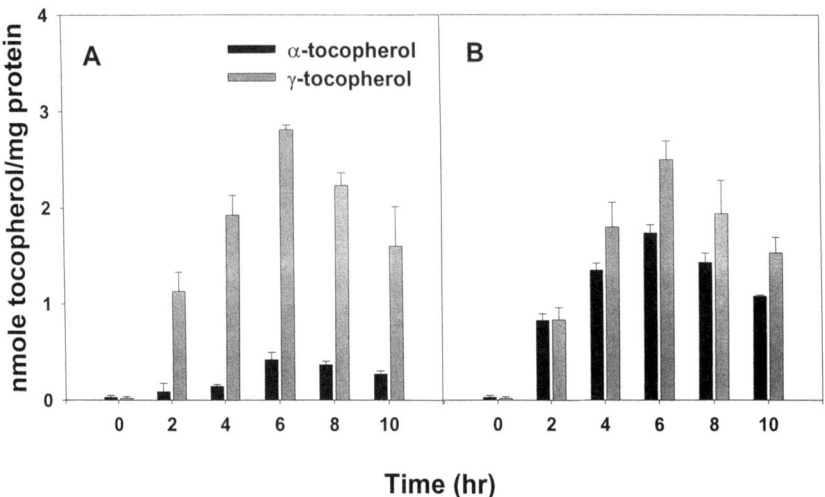

FIGURE 2. The uptake and depletion of α- and γ-tocopherol separately (**A**) and together (**B**) by RAW264.7 macrophages. Confluent RAW264.7 macrophages were incubated with either 5.6 mM α-tocopherol or 4.9 mM γ-tocopherol (**A**) or with both tocopherols (4.6 mM α- plus 5.2 mM γ-tocopherol) together (**B**) and the uptake of tocopherols measured during 6 hr of incubation. After 6 hr, the medium with tocopherols was removed and replaced with medium not containing tocopherols, and depletion of tocopherols followed for 4 hr. Tocopherols in the medium and cells were immediately determined by high-performance liquid chromatography with an electrochemical detector.[13] Each value is a mean ± SD of three wells. Each experiment was performed twice with excellent reproducibility.

were incubated with both α- and γ-tocopherols together, the cellular level of α-tocopherol was 70–80% (after 6 hr) that of γ-tocopherol (FIG. 2B). There were no marked changes in the levels of γ-tocopherol caused by the presence of α-tocopherol. Mass balance considerations suggest that products other than quinone were formed during the incubation of tocopherols with macrophages. In a separate study involving the colon cancer cell line SW 480, we observed a 20-fold increase in uptake of γ-tocopherol over α-tocopherol when incubated at the same concentration of VE in the medium.[14]

It is not known if the *in vitro* results of these studies are relevant to *in vivo* conditions. It is interesting, however, that in an animal model, graded levels of dietary γ-tocopherol in a diet containing a constant level of α-tocopherol were found to increase the levels of α-tocopherol in serum and most tissues.[15] This remarkable result in an animal model has yet to be reproduced in humans but certainly suggests an interaction between dietary γ-tocopherol and α-tocopherol similar to that reported here on the cellular level. The potential health related significance of γ-tocopherol is being increasingly recognized.[16–18]

Influence of Tocopherols on the Expression of Peroxisome Proliferator–Activated Receptors in SW 480 Human Colon Cancer Cell Line

Members of the nuclear receptor superfamily, peroxisome proliferator activated receptors (PPARs) factors are ligand-activated transcription factors that regulate

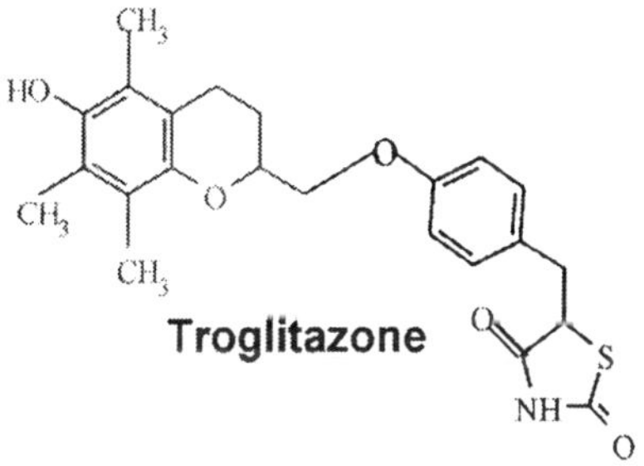

FIGURE 3. The structural comparison of the tocopherols (**A**) and troglitazone (**B**).

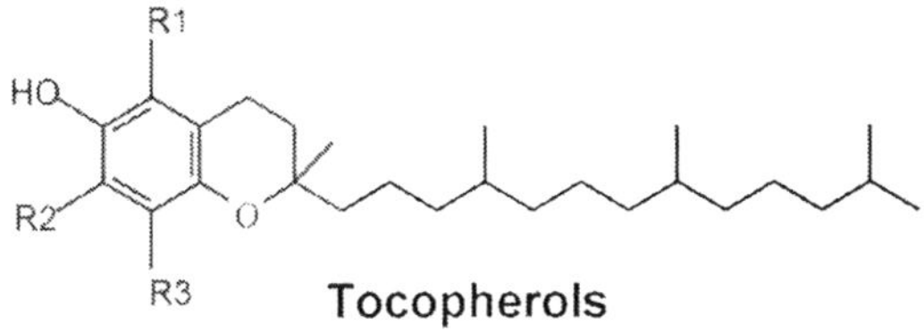

Form	R1	R2	R3
α-T	CH_3	CH_3	CH_3
β-T	CH_3	H	CH_3
γ-T	H	CH_3	CH_3
δ-T	H	H	CH_3

gene expression by binding to DNA. After heterodimerization with the 9-*cis* retinoic acid receptor X (RXR), PPARs bind to peroxisome proliferator responsive elements (PPREs) in the promoter region of several target genes. PPAR-γ has an important role in colon carcinogenesisis necessary for the normal growth and differentiation of colon epithelium.[19,20] Activation of PPAR-γ in colonic epithelial cells results in growth inhibition and an increase in differentiation markers.[20,21]

PPAR-γ ligands have been shown to be effective chemopreventive agents in a rat model of carcinogenesis and in azoxymethane-induced colon cancer in mice.[22] Because VE possesses structural similarities to the PPAR-γ ligand, troglitazone (FIG. 3), we studied the comparative effects of α- and γ-tocopherols on PPAR-γ expression in SW480 colon cancer cell lines.[14] FIGURE 4 shows the differences in mRNA expression as a result of treatment with 5 μM of either α- or γ-tocopherol as compared to vehicle- or troglitazone-treated cells. These data show that both α- and γ-tocopherol can upregulate mRNA expression when compared to vehicle. γ-Tocopherol was found, however, to be superior to α-tocopherol in this upregulation. Similarly, Western blot analyses indicated the α-tocopherol was superior to γ-tocopherol in upregulating the levels of PPAR-γ protein (data not shown here).

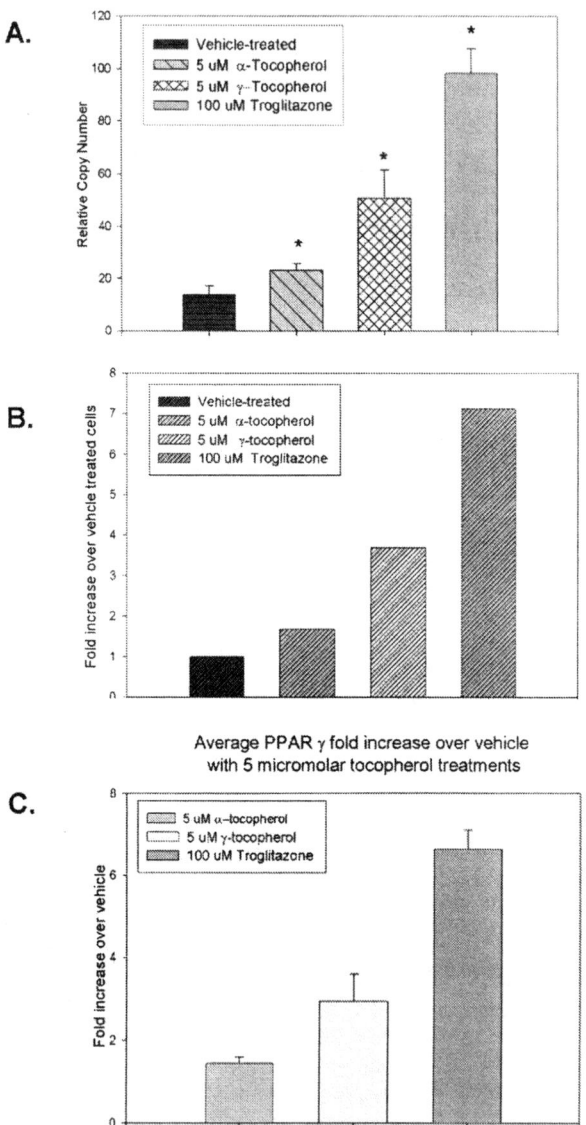

FIGURE 4. Tocopherol upregulation of PPAR-γ mRNA expression detected by QPCR after 24 hr of treatment with 5 μM tocopherol. Total RNA was isolated from SW480 colon cancer cells at 24 hr after treatment with α-tocopherol, γ-tocopherol (5 μM), or 100 μM troglitazone (positive control). The total RNA was reverse transcribed to cDNA. Changes in the mRNA expression were quantified using the cDNA and QPCR reaction with SYBR green. (**A**) Differences in mRNA expression as a result of treatment with 5 μM tocopherols compared to the vehicle and troglitazone-treated cells. (**B**) Data normalized to the vehicle treatment and expressed as a fold increase in PPAR-γ copy number. (**C**) Average of three treatments normalized to the vehicle treatment and expressed as a fold increase in PPAR-γ copy number.[14]

In Vivo *Studies*

Influence of α-Tocopherol or γ-Tocopherol and Dietary Iron on Oxidative Stress and ras-p21 Levels in the Rat Colon

It has been suggested that γ-tocopherol could be selectively sequestered in the colon compared to α-tocopherol.[23] Moreover, γ-tocopherol has a unique *in vitro* ability to detoxify peroxynitrite ($ONOO^-$), an ability which is not shared by α-tocopherol.[24–26] We were interested, therefore, in exploring the hypothesis that dietary γ-tocopherol, as well as α-tocopherol, could be effective in providing antioxidant protection to the epithelial cells of the colon and to fecal material. Work by Singh and colleagues[27] has also shown that some chemopreventive agents can diminish the expression of ras-p21 protein, which is a very useful intermediate biomarker for colon cancer. The ras-p21 protein is a 21-kDa guanine nucleotide binding protein with GTPase activity and is important in regulating cell growth.

Therefore, we investigated how dietary levels of α-tocopherol or γ-tocopherol and iron influence oxidative stress and ras-p21 levels in the rat colon.[8] Rats were fed diets deficient in tocopherols or supplemented with either α-tocopherol or γ-tocopherol. Half the rats in each of these groups received normal levels of dietary Fe, and the other half received Fe at eight times the normal level.

Our results (FIG. 5) indicated that γ-tocopherol levels were lower in plasma, liver, colonocytes, and feces compared to the levels found for α-tocopherol even though the dietary levels of α-tocopherol and γ-tocopherol were almost identical in the diets. The current model for VE absorption suggests that α-tocopherol and γ-tocopherol are absorbed from the intestine equally well and transported (via chylomicrons) to the liver, where α-tocopherol is selectively packaged into lipoproteins by the hepatic tocopherol binding protein, which has a much higher affinity for α-tocopherol than for γ-tocopherol. It has been suggested that the hepatic γ-tocopherol, not transferred

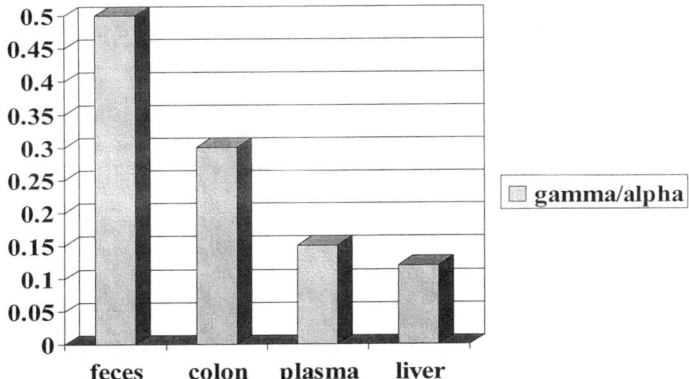

FIGURE 5. The ratio of γ-tocopherol (for rats fed RRR-γ-tocopherol) to α-tocopherol (for rats fed RRR-α-tocopherol) in feces, plasma, and liver. Half the rats in each tocopherol group were fed the recommended level of dietary iron (RFe), and the other half a high level of dietary iron (HFe).

to lipoproteins, is secreted via the bile back into the intestine and excreted, thereby accounting for the lower plasma and tissue levels of γ-tocopherol compared to α-tocopherol.[23] However, we found lower fecal levels of γ-tocopherol compared to α-tocopherol, suggesting that γ-tocopherol is also catabolized more rapidly than α-tocopherol.

Swanson and colleagues[28] have found that a major route of γ-tocopherol catabolism is via conversion (by phytyl-tail oxidation) to 2,7,8-trimethyl-2-(β-carboxyethyl)-6-hydroxychroman followed by glucuronide conjugation and urinary excretion. The data reported here support the view that γ-tocopherol is selectively catabolized by this phytyl-tail oxidation compared to α-tocopherol. Nevertheless, γ-tocopherol/α-tocopherol in plasma was not found to be predictive of the ratio in colonocytes or feces, where the ratio was 2–3 times higher. Moreover, we found that γ-tocopherol reduced the fecal level of lipid hydroperoxides and the expression of ras-p21 to a greater extent than α-tocopherol. The ras-p21 protein is an oncogenic protein expressed during azoxymethane-induced colon cancer[27,29] and is overexpressed in patients with advanced colorectal cancer.[30] There are no clinical trials in which a γ-tocopherol-enriched form of VE has been evaluated for its potential ability to reduce colonocyte proliferation or levels of ras-p21.

CONCLUSIONS

Epidemiologic studies relating colon cancer to VE have not yielded consistent results.[10,31–38] Some of this inconsistency may be related to differences in the chemical or stereochemical forms of the VE under investigation. Most studies relating VE to cancer have not paid sufficient attention to the different chemical forms/stereoisomers of VE. Increasing evidence suggests that the different forms of VE have distinct biopotencies and biokinetics[7–9,12,15–18,26,39–44] and different abilities to prevent neoplastic transformations.[45] Our *in vivo* data with rats suggest that γ-tocopherol in the human diet could make a major contribution to the antioxidant defense in the colon. Indeed, Nair and colleagues[46] have found that the concentration of γ-tocopherol in human colonic epithelial cells is higher than that of α-tocopherol.

Our *in vitro* data with RAW 264.7 macrophages suggests that γ-tocopherol could play a significant role in modulating intracellular antioxidant defense mechanisms. Moreover, we found the presence of γ-tocopherol dramatically influenced the cellular accumulation of α-tocopherol; that is, γ-tocopherol promoted the accumulation of α-tocopherol. If these results could be extrapolated to *in vivo* conditions, they would suggest that γ-tocopherol is selectively taken up by cells and removed from plasma more rapidly than α-tocopherol. This could contribute, in part, to the selective maintenance of α-tocopherol in plasma compared to γ-tocopherol. The colon cancer cell line, SW480, was also found to have a much greater uptake of γ-tocopherol compared to α-tocopherol.[14]

Our finding that γ-tocopherol was superior to α-tocopherol in upregulating the expression of PPAR-γ in a colon cancer cell line may have significant implications in chemoprevention.[9,14] Sato and colleagues have found that PPAR-γ activation induces growth inhibition in colon cancer cells by activation of apoptosis and together with G1 cell cycle arrest.[47] Moreover, work by Sarraf and colleagues[48] suggests that colon cancer in humans is associated with loss-of-function mutations in PPAR-γ. We are currently studying the comparative influence of α- and γ-tocopherol on apoptosis in a variety of colon and prostate cancer cell lines.

ACKNOWLEDGMENTS

This research was supported by grants from the U.S. Department of Agriculture (grant 9600976 to W.L.S.), the California Walnut Commission (to W.L.S.), the Department of Defense Prostate Cancer Research Program (PC030061 to W.L.S. and K.K.), the Cancer Research and Prevention Foundation of America (postdoctoral fellowship award to S.C.), the Ehrlmann Eagles Cancer Research Fund (to K.K.), and the Research and Development Committee of East Tennessee State University (to K.K.).

REFERENCES

1. NELSON, R.L. et al. 1994. Body iron stores and risk of colonic neoplasia. J. Natl. Cancer Inst. **86:** 455–460.
2. NELSON, R.L. 2001. Iron and colorectal cancer risk: human studies. Nutr. Rev. **59:** 140–148.
3. BABBS, C.F. 1990. Free radicals and the etiology of colon cancer. Free Radic. Biol. Med. **8:** 191–200.
4. SHARMA, R.A. et al. 2001. Cyclooxygenase-2, malondialdehyde and pyrimidopurinone adducts of deoxyguanosine in human colon cells. Carcinogenesis **22:** 1557–1560.
5. CHAUDHARY, A.K. et al. 1994. Detection of endogenous malondialdehyde-deoxyguanosine adducts in human liver. Science **265:** 1580–1582.
6. BIERI, J.G. & R.P. EVARTS. 1974. Gamma tocopherol: metabolism, biological activity and significance in human vitamin E nutrition. Am. J. Clin. Nutr. **27:** 980–986.
7. STONE, W.L. & A.M. PAPAS. 1997. Tocopherols and the etiology of colon cancer. J. Natl. Cancer Inst. **89:** 1006–1014.
8. STONE, W.L. et al. 2002. The influence of dietary iron and tocopherols on oxidative stress and ras-p21 levels in the colon. Cancer Detect. Prevent. **26:** 78–84.
9. CAMPBELL, S. et al. 2003. Development of gamma (gamma)-tocopherol as a colorectal cancer chemopreventive agent. Crit. Rev. Oncol./Hematol. **47:** 249–259.
10. KRISHNAN, K. et al. 2003. Cancer chemoprevention drug targets. Curr. Drug Target **4:** 45–54.
11. TRAN, K. & A.C. CHAN. 1992. Comparative uptake of alpha- and gamma-tocopherol by human endothelial cells. Lipids **27:** 38–41.
12. JIANG, Q. et al. 2000. gamma-tocopherol and its major metabolite, in contrast to alpha-tocopherol, inhibit cyclooxygenase activity in macrophages and epithelial cells. Proc. Natl. Acad. Sci. USA **97:** 11494–11499.
13. GAO, R. et al. 2002. The uptake of tocopherols by RAW 264.7 macrophages. Nutr. J. **1:** 2.
14. CAMPBELL, S.E. et al. 2003. Gamma (gamma) tocopherol upregulates peroxisome proliferator activated receptor (PPAR) gamma (gamma) expression in SW 480 human colon cancer cell lines. BMC Cancer **3:** 25.
15. CLEMENT, M. & J.M. BOURRE. 1997. Graded dietary levels of RRR-gamma-tocopherol induce a marked increase in the concentrations of alpha- and gamma-tocopherol in nervous tissues, heart, liver and muscle of vitamin-E-deficient rats. Biochim. Biophys. Acta **1334:** 173–181.
16. JIANG, Q. et al. 2001. gamma-tocopherol, the major form of vitamin E in the US diet, deserves more attention. Am. J. Clin. Nutr. **74:** 714–722.
17. JIANG, Q. et al. 2002. Gamma-tocopherol supplementation inhibits protein nitration and ascorbate oxidation in rats with inflammation. Free Radic. Biol. Med. **33:** 1534–1542.

18. JIANG, Q. & B.N. AMES. 2003. Gamma-tocopherol, but not alpha-tocopherol, decreases proinflammatory eicosanoids and inflammation damage in rats. FASEB J. **17:** 816–822.
19. JACKSON, L. et al. 2003. Potential role for peroxisome proliferator activated receptor (PPAR) in preventing colon cancer. Gut **52:** 1317–1322.
20. KITAMURA, S. et al. 1999. Peroxisome proliferator-activated receptor gamma induces growth arrest and differentiation markers of human colon cancer cells. Jpn. J. Cancer Res. (Gann) **90:** 75–80.
21. MANSEN, A. et al. 1996. Expression of the peroxisome proliferator-activated receptor (PPAR) in the mouse colonic mucosa. Biochem. Biophys. Res. Commun. **222:** 844–851.
22. KOHNO, H. et al. 2002. Dietary conjugated linolenic acid inhibits azoxymethane-induced colonic aberrant crypt foci in rats. Jpn. J. Cancer Res. (Gann) **93:** 133–142.
23. TRABER, M.G. & H.J. KAYDEN. 1989. Preferential incorporation of alpha-tocopherol vs gamma-tocopherol in human lipoproteins. Am. J. Clin. Nutr. **49:** 517–526.
24. WOLF, G. 1997. gamma-Tocopherol: an efficient protector of lipids against nitric oxide-initiated peroxidative damage. Nutr. Rev. **55:** 376–378.
25. HOGLEN, N.C. et al. 1997. Reactions of peroxynitrite with gamma-tocopherol. Chem. Res. Toxicol. **10:** 401–407.
26. CHRISTEN, S. et al. 1997. gamma-Tocopherol traps mutagenic electrophiles such as NO(X) and complements alpha-tocopherol: physiological implications. Proc. Natl. Acad. Sci. USA **94:** 3217–3222.
27. SINGH, J., R. HAMID & B.S. REDDY. 1997. Dietary fat and colon cancer: modulating effect of types and amount of dietary fat on ras-p21 function during promotion and progression stages of colon cancer. Cancer Res. **57:** 253–258.
28. SWANSON, J.E. et al. 1999. Urinary excretion of 2,7, 8-trimethyl-2-(beta-carboxyethyl)-6-hydroxychroman is a major route of elimination of gamma-tocopherol in humans. J. Lipid Res. **40:** 665–671.
29. SINGH, J., R. HAMID & B.S. REDDY. 1998. Dietary fish oil inhibits the expression of farnesyl protein transferase and colon tumor development in rodents. Carcinogenesis **19:** 985–989.
30. MIYAHARA, M. et al. 1991. Clinical significance of ras p21 overexpression for patients with an advanced colorectal cancer. Dis. Colon Rectum **34:** 1097–1102.
31. CASCINU, S. et al. 2000. Effects of calcium and vitamin supplementation on colon cell proliferation in colorectal cancer. Cancer Invest. **18:** 411–416.
32. NAIR, S. et al. 2001. Serum and colon mucosa micronutrient antioxidants: differences between adenomatous polyp patients and controls. Am. J. Gastroenterol. **96:** 3400–3405.
33. GIACOSA, A. et al. 1997. Vitamins and cancer chemoprevention. Eur. J. Cancer Prevent. **6**(Suppl. 1): S47–S54.
34. SLATTERY, M.L. et al. 1998. Vitamin E and colon cancer: is there an association? Nutr. Cancer **30:** 201–206.
35. SATIA-ABOUTA, J. et al. 2003. Associations of micronutrients with colon cancer risk in African Americans and whites: results from the North Carolina Colon Cancer Study. Cancer Epidemiology, Biomarkers, and Prevention: A Publication of the American Association for Cancer Research, Cosponsored By the American Society of Preventive Oncology. **12:** 747–754.
36. WU, K. et al. 2002. A prospective study on supplemental vitamin e intake and risk of colon cancer in women and men. Cancer Epidemiology, Biomarkers, and Prevention: A Publication of the American Association for Cancer Research, Cosponsored By the American Society of Preventive Oncology. **11:** 1298–1304.
37. BOSTICK, R.M. et al. 1993. Reduced risk of colon cancer with high intake of vitamin E: the Iowa Women's Health Study. Cancer Res. **53:** 4230–4237.
38. PATTERSON, R.E. et al. 1997. Vitamin supplements and cancer risk: the epidemiologic evidence. Cancer Causes Control **8:** 786–802.
39. CALVIELLO, G. et al. 2003. gamma-Tocopheryl quinone induces apoptosis in cancer cells via caspase-9 activation and cytochrome c release. Carcinogenesis **24:** 427–433.

40. SJOHOLM, A., P.O. BERGGREN & R.V. COONEY. 2000. gamma-tocopherol partially protects insulin-secreting cells against functional inhibition by nitric oxide. Biochem. Biophys. Res. Commun. **277:** 334–340.
41. COONEY, R.V. *et al.* 1995. Products of gamma-tocopherol reaction with NO2 and their formation in rat insulinoma (RINm5F) cells. Free Radic. Biol. Med. **19:** 259–269.
42. BERTRAM, J.S. *et al.* 1991. Diverse carotenoids protect against chemically induced neoplastic transformation. Carcinogenesis **12:** 671–678.
43. COONEY, R.V., P.D. ROSS & G.L. BARTOLINI. 1986. N-Nitrosation and N-nitration of morpholine by nitrogen dioxide: inhibition by ascorbate, glutathione and alpha-tocopherol. Cancer Lett. **32:** 83–90.
44. WILLIAMSON, K.S. *et al.* 2002. The nitration product 5-nitro-gamma-tocopherol is increased in the Alzheimer brain. Nitric Oxide **6:** 221–227.
45. COONEY, R.V. *et al.* 1993. Gamma-tocopherol detoxification of nitrogen dioxide: superiority to alpha-tocopherol. Proc. Natl. Acad. Sci. USA **90:** 1771–1775.
46. NAIR, P.P. *et al.* 1996. Uptake and distribution of carotenoids, retinol, and tocopherols in human colonic epithelial cells in vivo. Cancer Epidemiology, Biomarkers, and Prevention: A Publication of the American Association for Cancer Research, Cosponsored By the American Society of Preventive Oncology. **5:** 913–916.
47. SATO, H. *et al.* 2000. Expression of peroxisome proliferator-activated receptor (PPAR)gamma in gastric cancer and inhibitory effects of PPARgamma agonists. Br. J. Cancer **83:** 1394–1400.
48. SARRAF, P. *et al.* 1999. Loss-of-function mutations in PPAR gamma associated with human colon cancer. Mol. Cell **3:** 799–804.

Selenium and Vitamin E Cancer Prevention Trial

ERIC A. KLEIN

Section of Urologic Oncology, Glickman Urological Institute and Cleveland Clinic Lerner College of Medicine, Cleveland Clinic Foundation, Cleveland, Ohio 44195, USA

ABSTRACT: Preclinical, epidemiological, and phase III data from randomized, placebo-controlled clinical trials suggest that both selenium and vitamin E have potential efficacy in prostate cancer prevention. *In vitro* evidence suggests that selenium and vitamin E work synergistically to cause cell-cycle arrest, induce caspase-mediated apoptosis, and act as antiandrogens in arresting clonal expansion of nascent tumors. The Selenium and Vitamin E Cancer Prevention Trial (SELECT), sponsored by the National Cancer Institute, is an intergroup Phase III, randomized, double-blind, placebo-controlled, population-based clinical trial designed to test the efficacy of selenium and vitamin E alone and in combination in the prevention of prostate cancer. The study has a 2 × 2 factorial design with a target accrual of 32,400. Eligibility criteria include an age of at least 50 years for African Americans and of at least 55 years for Caucasians; a DRE not suspicious for cancer; a serum PSA no greater than 4 ng/mL; and a normal blood pressure. Randomization will be equally distributed among the four study arms, with intervention consisting of a daily oral dose of study supplement (200 μg l-selenomethionine or 400 mg of racemic α-tocopheryl) or matched placebo. Study duration is planned for 12 years, with a 5-year uniform accrual period and a minimum of 7 and maximum of 12 years of intervention. The primary endpoint for SELECT is the clinical incidence of prostate cancer as determined by a recommended routine clinical diagnostic work-up, including yearly DRE and serum PSA level. SELECT is the second large-scale study of chemoprevention for prostate cancer. Enrollment began in 2001, with final results anticipated in 2013.

KEYWORDS: prostate cancer; chemoprevention; selenium; vitamin E

The burden of prostate cancer, the most common nondermatologic malignancy in U.S. men since 1984, can be measured by its incidence, prevalence, and disease-related mortality. Although mortality from prostate cancer is decreasing, in the last 5 years alone more than 1 million men in the United States have been newly diagnosed with this disease.[1] Despite a PSA-induced stage migration, a high cure rate for localized disease, and an improved understanding of prostate cancer biology, most men who develop metastatic disease are still destined to die of prostate cancer, with almost half a million deaths in the United States between 1989 and 2001.[1] It is self-

Address for correspondence: Eric A. Klein, M.D., Head, Section of Urologic Oncology, Professor of Surgery, Glickman Urological Institute, Cleveland Clinic Foundation, 9500 Euclid Avenue, Cleveland, OH 44195. Voice: 216-444-5591.
kleine@ccf.org

evident that an effective prevention strategy would spare many men the burden of diagnosis and cure.

Recognition that androgens are important in the development of prostate cancer led to the first large-scale, population-based prevention study, the Prostate Cancer Prevention Trial (PCPT, SWOG-9217), a Phase III, double-blind, placebo-controlled, randomized trial to determine the efficacy of finasteride in reducing the period prevalence of prostate cancer. The PCPT was based on observations that androgens are required for the development of prostate cancer and that men with congenital deficiency of type 2 5-α reductase are unaffected by prostate cancer. In this trial, the 7-year period prevalence of prostate cancer was reduced by 24.8% (RR = 0.75), from 24.4 to 18.4% in those randomized to finasteride compared with placebo.[2] An unexpected finding of a slight increase in the risk of high-grade tumors in the finasteride arm has prevented widespread use of finasteride as a preventative agent and highlighted the need for alternative strategies.

Recent research suggests that selenium and vitamin E are promising candidates for prostate cancer prevention, based primarily on secondary analyses of large-scale chemoprevention trials for other cancers.[3,4] SELECT, the Selenium and Vitamin E Cancer Prevention Trial, is an intergroup Phase III, randomized, double-blind, placebo-controlled, population-based clinical trial designed to test the efficacy of selenium and vitamin E alone and in combination in the prevention of prostate cancer.

RATIONALE FOR STUDY AGENTS

Selenium

Selenium is a nonmetallic trace element recognized as a nutrient essential to human health. Selenium is an essential constituent of at least four extracellular and cellular glutathione peroxidases, three thyroidal and extrathyroidal iodothyronine 5′ deiodinases, thioredoxin reductase, and other selenoproteins. Selenium inhibits tumorigenesis in a variety of experimental models, and several potential mechanisms have been proposed for its anti-tumorigenic effects.[5] Much evidence suggests that selenium works by inhibiting important early steps in carcinogenesis and prevents clonal expansion. Dong and colleagues have demonstrated dose- and time-dependent growth inhibition and induction of apoptosis in the PC3 human prostate cancer cell line using methylselenic acid (MSA), and have identified 12 clusters of Se-responsive genes by oligonucleotide array.[6] A confirmatory study with LnCAP demonstrated that MSA affects transcriptional levels of many cell cycle regulated genes resulting in cell cycle arrest and decreased proliferation.[7] MSA also modulates expression of many androgen-regulated genes, suppresses androgen receptor expression, and decreases levels of secreted PSA. Combining vitamin E succinate (VES) and MSA produces a synergistic effect on cell growth suppression, primarily mediated by augmenting apoptosis.[8]

In vivo studies also support the antitumorigenic role of selenium in prostate cancer. In a dog model, Waters and colleagues demonstrated that oral selenium in various forms given over 7 months as a dietary supplement resulted in lower levels of DNA damage in prostatic epithelial cells and increased intraprostatic apoptosis compared with controls.[9] A study in men with normal pretreatment serum selenium levels demonstrated that 200 µg oral selenium per day resulted in statistically significant higher levels of selenium in prostatic tissue compared to placebo in men undergoing transurethral resection of the prostate for benign prostatic hypertrophy (BPH).[10] Together these studies demonstrate that orally ingested selenium reaches the prostate and modulates markers of oxidative stress.

Many epidemiologic studies suggest that selenium status is inversely related to the risk of prostate cancer.[5] A recent nested case-control study found that the risk of advanced prostate cancer was reduced by one-half to two-thirds for men with the highest selenium status.[11,12]

Enthusiasm for selenium in the prevention of prostate cancer comes from Nutrional Prevention of Cancer Study.[4] In this study, 1312 subjects with a prior history of skin cancer were randomized to receive 200 µg/day of selenium in the form of selenized yeast or placebo and had their progress followed for an average of 4.5 years for the development of basal or squamous cell carcinoma of the skin and other cancers. Although no difference was noted in rates of skin cancer, further analysis found that prostate cancer incidence was reduced by two-thirds among those in the selenium supplemented group. On the basis of a small number of cases, additional stratified analyses suggested a greater reduction in prostate cancer in those having low baseline selenium blood levels, in those aged than 65 years, and in those with low serum PSA values. In a subsequent report that added an additional 25 months of follow-up (mean of 7.45 years), re-analysis of the effect of selenium supplementation continues to show a marked reduction on the incidence of prostate cancer, with a HR of 0.48.[13] As in the initial analysis, the effect was strongest for those with a PSA < 4 ng/mL and those with the lowest serum selenium levels at study entry.

Vitamin E (α-Tocopherol)

Vitamin E is a family of naturally occurring, essential, fat-soluble vitamin compounds. Vitamin E functions as the major lipid-soluble antioxidant in cell membranes. It is a chain-breaking, free-radical scavenger, and it inhibits lipid peroxidation specifically, with biologic activity relevant to carcinogen-induced DNA damage.[14] The most active form of vitamin E is α-tocopherol; it is also among the most abundant forms. It is widely distributed in nature, and it is the predominant form in human tissues.[15,16]

α-Tocopherol may influence the development of cancer through several mechanisms. It has a strong inherent potential for antioxidation of highly reactive and genotoxic electrophiles, blocks nitrosamine formation, and inhibits protein kinase C activity and cell proliferation.[14,17–21] α-Tocopheryl succinate (VES), a derivative of vitamin E, is known to modulate prostate cancer cell growth. VES causes G1 cell cycle arrest by decreasing expression of the cell cycle regulatory proteins cyclin D1, D3, and E, and cdk2 and cdk4.[21] Thompson and Wilding have demonstrated that the chromanol moiety (PMCol) of vitamin E has antiandrogen activity. In LNCap, PMCol produced a growth curve similar to that produced by the androgen receptor antagonist bicalutamide, inhibited PSA secretion and androgen-induced promoter activation, and did not affect androgen receptor protein expression levels.[22]

Observational studies are inconsistent with regard to a beneficial association between serum vitamin E and prostate cancer. These studies have assessed cancer risk through estimated dietary intake or through determination of plasma or serum α-tocopherol concentrations. Of the few prospective studies having a sufficient number of prostate cancers for analysis, two reported no dose-response association, and one reported a statistically significant protective association.[23–25] A study of 2,974 subjects over a 17-year follow-up period found low α-tocopherol to be associated with higher prostate cancer risk.[26] One large-scale randomized, placebo-controlled trial, the Alpha-Tocopherol, Beta-Carotene Cancer Prevention Trial (ATBC), supports the role of vitamin E in the prevention of prostate cancer. ATBC was a randomized, double-blind, placebo-controlled trial of α-tocopherol (50 mg synthetic *dl*-α-tocopheryl acetate daily) and β-carotene (20 mg daily) (alone or in combination) among 29,133 male smokers aged 50–69 years at entry. During the median follow-up period of 6.1 years, there were 246 new cases and 64 deaths from prostate cancer. Among those assigned to the α-tocopherol arm ($n = 14{,}564$), there were 99 incident prostate cancers compared with 147 cases among those assigned to the non-α-tocopherol arm ($n = 14{,}569$).[3,27] This represented a statistically significant 32% reduction in prostate cancer incidence (95% confidence interval, 12% to 47%; $P = 0.002$). The observed preventive effect appeared stronger in clinically evident cases, where the incidence was decreased 40% in subjects receiving α-tocopherol (95% confidence interval, −20% to −55%). Prostate cancer mortality data, though based on fewer events, suggested a similarly strong effect of 41% lower mortality. An important post-intervention follow-up assessment of cancer incidence and mortality in this study was recently reported, with an overall posttrial relative risk (RR) for prostate cancer of 0.88 for those receiving α-tocopherol.[28] The study concluded that the beneficial effects of supplemental α-tocopherol (and the deleterious effects on lung cancer incidence of β-carotene) disappeared during postintervention follow-up, suggesting that these agents affect the risk of cancer in real time, and that their effects wash out after discontinuation.

Another randomized, double blind, placebo controlled lung cancer prevention trial, the β-Carotene and Retinol Efficacy Trial (CARET), lends support to the epidemiologic evidence that α-tocopherol may prevent prostate cancer. Analysis of serum micronutrients in CARET participants has demonstrated that low serum levels of α-tocopherol were associated with a higher risk of prostate cancer.[29] In contrast to some other studies,[30] no association between risk of prostate cancer and serum γ-tocopherol levels was found in CARET.

SELENIUM AND VITAMIN E CANCER PREVENTION TRIAL

The accumulated epidemiologic and biologic evidence that selenium and vitamin E may prevent prostate cancer led to the design and launch of the Selenium and Vitamin E Cancer Prevention Trial (SELECT).[31] SELECT, which is sponsored by the National Cancer Institute, is a Phase III, randomized, double-blind, placebo-controlled, population-based clinical trial designed to test the efficacy of selenium and vitamin E alone and in combination in the prevention of prostate cancer. The study has a 2×2 factorial design with a target accrual of 32,400. Eligibility criteria include age ≥ 50 years for African Americans, age ≥ 55 years for Caucasians, a digital rectal exam (DRE) not suspicious for cancer, a serum PSA ≤ 4 ng/mL, and a normal blood pressure (TABLE 1). Randomization will be equally distributed among four study arms (selenium + placebo, vitamin E + placebo, selenium + vitamin E, and pla-

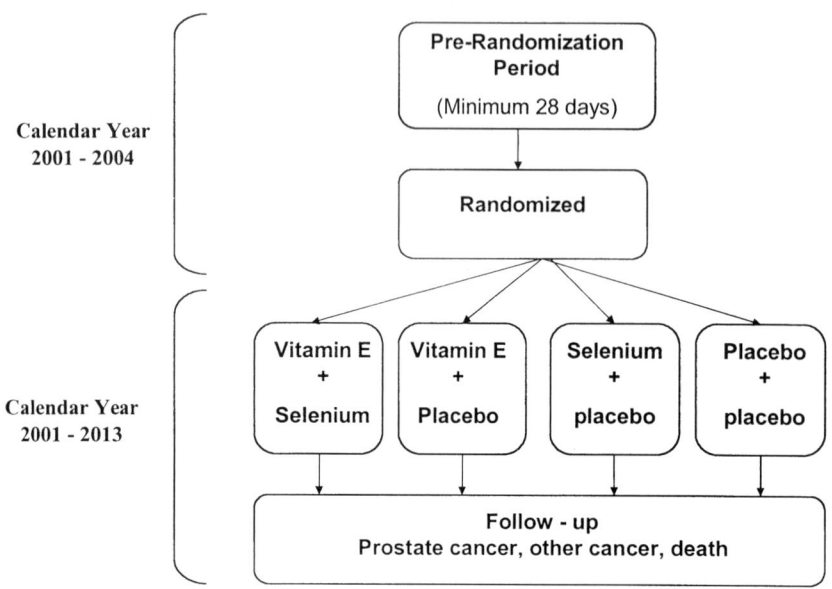

FIGURE 1. SELECT study schema.

cebo + placebo) (FIG. 1). Study duration is planned for 12 years, with a minimum of 7 and maximum of 12 years of intervention, depending on the time of randomization. The study supplements are 200 µg of l-selenomethionine, 400 mg of racemic α-tocopheryl, and an optional multivitamin containing no selenium or vitamin E.

Study Endpoints

The primary endpoint for the trial is the clinical incidence of prostate cancer as determined by a recommended routine clinical diagnostic work-up, including yearly DRE and serum PSA level. A centrally reviewed histologic diagnosis of prostate cancer will be required in all cases, except for those based on a total PSA > 50 ng/mL and a positive bone scan. Prostate biopsy will be performed at the discretion of study physicians according to local community standards. The study protocol recommends biopsy for study participants who have a DRE suspicious for cancer and/or for elevations in serum PSA. Unlike the PCPT, no biopsy will be required at the end of SELECT.

Secondary endpoints will include prostate cancer-free survival, all-cause mortality, and the incidence and mortality of other cancers and diseases potentially impacted by the chronic use of selenium and vitamin E. Other trial objectives will include periodic quality of life assessments, assessment of serum micronutrient levels and prostate cancer risk, and studies of the evaluation of biological and genetic markers with the risk of prostate cancer.

Accrual and Participant Characteristics

As of April 20, 2004, 32,400 men were enrolled and randomized on SELECT, representing 100% of planned accrual achieved 27 months sooner than planned. Of these enrollees, more than 95% have completed high school, and more than 80% have completed at least some college. Fourteen percent of the enrollees are African American, and an additional 4% represent other minorities and medically underserved populations.

Statistical Considerations

The primary analysis of the study includes five pre-specified comparisons: (1) vitamin E versus placebo; (2) selenium versus placebo; (3) combination (vitamin E + selenium) versus placebo; (4) combination versus vitamin E; and (5) combination versus selenium. The study design will permit detection of a 25% reduction in the incidence of prostate cancer for selenium or vitamin E alone, with an additional 25% reduction for the combination of selenium and vitamin E compared to either agent alone. The study allows for the potential interaction between vitamin E and selenium, and additional statistical analyses will include tests for vitamin E versus no vitamin E, selenium versus no selenium, and for interactions between the two agents.

The overall α level for is 5% (two-sided), with each of the five comparisons tested at the 1% level to maintain an overall 5% level for the study. With a sample size of 32,400, the estimated power for the comparison of a single agent versus placebo is 96%, and the power for the comparison of an effective single agent versus the combination of selenium and vitamin E is 89%. The median time under observation is estimated to be 8.8 years. The yearly prostate cancer incidence figures used in the sample-size calculations are derived from observations of the PCPT and SEER (Surveillance, Epidemiology, and End Results) databases. The estimated incidence of prostate cancer begins at 0% at randomization, reaches 0.14% at year 1, and rises steadily to 1.36% 12 years later. The expected incidence of prostate cancer in the placebo arm after 12 years is 6.6%.

It is assumed that the medication rate (an estimate of the percentage of participants who actually take the study supplements) will vary over time, with a decline from 100% after randomization to 51% at the end of 12 years of treatment. These estimates are based on observed rates in the PCPT. Compliance with daily medication use in SELECT may be higher than PCPT because finasteride has more side-effects than are known for selenium or vitamin E. The drop-in rate, defined as the rate of those randomized to placebo who obtain and take selenium and/or vitamin E on their own is assumed to be constant at 10% for the 12 years of treatment. Recent Heart Outcomes Prevention Evaluation (HOPE) data support this estimate.[32] The cumulative competing risk is defined to be the estimated cumulative all-cause mortality rate plus the cumulative lost-to-follow-up (LTFU) rate. The mortality rates used were taken from PCPT for the first 4 years of treatment and then adjusted upwards to the 1995 U.S. rates for all races. The LTFU rate was calculated to be 0.05% per year. The cumulative loss (death + LTFU) is expected to be 0.8% at the end of the first year of the study and 33.2% by the end of year 12.

In contrast to finasteride, the drugs being tested in SELECT are assumed to lack an affect on PSA or prostate size, either of which could bias the diagnosis of prostate cancer. PSA levels at baseline and after 2 years of vitamin E use were analyzed on a subsample of participants from the HOPE trial and after 3 years in the ATBC study.[3,27] There was no evidence of an effect on the PSA concentrations in these studies.

SUMMARY

Ample evidence exists from preclinical studies, epidemiologic observations, and controlled and uncontrolled clinical trials that selenium and vitamin E may prevent the development or progression of prostate cancer. SELECT is a large-scale, population-based, randomized, controlled trial that will directly test the effect of these agents alone and in combination on the incidence of prostate cancer in North American males.

REFERENCES

1. JEMAL, A., R.C. TIWARI, T. MURRAY, et al. 2004. Cancer statistics, 2004. CA Cancer J. Clin. **54:** 8–29.
2. THOMPSON, I.M., P.J. GOODMAN, C.M. TANGEN, et al. 2003. The influence of finasteride on the development of prostate cancer. N. Engl. J. Med. **17:** 215–224.
3. HEINONEN, O.P., D. ALBANES, J.K. HUTTUNEN, et al. 1998. Prostate cancer and supplementation with α-tocopherol and β-carotene: incidence and mortality in a controlled trial. J. Natl. Cancer Inst. **90:** 440–446.
4. CLARK, L.C., G.F. COMBS, JR., B.W. TURNBULL, et al. 1996. Effects of selenium supplementation for cancer prevention in patients with carcinoma of the skin: a randomized controlled trial. Nutritional Prevention of Cancer Study Group. J. Am. Med. Assoc. **276:** 1957–1963.
5. KLEIN, E.A. 2004. Selenium: epidemiology and basic science. J. Urol. **171:** S50–S53.
6. DONG, Y., H. ZHANG, L. HAWTHORNE, et al. 2003. Delineation of the molecular basis for Se-induced growth arrest in human prostate cancer cells by oligonucleotide array. Cancer Res. **63:** 52–59.
7. ZHAO, H., M.L. WHITFIELD, T. XU, et al. 2003. Diverse effects of methylseleninic acid on the transcriptional program of human prostate cancer cells. Mol. Biol. Cell. [Nov. 14 Epub, ahead of print.]
8. ZU, K & C. IP. 2003. Synergy between selenium and vitamin E in apoptosis induction is associated with activation of distinctive initiator caspases in human prostate cancer cells. Cancer Res. **63:** 6988–6995.
9. WATERS, D.J., S. SHEN, D.M. COOLEY, et al. 2003. Effects of dietary Se supplementation on DNA damage and apoptosis in canine prostate. J. Natl. Cancer Inst. **95:** 237–241.
10. GIANDUZZO, T.R., E.G. HOLMES, U. TINGGI, et al. 2003. Prostatic and peripheral blood selenium levels after oral supplementation. J. Urol. **170:** 870–873.
11. YOSHIZAWA, K., W.C. WILLETT, S.J. MORRIS, et al. 1998. Study of prediagnostic selenium level in toenails and the risk of advanced prostate cancer. J. Natl. Cancer Inst. **90:** 1219–1224.
12. LI, J.Y., P.R. TAYLOR, B. LI, et al. 1993. Nutrition intervention trials in Linxian, China: multiple vitamin/mineral supplementation, cancer incidence, and disease-specific mortality among adults with esophageal dysplasia. J. Natl. Cancer Inst. **85:** 1492–1498.
13. DUFFIELD-LILLICO, A.J., B.L. DALKIN, M.E. REID, et al. 2003. Se supplementation, baseline plasma Se status, and incidence of prostate cancer: an analysis of the complete treatment period of the Nutritional Prevention of Cancer Study Group. Br. J. Urol. Intl. **91:** 608–612.

14. BURTON, G.W. & K.U. INGOLD. 1981. Autoxidation of biological molecules. 1. The antioxidant activity of vitamin E and related chain-breaking phenolic antioxidants in vitro. J. Am. Chem. Soc. **103**: 6472.
15. MACHLIN, L.J. 1991. Vitamin E. In Handbook of Vitamins. 2nd edit. L.J. Machlin, Ed. :67–83. Marcel Dekker. New York, NY.
16. PAPPAS, A.M. 1998. Vitamin E: Tocopherols and Tocotrienols. In Antioxidant Status, Diet, Nutrition, and Health. A.M. Pappas, Ed. :460–478. CRC Press. Boca Raton, FL.
17. AZZI, A., D. BOSCOBOINIK, D. MARILLEY, et al. 1995. Vitamin E: a sensor and an information transducer of the cell oxidation state. Am. J. Clin. Nutr. **62**: 1337s–1346s.
18. MAHONEY, C.W. & A. AZZI. 1988. Vitamin E inhibits protein kinase C activity. Biochem. Biophys. Res. Commun. **154**: 694–697.
19. CHATELAIN, E., D.O. BOSCOBOINIK, G.M. BARTOLI, et al. 1993. Inhibition of smooth muscle cell proliferation and protein kinase C activity by tocopherols and tocotrienols. Biochim. Biophys. Acta **1176**: 83–89.
20. OTTINO, P. & J.R. DUNCAN. 1997. Effect of alpha-tocopherol succinate on free radical and lipid peroxidation levels in BL6 melanoma cells. Free Radic. Biol. Med. **22**: 1145–1151.
21. NI, J., M. CHEN, Y. ZHANG, et al. 2003. Vitamin E succinate inhibits human prostate cancer cell growth via modulating cell cycle regulatory machinery. Biochem. Biophys. Res. Commun. **300**: 357–363.
22. THOMPSON, T.A. & G. WILDING. 2003. Androgen antagonist activity by the antioxidant moiety of vitamin E, 2,2,5,7,8-pentamethyl-6-chromanol in human prostate carcinoma cells. Mol. Cancer Ther. **2**: 797–803.
23. DOLL, R. & R. PETO. 1981. The causes of cancer: quantitative estimates of avoidable risks of cancer in the United States. J. Natl. Cancer Inst. **66**: 1192–1308.
24. COMSTOCK, G.W., K.J. HELZLSOUER & T.L. BUSH. 1991. Prediagnostic serum levels of carotenoids and vitamin E as related to subsequent cancer in Washington County, Maryland. Am. J. Clin. Nutr. **53**: 260S–264S.
25. KNEKT, P., A. AROMAA, J. MAATALA, et al. 1988. Serum vitamin E and risk of cancer among Finnish men during a 10-year follow-up. Am. J. Epidemiol. **127**: 28–41.
26. HSING, A.W., G.W. COMSTOCK, H. ABBEY & B.F. POLK. 1990. Serologic precursors of cancer: retinol, carotenoids, and tocopherol and risk of prostate cancer. J. Natl. Cancer Inst. **82**: 941–946.
27. ATBC CANCER PREVENTION STUDY GROUP. 1994. The effect of vitamin E and beta carotene on the incidence of lung cancer and other cancers in male smokers. N. Engl. J. Med. **330**: 1029–1035.
28. VIRTAMO, J., P. PIETINEN, J.K. HUTTUNEN, et al. 2003. ATBC Study Group: incidence of cancer and mortality following alpha-tocopherol and beta-carotene supplementation: a postintervention follow-up. J. Am. Med. Assoc. **290**: 476–485.
29. GOODMAN, G.E., S. SCHAFFER, G.S. OMENN, et al. 2003. The association between lung and prostate cancer risk, and serum micronutrients: results and lessons learned from beta-carotene and retinol efficacy trial. Cancer Epidemiol. Biomarkers Prev. **12**: 518–526.
30. HUANG, H.Y., A.J. ALBERG, E.P. NORKUS, et al. 2003. Prospective study of antioxidant micronutrients in the blood and the risk of developing prostate cancer. Am. J. Epidemiol. **157**: 335–344.
31. KLEIN, E.A., I.M. THOMPSON, S.M. LIPPMAN, et al. 2003. The Selenium and Vitamin E Cancer Prevention Trial. World J. Urol. **21**: 21–27.
32. YUSUF, S., P. SLEIGHT, J. POGUE, et al. 2000. Effects of an angiotensin-converting-enzyme inhibitor, ramipril, on cardiovascular events in high-risk patients. The Heart Outcomes Prevention Evaluation Study. N. Engl. J. Med. **342**: 145–153.

Vitamin E in Preeclampsia

LUCILLA POSTON,[a] MAARTEN RAIJMAKERS,[a] AND FRANK KELLY[b]

[a]*Maternal and Fetal Research Unit, Division of Reproductive Health, Endocrinology and Development, King's College Hospital, St. Thomas' Hospital, London SE1 7EH, United Kingdom*

[b]*School of Health and Life Sciences, King's College, London SE1 9NN, United Kingdom*

> ABSTRACT: Preeclampsia is the disorder of pregnancy with the highest rate of both maternal and neonatal morbidity and mortality. The maternal syndrome is characterized by oxidative stress and activation of the vascular endothelium that may originate from placental release of lipid peroxidation products, cytokines, and microparticles leading to an acute inflammatory response. The current understanding of the etiology has allowed the improvement of predictive tests, tests that could make intervention possible from early pregnancy onwards. Although the large secondary intervention antioxidant trials in cardiovascular diseases did not show any beneficial effect of vitamin E and vitamin C, either alone or in combination, knowledge of the nature of the pathogenesis of preeclampsia offers hope for the beneficial use of antioxidants in the prevention of the disorder. Not only has our previous small trial shown that antioxidant prophylactics in high-risk women lowered the prevalence of preeclampsia, but also new evidence has demonstrated multiple other actions of α-tocopherol (such as anti-inflammation and inhibition of NAD(P)H oxidase activation) besides its antioxidant properties that could be advantageous in the prevention of the disorder. Several larger trials are under way to investigate the precise role that vitamins C and E can play in the prevention of preeclampsia.
>
> KEYWORDS: vitamin E; vitamin C; preeclampsia

Preeclampsia, a common and potentially serious complication of pregnancy, is responsible for the highest figures for maternal and fetal morbidity and mortality of all pregnancy complications. The World Health Organization has estimated that 0.4–2.8% of all pregnancies in developed countries are affected by this disorder, a figure that may rise to as much as 6.7% in developing countries. In total, as many as 8,370,000 cases worldwide occur every year.[1] The simple clinical definition [gestational hypertension (>90 mmHg diastolic) occurring after the 20th week of gestation with superimposed proteinuria (>300 mg/day)][2] belies the complexity of preeclampsia, which is often accompanied by multi-organ dysfunction. Maternal vascular endothelial activation and dysfunction is widely accepted as the common underlying

---

Address for correspondence: Professor Lucilla Poston, MFRU, Division of Reproductive Health, Endocrinology and Development, St.Thomas' Hospital, 10th Floor, North Wing, Lambeth Palace Road, London SE1 7EH, United Kingdom. Voice: (44) 207 188 3644; fax: (44) 207 620 1227.

lucilla.poston@kcl.ac.uk

defect.[3] In the cerebral circulation, this may lead to fits (that is, eclampsia) or stroke; in the liver, to intense vasoconstriction and hepatic necrosis; and in the lung, to development of pulmonary edema. In the kidney, glomerular endotheliosis, a lesion peculiar to preeclampsia, may obliterate the glomerular capillary lumen and lead to renal dysfunction and to proteinuria. Preeclampsia is considered to be a syndrome or constellation of pathologies, because involvement of the different vascular beds is highly variable from case to case. In developed countries, the greater part of antenatal care focuses upon early detection of preeclampsia (measurement of blood pressure and detection of proteinuria), and when diagnosis is made, the only cure is delivery. Because preeclampsia may occur at any time from the late second trimester onwards, it is one of the primary causes of pre-term delivery, accounting for as many as 25% of all early births.[1]

The last decade has witnessed acceleration in our understanding of the etiology of preeclampsia. In the current theory, oxidative stress plays a central role. The most crucial event during placental development is establishment of an effective maternal circulation, a process that requires conversion of the spiral arteries from highly tortuous and thick-walled vessels to flaccid conduits of low resistance.[4] Failure or only partial spiral artery conversion, as demonstrated by histological investigation of the placental bed post delivery, is evident in the placentas of many women with preeclampsia[5] and results in reduced placental blood flow and abnormally high uteroplacental resistance, which may be assessed by Doppler ultrasound of the uterine artery. Constriction and relaxation of the muscular walled spiral arteries or clot formation and dissolution may lead to ischemia/reperfusion insults and subsequent superoxide generation by the xanthine/xanthine oxidase pathway. The enzymes involved show increased expression in affected placentas.[6] Evidence for this pathogenic pathway was recently provided by Hung and colleagues,[7] who demonstrated that an *in vitro* ischemia/reperfusion stimulus enhanced nitrotyrosine staining in placental tissue and that this was prevented by addition of a free radical scavenger. Recent studies also implicate NAD(P)H oxidase as a source of superoxide. NAD(P)H oxidase activity is considerably enhanced in preeclamptic placentas,[8] which may arise from activation by a preeclampsia-specific angiotensin II receptor activating antibody.[9,10] Increased superoxide generation by these processes is held responsible for the frequently reported oxidative damage in placental trophoblast as shown by enhanced lipid peroxidation, nitrotyrosine staining, and protein carbonyl formation.[11–16]

Several different theories are proposed for transfer of the "preeclampsia signal" from the compromised placenta to the mother, all of which could be related to placental oxidative stress. These include deportation of placental apoptotic microparticles, lipid peroxides, placental cytokines, and activation of maternal leukocytes as the maternal blood perfuses the affected placenta.[17] Singly or together, these lead to the activation of the maternal vascular endothelium and circulating neutrophils, such that that the maternal disorder has all the hallmarks of an acute inflammatory state. While normal pregnancy is associated with a mild inflammatory response, in preeclampsia this seems to be exacerbated,[3] with enhanced neutrophil activation and an increased Th1:Th2 ratio.[18] There is extensive evidence that neutrophils isolated from women with preeclampsia synthesize more superoxide upon activation than those of normotensive pregnant women.[19–21] This appears to be mediated by NAD(P)H oxidase.[22] Increased superoxide generation not only leads to a vicious circle of endothelial cell and neutrophil activation, but results also in generalized oxidative stress, a hallmark of the disease. Indeed, several studies have reported elevation of makers of lipid peroxidation in the maternal circulation.[23]

ROLE OF ANTIOXIDANTS AND VITAMIN E IN PREECLAMPSIA

Numerous studies have investigated antioxidant capacity in the placenta or the maternal circulation in preeclampsia through investigation of total antioxidant capacity, the concentration of specific antioxidants, or the activity of antioxidant enzymes. The consensus opinion arising from these various studies suggests that antioxidant capacity is decreased in women with preeclampsia.[23] The investigations of antioxidant capacity in the maternal circulation have mainly been focused on the most important soluble antioxidants and have consistently reported a reduction in cellular and plasma glutathione concentrations[24,25] and in plasma concentrations of vitamin C.[26–29] In contrast, the findings on vitamin E are ambiguous, and reported concentrations vary widely amongst the different studies,[23] which may be explained by the fact that measurement of plasma vitamin E is a far from satisfactory estimate of the focal site of vitamin E activity, namely the cell membrane. Although elevation of total cholesterol and triglycerides is a characteristic of preeclampsia,[30] concentrations of lipid-soluble vitamin E have not always been adjusted for plasma cholesterol and triglyceride concentrations.[31,32] We and others have reported a modest increase in plasma vitamin E concentrations with gestation,[29] reflecting the pregnancy-related increase in plasma lipoproteins. It is striking, however, that in the reports describing either lowered or elevated levels of vitamin E in preeclamptic plasma, diversion from normal values correlated with severity of disease, with the largest difference from values in normotensive control women being found in women with more severe preeclampsia.[26,27,33,34] To our knowledge, there is no study in which red cell vitamin E concentrations have been estimated or indeed those in any other tissue in women with preeclampsia.

The substantive evidence for oxidative stress in preeclampsia has prompted the suggestion that antioxidant prophylaxis may have therapeutic benefit in the treatment of preeclampsia. Two early studies in which vitamin E was given either alone (100–300 mg/day)[35] or in association with vitamin C and allopurinol (800 IU/day, 1000 mg/day, and 200 mg/day, respectively)[36] showed no benefit in women with established preeclampsia. In the latter study, however, there was a trend for a reduction in plasma concentrations of uric acid, a biomarker of disease severity, probably caused by the inhibition of xanthine oxidase by allopurinol. We carried out a small, randomized trial[37] in which we combined 400 IU/day vitamin E (RRR-α-tocopherol) with 1000 mg/day vitamin C prompted by the reported synergy between these two antioxidants.[38] Women at known risk of preeclampsia, either on the basis of previous preeclampsia or because of a high resistance profile of the uterine artery Doppler waveform, entered the study at 16–22 weeks' gestation and took the antioxidant cocktail (or placebo) until delivery. The primary outcome measure of the study was endothelial cell activation, measured as the plasminogen activator inhibitor-1 and -2 (PAI-1/PAI-2) ratio, and the secondary outcome was the frequency of preeclampsia. The trial was stopped early, because interim analysis showed a highly significant difference between placebo and treatment groups for the primary outcome.

This was associated with a significant reduction in the number of cases of preeclampsia in the treatment vs. placebo group (8% vs. 26%, $P < 0.02$). We also reported that reduced plasma vitamin C concentrations compared to those of low-risk controls antedated the development of the disease. Moreover, antioxidant treatment resulted in a return to normal of vitamin C values, similar to those of low-risk controls, and reduced the abnormally raised plasma markers for oxidative damage (e.g., 8-epiprostaglandin $F_{2\alpha}$) and placental function (e.g., leptin).[39] As a result of this study, much larger trials using the same antioxidant regimen are under way in several other countries.

The use of α-tocopherol and vitamin C, either alone or in combination, in several clinical studies of cardiovascular disease, have shown ambiguous clinical outcomes. Although supplementation enhanced plasma vitamin status, meta-analysis failed to show a beneficial effect of the use of vitamin C and/or vitamin E in the amelioration of preexisting cardiovascular disease.[40,41] The largest secondary prevention study to date consists of 20,536 subjects with preexisting cardiovascular disease or diabetes that were randomized to antioxidants (600 mg vitamin E, 250 mg vitamin C, and 20 mg β-carotene daily) or matching placebo. Treatment for more than 5 years did not show an improvement in outcome in the vitamin group.[42] In the Women's Angiographic Vitamin and Estrogen (WAVE) trial, postmenopausal women with coronary disease who received two daily doses of 500 mg of vitamin C and 400 IU of vitamin E also showed no improvement in outcome compared to the placebo group; in fact treatment suggested a potential harm.[43] These studies contrast with the Antioxidant Supplementation in Arteriscleroses Prevention (ASAP) study, which documented a reduction in progression of arteriscleroses in subjects who received a combination of 250 mg slow release vitamin C and 136 IU vitamin E twice daily with a meal in a randomized trial of 520 subjects studied over a period of 6 years.[44] Moreover, it was shown that subjects who had low baseline plasma vitamin C concentrations benefited most from antioxidant supplementation.

Although these large secondary intervention trials in subjects with established cardiovascular disease have not provided convincing evidence in favor of vitamin supplementation, this does not rule out the possibility that primary antioxidant intervention may be effective in disorders that are more acute. For instance, small, randomized trials in heart transplant recipients have shown a reduction of transplant-associated arteriosclerosis in patient who received a combination of vitamin C and vitamin E.[45,46] Furthermore, one report has suggested that a combination of vitamin C and vitamin E may be effective in improving endothelial function as demonstrated in hyperlipidemic children taking part in the Endothelial Assessment of Risk from Lipids in Youth (EARLY) study.[47] These studies suggest that in the early pathogenic stages of cardiovascular diseases, the damaging effect of oxidative stress on endothelial dysfunction is reversible by antioxidants.

Although controversies of vitamin E and vitamin C prophylaxis are apparent in secondary intervention of cardiovascular diseases, antioxidant prophylaxis from early gestation onwards might be beneficial for the prevention of preeclampsia. Recent investigations have shown encouraging evidence in favor of the beneficial effect of vitamin E and vitamin C in the prevention of preeclampsia.[37,48,49] Two recent *in vitro* studies, of particular relevance to work from our unit, have been performed in placental tissue. Perfusion of preeclamptic placental tissue with 500 μM vitamin C returned elevated lipid peroxidation potential to values found in placental tissue of control women,[49] whereas another study demonstrated that vitamin C and vitamin E either alone or in combination achieved complete inhibition of lipid peroxidation in human placental mitochondria.[48] More important, this effect was much more pronounced when a combination of vitamins C and E was used, compared to the influence of each antioxidant alone.

In addition, the non-antioxidant properties of α-tocopherol have also become more widely appreciated. For example, it has been discovered that α-tocopherol may reduce inflammatory mediators, lower the expression of cell adhesion molecules, and increase peroxisome proliferator–activated receptor-γ (PPAR-γ) expression.[50,51] These properties are all highly relevant to women with preeclampsia in whom concentrations of several cytokines (such as IL-6 and TNFα)[3] and several soluble cell adhesion molecules are raised (such as sICAM-1 and sVCAM-1)[52] and in whom PPAR-γ is reduced.[53] The reported anti-apoptotic properties of α-tocopherol are also of interest in view of the suggestion that deportation of trophoblast in preeclampsia may occur as a result of activation of apoptotic pathways.[7] The report that α-tocopherol can prevent PKC activation and the translocation of the p47phox subunit of NAD(P)H oxidase to the plasma membrane, thereby preventing activation of the enzyme,[54] is pertinent to the recent recognition of the role this enzyme plays in superoxide generation in the preeclamptic placenta.[17] It will be of considerable interest to determine in the clinical trials under way whether biomarkers of inflammation as well as those of oxidative stress are reversed by the antioxidants. Two *in vitro* studies have already suggested that α-tocopherol can reverse inflammatory processes (activation of NFκB, ICAM-1, and IL-6) induced by incubation of preeclamptic plasma with cultured human umbilical venous endothelial cells.[55,56]

SUMMARY

Preeclampsia, a state of oxidative stress intimately associated with an inflammatory response, offers considerable potential for intervention with α-tocopherol. None of the trials in progress have a factorial design that would assess the potential value of vitamin E alone. Nonetheless, the studies will determine whether supplementation of vitamin E and vitamin C together may have a role to play in the prevention of preeclampsia.

REFERENCES

1. VILLAR, K. *et al.* 2003. Eclampsia and pre-eclampsia: a health problem for 2000 years. *In* Pre-eclampsia. H. Critchley, A.B. MacLean, L. Poston & J.J. Walker, Eds.: 189–207. RCOG Press. London.
2. BROWN, M.A. *et al.* 2001. The classification and diagnosis of the hypertensive disorders of pregnancy: statement from the International Society for the Study of Hypertension in Pregnancy (ISSHP). Hypertens. Pregnancy **20**: IX–XIV.
3. REDMAN, C.W.G. & I.L. SARGENT. 2003. Pre-eclampsia, the placenta and the maternal systemic inflammatory response: a review. Placenta **24**(Suppl. A): S21–S27.
4. PIJNENBORG, R. *et al.* 1983. Uteroplacental arterial changes related to interstitial trophoblast migration in early human pregnancy. Placenta **4**: 397–414.
5. PIJNENBORG, R. *et al.* 1991. Placental bed spiral arteries in the hypertensive disorders of pregnancy. Br. J. Obstet. Gynaecol. **98**: 648–655.

6. MANY, A. *et al.* 2000. Invasive cytotrophoblasts manifest evidence of oxidative stress in preeclampsia. Am. J. Pathol. **156:** 321–331.
7. HUNG, T.H. *et al.* 2002. Hypoxia-reoxygenation: a potent inducer of apoptotic changes in the human placenta and possible etiological factor in preeclampsia. Circ. Res. **90:** 1274–1281.
8. DECHEND, R. *et al.* 2003. AT1 receptor agonistic antibodies from preeclamptic patients stimulate NADPH oxidase. Circulation **107:** 1632–1639.
9. WALLUKAT, G. *et al.* 1999. Patients with preeclampsia develop agonistic autoantibodies against the angiotensin AT1 receptor. J. Clin. Invest. **103:** 945–952.
10. XIA, Y. *et al.* 2003. Maternal autoantibodies from preeclamptic patients activate angiotensin receptors on human trophoblast cells. J. Soc. Gynecol. Investig. **10:** 82–93.
11. GÜLMEZOGLU, A.M. *et al.* 1996. Placental malondialdehyde and glutathione levels in a controlled trial of antioxidant treatment in severe preeclampsia. Hypertens. Pregnancy **15:** 287–295.
12. MYATT, L. *et al.* 1996. Nitrotyrosine residues in placenta: evidence of peroxynitrite formation and action. Hypertension **28:** 488–493.
13. PORANEN, A.-K. *et al.* 1996. Lipid peroxidation and antioxidants in normal and preeclamptic pregnancies. Placenta **17:** 401–405.
14. GRATACOS, E. *et al.* 1998. Lipid peroxide and vitamin E patterns in pregnant women with different types of hypertension in pregnancy. Am. J. Obstet. Gynecol. **178:** 1072–1076.
15. WALSH, S.W. *et al.* 2000. Placental isoprostane is significantly increased in preeclampsia. FASEB J. **14:** 1289–1296.
16. ZUSTERZEEL, P.L.M. *et al.* 2001. Protein carbonyls in decidua and placenta of preeclamptic women as markers for oxidative stress. Placenta **22:** 213–219.
17. POSTON, L. & M.T.M. RAIJMAKERS. 2004. Trophoblast oxidative stress, antioxidants and pregnancy outcome. Placenta **S25:** S72–S78.
18. SAITO, S. *et al.* 1999. Quantitative analysis of peripheral blood Th0, Th1, Th2 and the Th1:Th2 cell ratio during normal human pregnancy and preeclampsia. Clin. Exp. Immunol. **117:** 550–555.
19. TSUKIMORI, K. *et al.* 1993. The superoxide generation of neutrophils in normal and preeclamptic pregnancies. Obstet. Gynecol. **81:** 536–540.
20. CROCKER, I.P. *et al.* 1999. Neutrophil function in women with pre-eclampsia. Br. J. Obstet. Gynaecol. **106:** 822–828.
21. LEE, V.M. *et al.* 2003. Neutrophil activation and production of reactive oxygen species in pre-eclampsia. J. Hypertens. **21:** 395–402.
22. LEE, V.M. *et al.* 2003. NADPH oxidase activity in preeclampsia with immortalized lymphoblasts used as models. Hypertension **41:** 925–931.
23. RAIJMAKERS, M.T.M. *et al.* 2004. Amino thiols, detoxficiation and oxidative stress in pre-eclampsia and other disorders of pregnancy. Curr. Pharm. Des.: in press.
24. KNAPEN, M.F.C.M. *et al.* 1998. Low whole blood glutathione levels in preganancies complicated by preeclampsia or the hemolysis, elevated liver enzymes, low platelets syndrome. Obstet. Gyn. **92:** 1012–1015.
25. KHARB, S. 2000. Low whole blood glutathione levels in pregnancies complicated by preeclampsia and diabetes. Clin. Chim. Acta **294:** 179–183.
26. MIKHAIL, M.S. *et al.* 1994. Preeclampsia and antioxidant nutrients: decreased plasma levels of reduced ascorbic acid, alpha-tocopherol, and beta-carotene in women with preeclampsia. Am. J. Obstet. Gynecol. **171:** 150–157.
27. SAGOL, S. *et al.* 1999. Impaired antioxidant activity in women with pre-eclampsia. Int. J. Gynaecol. Obstet. **64:** 121–127.
28. KHARB, S. 2000. Vitamins E and C in preeclampsia. Eur. J. Obstet. Gynecol. Reprod. Biol. **93:** 37–39.
29. CHAPPELL, L.C. *et al.* 2002. A longitudinal study of biochemical variables in women at risk of preeclampsia. Am. J. Obstet. Gynecol. **187:** 127–136.
30. SATTAR, N. *et al.* 2000. Lipoprotein (a) levels in normal pregnancy and in pregnancy complicated with pre-eclampsia. Atherosclerosis **148:** 407–411.
31. SCHIFF, E. *et al.* 1996. Dietary consumption and plasma concentrations of vitamin E in pregnancies complicated by preeclampsia. Am. J. Obstet. Gynecol. **175:** 1024–1028.

32. ZUSTERZEEL, P.L.M. *et al.* 2002. Ethene and other biomarkers of oxidative stress in hypertensive disorders of pregnancy. Hypertens. Pregnancy **21:** 39–49.
33. UOTILA, J.T. *et al.* 1993. Findings on lipid peroxidation and antioxidant function in hypertensive complications of pregnancy Br. J. Obstet. Gynaecol. **100:** 270–276.
34. MADAZLI, R. *et al.* 1999. Lipid peroxidation and antioxidants in preeclampsia. Eur. J. Obstet. Gynecol. Reprod. Biol. **85:** 205–208.
35. STRATTA, P. *et al.* 1994. Vitamin E supplementation in preeclampsia. Gynecol. Obstet. Invest. **37:** 246–249.
36. GÜLMEZOGLU, A.M. *et al.* 1997. Antioxidants in the treatment of severe pre-eclampsia: an explanatory randomised controlled trial. Br. J. Obstet. Gynaecol. **104:** 689–696.
37. CHAPPELL, L.C. *et al.* 1999. Effect of antioxidants on the occurrence of pre-eclampsia in women at increased risk: a randomised trial. Lancet **345:** 810–816.
38. CHAN, A.C. 1993. Partners in defense, vitamin E and vitamin C. Can. J. Physiol. Pharmacol. **71:** 725–731.
39. CHAPPELL, L.C. *et al.* 2002. Vitamin C and E supplementation in women at risk of preeclampsia is associated with changes in indices of oxidative stress and placental function. Am. J. Obstet. Gynecol. **187:** 777–784.
40. ASPLUND, K. 2002. Antioxidant vitamins in the prevention of cardiovascular disease: a systematic review. J. Intern. Med. **251:** 372–392.
41. STANNER, S.A. *et al.* 2004. A review of the epidemiological evidence for the "antioxidant hypothesis." Public Health Nutr. **7:** 407–422.
42. HEART PROTECTION STUDY COLLABORATIVE GROUP. 2002. MRC/BHF Heart Protection Study of antioxidant vitamin supplementation in 20,536 high-risk individuals: a randomised placebo-controlled trial. Lancet **360:** 23–33.
43. WATERS, D.D. *et al.* 2002. Effects of hormone replacement therapy and antioxidant vitamin supplements on coronary atherosclerosis in postmenopausal women: a randomized controlled trial. J. Am. Med. Assoc. **288:** 2432–2440.
44. SALONEN, R.M. *et al.* 2003. Six-year effect of combined vitamin C and E supplementation on atherosclerotic progression: the Antioxidant Supplementation in Atherosclerosis Prevention (ASAP) Study. Circulation **107:** 947–953.
45. FANG, J.C. *et al.* 2002. Effect of vitamins C and E on progression of transplant-associated arteriosclerosis: a randomised trial. Lancet **359:** 1108–1113.
46. LIU, L. & M. MEYDANI. 2002. Combined vitamin C and E supplementation retards early progression of arteriosclerosis in heart transplant patients. Nutr. Rev. **60:** 368–371.
47. ENGLER, M.M. *et al.* 2003. Antioxidant vitamins C and E improve endothelial function in children with hyperlipidemia: Endothelial Assessment of Risk from Lipids in Youth (EARLY) Trial. Circulation **108:** 1059–1063.
48. MILCZAREK, R. *et al.* 2000. The effects of ascorbate and alpha-tocopherol on the NADPH-dependent lipid peroxidation in human placental mitochondria. Mol. Cell. Biochem. **210:** 65–73.
49. PORANEN, A.K. *et al.* 1998. The effect of vitamins C and E on placental lipid peroxidation and antioxidative enzymes in perfused placenta. Acta Obstet. Gynecol. Scand. **77:** 372–376.
50. BRIGELIUS-FLOHE, R. *et al.* 2002. The European perspective on vitamin E: current knowledge and future research. Am. J. Clin. Nutr. **76:** 703–716.
51. MUNTEANU, A. *et al.* 2004. Anti-atherosclerotic effects of vitamin E: myth or reality? J. Cell. Mol. Med. **8:** 59–76.
52. AUSTGULEN, R. *et al.* 1997. Increased maternal plasma levels of soluble adhesion molecules (ICAM-1, VCAM-1, E-selectin) in preeclampsia. Eur. J. Obstet. Gynecol. Reprod. Biol. **71:** 53–58.
53. TAYLOR, R.N. *et al.* 1998. Circulating factors as a markers and mediators of endothelial cell dysfunction in preeclampsia. Semin. Reprod. Endocrinol. **16:** 17–31.
54. AZZI, A. *et al.* 2002. Non-antioxidant molecular functions of alpha-tocopherol (vitamin E). FEBS Lett. **519:** 8–10.
55. TAKACS, P. *et al.* 2001. Increased circulating lipid peroxides in severe preeclampsia activate NF-kappaB and upregulate ICAM-1 in vascular endothelial cells. FASEB J. **15:** 279–281.
56. TAKACS, P. *et al.* 2003. Increased vascular endothelial cell production of interleukin-6 in severe preeclampsia. Am. J. Obstet. Gynecol. **188:** 740–744.

Vitamin E in Neurodegenerative Disorders
Alzheimer's Disease

ANATOL KONTUSH[a] AND SVETLANA SCHEKATOLINA[b]

[a]*Dyslipoproteinemia and Atherosclerosis Research Unit (Unité 551), National Institute for Health and Medical Research (INSERM), Hôpital de la Pitié, Paris, France*

[b]*State Academy of Refrigeration, Odessa, Ukraine*

ABSTRACT: Oxidative stress is important in the pathogenesis of Alzheimer's disease (AD). The brain contains high levels of oxidizable lipids that must be protected by antioxidants. Low concentrations of vitamin E, quantitatively the major lipophilic antioxidant in the brain, are frequently observed in cerebrospinal fluid (CSF) of AD patients, suggesting that supplementation with vitamin E might delay the development of AD. In a placebo-controlled trial, vitamin E (2000 IU/day, 2 years) slowed (–53%) functional deterioration in patients with moderate AD (Sano *et al.*, N. Engl. J. Med. 336: 1216–1222, 1997). Recently, use of vitamin E and vitamin C supplements in combination was found to be associated with reduced prevalence (–78%) and incidence (–64%) of AD in elderly population (Zandi *et al.*, Arch. Neurol. 61: 82–88, 2004). These results are consistent with the ability of the supplementation with vitamin E (400 IU/day, 1 month) to increase its levels in CSF (+23%) and plasma (+45%) of AD patients and, in combination with vitamin C (1000 g/day), to decrease the susceptibility of CSF lipoproteins (up to –32%) to *in vitro* oxidation (Kontush *et al.*, Free Radic. Biol. Med. 31: 345–354, 2001). In addition, vitamin E reduced lipid peroxidation and amyloid deposition in a transgenic mice model of AD (Sung *et al.*, FASEB J. 18: 323–325, 2004). Computer modeling of the influence of vitamin E on lipoprotein oxidation reveals that the vitamin develops antioxidative activity in CSF lipoproteins in the presence of physiologically relevant, low amounts of oxidants. By contrast, under similar conditions, vitamin E behaves as a pro-oxidant in plasma lipoproteins, consistent with the model of tocopherol-mediated peroxidation (Stocker, Curr. Opin. Lipidol. 5: 422–433, 1994). This distinction is related to major differences in the levels of vitamin E (50 nM vs. 30 μM) and oxidizable lipids (4 μM vs. 2.5 mM) between CSF and plasma, which result in major differences in oxidative conditions (per unit of vitamin E) between CSF and plasma in the presence of similar amounts of oxidants. Altogether, these data suggest that vitamin E may be effective against *in vivo* oxidation of CSF lipoproteins and brain lipids, and offer new perspectives in the treatment of AD and other neurodegenerative disorders.

KEYWORDS: vitamin E; α-tocopherol; Alzheimer's disease; oxidative stress; amyloid-β; lipoproteins; cerebrospinal fluid; brain; transition metals; free radicals; computer modeling

Address for correspondence: Dr. Anatol Kontush, INSERM Unité 551, Pavillon Benjamin Delessert, Hôpital de la Pitié, 83 boulevard de l'Hôpital, 75651 Paris Cedex 13, France. Voice: 33-1-42177976; fax: 33-1-45828198.
kontush@chups.jussieu.fr

OXIDATIVE STRESS IN THE BRAIN PLAYS AN IMPORTANT ROLE IN THE PATHOGENESIS OF ALZHEIMER'S DISEASE

Several lines of evidence suggest that oxidative stress is an important event in the pathogenesis of Alzheimer's disease (AD).[1–3] The brain contains high levels of unsaturated lipids and accounts for 20–25% of the total body oxygen consumption, but for less than 2% of the total body weight. Such conditions favor oxidative damage to lipids and other biomolecules that must be adequately protected by antioxidants; there is ample evidence that such protection is impaired in AD.

Early studies documented elevated levels of products of lipid peroxidation, including thiobarbituric acid-reactive substances and 4-hydroxy-2-nonenal, in brain tissues of AD patients as compared to controls (reviewed in Arlt *et al.*[3]). These studies are supported by more recent publications that observe increased levels of F2-isoprostanes, stable products of non-enzymatic oxidation of arachidonic acid, and robust markers of oxidative stress *in vivo*, in brains of AD patients.[4] Interestingly, differences in F2-isoprostanes are highest in the temporal and frontal cortex, brain regions that are particularly affected in AD. Acrolein, another endproduct of lipid peroxidation, is also increased in AD brains.[5] Equally, other biomolecules, such as proteins and DNA, are oxidatively damaged in AD brains.[6] In addition, antioxidant enzymes are frequently elevated in brain tissues of AD patients, probably in response to elevated oxidative stress.[7] Moreover, accumulation of amyloid-β peptide, which in an aggregated form builds amyloid plaques, a pathological hallmark of AD, and in a monomeric form possesses properties of a potent meta-chelating antioxidant,[8,9] can be regarded as a protective response to elevated oxidative stress in aging.[10,11] Paradoxically, amyloid-β which is aggregated by transition metals initiates production of reactive oxygen species, behaves as a pro-oxidant, and may represent an important source of oxidative stress in AD brain.[2,10]

LEVELS OF VITAMIN E ARE FREQUENTLY DECREASED IN ALZHEIMER'S DISEASE

Vitamin E is quantitatively the major lipophilic antioxidant in the brain. It is thought that the major function of vitamin E is to protect lipids against oxidative stress. Elevated oxidative stress can theoretically result in accelerated consumption of vitamin E in AD brain, a process that should result in decreased levels of the vitamin in the brain and/or cerebrospinal fluid (CSF); several studies have attempted to assess this hypothesis.

Low concentrations of vitamin E have been observed in CSF of AD patients (TABLE 1). Tohgi and colleagues reported a significant 46% decrease in α-tocopherol levels in CSF of AD patients.[12] Jimenez-Jimenez and colleagues found a less pronounced 18% decrease,[13] whereas Schippling and colleagues observed a non-significant trend to reduced levels of α-tocopherol (−28%) in AD CSF.[14] Increased susceptibility of CSF to *in vitro* oxidation[14] and elevated CSF markers of *in vivo* lipid peroxidation (F2-isoprostanes)[15,16] paralleled the decreases in vitamin E levels in AD patients, suggesting a role of oxidative stress in the vitamin E depletion. Reactive oxygen and nitrogen species may account for the oxidation of vitamin E in AD brain, as suggested by a significant increase in the lipid nitration product 5-nitro-

TABLE 1. Levels of vitamin E in Alzheimer's disease

Fluid or Tissue	Levels of Vitamin E as Compared to Controls	References
CSF	Decreased (3 studies)	12–14
	Unchanged (1 study)	18
Serum or plasma	Decreased (10 studies)	13,16,23–30
	Unchanged (7 studies)	14,18,31–35
Brain cortex	Unchanged (1 study)	22

γ-tocopherol in affected regions of AD brain.[17] The only study that did not observe decreased levels of α-tocopherol in AD CSF was that of Quinn and colleagues.[18] However, most participants of this study took vitamin E supplements at doses ranging from 400 to 2,000 IU/day. These supplements should have potently influenced vitamin E levels (cf. Lonnrot et al.[19] and Kontush et al.[20]).

Consistent with these data, vitamin E concentrations were lowered (–66%) in brains of demented dogs as compared to age-matched, non-demented control animals.[21] By contrast, no difference in brain levels of vitamin E was found between AD patients and age-matched control subjects in an early study.[22]

The concept of local oxidative stress in AD brain implies that levels of vitamin E in plasma or serum should be affected by the disease to a lesser extent. Indeed, only 10 of 17 published studies found decreased levels of vitamin E in the circulation of AD patients as compared to controls,[13,16,23–30] whereas the other 7 studies reported no difference[14,18,31–35] (TABLE 1). Such conflicting results suggest that vitamin E should be measured in CSF, rather than in plasma or serum, in order to reliably assess its deficiency in AD.

SUPPLEMENTATION WITH VITAMIN E IS ABLE TO BENEFICIALLY INFLUENCE THE DEVELOPMENT OF ALZHEIMER'S DISEASE

If vitamin E is deficient in AD, and if it protects against oxidative stress in this disorder, then supplementation with vitamin E might delay the development of AD. This intriguing possibility was addressed in several interventional and prospective studies (TABLE 2).

In the only large interventional trial performed to date, vitamin E (2000 IU/day for 2 years) slowed functional deterioration in patients with moderate AD.[36] This double-blind, placebo-controlled, randomized, multi-center trial was conducted in 341 patients who received the selective monoamine oxidase inhibitor selegiline (10 mg/day), racemic α-tocopherol (2000 IU/day), both selegiline and α-tocopherol, or placebo for 2 years. Patients treated with α-tocopherol (risk ratio: 0.47), selegiline (risk ratio: 0.57), or combination therapy (risk ratio: 0.69) revealed significant delays in the time to the primary outcome (death, institutionalization, loss of the ability to perform basic activities of daily living, or severe dementia) as compared to the placebo group.

By contrast, no beneficial effect of vitamin E was found in a small trial conducted in 60 AD patients. Neuropsychological test scores significantly worsened in AD pa-

TABLE 2. Interventional and prospective studies on vitamin E in Alzheimer's disease

Studies and Subjects	Number of Subjects	Follow-up (yr)	Daily Dose	Effect	Comments	Ref.
Interventional studies						
Moderate AD	341	2.0	2000 IU	Beneficial (RR 0.47)		36
Mild to moderate AD	60	0.5	2000 IU	Deleterious[a]		37
Prospective studies						
Elderly subjects, Cache County, Utah, USA	4740	6.0		Beneficial (OR 0.22)	In combination with vitamin C	38
Elderly subjects, WICAP, New York City, USA	980	4.0		No		43
Elderly subjects, Chicago, USA	815	3.9		Beneficial (RR 0.36)	E from foods; apoE4-negative	40
Elderly subjects, Rotterdam, the Netherlands	5395	6.0		Beneficial	Particularly in smokers	41
Elderly Japanese-American men, Hawaii, USA	3385			No		44
Elderly subjects, Chicago, USA	633	4.3		Beneficial		42

ABBREVIATIONS: RR, relative risk; OR, odds ratio; WICAP, Washington Heights-Inwood Columbia Aging Project.
[a] vs. treatment with donepezil.

tients given vitamin E (2000 IU/day for 6 months).[37] The scores improved in patients given the acetylcholine esterase inhibitor donepezil as well as in patients on a combination vitamin E + donepezil therapy.

Six prospective studies performed to date studied the relationship between vitamin E intake and risk of AD in a total of 15,948 elderly subjects (TABLE 2). Beneficial association between vitamin E intake and risk of AD was found in four studies, whereas two studies failed to confirm this conclusion. Most recently, use of vitamin E and vitamin C supplements in combination was found to be associated with reduced prevalence (adjusted odds ratio: 0.22) and incidence (adjusted hazard ratio: 0.36) of AD in 4,740 elderly county residents in Utah.[38] A trend towards lower AD risk was also evident in users of vitamin E and multivitamins containing vitamin C. By contrast, no evidence of a protective effect with use of vitamin E or vitamin C supplements alone, or with multivitamins alone, was obtained. Analyses of prevalent and incident AD yielded similar results. It is highly relevant in this context that vitamin C can serve as a co-antioxidant for vitamin E, regenerating the latter from its oxidized radical form.[39]

The relationship between AD and the intake of vitamin E was equally studied in 815 elderly residents of Chicago (IL, USA) who were free of AD at baseline.[40] Increased vitamin E intake from foods was associated with decreased risk of developing AD; relative risks from lowest to highest quintiles of the intake were 1.00, 0.71, 0.62, 0.71, and 0.30. After adjustment for baseline memory score, the relative risk was 0.36. Unexpectedly, the protective effect of vitamin E was observed only among persons who did not carry the apolipoprotein E4 (apoE4) allele. By contrast, intake of vitamin E from supplements was not significantly associated with risk of AD. Similarly, no protective effect of β-carotene or vitamin C intake was observed.

The Rotterdam Study, a population-based, prospective cohort study conducted in the Netherlands, analyzed the association between intake of antioxidant vitamins and risk of AD in 5,395 elderly participants who were free of AD at baseline.[41] The study found that high intake of vitamin C and vitamin E was associated with low risk of AD; the rate ratio per 1SD increase in intake was 0.82 for either vitamin. Among current smokers, this relationship was most pronounced (the rate ratios were 0.65 and 0.58 for vitamin C and vitamin E intake, respectively), and it was also present for intake of β-carotene and flavonoids.

Another study prospectively examined the relationship between use of vitamin E and vitamin C and incident AD in 633 AD-free elderly persons.[42] After an average follow-up period of 4.3 years, 91 subjects met accepted criteria for the diagnosis of AD. Interestingly, none of 27 vitamin E supplement users developed AD as compared to the 3.9 predicted on the basis of the crude observed incidence among non-users and the 2.5 predicted on the basis of age, sex, years of education, and length of follow-up interval. Similarly, none of 23 vitamin C supplement users developed AD as compared to the 3.3 predicted on the basis of the crude observed incidence among non-users and the 3.2 predicted on the basis of adjustments for age, sex, education, and follow-up interval. There was no relation between AD and use of multivitamins.

The relationship between AD and the intake vitamin E was equally studied in 980 elderly subjects in the Washington Heights-Inwood Columbia Aging Project.[43] No association between the intake of vitamin E in supplemental or dietary form (or in both forms) and AD risk was found. In this study, similar negative results were obtained for the intake of carotenes and vitamin C. Finally, the Honolulu-Asia Aging Study did not reveal any protective effect of either vitamin E or vitamin C supplements on the risk of AD in 3,385 elderly Japanese-American men in Hawaii.[44] By contrast, a significant protective effect of both vitamin E and vitamin C supplements was found for vascular dementia. In addition, use of either vitamin E or vitamin C supplements alone at baseline was associated with better cognitive performance at follow-up in subjects who were free of dementia at baseline.

This brief review of available data shows that vitamin E appears to be able to beneficially influence the development of AD; protective associations between vitamin E intake and risk of AD were documented in several studies. Some studies, however, brought about negative results; therefore, evidence of the efficacy of vitamin E in the treatment of AD remains insufficient. In addition, although supplemental vitamin E appears to be safe at doses up to 2000 IU/day for periods up to 2 years, safety of vitamin E over periods of many years in the treatment of such chronic diseases as AD has not been adequately explored.[45] Large-scale interventional trials on vitamin E in AD are urgently needed to address these critical questions.

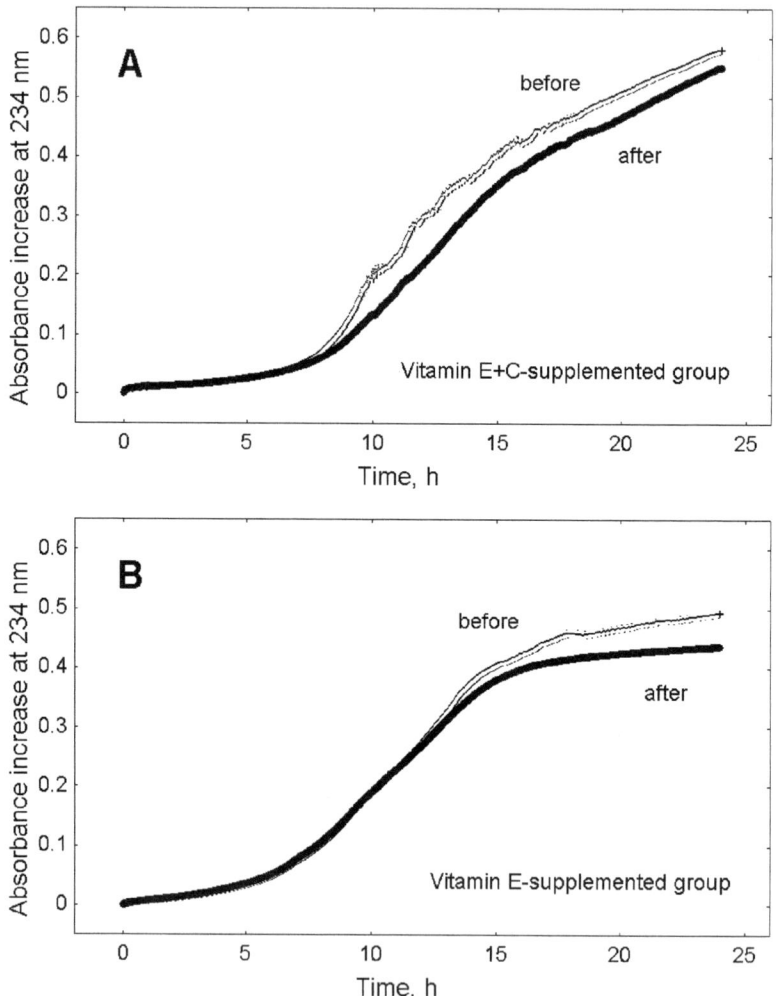

FIGURE 1. Kinetics of CSF oxidation before and after supplementation with vitamin E. (From Kontush *et al.*[20] Reproduced by permission.) Absorbance increases are shown at 234 nm during AAPH-induced oxidation of CSF of AD patients receving supplementation for 1 month with vitamins E and C ($n = 10$; **A**) or vitamin E alone ($n = 10$; **B**). The results for oxidation kinetics were averaged for all 10 subjects in each group. Time points were taken every 5 min. CSF was diluted 10-fold with PBS and incubated at 37°C in the presence of AAPH (100 µM).

SUPPLEMENTATION WITH VITAMIN E INCREASES ITS LEVELS IN CSF AND PLASMA AND BENEFICIALLY INFLUENCES OXIDATIVE STRESS IN AD

Effective supplementation with vitamin E aimed at the prevention and/or treatment of AD implies that the vitamin must reach its target tissue, that is, the brain. Data on the ability of supplemental vitamin E to accumulate in brain tissues in humans, however, are lacking. It appears reasonable to assume that levels of vitamin E in CSF reflect its levels in the brain.

On the basis of this assumption, we studied whether supplementation with vitamin E, alone or in combination with vitamin C, was able to increase its CSF concentration in AD patients.[20] Two groups, each consisting of 10 patients with AD, received daily supplementation for 1 month with either 400 IU vitamin E alone, or a combination of 400 IU vitamin E and 1000 mg vitamin C. The supplementation with vitamin E alone significantly increased its levels in CSF (+23%) and plasma (+45%); significant increases in the vitamin E levels in CSF and plasma were equally observed following combined supplementation with vitamins E and C (+56 and +35%, respectively). In addition, abnormally low concentrations of vitamin C observed in both CSF and plasma of AD patients before the supplementation as compared to controls[14] were returned to normal levels after combined treatment with vitamins E and C.

Importantly, combined supplementation with vitamins E and C significantly decreased the susceptibility of CSF lipoproteins (up to −32%) to *in vitro* oxidation in the presence of physiologically relevant, low amounts of oxidants (autoxidation or oxidation by low concentrations of AAPH; FIG. 1).[20] By contrast, beneficial impact of the supplementation with vitamin E alone on lipoprotein oxidizability was weaker and did not reach significance. These finding are consistent with decreased *in vitro* oxidizability of temporal cortex tissue of an AD patient who took daily vitamin E supplements for 4 years as compared to AD patients who did not take vitamin E.[46]

Lipoproteins are major carriers of amyloid-β and apoE in CSF and participate in the clearance of amyloid-β from the brain[47]; in addition, lipoproteins appear to supply amyloid-β and other components to growing amyloid plaques.[48] CSF lipoproteins are highly susceptible to *in vitro* oxidation[49,50]; oxidized lipoproteins are toxic to neuronal cells[49] and possess altered composition and structure.[50] It is plausible to speculate that oxidation of brain lipoproteins can result in major impairments in the transport and metabolism of amyloid-β, resulting in the accumulation of the peptide in the brain and formation of amyloid plaques. Hence, decreased susceptibility of CSF lipoproteins to oxidation as a result of antioxidant supplementation may have physiological significance, reflecting diminished oxidative stress in the brain.

Consistent with this mechanism, vitamin E reduced both oxidative stress and amyloid deposition in the brain in a transgenic mice model of AD.[51] When young Tg2576 mice (aged 5 months) were given vitamin E, significant reductions in both brain amyloid-β levels and amyloid deposition were observed. By contrast, mice receiving the diet supplemented with vitamin E at a later age (14 months) did not show any significant difference in either marker when compared with placebo. Brain levels of F2-isoprostanes were significantly reduced in both groups of mice receiving vitamin E compared with placebo. These results support the hypothesis that oxidative stress is an important early event in AD pathogenesis that precedes amyloid deposition and can be decreased by antioxidants; thus, antioxidant therapy may be beneficial if given at an early stage of the disease. It is important to mention that antioxidative activity is not the only biological activity of vitamin E that can have a beneficial impact on AD; the vitamin is also able to exert important anti-apoptotic actions via inhibition of protein kinase C.[52]

In summary, these findings suggest that supplementation with vitamin E, particularly in combination with its co-antioxidant vitamin C and at an early stage of the disease, represents a promising strategy to combat elevated oxidative stress in AD and to delay the disease progression.

IS ANTIOXIDATIVE ACTION OF VITAMIN E MORE POTENT IN THE BRAIN THAN IN PLASMA?

Plausible beneficial effect of vitamin E on the development of AD in the brain is in sharp contrast with the lack of such effect on the development of atherosclerosis in the vascular wall observed in large-scale clinical trials.[53] Which biochemical mechanisms can account for this important difference?

Several lines of evidence suggest that the activity of vitamin E towards oxidation of plasma lipoproteins critically depends on oxidative conditions. Vitamin E consistently inhibits oxidation under strong oxidative conditions (that is, at high fluxes of free radicals as compared to the concentration of the vitamin).[54] By contrast, under mild oxidative conditions, vitamin E behaves as a pro-oxidant and accelerates oxidation by a mechanism of tocopherol-mediated peroxidation.[54] The pro-oxidative activity of vitamin E at low concentrations of various oxidants has been widely documented in plasma lipoproteins.[39,54,55]

Interestingly, our studies suggested that vitamin E might function as an antioxidant for CSF lipoproteins under conditions that are normally referred to as mild in the case of the oxidation of plasma lipoproteins (FIG. 1; see the preceding text). This distinction between plasma and CSF lipoproteins can be related to major

TABLE 3. Levels of major antioxidants, pro-oxidants, and oxidizable lipids in human CSF and plasma[10,14,19,20]

Antioxidant	Level in CSF (µM)	Plasma Level (µM)
Lipophilic antioxidants		
α-Tocopherol	0.050	30
Ubiquinol-10	0.005	0.6
Hydrophilic antioxidants		
Ascorbate	200	50
Urate	30	230
Pro-oxidants		
Redox-active copper	<0.1?	<1.0[57]
Redox-active iron	<0.1?	<0.4[58]
Oxidizable lipids	4.0	2500

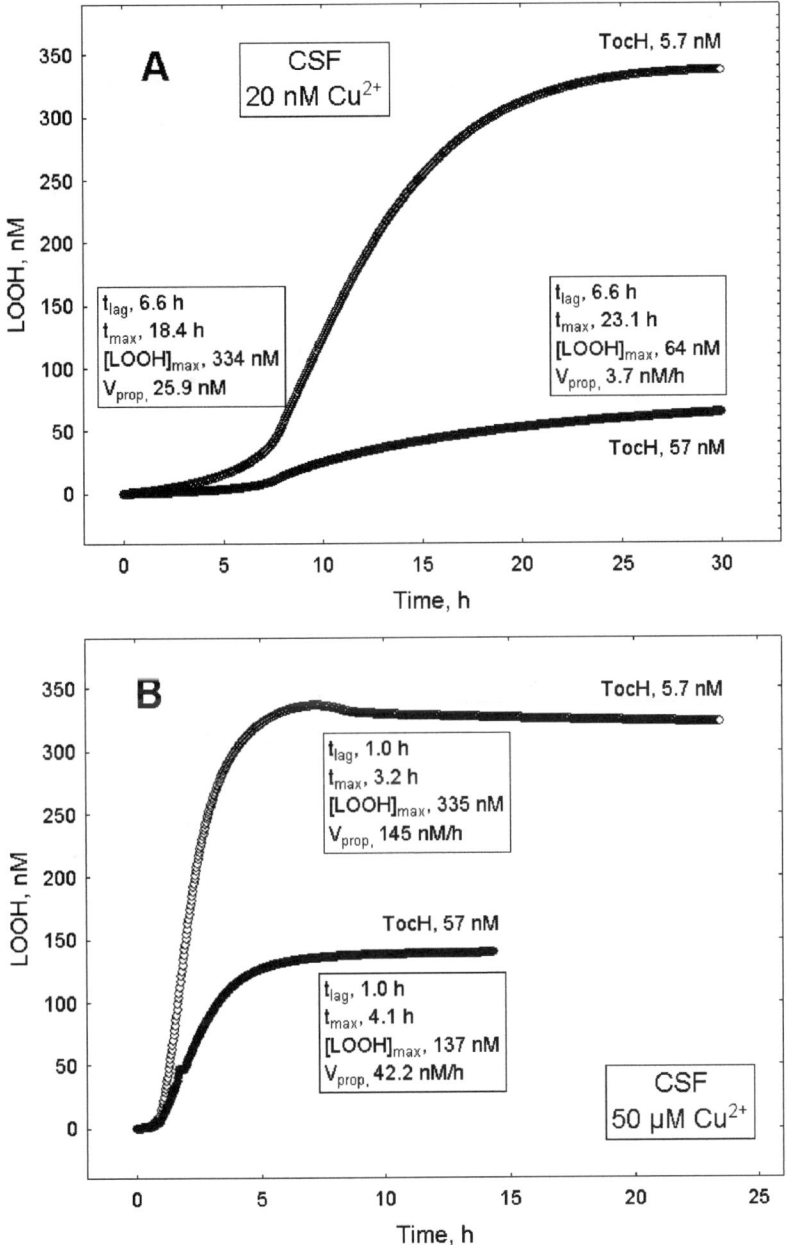

FIGURE 2. Computer modeling of the influence of α-tocopherol on the kinetics of lipoprotein oxidation in CSF (**A** and **B**) and plasma (**C** and **D**). Accumulation of lipid hydroperoxides (LOOH) shown under conditions of mild (20 nM Cu^{2+}; **A** and **C**) and strong (5 μM Cu^{2+}; **B** and **D**) oxidation by copper ions. Consistent with experimental conditions

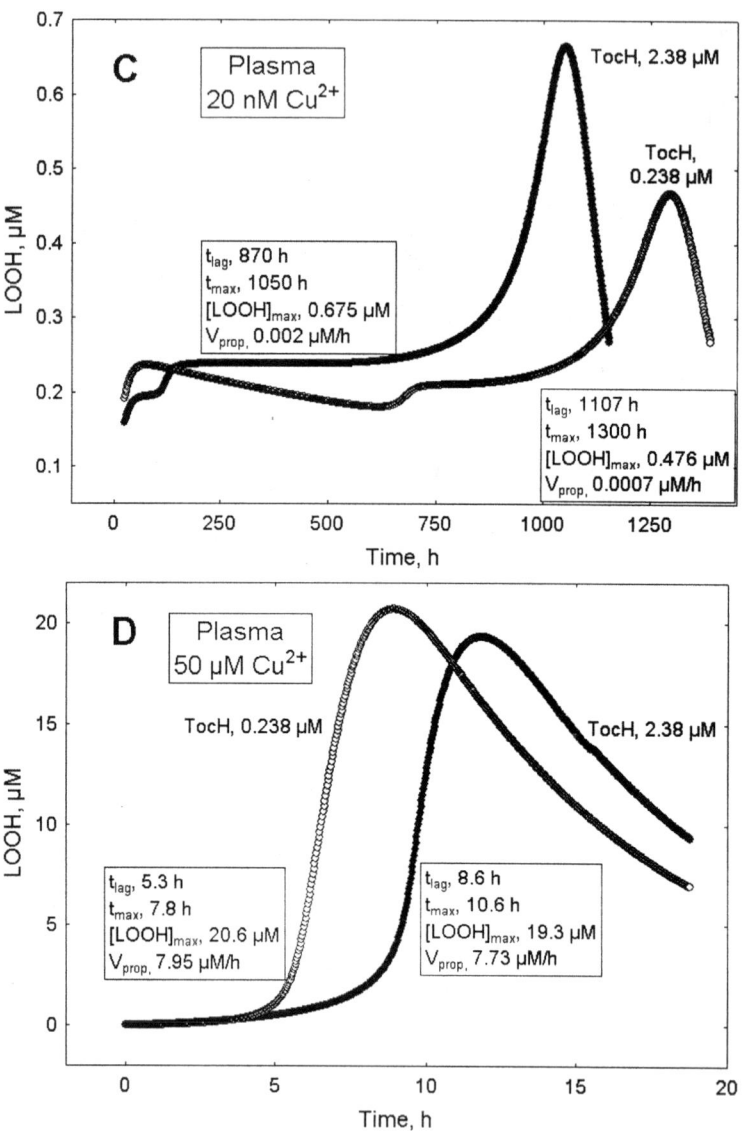

used in our studies, oxidation time-courses were calculated for 150-fold diluted plasma and 10-fold diluted CSF.[14,20] Two different concentrations of α-tocopherol, corresponding to 36 μM (*open circles*) and 360 μM (*solid circles*) in undiluted plasma, and 57 nM (*open circles*) and 570 nM (*solid circles*) in undiluted CSF, were studied in each model. Insets show calculated parameters of lipoprotein oxidation for each LOOH curve: t_{lag}, duration of the lag-phase; t_{max}, duration of the propagation phase; $[LOOH]_{max}$, maximal concentration of lipid hydroperoxides; and V_{prop}, mean oxidation rate in the propagation phase.

differences in the levels of vitamin E (50 nM vs. 30 µM) and oxidizable lipids (4 µM vs. 2.5 mM) between CSF and plasma (TABLE 3), which should result in major differences in oxidative conditions (per unit of vitamin E) between CSF and plasma in the presence of similar amounts of oxidants. Thus, free radical fluxes that correspond to mild oxidative conditions relative to plasma lipoproteins (for example, nanomolar concentrations of transition metal ions) should nevertheless correspond to strong oxidative conditions relative to CSF lipoproteins; the antioxidative action of α-tocopherol should, therefore, be more potent in CSF than in plasma.

In order to assess this hypothesis, we developed a two-compartmental computer model of lipid peroxidation in CSF and plasma lipoproteins. In this model, lipoprotein oxidation is initiated by copper ions or exogenous free radicals and is inhibited by water-soluble (ascorbate and urate) and lipid-soluble (α-tocopherol and ubiquinol-10) antioxidants. Computer modeling of the influence of vitamin E on lipoprotein oxidation (characterized as an accumulation of lipid hydroperoxides) reveals that the vitamin develops antioxidative activity in CSF lipoproteins in the presence of physiologically relevant, low amounts of oxidants (low concentrations of transition metal ions, <100 nM; low fluxes of exogenous free radicals, <100 nM/min; FIG. 2A). Under similar conditions, vitamin E behaves as a pro-oxidant in plasma lipoproteins (FIG. 2C), consistent with the model of tocopherol-mediated peroxidation.[54] By contrast, at high concentrations of transition metal ions or high fluxes of exogenous free radicals, vitamin E develops antioxidative activity both in CSF (FIG. 2B) and plasma (FIG. 2D) lipoproteins. Mild oxidation of lipoproteins should better reflect their hypothetical *in vivo* oxidation than strong oxidation (see Stocker[39] for discussion); low concentrations of oxidants should, therefore, be more physiologically relevant than high and the antioxidative action of vitamin E more potent in the brain than in the vascular wall.

In brain lipoproteins, vitamin E appears to act in concert with other antioxidants, such as ubiquinol-10, vitamin C, or monomeric amyloid-β, to protect against oxidative damage. Whereas monomeric amyloid-β can function as a preventive antioxidant by chelating redox-active transition metal ions,[56] both ubiquinol-10 and vitamin C are able to recycle α-tocopheroxyl radicals back to α-tocopherol, regenerating the vitamin[53]; in addition, ubiquinol-10 and vitamin C are potent chain-breaking antioxidants that inactivate various free radical species. Such combination of chain-breaking and preventive antioxidants could be critical to protect brain lipoproteins and lipids against oxidative stress. Altogether, these data suggest that vitamin E may be effective against *in vivo* oxidation of CSF lipoproteins and brain lipids, and offer new perspectives in the treatment of AD and other neurodegenerative disorders.

REFERENCES

1. PRATICO, D. & N. DELANTY. 2000. Oxidative injury in diseases of the central nervous system: focus on Alzheimer's disease. Am. J. Med. **109:** 577–585.
2. BUTTERFIELD, D.A. 2002. Amyloid beta-peptide (1-42)-induced oxidative stress and neurotoxicity: implications for neurodegeneration in Alzheimer's disease brain: a review. Free Radic. Res. **36:** 1307–1313.
3. ARLT, S., U. BEISIEGEL & A. KONTUSH. 2002. Lipid peroxidation in neurodegeneration: new insights into Alzheimer's disease. Curr. Opin. Lipidol. **13:** 289–294.

4. PRATICO, D., M.Y.L. V, J.Q. TROJANOWSKI, et al. 1998. Increased F2-isoprostanes in Alzheimer's disease: evidence for enhanced lipid peroxidation in vivo. FASEB J. **12:** 1777–1783.
 5. LOVELL, M.A., C. XIE, W.R. MARKESBERY. 2001. Acrolein is increased in Alzheimer's disease brain and is toxic to primary hippocampal cultures. Neurobiol Aging **22:** 187–194.
 6. SMITH, M.A., C.A. ROTTKAMP, A. NUNOMURA, et al. 2000. Oxidative stress in Alzheimer's disease. Biochim. Biophys. Acta **1502:** 139–144.
 7. MARKESBERY, W.R. 1997. Oxidative stress hypothesis in Alzheimer's disease. Free Radic. Biol. Med. **23:** 134–147.
 8. KONTUSH, A., C. BERNDT, W. WEBER, et al. 2001. Amyloid-beta is an antioxidant for lipoproteins in cerebrospinal fluid and plasma. Free Radic. Biol. Med. **30:** 119–128.
 9. ZOU, K., J.S. GONG, K. YANAGISAWA, et al. 2002. A novel function of monomeric amyloid beta-protein serving as an antioxidant molecule against metal-induced oxidative damage. J. Neurosci. **22:** 4833–4841.
10. KONTUSH, A. 2001. Amyloid-beta: an antioxidant that becomes a pro-oxidant and critically contributes to Alzheimer's disease. Free Radic. Biol. Med. **31:** 1120–1131.
11. ATWOOD, C.S., M.E. OBRENOVICH, T. LIU, et al. 2003. Amyloid-beta: a chameleon walking in two worlds: a review of the trophic and toxic properties of amyloid-beta. Brain Res. Brain Res. Rev. **43:** 1–16.
12. TOHGI, H., T. ABE, M. NAKANISHI, et al. 1994. Concentrations of alpha-tocopherol and its quinone derivative in cerebrospinal fluid from patients with vascular dementia of the Binswanger type and Alzheimer type dementia. Neurosci. Lett. **174:** 73–76.
13. JIMENEZ-JIMENEZ, F.J., F. DE BUSTOS, J.A. MOLINA, et al. 1997. Cerebrospinal fluid levels of alpha-tocopherol (vitamin E) in Alzheimer's disease. J. Neural Transm. **104:** 703–710.
14. SCHIPPLING, S., A. KONTUSH, S. ARLT, et al. 2000. Increased lipoprotein oxidation in Alzheimer's disease. Free Radic. Biol. Med. **28:** 351–360.
15. MONTINE, T.J., M.F. BEAL, M.E. CUDKOWICZ, et al. 1999. Increased CSF F2-isoprostane concentration in probable AD. Neurology **52:** 562–565.
16. PRATICO, D. & S. SUNG. 2004. Lipid peroxidation and oxidative imbalance: early functional events in Alzheimer's disease. J. Alzheimers Dis. **6:** 171–175.
17. WILLIAMSON, K.S., S.P. GABBITA, S. MOU, et al. 2002. The nitration product 5-nitrogamma-tocopherol is increased in the Alzheimer brain. Nitric Oxide **6:** 221–227.
18. QUINN, J., J. SUH, M.M. MOORE, et al. 2003. Antioxidants in Alzheimer's disease: vitamin C delivery to a demanding brain. J. Alzheimers Dis. **5:** 309–313.
19. LONNROT, K., T. METSA KETELA, G. MOLNAR, et al. 1996. The effect of ascorbate and ubiquinone supplementation on plasma and CSF total antioxidant capacity. Free Radic. Biol. Med. **21:** 211–217.
20. KONTUSH, A., U. MANN, S. ARLT, et al. 2001. Influence of vitamin E and C supplementation on lipoprotein oxidation in patients with Alzheimer's disease. Free Radic. Biol. Med. **31:** 345–354.
21. SKOUMALOVA, A., J. ROFINA, Z. SCHWIPPELOVA, et al. 2003. The role of free radicals in canine counterpart of senile dementia of the Alzheimer type. Exp. Gerontol. **38:** 711–719.
22. METCALFE, T., D.M. BOWEN & D.P. MULLER. 1989. Vitamin E concentrations in human brain of patients with Alzheimer's disease, fetuses with Down's syndrome, centenarians, and controls. Neurochem. Res. **14:** 1209–1212.
23. RINALDI, P., M.C. POLIDORI, A. METASTASIO, et al. 2003. Plasma antioxidants are similarly depleted in mild cognitive impairment and in Alzheimer's disease. Neurobiol. Aging **24:** 915–919.
24. MECOCCI, P., M.C. POLIDORI, A. CHERUBINI, et al. 2002. Lymphocyte oxidative DNA damage and plasma antioxidants in Alzheimer disease. Arch. Neurol. **59:** 794–798.
25. POLIDORI, M.C. & P. MECOCCI. 2002. Plasma susceptibility to free radical-induced antioxidant consumption and lipid peroxidation is increased in very old subjects with Alzheimer disease. J. Alzheimers Dis. **4:** 517–522.
26. BOURDEL-MARCHASSON, I., M.C. DELMAS-BEAUVIEUX, E. PEUCHANT, et al. 2001. Antioxidant defences and oxidative stress markers in erythrocytes and plasma from normally nourished elderly Alzheimer patients. Age Ageing **30:** 235–241.

27. Foy, C.J., A.P. Passmore, M.D. Vahidassr, et al. 1999. Plasma chain-breaking antioxidants in Alzheimer's disease, vascular dementia and Parkinson's disease. Q.J.M. **92:** 39–45.
28. Sinclair, A.J., A.J. Bayer, J. Johnston, et al. 1998. Altered plasma antioxidant status in subjects with Alzheimer's disease and vascular dementia. Int. J. Geriatr. Psychiatry **13:** 840–845.
29. Zaman, Z., S. Roche, P. Fielden, et al. 1992. Plasma concentrations of vitamins A and E and carotenoids in Alzheimer's disease. Age Ageing **21:** 91–94.
30. Jeandel, C., M.B. Nicolas, F. Dubois, et al. 1989. Lipid peroxidation and free radical scavengers in Alzheimer's disease. Gerontology **35:** 275–282.
31. Charlton, K.E., T.L. Rabinowitz, L.N. Geffen, et al. 2004. Lowered plasma vitamin C, but not vitamin E, concentrations in dementia patients. J. Nutr. Health Aging **8:** 99–107.
32. Ryglewicz, D., M. Rodo, P.K. Kunicki, et al. 2002. Plasma antioxidant activity and vascular dementia. J. Neurol. Sci. **203–204:** 195–197.
33. Fernandes, M.A., M.T. Proenca, A.J. Nogueira, et al. 1999. Influence of apolipoprotein E genotype on blood redox status of Alzheimer's disease patients. Int. J. Mol. Med. **4:** 179–186.
34. Riviere, S., I. Birlouez-Aragon, F. Nourhashemi, et al. 1998. Low plasma vitamin C in Alzheimer patients despite an adequate diet. Int. J. Geriatr. Psychiatry **13:** 749–754.
35. Ahlskog, J.E., R.J. Uitti, P.A. Low, et al. 1995. No evidence for systemic oxidant stress in Parkinson's or Alzheimer's disease. Mov. Disord. **10:** 566–573.
36. Sano, M., C. Ernesto, R.G. Thomas, et al. 1997. A controlled trial of selegiline, alpha-tocopherol, or both as treatment for Alzheimer's disease: The Alzheimer's Disease Cooperative Study. N. Engl. J. Med. **336:** 1216–1222.
37. Onofrj, M., A. Thomas, A.L. Luciano, et al. 2002. Donepezil versus vitamin E in Alzheimer's disease. Part 2. Mild versus moderate-severe Alzheimer's disease. Clin. Neuropharmacol. **25:** 207–215.
38. Zandi, P.P., J.C. Anthony, A.S. Khachaturian, et al. 2004. Reduced risk of Alzheimer disease in users of antioxidant vitamin supplements: the Cache County study. Arch. Neurol. **61:** 82–88.
39. Stocker, R. 1994. Lipoprotein oxidation: mechanistic aspects, methodological approaches and clinical relevance. Curr. Opin. Lipidol. **5:** 422–433.
40. Morris, M.C., D.A. Evans, J.L. Bienias, et al. 2002. Dietary intake of antioxidant nutrients and the risk of incident Alzheimer disease in a biracial community study. J. Am. Med. Assoc. **287:** 3230–3237.
41. Engelhart, M.J., M.I. Geerlings, A. Ruitenberg, et al. 2002. Dietary intake of antioxidants and risk of Alzheimer disease. J. Am. Med. Assoc. **287:** 3223–3229.
42. Morris, M.C., L.A. Beckett, P.A. Scherr, et al. 1998. Vitamin E and vitamin C supplement use and risk of incident Alzheimer disease. Alzheimer Dis. Assoc. Disord. **12:** 121–126.
43. Luchsinger, J.A., M.X. Tang, S. Shea, et al. 2003. Antioxidant vitamin intake and risk of Alzheimer disease. Arch. Neurol. **60:** 203–208.
44. Masaki, K.H., K.G. Losonczy, G. Izmirlian, et al. 2000. Association of vitamin E and C supplement use with cognitive function and dementia in elderly men. Neurology **54:** 1265–1272.
45. Vatassery, G.T., T. Bauer & M. Dysken. 1999. High doses of vitamin E in the treatment of disorders of the central nervous system in the aged. Am. J. Clin. Nutr. **70:** 793–801.
46. McIntosh, L.J., M.A. Trush & J.C. Troncoso. 1997. Increased susceptibility of Alzheimer's disease temporal cortex to oxygen free radical-mediated processes. Free Radic. Biol. Med. **23:** 183–190.
47. Bassett, C.N., K.S. Montine, M.D. Neely, et al. 2000. Cerebrospinal fluid lipoproteins in Alzheimer's disease. Microsc. Res. Tech. **50:** 282–286.
48. Burns, M.P., W.J. Noble, V. Olm, et al. 2003. Co-localization of cholesterol, apolipoprotein E and fibrillar Abeta in amyloid plaques. Brain Res. Mol. Brain Res. **110:** 119–125.

49. BASSETT, C.N., M.D. NEELY, K.R. SIDELL, *et al.* 1999. Cerebrospinal fluid lipoproteins are more vulnerable to oxidation in Alzheimer's disease and are neurotoxic when oxidized ex vivo. Lipids **34:** 1273–1280.
50. ARLT, S., B. FINCKH, U. BEISIEGEL, *et al.* 2000. Time-course of oxidation of lipids in human cerebrospinal fluid in vitro. Free Radic. Res. **32:** 103–114.
51. SUNG, S., Y. YAO, K. URYU, *et al.* 2004. Early vitamin E supplementation in young but not aged mice reduces Abeta levels and amyloid deposition in a transgenic model]of Alzheimer's disease. FASEB J. **18:** 323–325. [e-pub 2003, print Dec. 2004.
52. NEUZIL, J., C. WEBER & A. KONTUSH. 2001. The role of vitamin E in atherogenesis: linking the chemical, biological and clinical aspects of the disease. Atherosclerosis **157:** 257–283.
53. UPSTON, J.M., L. KRITHARIDES & R. STOCKER. 2003. The role of vitamin E in atherosclerosis. Prog. Lipid Res. **42:** 405–422.
54. BOWRY, V.W. & R. STOCKER. 1993. Tocopherol-mediated peroxidation: the prooxidant effect of vitamin E on the radical-initiated oxidation of human low-density lipoprotein. J. Am. Chem. Soc. **115:** 6029–6044.
55. KONTUSH, A., B. FINCKH, B. KARTEN, *et al.* 1996. Antioxidant and prooxidant activity of alpha-tocopherol in human plasma and low-density lipoprotein. J. Lipid Res. **37:** 1436–1448.
56. KONTUSH, A. 2001. Alzheimer's amyloid-beta as a preventive antioxidant for brain lipoproteins. Cell. Mol. Neurobiol. **21:** 299–315.
57. EVANS, P.J., A. BOMFORD & B. HALLIWELL. 1989. Non-caeruloplasmin copper and ferroxidase activity in mammalian serum: ferroxidase activity and phenanthroline-detectable copper in human serum in Wilson's disease. Free Radic. Res. Commun. **7:** 55–62.
58. DURKEN, M., P. NIELSEN, S. KNOBEL, *et al.* 1997. Nontransferrin-bound iron in serum of patients receiving bone marrow transplants. Free Radic. Biol. Med. **22:** 1159–1163.

Vitamin E in Neural and Visual Function

S.M. HAYTON[a] AND D.P.R. MULLER

Biochemistry, Endocrinology, and Metabolism Unit, and [a]Visual Sciences Unit, Institute of Child Health, University College London, London WC1N 1EH, United Kingdom

ABSTRACT: A rat model of vitamin E (α-tocopherol) deficiency with similar "clinical," electrophysiological, and neuropathological abnormalities to those seen in man was used to investigate the effects of various amounts and forms of α-tocopheryl acetate (αTA) on neural and visual function. Electrophysiological techniques provide an objective, non-invasive measure of neural and visual function. These techniques were used in the animal model to determine the minimum dietary requirement of vitamin E necessary to prevent neural and visual abnormalities. They were also used to compare the biological activities of the natural (RRR-) and synthetic (all-rac-) forms of α-tocopherol in neural tissues. The results were as follows: (1) Significant differences in neural and visual function were observed between deficient and control rats after approximately 8 months. (2) An intake of 1.0 mg/kg all-rac- or 0.75 mg/kg RRR-αTA was observed to marginally protect nerves from vitamin E deficiency. (3) The biological activity of all-rac-α-tocopherol in neural tissues was approximately 75% of RRR-α-tocopherol. (4) The concentration of free malondialdehyde (an indicator of lipid peroxidation) was significantly increased in tissues from the deficient compared to the control animals. These results are consistent with a deficiency of α-tocopherol causing increased lipid peroxidation leading to abnormal neural electrophysiology. They could also be explained by more specific but as yet undefined function(s) of α-tocopherol in neural tissues.

KEYWORDS: α-tocopherol; vitamin E; somatosensory evoked potential; electroretinogram; visual evoked potential; neural function; visual function; oxidative stress

INTRODUCTION

It is now established that a severe and chronic deficiency of vitamin E (α-tocopherol) is associated with a progressive neurological syndrome in man,[1–3] a syndrome that includes both neural and visual features. These neural and visual features are associated with electrophysiological abnormalities,[3] including abnormalities of the somatosensory evoked potentials (SEPs), flash electroretinograms (ERGs), and visual evoked potentials (VEPs). Similar neural and visual electrophysiological abnormalities have been reported in the vitamin E-deficient rat[4,5]; therefore, longitu-

---

Address for correspondence: Professor David Muller, Biochemistry, Endocrinology, and Metabolism Unit, Institute of Child Health, University College London, 30 Guilford Street, London WC1N 1EH, United Kingdom. Voice: +44 (0)20 7905 2631; fax: +44 (0)20 7404 6191.
d.muller@ich.ucl.ac.uk

dinal electrophysiological changes can be used as an objective measure of vitamin E status and function.

In this paper, electrophysiological techniques have been used to monitor SEPs, ERGs, and VEPs longitudinally over 14 months in rats receiving different amounts and forms of vitamin E in order to (*a*) determine the minimum dietary requirements of vitamin E necessary to prevent neural and visual dysfunction and (*b*) compare the biological activities of natural (RRR-) and synthetic (all-rac-) α-tocopherol.

METHODS

Details of the animals, their diets, the electrophysiological techniques, and the biochemical methods used have been described in detail previously.[6,7] In summary, weanling (21 ± 7 days) male Wistar rats were obtained from B & K Universal (Hull, United Kingdom). The rats ($n = 12$/group) were fed a synthetic vitamin E-deficient diet (Machlin/Draper-HLR 814, Dyets, Bethlehem, PA, USA) to which various amounts and forms of α-tocopheryl acetate (RRR- and all-rac-) were added. The diets, which were distinguished by the addition of inert dyes, contained either (*a*) 0-mg/kg α-tocopheryl acetate; (*b*) 0.4-, 0.75-, and 5.0-mg/kg RRR-α-tocopheryl acetate; or (*c*) 1.0-mg/kg all-rac-α-tocopheryl acetate. Diets containing 0.75-mg/kg RRR- and 1.0-mg/kg all-rac-α-tocopheryl acetate were chosen because they would be expected to have similar biological activities if the common conversion factor of 1.36 were used. The animals were weighed weekly. The electrophysiological recordings were made monthly from 5 to 14 months, after which the animals were killed and tissues stored at –70°C until the biochemical analyses were carried out.

Prior to the electrophysiological studies, the rats were anesthetized with a combination of fentanyl/fluanisone (Hypnorm, Janssen, High Wycombe, United Kingdom) and midazolam (Hypnovel, Roche, Welwyn Garden City, United Kingdom) as described by Hayton and colleagues.[6] This anesthetic regime has minimal and reproducible effects on evoked potentials.[6] Neural function was assessed by measuring the conduction velocity and amplitude of peripheral and central SEPs following stimulation of the lower limb as previously described.[6] Visual function (latency and amplitude of ERGs and VEPs) was assessed following stimulation by white light in fully darkened conditions after a minimum period of 16-hr dark adaptation as described previously.[7]

Concentrations of α-tocopherol were measured in various neural and non-neural tissues from each group ($n = 6$/group) using high-performance liquid chromatography (HPLC) with fluorimetric detection, by a modification[8] of the method of Buttriss and Diplock.[9] The inter- and intra-assay coefficients of variation were <5%. The detection limit was approximately 2 pmol. Free malondialdehyde (MDA) was estimated in the deficient and control groups ($n = 9$/group) by a modification[10] of the specific method of Esterbauer and colleagues[11] that used HPLC. The assay was linear up to at least 120 pmol/20 µl injection volume and 1–2 pmol could be detected per injection.

Unless stated otherwise, each result is expressed as a mean ± 1 SEM. The significance of difference between mean values was calculated by the Student's unpaired *t*-test, with significance being taken as $P < 0.05$.

The experiments were performed under appropriate personal and project licenses issued by the Home Office and following local ethical approval.

RESULTS

Growth and Physical Condition

A rapid increase in weight was observed in all the groups ($n = 12$/group) during the first 16 weeks, which was followed by a second phase of slower weight gain. Deficient animals (that is, those receiving a diet with no added vitamin E) or those fed a diet containing 0.4-mg/kg RRR-α-tocopheryl acetate did not show an appreciable increase in weight after week 16. There was a progressive deterioration in the general condition of the deficient rats and those receiving 0.4 mg/kg after 20 weeks. The first signs of neural deficit (impaired balance and irregular gait) were seen in the deficient rats and those receiving 0.4 mg/kg at 43 weeks, and after 48 weeks in the 0.75-mg/kg group. Rats fed a diet containing 1-mg/kg all-rac-α-tocopheryl acetate started to display neural signs after 50 weeks. The control group (5 mg/kg) did not show any signs of neural deficit or deterioration in appearance for the duration of the studies.

Neural Function (Somatosensory Evoked Potentials)

The group mean peripheral conduction velocities were similar throughout the study (data not shown), and there were no significant differences between the different dietary groups at any time point. The group mean central conduction velocities are shown in FIGURE 1. No significant differences were seen between the deficient,

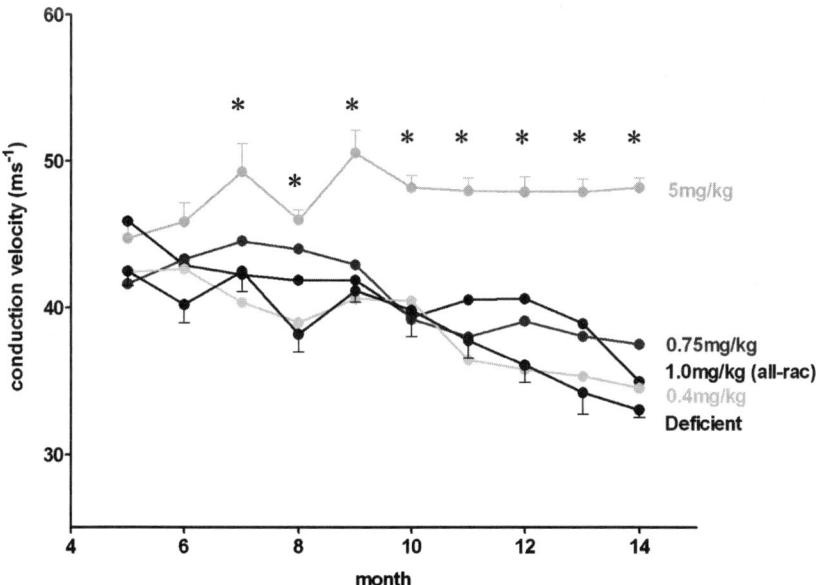

FIGURE 1. The group mean SEP central conduction velocities (± 1 SEM for the deficient and 5-mg/kg groups). *: significant differences ($P < 0.05$) between the 5-mg/kg group and the deficient, 0.4-mg/kg, and 1.0-mg/kg groups.

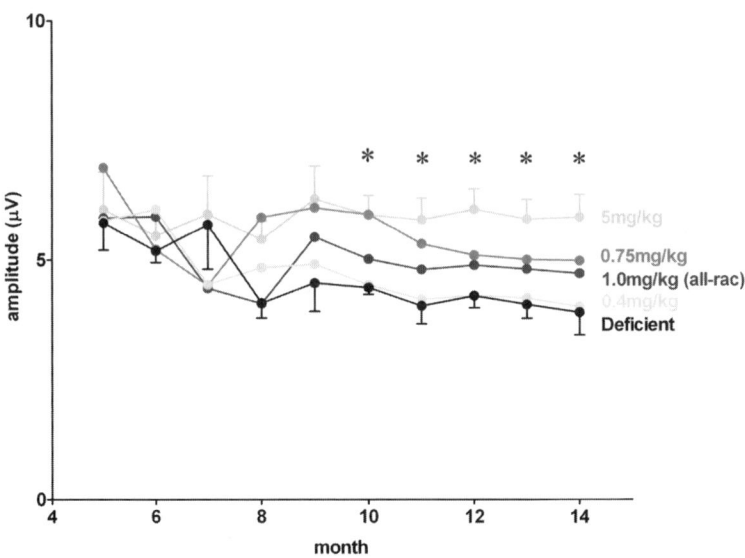

FIGURE 2. The group mean SEP peripheral amplitudes (± 1 SEM for the deficient and 5-mg/kg groups). *: significant differences ($P < 0.05$) between the 5-mg/kg group and the deficient and 0.4-mg/kg groups.

0.4-mg/kg, 0.75-mg/kg, and 1.0-mg/kg groups at any time point during the study. However, the mean central conduction velocities of the 5-mg/kg group was consistently significantly greater than the deficient group and the 0.4- and 1.0-mg/kg groups after 7 months and significantly greater than the 0.75-mg/kg group after 9 months.

The group mean amplitudes of the peripheral responses are shown in FIGURE 2. The amplitudes of the 5-mg/kg group became consistently significantly different from the deficient and 0.4-mg/kg groups after 10 months but did not differ significantly from either the 0.75-mg/kg or 1.0-mg/kg groups. There were no significant differences between the deficient, 0.4-mg/kg, 0.75-mg/kg, or 1.0-mg/kg groups at any time point during the study. FIGURE 3 shows the group mean central somatosensory evoked potential (SEP) amplitudes. The mean amplitudes of the 5-mg/kg group were consistently significantly higher than the deficient group after 12 months, the 0.4-mg/kg group after 10 months, and the 0.75- and 1.0-mg/kg groups after 14 months. No significant differences were observed between the deficient, 0.4-mg/kg, 0.75-mg/kg, and 1.0-mg/kg groups at any time point.

Visual Function

The effects of different amounts and forms of vitamin E on visual function have been described in detail elsewhere.[7] The 5-mg/kg group had significantly shorter ERG latencies than the deficient and 0.4-mg/kg groups after 8 months, the 0.75-mg/kg

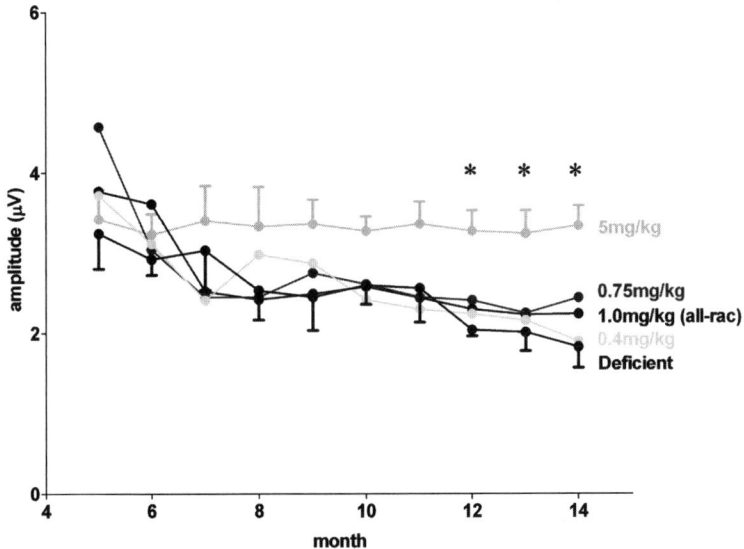

FIGURE 3. The group mean SEP central amplitudes (± 1 SEM for the deficient and 5-mg/kg groups). *: significant differences ($P < 0.05$) between the 5-mg/kg group and the deficient group.

group after 9 months, and the 1.0-mg/kg group after 11 months. After 14 months, the mean ERG latencies of the deficient group were significantly longer than those of the 0.4-, 0.75-, and 1.0-mg/kg groups. The 5-mg/kg group had significantly higher mean ERG amplitudes than the deficient and 0.75-mg/kg groups after 6 months and the 0.4-mg/kg and 1.0-mg/kg groups after 8 months.

After 6 months, the 5-mg/kg group was found to have significantly shorter VEP onset latencies than the other groups. No statistically significant differences were found between the deficient, 0.4-mg/kg, 0.75-mg/kg, and 1.0-mg/kg groups. The VEP amplitudes of the 5-mg/kg group became significantly greater than the deficient, 0.4-mg/kg, and 0.75-mg/kg groups after 13 months and from the 1.0-mg/kg group after 14 months.

Biochemical Studies

Tissue α-tocopherol concentrations showed the expected increase with increasing dietary intake ($n = 6$/group). The concentrations found in the neural tissues are shown in TABLE 1. α-Tocopherol was undetectable or barely detectable in all tissues studied from the deficient group with the exception of the thoracic cord and cerebral cortex, which had mean concentrations of 0.69 and 0.47 µg/g wet weight of tissue, respectively. All tissues from the 0.4-, 0.75-, 1.0-mg/kg groups were found to contain much lower concentrations of α-tocopherol than the 5-mg/kg group. Similar

TABLE 1. Concentrations of α-tocopherol in neural tissues (mean ± 1 SEM) after 14 months on the various diets ($n = 6$/group)

Diet (mg/kg)	Sciatic Nerve (μg/g wet wt)	Thoracic Cord (μg/g wet wt)	Cerebral Cortex (μg/g wet wt)	Eye (μg/g wet wt)
Deficient	0	0.69 ± 0.04	0.47 ± 0.08	0
0.4	0	1.10 ± 0.10	0.92 ± 0.08	0.08 ± 0.01
0.75	0.21 ± 0.13	1.38 ± 0.06	1.52 ± 0.07	0.09 ± 0.02
1.0	0.13 ± 0.07	1.49 ± 0.10	1.63 ± 0.14	0.12 ± 0.02
5.0	7.26 ± 1.37	6.47 ± 0.23	7.81 ± 0.21	1.13 ± 0.13

concentrations of α-tocopherol were found in tissues from the groups receiving 0.75-mg/kg (RRR-) and 1.0-mg/kg (all-rac-) α-tocopheryl acetate.

Free MDA concentrations were determined in several neural and non-neural tissues from the deficient and control groups ($n = 9$ for each group). Significant increases were seen in the concentrations of free MDA in all the tissues from the deficient compared with the control group. The differences were greater in the non-neural tissues than the cerebral cortex and eye.

DISCUSSION

The growth patterns and physical signs (poor coat condition, muscle wasting, kyphoscoliosis, and ataxia) seen in the deficient and low-tocopherol-intake groups in the present studies were similar to those previously reported.[4,12,13]

The electrophysiological results of neural and visual function observed in the deficient animals (that is, significantly decreased SEP central conduction velocities and central and peripheral amplitudes, increased ERG and VEP latencies and decreased amplitudes) were similar to those reported previously.[4,5] There were no significant changes in the peripheral SEP conduction velocities; this observation also agrees with other published studies.[4,13,14] Consistent significant electrophysiological abnormalities were recorded approximately 3 months before "clinical" signs of neural deficit were observed, suggesting that this technique provides an early indication of neural problems. The changes in neural and visual electrophysiology observed in vitamin E-deficient rats are similar to those observed in vitamin E-deficient man (see Muller and Goss-Sampson[3] and Goss-Sampson and colleagues[7]). These similarities confirm the validity of the rat model.

Decreased SEP conduction velocities and increased ERG and VEP latencies are likely to result from demyelination, whereas a reduction in SEP, ERG, and VEP amplitudes reflects a decrease in the total number of functioning axons. These findings are consistent with the known neuropathology of vitamin E deficiency. This is described as a "dying back" axonal neuropathy with secondary demyelination, which is more severe in the central than the peripheral nervous system.[15]

In a recent study of visual function in groups of animals receiving different amounts of vitamin E, we reported that a diet containing 1.25-mg/kg all-rac-α-tocopheryl acetate marginally protected against visual dysfunction.[7] This observation is confirmed in this study, where diets containing 1.0-mg/kg all-rac- and 0.75-mg/kg RRR-α-tocopheryl acetate marginally protected against both neural and visual dysfunction. A dietary intake of 0.4-mg/kg α-tocopheryl acetate did not protect against either neural or visual dysfunction. In the deficient animals, only the cerebral cortex and thoracic cord contained detectable amounts of the vitamin, confirming previous observations that neural tissues retain α-tocopherol more effectively than non-neural tissues.[13,16]

Using the common conversion factor of 1.36, the dietary intakes of 0.75-mg/kg RRR- and 1.0-mg/kg all-rac-a-tocopheryl acetate would have been expected to have similar biological activities and, therefore, result in similar electrophysiological results. This was generally the case. This suggests that a ratio of approximately 1.3 is appropriate for this functional assay in the rat, which is more relevant to the characteristic neurological syndrome seen in vitamin E-deficient man than the classical fetal resorption assay.

Free MDA concentrations were significantly increased in all tissues from the rats receiving the deficient compared to the control diet. These results are in agreement with previous observations[10] and indicate that a reduced or absent tissue concentration of α-tocopherol affords less protection from lipid peroxidation.

The results from the present study, therefore, suggest that vitamin E deficiency could lead to increased oxidative stress in nerves and the retina with increased lipid peroxidation and a loss of long-chain PUFA. Southam and colleagues[17] suggested that the neural abnormalities could result from damage to mitochondria and other intra-axonal membranous structures. The membranes of mitochondria and smooth endoplasmic reticulum contain a high proportion of polyunsaturated fatty acyl chains and may well, therefore, be more susceptible to damage during vitamin E deficiency. In addition, there is a continuous production of oxygen-derived free radicals in mitochondria as a result of oxidative phosphorylation. A disturbance of the axonal mitochondria could then lead to the reported abnormalities in fast retrograde transport,[17] which in turn could result in the characteristic "dying back" axonal neuropathy. Increased oxidative stress in the retina could affect the membrane-bound proteins involved in ion transport, which could then alter phototransduction by impairing the ability of photoreceptors to hyperpolarize and depolarize. Changes in the membrane microenvironment could also affect phototransduction by altering the light-induced movement of rhodopsin within the membrane.

It is now clear, however, that in addition to its antioxidant properties, α-tocopherol has highly specific functions, including an involvement in cell signaling.[18] Thus, α-tocopherol may also have more specific role(s) in neural and visual function with a deficiency resulting in the observed electrophysiological abnormalities.

ACKNOWLEDGMENTS

S.M.H. thanks Roche Vitamins Ltd. for financial assistance, and we thank the staff of the Western Laboratories (Institute of Child Health) for valuable technical assistance. We also thank Dr. Tony Kriss, who died shortly after the completion of these studies, for his help in establishing the electrophysiological methods.

REFERENCES

1. MULLER, D.P.R., J.K. LLOYD & O.H. WOLFF. 1983. Vitamin E and neurological function. Lancet **1**: 225–228.
2. HARDING, A.E. 1987. Vitamin E and the nervous system. Crit. Rev. Neurobiol. **3**: 89–103.
3. MULLER, D.P.R. & M.A. GOSS-SAMPSON. 1990. Neurochemical, neurophysiological, and neuropathological studies in vitamin E deficiency. Crit. Rev. Neurobiol. **5**: 239–263.
4. GOSS-SAMPSON, M.A., A.KRISS & D.P.R. MULLER. 1990. A longitudinal study of somatosensory, brainstem auditory and peripheral sensory-motor conduction during vitamin E deficiency in the rat. J. Neurol. Sci. **100**: 79–84.
5. GOSS-SAMPSON, M.A., T. KRISS & D.P.R. MULLER. 1998. Retinal abnormalities in experimental vitamin E deficiency. Free Radic. Biol. Med. **25**: 457–462.
6. HAYTON, S.M., A. KRISS & D.P.R. MULLER. 1999. Comparison of the effects of four anaesthetic agents on somatosensory evoked potentials in the rat. Lab. Anim. **33**: 243–251.
7. HAYTON, S.M., A. KRISS, A. WADE & D.P.R. MULLER. 2003. The effects of different levels of all-rac- and RRR-α-tocopheryl acetate (vitamin E) on visual function in rats. Clin. Neurophysiol. **114**: 2124–2131.
8. METCALFE, T., D.M. BOWEN & D.P.R. MULLER. 1989. Vitamin E concentrations in human brain of patients with Alzheimer's disease, fetuses with Down's syndrome, centenarians and controls. Neurochem. Res. **14**: 1209–1212.
9. BUTTRISS, J.L. & A.T. DIPLOCK. 1984. High-performance liquid chromatography methods for vitamin E in tissues. Methods Enzymol. **105**: 131–138.
10. MACEVILLY, C.J. & D.P.R. MULLER. 1996. Lipid peroxidation in neural tissues and fractions from vitamin E-deficient rats. Free Radic. Biol. Med. **20**: 639–648.
11. ESTERBAUER, H., J.J. LANG, S. ZADDRAVEC & T.F. SLATER. 1984. Detection of malonaldehyde by high-performance liquid chromatography. Methods Enzymol. **105**: 319–328.
12. MACHLIN, L.J., R. FILIPSKI, J.S. NELSON, L.R. HORN & M. BRIN. 1977. Effects of a prolonged vitamin E deficiency. J. Nutr. **107**: 1200–1208.
13. GOSS-SAMPSON, M.A., C.J. MACEVILLY & D.P.R. MULLER. 1988. Longitudinal studies of the neurobiology of vitamin E and other antioxidant systems, and neurological function in the vitamin E deficient rat. J. Neurol. Sci. **87**: 25–35.
14. GOSS SAMPSON, M.A., A. KRISS, J.R. MUDDLE, P.K. THOMAS & D.P. MULLER. 1988. Lumbar and cortical somatosensory evoked potentials in rats with vitamin E deficiency. J. Neurol. Neurosurg. Psychiatry **51**: 432–435.
15. NELSON, J.S., C.D. FITCH, V.W. FISCHER, G.O. BROUN & A.C. CHOU. 1981. Progressive neuropathologic lesions in vitamin E deficient Rhesus monkeys. J. Neuropath. Exp. Neurol. **40**: 166–186.
16. INGOLD, K.U., G.W. BURTON, D.O. FOSTER, L. HUGHES, D.A. LINDSAY & A. WEBB. 1987. Biokinetics of and discrimination between dietary RRR- and SRR- α-tocopherols in the male rat. Lipids **22**: 163–172.
17. SOUTHAM, E., P.K. THOMAS, R.H.M. KING, M.A. GOSS-SAMPSON & D.P.R. MULLER. 1991. Experimental vitamin E deficiency in rats: morphological and functional evidence of abnormal axonal transport secondary to free radical damage. Brain **114**: 915–936.
18. BRIGELIUS-FLOHE, R., F.J. KELLY, J.T. SALONEN, J. NEUZIL, J.M. ZINGG & A. AZZI. 2002. The European perspective on vitamin E: current knowledge and future research. Am. J. Clin. Nutr. **76**: 703–716.

Vitamin E Modulation of Cardiovascular Disease

MOHSEN MEYDANI

Vascular Biology Laboratory, Jean Mayer USDA Nutrition Research Center on Aging at Tufts University, Boston, Massachusetts, 02111 USA

ABSTRACT: Endothelium in the vascular system is an important modulator of vasomotor tone and coagulation, and it plays a crucial role in the inhibition of adhesion and activation of platelets and leukocytes. Evidence indicates that dietary antioxidants may modulate these endothelium-dependent vascular functions through several mechanisms and may contribute to the prevention of vascular diseases such as atherosclerosis. Several cell cultures as well as animal and human clinical and observational studies have tested the efficacy of vitamin E on vascular function and the prevention of atherosclerosis. Our cell culture studies have indicated that vitamin E (α-tocopherol) inhibits the activation of endothelial cells stimulated by high levels of low-density lipoprotein cholesterol and pro-inflammatory cytokines. This inhibition is associated with the suppression of chemokines, the expression of cell surface adhesion molecules, and the adhesion of leukocytes to endothelial cells, all of which contribute to the development of lesions in the arterial wall. The molecular mechanisms by which α-tocopherol and other tocopherols modulate endothelial cells and smooth muscle functions have been delineated. We, and others, have also demonstrated a positive effect of dietary vitamin E on endothelium and vascular function in animal models of atherosclerosis. Several human clinical trials have also shown an improvement in the surrogate markers of atherosclerosis and vascular function by vitamin E supplementation. However, these findings have been contradicted by several vitamin E supplementation trials for the prevention of secondary cardiovascular events showing null effect. Intervention at a relatively late stage of disease and the single use of vitamin E rather than in combination with other antioxidants might have contributed to these contradictory findings. Evidence from cell cultures, as well as animal and human clinical and observational studies, strongly supports the contribution of dietary vitamin E to the maintenance of vascular function and health, in particular when it is used in combination with other dietary antioxidants, which are found in fruits, vegetables, and nuts.

KEYWORDS: α-tocopherol; cardiovascular disease; atherosclerosis; cell culture; animal model

Address for correspondence: Mohsen Meydani, DVM, PhD., Professor of Nutrition and Director, Vascular Biology Laboratory, Jean Mayer U.S. Department of Agriculture Human Nutrition Center on Aging at Tufts University, 711 Washington Street, Boston MA 02111. Voice: 617-556-3126; fax: 617-556-3224.
mohsen.meydani@tufts.edu

Cardiovascular disease (CVD) is the major cause of morbidity and mortality in Western countries. It is a multi-factorial disease in which the presence of high levels of lipids in the circulation has been well established to be the major contributing factor. Inflammation of the coronary artery and associated oxidative stress, together with the accumulation of lipids, leads to the formation of arterial lesions known as atheroma. In addition, high levels of plasma lipids lead to endothelium activation and increased adhesion of immune cells to the endothelium, which in turn results in endothelium dysfunction. When the atherosclerotic lesions rupture, several chemotactic factors are released, resulting in platelet aggregation and thrombosis of the coronary artery and heart attack.

Experimental and epidemiological evidence suggests that dietary antioxidants may reduce the risk of CVD through modulation of several of these factors. This concept is generated from findings that the consumption of fruits and vegetables, which increase antioxidant nutrient levels in plasma, is associated with a reduced risk of CVD.[1] Most recently, Joshipura and colleagues,[2] in a follow-up study of 42,148 men for 8 years from the Health Professionals' Study and 84,251 women for 14 years from the Nurses' Health Study, confirmed that the consumption of fruits and vegetables is associated with a reduced risk of CVD. They suggested that the consumption of green leafy vegetables and fruits and vegetables rich in vitamin C protects against coronary heart disease (CHD). Fruits and vegetables have also been reported to protect against the risk of ischemic and hemorrhagic stroke in men.[3] The healthful benefits of fruits and vegetables are thought to be due to their high antioxidant content, in particular vitamins C and E and carotenoids. In addition, the presence of phytochemicals in fruits and vegetables, which are not classified as micronutrients, contributes significantly to the total antioxidant capacity of fruits and vegetables. For example, the inclusion of 10 servings of fruits and vegetables per day for 15 days increased the total antioxidant level in plasma by 50–80 µM Trolox equivalent as measured by ORAC (oxygen radical absorbance capacity) assay.[4] In this context, several observational studies have demonstrated the association of antioxidant vitamins with a reduced risk of CVD, which in part supports the oxidative hypothesis of CVD. Gey and colleagues,[5] in cross-cultural studies of 16 European countries, reported an inverse association of high plasma content of α-tocopherol with ischemic heart disease mortality. The Health Professionals' and Nurses' Health studies cited above also indicated that supplemental intake of vitamin E was associated with a reduced risk of CVD.[6,7] TABLE 1 lists the studies where vitamin E intake or plasma levels of vitamin E or vitamin E supplementation were reported to be associated with a reduced risk of CVD diseases. A few small clinical studies have also demonstrated that supplemental intake of vitamin E alone or in combination with drugs or other antioxidants such as vitamin C was effective in the secondary prevention of CHD.[8–10] However, several observational and large clinical trials reported that vitamin E supplementation was not effective in secondary or primary prevention of coronary vascular events and mortality (TABLE 2).[11–13] Despite these inconclusive clinical results, experimental evidence and observation studies strongly support the concept that vitamin E may contribute to the prevention of CHD.

According to the oxidative hypothesis of atherosclerosis, oxidative stress induced by oxidation of low-density lipoprotein (LDL) results in the inflammation of the coronary artery leading to the formation of atherosclerotic lesions, which can cause heart attacks. It is well established that oxidative stress contributes to this process;

TABLE 1. Studies showing beneficial effects of dietary or high serum vitamin E on CVD

Cross-cultural survey of 4 European populations[45]
Edinburgh Case-Controlled Study[46]
Cross-cultural survey of 16 European populations[47]
Basel Prospective Study[47]
Nurses' Health Study, USA[7]
Health Professionals' Follow-Up Study[6]
Linxian China Study[48]
Finnish Men's and Women's Follow-Up Study[49]
Cambridge Heart Antioxidant Study (CHAOS)[9]
Vitamin E and Lesion Progression Study[8]
Antioxidant Vitamins and CHD in Women[50]
Vitamin E and Coronary Mortality in Elderly[51]
Atherosclerosis Risk in Communities Study (ARIC)[52]
Secondary Prevention with Antioxidants of Cardiovascular Disease in End Stage Renal Disease (SPACE)[53]
Vitamins E and C on progression of transplant associated atherosclerosis[10]

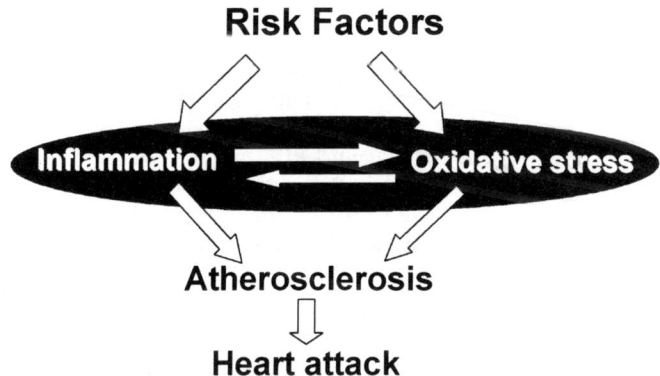

FIGURE 1. The association of risk factors with arterial inflammation, oxidative stress, and atherosclerosis.

however, it is not known whether it is the cause of or the result of the inflammation of the arterial wall (FIG. 1). Nevertheless, there is convincing evidence that lipid oxidation is involved in this process. It has been shown that the level of hydroperoxides is higher in the plasma of individuals with high levels of cholesterol.[14] Several studies have also corroborated the presence of oxidatively modified LDL in this process, including the presence of epitopes of oxidized LDL in atherosclerotic lesions,[15] elevated titers of circulating auto-antibodies against oxidized LDL in patients with carotid atherosclerosis,[16] and knockout of scavenger receptors or 12/15 lipoxygenase in animal model ameliorated atherosclerosis.[17] Accordingly, lipid-soluble antioxidants such as vitamin E are believed to protect oxidative modifications of LDL. Al-

TABLE 2. Studies showing no clear association between CVD and antioxidant supplementation or serum vitamin E levels

Eastern Finland Heart Survey[54]
Dutch Case–Control Follow-Up[55]
Nested Case–Control Study (MONICA Augsburg Project)[56]
Gruppo Italiano per lo Studio Della Sopravivnza Nell'Infarto (GISSI-prevention trial)[11]
Heart Outcomes Prevention Evaluation (HOPE)[57]
Primary Prevention Project (PPP)[58]
Antagonist effect of antioxidants (vitamins E, C and beta-carotene selenium) on simvastatin–niacin on HDL level in CADs[37]
Heart Protection Study (MRC/BHF-UK)[59]

though vitamin E supplementation in a dose-responsive manner inhibited *in vitro* LDL oxidation, it was found that it was not correlated to the clinical endpoints of CVD. Moreover, it has been suggested that high levels of vitamin E supplementation may increase oxidation of LDL *in vivo*[18,19] and increase accumulation of oxidized lipids in atherosclerosis.[20] However, vitamin E is incorporated not only into LDL, but also into other tissues including the endothelial cell lining of arteries and cells of the immune system, which are involved in the inflammation of the arterial wall. Oxidized lipids and inflammatory cytokines cause the activation of endothelium leading to the generation of reactive oxygen species in the endothelial cells, which in turn leads to activation of NF-κB, a nuclear transcription factor that targets activation of several genes such as adhesion molecules, tissue factors, inflammatory cytokines, and chemokines.[21,22] In addition, vitamin E is incorporated into immune cells, smooth muscle cells, and platelets. In immune cells, vitamin E has been reported to modulate the expression of ligands for adhesion molecules and the production of cytokines and lipid mediators.[23] It influences smooth muscle cell proliferation[24] and vaso-relaxation of arteries [25] and inhibits platelet aggregation.[26]

Using human endothelial cell monolayers in culture, we have investigated the effect of increasing levels of exposure to native LDL[27] and the cytokine, interleukin-1β (IL-1β),[28] on the adhesion of monocytes and expression of adhesion molecules when cells were supplemented with vitamin E. The endothelial cells were supplemented with vitamin E at the concentration that is achievable in plasma (40–60 μM) by supplemental intake of vitamin E at doses of 400–800 IU/day. This increased the concentration of α-tocopherol in the cells to 60–90 nM/10^6 cells over a 24-hr supplementation period. The enrichment of endothelial cells with vitamin E resulted in the inhibition of LDL- and IL-1β-induced monocyte adhesion to the endothelial cell monolayer in a dose-responsive manner. The inhibition of monocyte adhesion to the monolayer of endothelial cells by vitamin E supplementation was mediated by the decrease in endothelial cell expression of adhesion molecules such as intracellular adhesion molecule-1 (ICAM-1), vascular cell adhesion molecule-1 (VCAM-1), and E-selectin. Vitamin E supplementation also resulted in the suppression of a pro-inflammatory cytokine such as IL-6 and chemokines such as IL-8 and monocytes chemotactic protein-1 (MCP-1). In addition, vitamin E increased the production of prostacycline (PGI_2), which has vasodilatory and platelet antiaggregatory properties.

These effects of vitamin E in cell culture systems were further examined in animal models.[29] New Zealand white rabbits were fed a semi-purified diet containing 30 (control) or 1000 IU/kg vitamin E. After 4 weeks, both groups' diets were switched to an atherogenic diet (0.3% cholesterol, 9% hydrogenated coconut oil, and 1% corn oil) containing the respective levels of vitamin E and fed for another 2, 4, and 6 weeks. Vitamin E-supplemented rabbits had significantly higher levels of vitamin E in their plasma and aortas. Frozen aorta sections were examined by immunohistochemistry techniques using monoclonal antibodies against rabbit ICAM-1, VCAM-1, and rabbit macrophages (RAM-11), and von Willebrand factor for endothelial cells. The aortas of rabbits treated with the atherogenic diet but supplemented with vitamin E showed a trend towards a lower score of ICAM-1 expression by endothelial cells compared to the aortas of control rabbits. At 4 and 6 weeks on the atherogenic diet, vitamin E supplementation also significantly inhibited the accumulation of macrophages in the aortas. Our findings also concurred with the findings of Fruebis and colleagues,[30] who reported that 1000 IU of vitamin E was effective in reducing atherosclerosis and the expression of VCAM-1 in hypercholesterolemic rabbits. Sirikci and colleagues[31] also reported a reduction of smooth muscle proliferation in rabbits supplemented with vitamin E. These observations in animal models support the concept that down-regulation of adhesion molecule expression, suppression of monocyte/macrophage activation, and inhibition of smooth muscle proliferation by vitamin E are some of the potential mechanisms by which vitamin E may suppress the development of atherosclerosis. The suppressive effect of supplemental levels of vitamin E (2000 IU/kg diet) on atherosclerosis has also been demonstrated in other animal models of atherosclerosis including ApoE null mice[32] and in LDL-receptor-deficient mice with or without established vascular lesions.[33,34] Currently, we are investigating whether vitamin E supplementation begun at an early age is more effective than vitamin E supplementation initiated at middle age or late age in LDL-receptor-deficient mice.

Although the effects of vitamin E supplementation on several of the endpoint measurements of clinical trials for primary and secondary prevention of CVD have been inconclusive, data on several clinical markers of CVD such as flow mediated dilation (FMD) and carotid artery intima-media ratio as well as C-reactive protein (CRP) levels, soluble adhesion molecules, antibody against oxLDL, and plasma levels of nitric oxide and F_2-isoprostanes have been promising. Desideri and colleagues[35] reported that supplementing the hypercholesterolemic patients with either 400 IU or 800 IU of vitamin E for 4 and 8 weeks decreased plasma levels of soluble adhesion molecules sVCAM-1 and von Willebrand factor and increased the total nitrite and nitrate levels as an index of NO production. An increase in plasma vitamin E levels significantly correlated to an increase of NO and inversely was associated with levels of sVCAM-1. These investigators also found that vitamin E supplementation (400 IU/day) further reduced indexes of endothelial activation and lipid peroxidation in patients treated with simvastatin.[36] Furthermore, they reported that changes in sVCAM-1 levels in the circulation were directly correlated to changes in total F_2-isoprostane concentration in simvastatin-treated patients receiving vitamin E supplements. However, they did not observe any effect of vitamin E on the levels of LDL or HDL on treated patients. This refutes the notion that vitamin E is contraindicated to Simvastatin, as earlier reported by Cheung and colleagues,[37] who showed that an increase in HDL levels combined with Simvastatin and niacin treatment was attenuated when a cocktail of antioxidants (vitamin E: 400 IU; vitamin C: 500 mg; β-carotene: 12.5mg; and selenium: 50 mg) was included in the treatment of hypercholesterolemia of CHD patients.

It has been suggested that an increase in oxidative stress is associated with endothelial dysfunction in patients with risk factors for CVD. In this regard, FMD has been used to examine the effect of dietary antioxidants on endothelial function. Although vitamin E supplementation in hypercholesterolemic animal models has been shown to be effective in preserving endothelial vasodilator function,[25] the effect of vitamin E supplementation on FMD in humans has been equivocal.[38–41] However, when vitamin E is consumed with vitamin C, it appears to be effective in reducing FMD. For example, when vitamin E (800 IU/day) was included with vitamin C (2 g/day) supplementation, it further increased the improvement of FMD in chronic smokers.[42] Vitamin E at the dose of 400 IU/day together with 500 mg vitamin C/day also improved endothelial function in children with hyperlipidemia.[43] However, in coronary artery disease patients, the administration of 1 g vitamin C and 800 IU vitamin E per day for 6 months was not effective in improving FMD.[44] In contrast, combined vitamin E (400 IU, 2 times/day) and C (500 mg, 2 times/day) supplementation for 1 year reduced the progression of arteriosclerosis in heart transplant patients.[10]

In conclusion, it is now well established that atherosclerosis is an inflammatory disease of the arterial walls, and its association with oxidative stress is well investigated. Evidence from cell culture and animal studies indicates that vitamin E may prevent the development of this disease, a finding that concurs with several observational and clinical studies using surrogate markers. However, several large secondary and primary prevention studies, conducted mainly on middle-aged and older patients, showed no benefit from vitamin E supplementation. It appears that combining vitamin E with vitamin C given their synergistic and recycling interactions may be one possible dietary intervention, as they are present in selected foods including fruits, vegetables, and nuts containing high levels of these vitamins. Including a dietary regimen rich in vitamin E and other natural antioxidants through the consumption of fruits and vegetables from early age may be a better strategy to prevent the development of CVD in later life when the clinical symptoms are commonly manifested. This concept is currently under investigation in our laboratory.

ACKNOWLEDGMENTS

This material is based upon work supported by the U.S. Department of Agriculture (agreement 58-1950-9-001). Any opinions, findings, conclusions, or recommendations expressed in this publication are those of the author(s) and do not necessary reflect the view of the U.S. Department of Agriculture. The author thanks Stephanie Marco for her assistance in the preparation of the manuscript.

REFERENCES

1. NESS, A.R. & J.W. POWLES. 1997. Fruit and vegetables, and cardiovascular disease: a review. Int. J. Epidemiol. **26:** 1–13.

2. JOSHIPURA, K.J., F.B. HU, J.E. MANSON, et al. 2001. The effect of fruit and vegetable intake on risk for coronary heart disease. Ann. Intern. Med. **134:** 1106–1114.
3. GILLMAN, M.W., L.A. CUPPLES, D. GAGNON, et al. 1995. Protective effect of fruits and vegetables on development of stroke in men. J. Am. Med. Soc. **273:** 1113–1117.
4. CAO, G., S.L. BOOTH, J.A. SADOWSKI & R.L. PRIOR. 1998. Increases in human plasma antioxidant capacity following consumption of controlled diet high in fruits and vegetables. Am. J. Clin. Nutr. **68:** 1081–1087.
5. GEY, K.F., P. PUSKA, P. JORDAN & U.K. MOSER. 1991. Inverse correlation between plasma vitamin E and mortality from ischemic heart disease in cross-cultural epidemiology. Am. J. Clin. Nutr. **53:** 326S–334S.
6. RIMM, E.B., M.J. STAMPFER, A. ASCHERIO, et al. 1993. Vitamin E consumption and the risk of coronary heart disease in men. N. Engl. J. Med. **328:** 1450–1456.
7. STAMPFER, M.J., C.H. HENNEKENS, J.E. MANSON, et al. 1993. Vitamin E consumption and the risk of coronary disease in women. N. Engl. J. Med. **328:** 1444–1449.
8. HODIS, H.N., W.J. MACK, L. LABREE, et al. 1995. Serial coronary angiographic evidence that antioxidant vitamin intake reduces progression of coronary artery atherosclerosis. J. Am. Med. Assoc. **273:** 1849–1854.
9. STEPHENS, N.G., A. PARSONS, P.M. SCHOFIELD, et al. 1996. Randomized, controlled trial of vitamin E in patients with coronary disease: Cambridge Heart Antioxidant Study (CHAOS). Lancet **347:** 781–786.
10. FANG, J.C., S. KINLAY, J. BELTRAME, et al. 2002. Effect of vitamins C and E on progression of transplant-associated arteriosclerosis: a randomized trial. Lancet **359:** 1108–1113.
11. GISSI-Prevenzione Investigators. 1999. Dietary supplementation with n-3 polyunsaturated fatty acids and vitamin E after myocardial infarction: results of the GISSI-Prevenzione trial. Lancet **354:** 447–455.
12. THE HEART OUTCOMES PREVENTION EVALUATION STUDY. 1999. Vitamin E supplementation and cardiovascular events in high-risk patients. N. Engl. J. Med. **342:** 154–160.
13. DE GAETANO, G. 2001. Low-dose aspirin and vitamin E in people at cardiovascular risk: a randomised trial in general practice. Collaborative Group of the Primary Prevention Project. Lancet **357:** 89–95.
14. KINOSHITA, M., S. OIKAWA, K. HAYASAKA, et al. 2000. Age-related increases in plasma phosphatidylcholine hydroperoxide concentrations in control subjects and patients with hyperlipidemia. Clin. Chem. **46:** 822–828.
15. YLA-HERTTUALA, S., W. PALINSKI, M.E. ROSENFELD, et al. 1989. Evidence for the presence of oxidatively modified LDL in human atherosclerotic lesions. Circulation **80:** II-160.
16. SALONEN, J.T., S. YLA-HERTTUALA, R. YAMAMATO, et al. 1992. Autoantibody against oxidized LDL and progression of carotid atherosclerosis. Lancet **339:** 883–887.
17. WITZTUM, J.L. & D. STEINBERG. 1991. Role of oxidized low-density lipoprotein in atherogenesis. J. Clin. Invest. **88:** 1785–1792.
18. THOMAS, S.R. & R. STOCKER. 2000. Molecular action of vitamin E in lipoprotein oxidation: implications for atherosclerosis. Free Radic. Biol. Med. **28:** 1795–1805.
19. UPSTON, J.M., A.C. TERENTIS & R. STOCKER. 1999. Tocopherol-mediated peroxidation of lipoproteins: implications for vitamin E as a potential antiatherogenic supplement. FASEB J. **13:** 977–994.
20. UPSTON, J.M., A.C. TERENTIS, K. MORRIS, et al. 2002. Oxidized lipid accumulates in the presence of α-tocopherol in atherosclerosis. Biochem. J. **363:** 753–760.
21. BEVILACQUA, M.P., J.S. POBER, M.E. WHEELER, et al. 1985. Interleukin-1 acts on cultured human vascular endothelium to increase the adhesion of polymorphonuclear leukocytes, monocytes, and related leukocyte cell lines. J. Clin. Invest. **76:** 2003–2011.
22. PARHAMI, F., Z.T. FANG, A.M. FOGELMAN, et al. 1993. Minimally modified low-density lipoprotein-induced inflammatory responses in endothelial cells are mediated by cyclic adenosine monophosphate. J. Clin. Invest. **92:** 471–478.
23. DEVARAJ, S., D. LI & I. JIALAL. 1996. The effects of α-tocopherol supplementation on monocyte function: decreased lipid oxidation, interleukin-1β secretion, and monocyte adhesion to endothelium. J. Clin. Invest. **98:** 756–763.

24. Azzi, A., E. Aratri, D. Boscoboinik, *et al.* 1998. Molecular basis of alpha-tocopherol control of smooth muscle cell proliferation. Biofactors **7:** 3–14.
25. Keaney, J.F., Jr., J.M. Gaziano, A. Xu, *et al.* 1994. Low-dose α-tocopherol improves and high-dose α-tocopherol worsens endothelial vasodilator function in cholesterol-fed rabbits. J. Clin. Invest. **93:** 844–851.
26. Freedman, J.E. & J.F. Keaney, Jr. 2001. Vitamin E inhibition of platelet aggregation is independent of antioxidant activity. J. Nutr. **131:** 374S–377S.
27. Martin, A., T. Foxall, J.B. Blumberg & M. Meydani. 1997. Vitamin E inhibits low-density lipoprotein-induced adhesion of monocytes to human aortic endothelial cells in vitro. Arterioscler. Thromb. Vasc. Biol. **17:** 429–436.
28. Wu, D., T. Koga, K.R. Martin & M. Meydani. 1999. Effect of vitamin E on human aortic endothelial cell production of chemokines and adhesion to monocytes. Atherosclerosis **147:** 297–307.
29. Koga, T., P. Kwan, L. Zubik, *et al.* 2004. Vitamin E supplementation suppresses macrophage accumulation and endothelial sell expression of adhesion molecules in the aorta of hypercholesterolemic rabbits. Atherosclerosis **176:** 265–272.
30. Fruebis, J., M. Silvestre, D. Shelton, *et al.* 1999. Inhibition of VCAM-1 expression in the arterial wall is shared by structurally different antioxidants that reduce early atherosclerosis in NZW rabbits. J. Lipid Res. **40:** 1958–1966.
31. Sirikci, O., N.K. Ozer & A. Azzi. 1996. Dietary cholesterol-induced changes of protein kinase C and the effect of vitamin E in rabbit aortic smooth muscle cells. Atherosclerosis **126:** 253–263.
32. Pratico, D., R.K. Tangirala, D.J. Rader, *et al.* 1998. Vitamin E suppresses isoprostane generation in vivo and reduces atherosclerosis in ApoE-deficient mice. Nature Med. **4:** 1189–1192.
33. Cyrus, T., L.X. Tang, J. Rokach, *et al.* 2001. Lipid peroxidation and platelet activation in murine atherosclerosis. Circulation **104:** 1940–1945.
34. Cyrus, T., Y. Yao, J. Rokach, *et al.* 2003. Vitamin E reduces progression of atherosclerosis in low-density lipoprotein receptor-deficient mice with established vascular lesions. Circulation **107:** 521–523.
35. Desideri, G., M.C. Marinucci, G. Tomassoni, *et al.* 2002. Vitamin E supplementation reduces plasma vascular cell adhesion molecule-1 and von Willebrand factor levels and increases nitric oxide concentrations in hypercholesterolemic patients. J. Clin. Endocrinol. Metab. **87:** 2940–2945.
36. Desideri, G., G. Croce, M. Tucci, *et al.* 2003. Effects of bezafibrate and simvastatin on endothelial activation and lipid peroxidation in hypercholesterolemia: evidence of different vascular protection by different lipid-lowering treatments. J. Clin. Endocrinol. Metab. **88:** 5341–5347.
37. Cheung, M.C.Z., X.Q. Chait, A. Albers, *et al.* 2001. Antioxidant supplements block the response of HDL to Simvastatin-niacin therapy in patients with coronary artery disease and low HDL. Arterio. Thrombo. Vascul. Biol. **21:** 1320–1326.
38. Kinlay, S., J.C. Fang, H. Hikita, *et al.* 1999. Plasma α-tocopherol and coronary endothelium-dependent vasodilator function. Circulation **100:** 219–221.
39. Jorge, P.A., M.R. Osaki, E. de Almeida, *et al.* 1996. Effects of vitamin E on endothelium-dependent coronary flow in hypercholesterolemic dogs. Atherosclerosis **126:** 43–51.
40. Simons, L.A., M. von Konigsmark, J. Simons, *et al.* 1999. Vitamin E ingestion does not improve arterial endothelial dysfunction in older adults. Atherosclerosis **143:** 193–199.
41. Elliott, T.G., J.D. Barth & G.B. Mancini. 1995. Effects of vitamin E on endothelial function in men after myocardial infarction. Am. J. Cardiol. **76:** 1188–1190.
42. Tousoulis, D., C. Antoniades, C. Tentolouris, *et al.* 2003. Effects of combined administration of vitamins C and E on reactive hyperemia and inflammatory process in chronic smokers. Atherosclerosis **170:** 261–267.
43. Engler, M.M., M.B. Engler, M.J. Malloy, *et al.* 2003. Antioxidant vitamins C and E improve endothelial function in children with hyperlipidemia: Endothelial Assessment of Risk from Lipids in Youth (EARLY) Trial. Circulation **108:** 1059–1063.

44. KINLAY, S., D. BEHRENDT, J.C. FANG, et al. 2004. Long-term effect of combined vitamins E and C on coronary and peripheral endothelial function. J. Am. Coll. Cardiol. **43:** 629–634.
45. RIEMERSMA, R.A., M. OLIVER, R.A. ELTON, et al. 1990. Plasma antioxidants and coronary heart disease: vitamins C and E and selenium. Eur. J. Clin. Nutr. **44:** 143–150.
46. RIEMERSMA, R.A., D.A. WOOD, C.C.H. MACINTYRE, et al. 1991. Risk of angina pectoris and plasma concentrations of vitamins A, C, and E and carotene. Lancet **337:** 1–5.
47. GEY, K.F. 1993. Prospects for the prevention of free radical disease, regarding cancer and cardiovascular disease. Br. Med. Bull. **49:** 679–699.
48. BLOT, W.J., J.-Y. LI, P.R. TAYLOR, et al. 1995. The Linxian Trials: mortality rates by vitamin-mineral intervention group. Am. J. Clin. Nutr. **62**(Suppl.).
49. KNEKT, P., A. REUNANEN, R. JARVINEN, et al. 1994. Antioxidant vitamin intake and coronary mortality in a longitudinal population study. Am. J. Epidemiol. **139:** 1180–1189.
50. KUSHI, L.H., A.R. FOLSOM, R.J. PRINEAS, et al. 1996. Dietary antioxidant vitamins and death from coronary heart disease in postmenopausal women. N. Engl. J. Med. **334:** 1156–1162.
51. LOSONCZY, K.G., T.B. HARRIS & R.J. HAVLIK. 1996. Vitamin E and vitamin C supplementation use and risk of all-cause and coronary heart disease mortality in older persons: the Established Populations for Epidemiologic Studies of the Elderly. Am. J. Clin. Nutr. **64:** 190–196.
52. KRITCHEVSKY, S.B., T. SHIMAKAWA, G.S. TELL, et al. 1995. Dietary antioxidants and carotid artery wall thickness: the ARIC Study. Circulation **92:** 2142–2150.
53. BOAZ, M., S. SMETANA, T. WEINSTEIN, et al. 2000. Secondary prevention with antioxidants of cardiovascular disease in endstage renal disese (SPACE): randomised placebo-controlled trial. Lancet **356:** 1213–1218.
54. SALONEN, J.T., R. SALONEN, I. PENTTILA, et al. 1985. Serum fatty acids, apolipoproteins, selenium and vitamin antioxidants and risk of death from coronary artery disease. Am. J. Cardiol. **56:** 226–231.
55. KOK, F.J., A.M. DE BRUIJN, R. VERMEEREN, et al. 1987. Serum selenium, vitamin antioxidants and cardiovascular mortality. Am. J. Clin. Nutr. **45:** 462–468.
56. HENSE, H.W., M. STENDER, W. BORS & U. KEIL. 1993. Lack of an association between serum vitamin E and myocardial infarction in a population with high vitamin E levels. Atherosclerosis **103:** 21–28.
57. MANCINI, G.B. & D.J. STEWART. 2001. Why were the results of the Heart Outcomes Prevention Evaluation (HOPE) trial so astounding? Can. J. Cardiol. **17**(Suppl. A): 15A–17A.
58. PALUMBO, G., F. AVANZINI, C. ALLI, et al. 2000. Effects of vitamin E on clinic and ambulatory blood pressure in treated hypertensive patients: Collaborative Group of the Primary Prevention Project (PPP)—Hypertension Study. Am. J. Hyperten. **13:** 564–567.
59. HEART PROTECTION STUDY COLLABORATIVE GROUP. 2002. MRC/BHF Heart Protection Study of antioxidant vitamin supplementation in 20,536 high-risk individuals: a randomised placebo-controlled trial. Lancet **360:** 23–33.

Vitamin E and Cardiovascular Disease

Observational Studies

J. MICHAEL GAZIANO

Divisions of Aging and Preventive Medicine, Department of Medicine, Brigham and Women's Hospital and Harvard Medical School, Boston, Massachusetts, USA

VA Boston Health Care System, Boston, Massachusetts, USA

ABSTRACT: Basic research suggests that oxidative stress may play an important role in many chronic diseases and provides plausible mechanisms by which natural antioxidants such as vitamin E may delay or prevent steps in atherogenesis. Dietary research has shown that those who consume higher amounts of fruits and vegetables have lower rates of heart disease and stroke, raising the possibility that antioxidants are protective. Results from large-scale human observational studies suggest that antioxidant consumption reduces the risk of developing cardiovascular disease (CVD). Both case-control and prospective cohort studies have carefully explored the relationship between vitamin E intake and plasma and tissue vitamin E levels and the risk of CVD. In many, but not all, of these studies vitamin E intake over an extended period was associated with decreased risk of cardiovascular events. Results from studies of blood levels are more limited and less consistent. This presentation summarizes data from the major observational studies. Overall, they support the possibility that vitamin E intake either from food or supplements may reduce risk of CVD; however, these studies have important limitations. For example, uncontrolled confounding can be similar in magnitude to the observed health effects, and antioxidant consumption may be merely a marker for a different cardioprotective factor (such as exercise or diet) that is responsible for these effects. In the search for small to moderate effects, randomized trials may be helpful, although to date, data from large-scale trials have been inconsistent. Several large-scale trials currently under way will help identify the potential benefits of vitamin E in the primary prevention of CVD and other chronic illness. Some are designed to test vitamin E alone as well as in combination with other antioxidant supplements because it is possible that antioxidants may be most effective if taken in particular combinations. Currently, the American Heart Association maintains that there are insufficient efficacy data from completed randomized trials to justify population-wide recommendations for use of vitamin E supplements in disease prevention.

KEYWORDS: antioxidant; cardiovascular disease; vitamin E

Address for correspondence: J. Michael Gaziano, M.D., Brigham and Women's Hospital, Division of Aging, 1620 Tremont Street, Boston MA 02120. Voice: 617-525-7631; fax: 617-525-7739.
jmgaziano@partners.org

INTRODUCTION

One of the most consistent findings in dietary research is that those who consume higher amounts of fruits and vegetables have lower rates of heart disease and stroke, raising the possibility that antioxidants are protective. The exact mechanism for these apparent protective effects is not entirely clear, although basic research has identified plausible mechanisms by which natural antioxidants may delay or prevent steps in atherogenesis. The oxidation of low-density lipoprotein (LDL) cholesterol is suspected to occur at the initial stages of atherosclerosis, and vitamin E has been shown to inhibit this oxidative reaction.

Many cross-sectional, case-control, and cohort studies have found an association between antioxidant consumption and a reduced risk of developing heart disease, with the strongest data in favor of vitamin E. Conversely, several large-scale, randomized trials of antioxidant supplements have now been completed, but their results are not entirely consistent. In this paper, I will focus on the observational study results, and then briefly put these in the context of the results of the completed large-scale trials as well as review the status of ongoing studies.

BASIC LABORATORY RESEARCH

Oxidative processes may play an important role in the pathogenesis of many chronic diseases, including atherosclerosis, cancer, arthritis, eye disease, and reperfusion injury during myocardial infarction. Data from *in vitro* and *in vivo* studies suggest that oxidative damage to LDL promotes several steps in atherogenesis,[1] including endothelial cell damage,[2,3] foam cell accumulation,[4–6] and growth[7,8] and synthesis of autoantibodies.[9] In addition, animal studies suggest that free radicals may directly damage arterial endothelium,[10] promote thrombosis,[11] and interfere with normal vasomotor regulation.[12] Oxidative damage may enhance atherogenesis by a cascade of reactions. Several systems have evolved in aerobic organisms to minimize the damaging effects of uncontrolled oxidation. Mechanisms exist to prevent the formation of unintended free radicals, and oxidative metabolism is carefully compartmentalized with oxygen and its highly reactive species tightly bound to enzymes. Metal ions such as copper and iron are bound to storage or transport proteins to prevent catalytic reactions with oxygen species that could lead to the formation of free radicals. In addition, enzymatic antioxidants (such as superoxide dismutase, catalase, and glutathione peroxidase) and nonenzymatic antioxidants (such as vitamin E) scavenge free radicals, thereby minimizing the damage they can cause once formed. Lastly, there are mechanisms for repairing the damage resulting from unintended oxidative reactions.

Antioxidant vitamins represent one of the many nonenzymatic antioxidant defense mechanisms. Vitamin E (of which α-tocopherol is the major component) is among the most abundant and most widely studied natural antioxidants. However, there are hundreds or thousands of other dietary compounds that may function as antioxidants. *In vitro* data have demonstrated the possible role of these antioxidants in preventing or slowing various steps in atherogenesis by inhibiting the oxidation of LDL or other free radical reactions. These antioxidants have also been shown to prevent experimental atherogenesis in many but not all animal models of atherosclerosis.[13–17]

OBSERVATIONAL EPIDEMIOLOGY

Basic research provides insight into the mechanisms underlying atherogenesis and helps elucidate potential interventions to modify these effects. But to establish cause and effect, data from complementary methods of population research are needed, including descriptive, analytical, and intervention studies. Each has strengths and weaknesses.

Descriptive studies (case reports, cross-sectional surveys, and cross-cultural analyses) are valuable primarily for their ability to generate hypotheses. However, their design prevents adequate control for potential factors that may confound apparent associations. Observational studies (case-control and prospective cohort studies) give researchers greater control over potential confounders. They are extremely useful in establishing risk attributable to a single factor, particularly when the effect of a given factor is large, as in the case for smoking and lung cancer. But in the search for small-to-moderate effects, the amount of uncontrolled confounding in observational studies may be as large as the probable risk reduction itself. In such cases, randomized trials are essential for confirming causation. Even when causality is not in question, trials help quantify the magnitude of an intervention's effect. And although logistically difficult and expensive to conduct, randomized trials generally provide the best data on the magnitude of benefit and risk from a given intervention, which is essential for assessing cost efficacy and developing preventive strategies.

Descriptive Epidemiologic Studies

Some of the early data supporting the hypothesis that vitamin E was protective against cardiovascular disease (CVD) came the MONICA (Multinational MONitoring of trends and determinants in CArdiovascular disease) cross-cultural studies; of the16 populations of men and women that had been analyzed, lipid-standardized α-tocopherol levels were inversely associated ($RR = 0.49$; $P = .01$) with mortality rates due to ischemic heart disease.[18] In the partial regression analysis, lipid-standardized vitamin E exhibited an even stronger inverse correlation with ischemic heart disease mortality ($RR = 0.69$; $P < .001$). However, a similar study of four European populations of men between 40 and 49 found a nonsignificant inverse association between vitamin E intake and cardiovascular mortality.[19]

Case–Control Studies

Two separate studies of subsets of the same population of 6,000 Scottish men aged 35 to 54 identified a significant inverse association between plasma antioxidant levels and CVD. Lipid-standardized concentrations of vitamin E in patients with angina (as identified by a questionnaire) were lower than in controls. The first study included 125 men with angina and 430 controls; the vitamin E/cholesterol molar ratio was lower in those with angina than in the controls.[20] The relative risk of angina for those in the lowest versus those in the highest quintile of the vitamin E/cholesterol ratio was 2.2:1. In the second study, 110 men with angina were compared with 394 controls, and Vitamin E was independently and inversely related to the risk of angina after adjusting for age, smoking, blood pressure, lipids, and relative weight.[21]

A large case-control study, the EURAMIC (European Community Multicenter Study on Antioxidants, Myocardial Infarction, and Breast Cancer) study, compared vitamin E concentrations in adipose tissue samples of 683 people with acute myocardial infarction (MI) and 727 hospital-based controls.[22] The mean α-tocopherol concentrations were virtually the same in both groups; low levels were not associated with increased risk of MI. Supplemental vitamin E appeared to be associated with lower risk of MI, a finding consistent with other studies. Adipose levels of β-carotene were also measured, and it appeared to have a protective effect; vitamin E strengthened the inverse association of with MI, which was the greatest at the highest α-tocopherol concentrations.

Prospective Cohort Studies

Although case-control studies are often efficient and less costly than cohort studies, prospective cohort studies are less subject to selection and recall bias because information is collected before disease develops. Many large cohort studies have evaluated the relationship between vitamin E intake and the incidence of coronary disease. These studies are summarized in TABLE 1.

Nurses' Health Study. The largest of the prospective cohort studies is the Nurses' Health Study (NHS), an investigation in which the association between vitamin E and CVD was analyzed among more than 87,000 U.S. female nurses between 34 and 59 years old with no history of CVD.[23] Dietary antioxidant intake and use of antioxidant vitamin supplements were determined using a semi-quantitative food frequency questionnaire administered at baseline; information on vitamin E intake and antioxidant supplements was updated biennially. After 8 years, women in the highest quintile of vitamin E intake had a 34% lower risk of coronary disease (nonfatal MI and fatal coronary heart disease) compared with those in the lowest quintile (P for trend < .001). When vitamin E intake was examined separately by source (food or supplements), an inverse association emerged only for supplements. Women who took at least 100 IU of vitamin E supplements per day for more than 2 years experienced reductions of 40% or more in the risk of coronary disease, after adjustment for age and cardiac risk factors.

Health Professionals Follow-up Study. The NHS findings were mirrored in the Health Professionals Follow-up Study (HPFS) of nearly 40,000 U.S. male health professionals aged 40 to 75 who did not have coronary heart disease (CHD), diabetes, or hypercholesterolemia at baseline.[24] After adjustment for cardiac risk factors, the relative risk of major coronary disease for those in the highest versus the lowest quintile of vitamin E intake was 0.60 (95% confidence interval (CI), 0.44–0.81; P for trend = .01). Further analysis revealed that the protective association was strongest for vitamin E consumed in supplements. Men who took at least 100 IU per day for at least 2 years had a multivariate risk of coronary disease of 0.63 (95% CI, 0.47–0.84) compared with men who did not take vitamin E supplements. A weak association was found for dietary vitamin E intake alone; among men who did not take vitamin supplements, the relative risk comparing the extreme quartiles was 0.79 (95% CI, 0.54–1.15, P for trend = .11).

Iowa Women's Health Study. The Iowa Women's Health Study evaluated the association between antioxidant vitamin intake and CHD mortality over 7 years among 34,486 postmenopausal women with no history of CVD.[25] In contrast to the NHS and HPFS findings, vitamin E intake from food but not from supplements was strongly associated with a lower risk of CHD mortality. Women in the highest quin-

TABLE 1. Prospective cohort studies of vitamin E intake in the prevention of cardiovascular disease (CVD)

Study	Population and Age (yr)	Exposure	Duration (yr)	Endpoint	Risk Reduction from Vit. E
Nurses' Health Study (1993)	87,245 U.S. female nurses, 34–59	Dietary vitamin E & antioxidant supplements	8	Coronary disease (nonfatal MI and fatal CHD)	Yes
Health Professionals Follow-up (1993)	39,910 U.S. male health professionals, 40–75	Dietary vitamin E and vitamin E supplements	4	Major coronary disease (fatal coronary disease, nonfatal MI, bypass, angioplasty)	Yes
Iowa Women's Health Study (1996)	34,486 postmenopausal women, 55–69	Dietary vitamin E and antioxidant supplements	7	CHD mortality	Yes
Finnish Cohort (1994)	5,133 men, 30–69	Dietary	12–16	CHD mortality	Yes
French Canadian Men (1996)	2,313 middle-aged men	Vitamin supplements	5	Ischemic heart disease (IHD death, new IHD event, MI, angina)	Yes
Multiple Risk Factor Intervention (1996)	734 U.S. men, 35–57	Blood samples taken at baseline and frozen for 20 years	20	Nonfatal MI or coronary death	No
Established Populations for Epidemiologic Studies of the Elderly (1996)	11,178 U.S. men and women, 67–105	Vitamin E supplements and vitamin C supplements	9	Coronary disease mortality, CHD mortality, all-cause mortality	Yes
Rotterdam	4,802 Dutch men and women, 55–95	Dietary antioxidants	4	Myocardial infarction	No

tile of dietary vitamin E intake, without any supplementation, had a relative risk of 0.38 compared to those in the lowest quintile (P for trend = 0.004). Controlling for other dietary factors associated with vitamin E intake, such as intake of linoleic acid, folate, and fiber, did not affect the results.

Finnish Cohort Study. Similarly, a 14-year Finnish study also found a significant inverse association between dietary intake of vitamin E and coronary mortality among 5,133 men and women 30 to 69 years of age and initially free of heart disease.[26] Among women, those in the highest tertile of vitamin E usage versus those in the lowest had a relative risk of death from heart disease of 0.35 (P for trend < .01). In men, this relative risk was 0.66 (P for trend = .01).

Study of Middle-Aged French-Canadian Men. This study assessed the relationship between use of vitamin and mineral supplements in a cohort of 2,313 men from Quebec who provided baseline information on supplement use and risk factors for ischemic heart disease.[27] A total of 23% reported taking supplements, with 5.1% of these men receiving vitamin E from supplements. Their progress was followed for 5 years, and, in general, men taking supplements had a statistically significant lower risk of ischemic heart disease and MI. In particular, vitamin E appeared to be more strongly and more consistently associated with a lower incidence of ischemic heart disease events.

Multiple Risk Factor Intervention Trial. This nested case-control study consisted of 734 U.S. men age 35–57 at risk for CVD and enrolled in the Multiple Risk Factor Intervention Trial (MRFIT). Blood samples were taken at baseline and frozen for 20 years before being analyzed; there was no association between serum vitamin E levels and risk of nonfatal MI or coronary death.

Elderly Cohort Studies. The relationship between vitamin E and CVD has also been examined in two elderly cohorts, the Established Populations for Epidemiologic Studies of the Elderly (EPESE) program, and the Rotterdam Study. EPESE, a National Institute on Aging study of 11,178 U.S. men and women aged 67 to 105 years, found a decreased risk of CHD mortality (RR = 0.53; 95% CI, 0.34–0.84) and overall mortality (RR = 0.66%; 95% CI, 0.53–0.83) among those taking vitamin E supplements (not as part of a multivitamin) over a 9-year period.[28]

The Rotterdam Study also assessed an older population, 4,802 Dutch men and women aged 55 to 95 years with no history of MI. However, unlike the EPESE study, it was limited to dietary antioxidants, as determined using the semi-quantitative food frequency questionnaire. After a follow-up period of 4 years, no association between vitamin E intake and myocardial infarction (MI) was observed.[29]

Limitations of Observational Studies

Observational results suggest that antioxidants may have protective effects, but these studies have important limitations. For example, uncontrolled confounding from unknown or unmeasured confounders can be similar in magnitude to the observed health effects, and antioxidant consumption may be merely a marker for a different cardioprotective factor (such as exercise and diet) that is responsible for the observed health benefits. In addition, intakes of individual dietary antioxidants tend to be highly correlated with each other, making it difficult to determine the specific benefit of a particular antioxidant.

Antioxidant vitamins are commonly used nutritional supplements. Evaluation of the benefits and risks of antioxidants is essential for determining the place of these supplements in clinical medicine. As far back as 1991, the U.S. National Heart, Lung, and Blood Institute's (NHLBI's) conference "Antioxidants in the Prevention of Human Atherosclerosis" concluded that data from large-scale randomized trials, which by design can limit the amount of confounding because subjects are randomly assigned to treatment or placebo, were required to test the hypothesis that dietary antioxidants reduce the risk of CVD. Several large-scale randomized trials have now been completed, and more are currently under way.

COMPLETED RANDOMIZED CLINICAL TRIALS

Primary Prevention

With the completion of the SUpplémentation en VItamines et Minéraux AntioXydants (SU.VI.MAX) study, more detailed data examining the role of antioxidants in reducing CAD should soon be available. The SU.VI.MAX trial evaluated for 8 years the efficacy of a balanced combination of antioxidants (including 30 mg of vitamin E) and minerals in the primary prevention of cancer and CVD in 12,375 French men and women age 35 to 60.[30] The results are slated to be published in the *Archives of Internal Medicine* this year (2004); however, according to information released prior to publication, there was no reduction in CVD risk among those taking the vitamin cocktail.

Although lung cancer was the primary endpoint of the Alpha-Tocopherol, Beta-Carotene (ATBC) trial, this trial also provided data on antioxidants and heart disease in more than 20,000 male Finnish smokers. After a median treatment period of 6.1 years, supplementation with synthetic vitamin E (50 mg/day) did not reduce the incidence of lung cancer,[31] and there was no clear reduction in risk of death due to ischemic heart disease ($RR = 0.84$; 95% CI, 0.59–1.19). However, the risk of developing angina was lower among those taking vitamin E ($RR = 0.91$; 95% CI, 0.83–0.99).[32] Initially, it was thought that the lack of convincing beneficial effect may have been due to inadequate dosing of vitamin E or short follow-up time, but post-trial results with 8 more years of follow-up found no effect of α-tocopherol on total mortality ($RR = 1.01$; 95% CI, 0.96–1.05).[33]

Two other primary prevention trials, the Primary Prevention Project (PPP)[34] and the Vitamin E Atherosclerosis Prevention Study (VEAPS),[35] involved larger doses of vitamin E. The PPP was an open-label 2 × 2 factorial trial of 300 mg of synthetic vitamin E and/or 100 mg of low-dose aspirin daily in 4,495 Italian men and women with at least one major risk factor for heart disease. Because of a strong treatment effect for aspirin, the trial was stopped early after a mean follow-up of 3.6 years, but at that time, vitamin E had no effect on reducing the incidence of pre-specified cardiovascular events. It has been suggested that the null findings may have been due to insufficient statistical power.

VEAPS followed the progress of 353 men and women who had LDL cholesterol levels of greater than 130 mg/dL and no clinical symptoms of CVD at baseline for 2 years, 258 of whom continued follow-up for an additional year. The primary endpoint was the rate of change in the common carotid artery far-wall intima-media thickness; there was no difference in the progression of intima-media thickness in those randomized to 400 IU of vitamin E daily versus those randomized to placebo.

Secondary Prevention

The Cambridge Heart Antioxidant Study (CHAOS) assessed 2,002 patients with coronary artery disease who were randomly assigned to receive vitamin E (either 400 or 800 IU/day) or placebo for a median of 510 days.[36] Those taking vitamin E had a lower risk of nonfatal MI ($RR = 0.23$; 95% CI, 0.11–0.47), but they also had a nonsignificant increase in cardiovascular deaths ($RR = 1.18$; 95% CI, 0.62–2.27). The primary endpoint was combined nonfatal MI and CVD death, and vitamin E reduced this risk ($RR = 0.53$; 95% CI, 0.34–0.83). There is no clear explanation for the striking difference between nonfatal and fatal cardiovascular outcomes; however, because of the relatively small number of participants, the placebo group had more men, lower total cholesterol levels, and lower systolic blood pressures, as well as fewer diabetics.

In the Gruppo Italiano per lo Studio della Sopravvivenza nell'Infarto miocardico (GISSI) Prevention Trial, 11,324 patients with a history of acute MI within the last 3 months were randomized in an open-label design to vitamin E (300 mg daily), n-3 polyunsaturated fatty acids (1 g daily), both, or neither over 3.5 years.[37] The primary analysis included cardiovascular death, nonfatal MI, and nonfatal stroke, and vitamin E did not have an effect on this combined endpoint ($RR = 0.98$; 95% CI 0.87–1.10). However, in contrast to the CHAOS study, vitamin E supplementation did have a statistically significant effect on the secondary endpoint of cardiovascular death ($RR = 0.80$; 95% CI 0.65–0.99).

The Heart Outcomes Prevention Evaluation (HOPE) Study randomized 9,541 participants with CVD or diabetes and at least one other cardiovascular risk factor into a study of 400 IU of vitamin E daily, the angiotensin-converting enzyme inhibitor ramipril, both agents, or neither.[38] The study was stopped early after a mean of 4.5 years because of the beneficial effects of ramipril. Vitamin E had no effect on the primary combined endpoint of MI, stroke, and cardiovascular death ($RR = 1.05$; 95% CI 0.95–1.16), and secondary analysis of various cardiovascular endpoints also failed to show any reduced risk with vitamin E. With high rates of compliance and large doses of vitamin E, this study cast doubt on the clinical usefulness of vitamin E supplementation in patients at relatively high risk for a cardiovascular event.

Ongoing Randomized Clinical Trials

Results from the Women's Health Study (WHS), which assessed the effect of 600 IU of vitamin E every other day and low-dose aspirin in nearly 40,000 women over a 12-year period, should be available this year (2004).[39] Another primary prevention trial, the Physicians' Health Study II (PHS II), is evaluating several antioxidants, including 400 IU of vitamin E every other day for 8 years.[40]

The Women's Antioxidant Cardiovascular Study (WACS), scheduled to end in 2005,[41] and the Selenium and Vitamin E Cancer Prevention Trial (SELECT),[42] which has randomized over 30,000 men, are looking at secondary prevention. In WACS, approximately 8,000 high-risk professionals with preexisting CVD or with several coronary risk factors were randomized to 600 IU of natural vitamin E every other day or placebo. The main focus of the SELECT trial is prostate cancer, but it will also evaluate any cardiovascular impact associated with taking 400 IU of vitamin E every other day.

SUMMARY AND CONCLUSIONS

Potential biological mechanisms by which vitamin E supplementation may inhibit atherosclerosis have been identified, and, overall, human observational data are compatible with the possibility that vitamin E intake either from food or supplements may reduce the risk of CVD. Many but not all of the prospective cohort studies examining the role of dietary intake of this antioxidant and CVD suggest an inverse association. However, these studies have important limitations, and caution should be exercised when interpreting the data. For example, bias is inherent in the selection of participants. It is possible that the low incidence of heart disease was actually the result of uncontrolled confounding. People who consume large amounts of fruits and vegetables may have more healthy lifestyles, and diets rich in antioxidants are lower in saturated fat and cholesterol and higher in fiber, which could possibly account for the observed health effects.

Clinical trials of vitamin E alone for primary prevention have not generally supported the observational results. The discrepancy between the observational studies could be the result of some of the limitations of the trials with respect to the dose, the duration, and the specific preparations. The ATBC study was restricted to smokers and may have used a subtherapeutic dose, whereas the follow-up time may have been inadequate in the PPP trial, which was stopped early. Secondary prevention trials have tended to show minimal benefit from vitamin E supplementation. The promising findings of the seminal CHAOS trial have generally not been confirmed in subsequent large trials.

No randomized trial has addressed whether antioxidant vitamins from natural food sources are cardioprotective. Dietary vitamin E is a mixture of tocopherols and tocotrienols, whereas vitamin E supplements generally contain only α-tocopherol. It has been suggested that the absence of other tocopherols, particularly γ-tocopherol, may explain some of the disappointing trial results.[43–45]

Several large-scale trials currently under way will provide additional data to help identify the potential benefits of vitamin E in the primary prevention of CVD as well as other chronic illness. Some of these studies are specifically designed to test the effect of vitamin E alone as well as in combination with other antioxidant supplements because it is possible that antioxidants may be most effective when taken in particular combinations.

At present, according to the American Heart Association (AHA), there is insufficient efficacy data from completed randomized trials to justify establishment of population-wide recommendations regarding the use of vitamin E for disease prevention. Instead, the AHA's dietary guidelines recommend a balanced diet with an emphasis on antioxidant-rich fruits and vegetables and whole grains. The U.S. Preventive Services Task Force indicates that it is "neither for nor against taking vitamins A, C, or E; multivitamins with folic acid; or combinations of these vitamins for the primary purpose of preventing CVD or cancer."[46] In 2002, the influential Institute of Medicine concurred with this recommendation and concluded that available empirical evidence indicates that the relationship between vitamin E supplement use and CHD is "uncertain."

Even if future clinical trials demonstrate that vitamin E supplementation reduces the risk of CVD, the use of these supplements should be considered an adjunct, not an alternative, to other established cardioprotective measures, such as smoking abstension, avoidance of obesity, adequate physical activity, and control of high blood pressure and dyslipidemia.

REFERENCES

1. STEINBERG, D. et al. 1989. Beyond cholesterol: modifications of low-density lipoprotein that increase its atherogenicity. N. Engl. J. Med. **320:** 915–924.
2. HESSLER, J.R. et al. 1983. Lipoprotein oxidation and lipoprotein-induced cytotoxicity. Arteriosclerosis **3:** 215–222.
3. YAGI, K. 1984. Increased serum lipid peroxides initiate atherogenesis. Bioassays **1:** 58–60.
4. GERRITY, R.G. 1981. The role of the monocyte in atherogenesis. I. Transition of blood-borne monocytes into foam cells in fatty lesions. Am. J. Pathol. **103:** 181–190.
5. QUINN, M.T., S. PARTHASARATHY & D. STEINBERG. 1985. Endothelial cell-derived chemotactic activity for mouse peritoneal macrophages and the effects of modified forms of low-density lipoprotein. Proc. Natl. Acad. Sci. USA **82:** 5949–5953.
6. SCHAFFNER, T. et al. 1980. Arterial foam cells with distinctive immunomorphologic and histochemical features of macrophages. Am. J. Pathol. **100:** 57–80.
7. GOLDSTEIN, J.L. et al. 1979. Binding site on macrophages that mediates uptake and degradation of acetylated low-density lipoprotein, producing massive cholesterol deposition. Proc. Natl. Acad. Sci. USA **76:** 333–337.
8. FOGELMAN, A.M. et al. 1980. Malondialdehyde alteration of low-density lipoproteins leads to cholesteryl ester accumulation in human monocyte-macrophages. Proc. Natl. Acad. Sci. USA **77:** 2214–2218.
9. SALONEN, J.T. et al. 1992. Autoantibody against oxidised LDL and progression of carotid atherosclerosis. Lancet **339:** 883–887.
10. BECKMAN, J.S. et al. 1990. Apparent hydroxyl radical production by peroxynitrite: implications for endothelial injury from nitric oxide and superoxide. Proc. Natl. Acad. Sci. USA **87:** 1620–1624.
11. MARCUS, A.J. et al. 1977. Superoxide production and reducing activity in human platelets. J. Clin. Invest. **59:** 149–158.
12. SARAN, M., C. MICHEL & W. BORS. 1990. Reaction of NO with O_2^-: implications for the action of endothelium-derived relaxing factor (EDRF). Free Radic. Res. Commun. **10:** 221–226.
13. WOJCICKI, J. et al. 1991. Effect of selenium and vitamin E on the development of experimental atherosclerosis in rabbits. Atherosclerosis **87:** 9–16.
14. WILLIAMS, R.J. et al. 1992. Dietary vitamin E and the attenuation of early lesion development in modified Watanabe rabbits. Atherosclerosis **94:** 153–159.
15. KEANEY, J.F., JR. et al. 1994. Low-dose alpha-tocopherol improves and high-dose alpha-tocopherol worsens endothelial vasodilator function in cholesterol-fed rabbits. J. Clin. Invest. **93:** 844–851.
16. SMITH, T.L. & F.A. KUMMEROW. 1989. Effect of dietary vitamin E on plasma lipids and atherogenesis in restricted ovulator chickens. Atherosclerosis **75:** 105–109.
17. VERLANGIERI, A.J. & M.J. BUSH. 1992. Effects of d-alpha-tocopherol supplementation on experimentally induced primate atherosclerosis. J. Am. Coll. Nutr. **11:** 131–138.
18. GEY, K.F. & P. PUSKA. 1989. Plasma vitamins E and A inversely correlated to mortality from ischemic heart disease in cross-cultural epidemiology. Ann. N.Y. Acad. Sci. **570:** 268–282.
19. RIEMERSMA, R.A. et al. 1990. Plasma antioxidants and coronary heart disease: vitamins C and E, and selenium. Eur. J. Clin. Nutr. **44:** 143–150.

20. RIEMERSMA, R.A. *et al.* 1989. Low plasma vitamins E and C: increased risk of angina in Scottish men. Ann. N.Y. Acad. Sci. **570:** 291–295.
21. RIEMERSMA, R.A. *et al.* 1991. Risk of angina pectoris and plasma concentrations of vitamins A, C, and E and carotene. Lancet **337:** 1–5.
22. KARDINAAL, A.F. *et al.* 1993. Antioxidants in adipose tissue and risk of myocardial infarction: the EURAMIC Study. Lancet **342:** 1379–1384.
23. STAMPFER, M.J. *et al.* 1993. Vitamin E consumption and the risk of coronary disease in women. N. Engl. J. Med. **328:** 1444–1449.
24. RIMM, E.B. *et al.* 1993. Vitamin E consumption and the risk of coronary heart disease in men. N. Engl. J. Med. **328:** 1450–1456.
25. KUSHI, L.H. *et al.* 1996. Intake of vitamins A, C, and E and postmenopausal breast cancer: the Iowa Women's Health Study. Am. J. Epidemiol. **144:** 165–174.
26. KNEKT, P. *et al.* 1994. Antioxidant vitamin intake and coronary mortality in a longitudinal population study. Am. J. Epidemiol. **139:** 1180–1189.
27. MEYER, F., I. BAIRATI & G.R. DAGENAIS. 1996. Lower ischemic heart disease incidence and mortality among vitamin supplement users. Can. J. Cardiol. **12:** 930–934.
28. LOSONCZY, K.G., T.B. HARRIS & R.J. HAVLIK. 1996. Vitamin E and vitamin C supplement use and risk of all-cause and coronary heart disease mortality in older persons: the Established Populations for Epidemiologic Studies of the Elderly. Am. J. Clin. Nutr. **64:** 190–196.
29. KLIPSTEIN-GROBUSCH, K. *et al.* 1999. Dietary antioxidants and risk of myocardial infarction in the elderly: the Rotterdam Study. Am. J. Clin. Nutr. **69:** 261–266.
30. HERCBERG, S. *et al.* 1998. A primary prevention trial using nutritional doses of antioxidant vitamins and minerals in cardiovascular diseases and cancers in a general population: the SU.VI.MAX study—design, methods, and participant characteristics. SUpplementation en VItamines et Mineraux AntioXydants. Control Clin. Trials **19:** 336–351.
31. The Alpha-Tocopherol Beta Carotene Cancer Prevention Study Group. 1994. The effect of vitamin E and beta-carotene on the incidence of lung cancer and other cancers in male smokers: the Alpha-Tocopherol, Beta-Carotene Cancer Prevention Study Group. N. Engl. J. Med. **330:** 1029–1035.
32. RAPOLA, J.M. *et al.* 1996. Effect of vitamin E and beta-carotene on the incidence of angina pectoris: a randomized, double-blind, controlled trial. J. Am. Med. Assoc. **275:** 693–698.
33. VIRTAMO, J. *et al.* 2003. Incidence of cancer and mortality following alpha-tocopherol and beta-carotene supplementation: a postintervention follow-up. J. Am. Med. Assoc. **290:** 476–485.
34. DE GAETANO, G. 2001. Low-dose aspirin and vitamin E in people at cardiovascular risk: a randomised trial in general practice. Collaborative Group of the Primary Prevention Project. Lancet **357:** 89–95.
35. HODIS, H.N. *et al.* 2002. Alpha-tocopherol supplementation in healthy individuals reduces low-density lipoprotein oxidation but not atherosclerosis: the Vitamin E Atherosclerosis Prevention Study (VEAPS). Circulation **106:** 1453–1459.
36. STEPHENS, N.G. *et al.* 1996. Randomised controlled trial of vitamin E in patients with coronary disease: Cambridge Heart Antioxidant Study (CHAOS). Lancet **347:** 781–786.
37. The GISSI-Prevenzione Investigators. 1999. Dietary supplementation with n-3 polyunsaturated fatty acids and vitamin E after myocardial infarction: results of the GISSI-Prevenzione trial. Gruppo Italiano per lo Studio della Sopravvivenza nell'Infarto miocardico. Lancet **354:** 447–455.
38. YUSUF, S. *et al.* 2000. Vitamin E supplementation and cardiovascular events in high-risk patients: the Heart Outcomes Prevention Evaluation Study Investigators. N. Engl. J. Med. **342:** 154–160.
39. BURING, J.E. & C.H. HENNEKENS (for the Women's Health Study Research Group). 1992. The Women's Health Study: summary of the study design. J. Myocard. Isch. **4:** 27–29.
40. CHRISTEN, W.G., J.M. GAZIANO & C.H. HENNEKENS. 2000. Design of Physicians' Health Study II: a randomized trial of beta-carotene, vitamins E and C, and multivi-

tamins, in prevention of cancer, cardiovascular disease, and eye disease, and review of results of completed trials. Ann. Epidemiol. **10:** 125–134.
41. MANSON, J.E. *et al.* 1995. A secondary prevention trial of antioxidant vitamins and cardiovascular disease in women: rationale, design, and methods. The WACS Research Group. Ann. Epidemiol. **5:** 261–269.
42. KLEIN, E.A. *et al.* 2001. SELECT: the next prostate cancer prevention trial. Selenum and Vitamin E Cancer Prevention Trial. J. Urol. **166:** 1311–1315.
43. JIANG, Q. *et al.* 2001. Gamma-tocopherol, the major form of vitamin E in the U.S. diet, deserves more attention. Am. J. Clin. Nutr. **74:** 714–722.
44. LIU, M. *et al.* 2003. Mixed tocopherols inhibit platelet aggregation in humans: potential mechanisms. Am. J. Clin. Nutr. **77:** 700–706.
45. DEVARAJ, S. & M.G. TRABER. 2003. Gamma-tocopherol, the new vitamin E? Am. J. Clin. Nutr. **77:** 530–531.
46. 2003. Summaries for patients taking vitamin supplements to prevent cardiovascular disease and cancer: recommendations from the U.S. Preventive Services Task Force. Ann. Intern. Med. **139:** I-76.

Vitamin E for the Treatment of Cardiovascular Disease

Is There a Future?

FRANCESCO VIOLI,[a] ROBERTO CANGEMI,[a] GIUSEPPE SABATINO,[b] AND PASQUALE PIGNATELLI[a]

[a]*IV Division of Clinical Medicine, Department of Experimental Medicine and Pathology, University of Rome "La Sapienza," Italy*

[b]*University of Chieti "G. D'Annunzio," Italy*

ABSTRACT: Oxidative stress seems to play a key role in the pathogenesis of atherosclerosis. Agents that protect low-density lipoprotein from oxidation have been shown in a range of *in vitro* and animal models to reduce the development and progression of atherosclerosis. These agents include antioxidant micronutrients such as vitamin E. They have gained wide interest because of the potential for prevention of atherosclerotic vascular disease in humans. In the last decade, many trials with antioxidants have been carried out in patients with cardiovascular disease, but the results are equivocal. The reason for the disappointing findings is unclear, but one possible explanation is the lack of identification criteria of patients who are potential candidates for antioxidant treatment. This review analyses the data reported so far to determine whether they clearly support the premise that patients at risk of cardiovascular disease may be candidates for antioxidant treatment.

KEYWORDS: oxidative stress; atherosclerosis; vitamin E; antioxidant; cardiovascular disease.

INTRODUCTION

Oxidative stress is believed to play a crucial role in the initiation and progression of atherosclerosis. Oxidation of low-density lipoprotein (LDL) within the vessel wall represents a key step in the accumulation of LDL by resistant macrophages that ultimately become the foam cells of atherosclerotic plaque.[1] Oxidation of LDL, whether enzymatic or non-enzymatic, seems to be involved in this process; however, its relevance in the evolution of human atherosclerosis is still unclear.[1] An important consideration is the evident discrepancy between experimental and clinical trials with antioxidants, trials that have provided divergent results. Most trials with antioxidants in experimental models of atherosclerosis have demonstrated that this treatment is able to retard the progression of atherosclerosis, whereas the results of

---

Address for correspondence: Professor Francesco Violi, IV Divisione di Clinica Medica, Viale del Policlinico 155, Roma, 00161, Italy. Voice: +39-064461933; fax +39-0649970102.
francesco.violi@uniroma1.it

clinical trials are conflicting,[1] inasmuch as positive as well as negative effects have been reported. Investigation of antioxidants for prevention of atherosclerosis stems from observational trials that demonstrated the existence of an inverse relation between the consumption of antioxidant vitamins and the risk of cardiovascular events. However, meta-analysis of the observational studies indicated that among antioxidant vitamins, vitamin E was the only one that exerted a beneficial effect against atherosclerotic complications.[2] On the basis of these data, almost all the trials have assumed that supplementation with vitamin E would represent a useful approach for preventing cardiovascular disease (CVD). However, candidates for antioxidant treatment were not accurately defined: any patient at risk of cardiovascular events has been indiscriminately enrolled in those trials. We argue, on the contrary, that as antioxidant status represents an important marker of oxidative stress,[3] its determination may useful for better identifying candidates for antioxidant treatment. To substantiate this hypothesis, data inherent to oxidative stress and antioxidant status in patients at risk for CVD and in patients included in observational and interventional trials have been reviewed. The antioxidant vitamin E has been the subject of the most important research in this field. Our analysis is essentially concentrated on the clinical relevance of this vitamin in patients with CVD.

CVD RISK FACTORS AND OXIDATIVE STRESS

The Framingham studies have demonstrated how hypercholesterolemia, hypertension, diabetes mellitus, cigarette smoking, elevated plasma homocysteine concentrations, aging, and their combination are associated with the atherosclerotic diseases.[4] We should like to pay attention to the association of all these CVD risk factors with oxidative stress.

Free radical formation can mediate some of the effects of hypertension. Several studies strongly suggested that enhanced oxidative stress might represent an important trigger for atherogenesis elicited by angiotensin II. Angiotensin II, which is often present in elevated concentrations in patients with hypertension, is a potent vasoconstrictor. It also increases smooth-muscle hypertrophy and lipoxygenase activity that, in turn, can increase inflammation and the oxidation of LDL.

Griendling and colleagues[5] examined the effect of angiotensin II on superoxide anion (O_2^-) production by smooth muscle cells and demonstrated that exposure of these cells to angiotensin II elicited enhanced production of O_2^-. This effect was mediated by NADH and NADPH oxidase activation, probably via intracellular mobilization of fatty acids such as arachidonic acid. These data have important pathophysiologic implications due to the effect of O_2^- on vascular motility. The oxidative stress may have a role in hypertensive patients, in whom a reduced vasodilating response to acetylcholine has been demonstrated. Thus, in patients with hypertension, the administration of the antioxidant vitamin C has been able to restore acetylcholine-induced vasorelaxation, suggesting a role for oxygen free radicals in inducing vascular dysfunction in patients with hypertension.[6]

Blood analysis of lipid peroxides or measurement of urinary excretion of isoprostanes provided evidence that oxidative stress is enhanced in patients with diabetes.[7] The impact of these data in the context of atherosclerosis progression is still unclear, but there is some evidence supporting a role for oxidative stress in contributing to deteriorative vascular disease. For instance, an important finding is the demonstration that endothelium-dependent vasodilation is reduced in patients with diabetes and that vitamin C is able to prevent it.[8]

Hyperglycemia may enhance oxidative stress and in turn induce vascular damage via several pathways, including the formation of the advanced glycated end products that are proatherogenic and prothrombotic substance. Furthermore, glucose may alter the balance between free radicals such as O_2^- and NO in endothelial cells; thus, NO exerts its vasodilatory and antioxidant effect unless it is converted to ONOO$^-$ by interaction with O_2^0. This deleterious effect occurs in endothelial cells exposed to glucose. In fact, it favors the formation of O_2^- and in turn promotes oxidation.[9]

Hyperglycemia was shown to enhance endothelial O_2^- generation via activation of the cyclooxygenase pathway, which is believed to generate reactive oxygen species (ROS) with a mechanism involving NAD(P)H oxidase.[10] Guzik and colleagues found vascular expression of NAD(P)H oxidase subunits p22 phox and p47 phox were overexpressed in diabetic patients.[11]

Both experimental and clinical results indicate that hypercholesterolemia is associated with enhanced oxidative stress. Elevated levels of oxygen free radicals, such as O_2^-, and F_2-isoprostanes, have been found in the artery of hypercholesterolemic animals and in the urine of patients with high serum cholesterol, respectively.[12,13]

Two hypotheses may help explain why hypercholesterolemia enhances oxidative stress. Cholesterol has been recently shown to activate the metabolism of the arachidonic acid pathway.[14] This pathway, in turn, seems to be associated with NAD(P)H oxidase activation.[10] The cascade of cholesterol biosynthesis may represent another pathway leading to enhanced oxidative stress. Intracellular metabolism of mevalonate leads, in fact, to the formation of protein isoprenylation, which has a key role in the production of proinflammatory and pro-oxidant cytokines such as tumor necrosis factor-α (TNF-α).[15] Accordingly, treatment of hypercholesterolemic patients with an inhibitor of HMG-CoA-reductase was associated with reduced monocyte formation of TNF-α[16] and reduced the urinary excretion of 8-iso-prostaglandin $F_{2\alpha}$,[17] suggesting a relationship between cholesterol and intracellular formation of pro-oxidant cytokines. Cigarette smoke contains large amounts of free radicals that may degrade nitric oxide release from the endothelium and also produce highly reactive intermediates resulting in endothelial injury. Morrow and colleagues[18] found that the plasma concentrations and urinary excretion of F_2-isoprostane were significantly higher in smokers than in nonsmokers and that cessation of smoking was associated with a significant decrease of isoprostanes.[18]

CVD RISK FACTORS AND ANTIOXIDANT STATUS

Several studies[19-24] measured the circulating concentrations of vitamins E in patients with risk factors for atherosclerosis. However, data are extremely variable and difficult to interpret because of the lack of control groups. Vitamin E has been measured in smokers with hypertension, diabetes, and hypercholesterolemia. In patients with risk factors for atherosclerosis, a wide variability of values was found also within the same category of patients. Considering the fact that values > 5 µmol/mmol cholesterol are found in healthy people, the patients with risk factors showed values ranging from 1.6 to 5.8.[25] The reason for this large variability cannot be explained as yet, but it is possible that oxidative stress may condition the rate of vitamin consumption. This hypothesis may be supported by a previous study showing an inverse correlation between F_2-isoprostanes and circulating concentrations of vitamin E,[26] but we are not certain that elevated markers of oxidative stress are always associated with low antioxidant status.

Recently, plasma levels of vitamin E and urinary isoprostane have been reported in a population with and without type 2 diabetes.[27] Compared with patients without diabetes ($n = 650$), those with diabetes ($n = 112$) had lower plasma levels of vitamin E and higher urinary isoprostanes. A surprising finding of the study was the absence of any correlation between vitamin E and oxidative stress. Also surprising was the demonstration that in the early stage of diabetes, vitamin E was low whereas oxidative stress was not; conversely, in the late stage of diabetes, vitamin E was normal whereas oxidative stress was elevated. The clinical and biological plausibility of these data is unclear; therefore, further study is necessary to explore antioxidant status and oxidative stress in diabetes patients.

A recent report showed that in animals with cardiovascular aging, which is associated with enhanced oxidative stress, circulating and tissue concentrations of vitamin E were elevated.[28] If it may be assumed that this might also occur in human atherosclerosis, the evidence of enhanced oxidant stress alone perhaps does not imply the existence of low antioxidant status or justify supplementation with antioxidant vitamins.

Unfortunately, the majority of previous studies exploring oxidative stress in patients with classic risk factors for atherosclerosis included very little information regarding vitamin E plasma concentrations and antioxidant status in control populations. This limits the clinical usefulness of those studies because we are not certain that, in the case of enhanced oxidative stress, antioxidant treatment is warranted. The reason for the wide variation of antioxidant status in patients at risk of CVD is unclear, but it should be carefully investigated to justify the use of antioxidant supplements in this context.

OBSERVATIONAL STUDIES

CVD and Antioxidant Plasma Levels

Many observational epidemiologic studies have evaluated potential relationships between antioxidant status and CVD. To this purpose, in the past 10 years, studies to assess the relationship between CVD and plasma levels of different antioxidants, such as vitamins E and C and β-carotene, were performed (TABLE 1).

The WHO/MONICA (Monitoring of Trends and Determinants in Cardiovascular Disease) project has been one of the largest studies that analyzed the behavior of these vitamins in populations with different incidence values of coronary heart disease (CHD) mortality.[29] In populations with similar values of serum cholesterol and blood pressure, an inverse correlation between CHD mortality and vitamin E plasma levels was observed; conversely, no relation existed between CHD mortality and other vitamins. In areas with low and medium coronary mortality, plasma levels of vitamin E were 26–28 µM; in areas with frequent CHD mortality, plasma levels were 20–21.5 µM. Gey et al. also estimated that the threshold risk for CVD would be

TABLE 1. Observational studies: cardiovascular disease and antioxidant plasma levels

Observational Studies	Patients' Characteristics	Year	Data Analyzed
WHO/ MONICA Project[29]	More than 100,000 middle-aged men	1991	CHD mortality and vitamin E plasma levels
Riemersma et al.[32]	110 cases of angina, 394 controls	1991	History of angina and plasma concentrations of vitamins
Singh et al.[33]	Cross-sectional survey within a random sample of 595 elderly people (72 with CHD)	1995	Coronary artery disease and plasma levels of vitamins
Feki at al.[34]	62 angiographically confirmed coronary atherosclerotic patients and 65 age- and sex-matched controls	2000	Coronary artery disease and vitamin E plasma levels
Mezzetti et al.[35]	102 apparently healthy subjects age 80 and older, followed-up for 47.4 months	2002	Cardiovascular events and vitamin E plasma levels

<25 µM. In this particular population, that threshold corresponds to <4.3 µmol vitamin E/mmol cholesterol. This finding is consistent with other studies showing an inverse correlation between vitamin E plasma levels and cardiovascular mortality.[30] It was noticed, in particular, that in persons with high risk for cardiovascular mortality the vitamin E/cholesterol ratio was 3.5, whereas in persons with low risk the ratio was almost 5.[31] The inverse correlation between vitamin E levels and CHD was also noted in another observational study. In this study, 110 patients with angina were compared to 394 controls.[32] The study demonstrated that patients with a history of angina had a lower vitamin E/cholesterol ratio than controls with a significant adjusted odds ratio for angina between patients in the lowest and highest quartiles.

In a cross-sectional survey within a random sample of a single urban setting in India, the relation between risk of coronary artery disease (CAD) and plasma levels of vitamins A, C, and E and β-carotene was examined in 595 elderly subjects. Plasma levels of vitamins C and E appeared significantly inversely related to CAD. The adjusted odds ratio for CAD between the lowest and the highest quintiles of vitamin E levels was 2.53 after adjustment for confounding variables.[33]

Another study, designed to assess the degree of association between vitamin E and CHD in a sample of the Tunisian population, included 62 angiographically confirmed coronary atherosclerotic patients and 65 age- and sex-matched controls. A trend towards a meaningful decrease of plasma tocopherol was observed in affected patients compared with controls ($P = .06$). This association between vitamin E and CHD remained unchanged independent of age, sex, smoking habit, hypertension, and diabetes.[34]

These findings have been further corroborated by another study, one in which the progress of 102 apparently healthy subjects was followed for 47.4 months.[35] A higher risk of cardiovascular events in subjects in the lowest quartile of vitamin E plasma levels compared to those in the highest was shown.

Atherogenesis and Antioxidant Plasma Levels

Few data are available on the importance of antioxidant vitamins in the earlier stages of atherogenesis. Gale and colleagues[36] investigated the relation between antioxidant vitamin status and carotid atherosclerosis in a group of 468 elderly people. Compared with those with high levels of vitamin E, men with low blood concentrations of cholesterol-adjusted vitamin E were 2.5 times as likely to have carotid stenosis of >30%. The results of a few similar studies provided limited support for the hypothesis that increased plasma tocopherol may decrease the risk of atherosclerosis.[37,38]

In a more recent study, the association between preclinical carotid atherosclerosis (accounting for both the intake and plasma concentrations of antioxidant vitamins) was evaluated. Among the 5,062 participants in Progetto Atena, a population-based study on the etiology of CVD and cancer in women, 310 women were examined by B-mode ultrasound to detect early signs of carotid atherosclerosis. The participants answered a food-frequency questionnaire, and their plasma concentrations of vitamins were measured. Both vitamin E intake and the ratio of plasma vitamin E to plasma cholesterol were inversely associated with occurrence of atherosclerotic plaques at the carotid bifurcation. No association was found with the intake of other antioxidant vitamins or their plasma concentrations.[39]

These findings are at variance with a recent study that measured antioxidant status and carotid intima-media thickness in a population that was free of CVD.[40] After 18 months of follow-up, progression of intima-media thickness was inversely related to three oxygenated carotenoids and to α-carotene. In this study, neither vitamin C nor vitamin E was associated with atherosclerosis progression. However, plasma levels of these two vitamins raise some doubt over the validity of these findings. For instance, the highest quintiles of vitamin E (from 38 to 100 μM) and C (from 43 to 200 μM) are hardly achievable even after supplementation with high doses of these vitamins.

Taken together, these data suggest that vitamin E may be an important predictor of CHD and may represent an independent risk factor for atherosclerosis and its complication. Because of the lack of standardization and a somewhat large dispersion of vitamin E/cholesterol ratio values, accurate analysis of vitamin E levels in patients and healthy subjects is crucial in order to have a reliable use of this variable in clinical practice and interventional trials. The increasing interest in antioxidant vitamins for the assessment of risk for CVD strongly suggests a need for standardization assays.

INTERVENTIONAL TRIALS

Although most epidemiologic studies have demonstrated that dietary intake of vitamin E is inversely related to coronary heart complications, supplementation studies have given conflicting results. Clinical trials with antioxidants have been done in patients with or without previous history of CVD. Surrogate endpoints, such as anal-

TABLE 2. Randomized trials of vitamin E treatment

Trial	Patients' Characteristics	Number in Treatment Group		Dose	Follow-up (yr)	Results
		Antioxidant	Control			
ATBC[42]	1862 male smokers, 50–69 yrs old, who had a previous MI	963	799	Vit E, 50 mg	5.3	Vitamin E showed no effect
CHAOS[43]	Median age 62 yr; angiographically proven CAD; 84% male ($n=2002$)	1035	967	Vit E, 400–800 IU	1.4	Vitamin E treatment substantially reduced rate of non-fatal MI
GISSI[45]	Survivors of recent MI (<3 months); 85% male ($n=11,324$)	5660	5664	Vit E, 300 mg	3.5	Vitamin E showed no effect
HOPE[46]	Mean age 66 yr; known cardiovascular disease or diabetes; 73% male ($n=9541$)	4761	4780	Vit E, 400 IU	4.5	Vitamin E showed no effect
SPACE[47]	Hemodialysis patients with pre-existing cardiovascular disease ($n=196$) aged 40–75 years	97	99	Vit E, 800 IU	1.4	Vitamin E reduced composite CVD endpoints and MI
HPS[50]	Age range 40–80 years; known vascular disease or at-risk of vascular disease; 75% male ($n=20\,536$)	10269	10267	Vit E, 600 mg; Vit C, 250 mg	5	Vitamin E showed no effect
PPP[51]	Primary prevention in patients with at least one risk factor; age range 55–80 years; ($n=4495$)	2231	2264	Vit E 300 mg	3,6	Results on vitamin E are not conclusive
Fang et al.[52]	40 patients (0-2 years after cardiac transplantation)	19	21	Vit E, 800 IU; Vit C, 1 g	1	Antioxidants retarded early progression of transplant-associated coronary arteriosclerosis
ASAP[53]	520 men and postmenopausal women aged 45 to 69 yr with serum cholesterol ≥5.0 mmol/L	390	130	Vit E, 272 IU; Vit C, 500 mg	6	Vitamins C and E retard atherosclerotic progression

ysis of atherosclerosis progression, or hard endpoints, such as vascular death and myocardial infarction, have been examined for evaluating the clinical benefit of antioxidant vitamins (TABLE 2). The ATBC[41] prevention study was a randomized, placebo-controlled, primary-prevention trial to determine whether daily supplementation with α-tocopherol, β-carotene, or both reduced the incidence of lung cancer over 29,133 male smokers. The result of this trial showed no beneficial effect of supplemental vitamin E (α-tocopherol) or β-carotene in terms of the prevention of lung cancer, but the authors observed a reduction for death due to cardiovascular events in the group treated with α-tocopherol. For this reason, the authors extended their analysis to study the clinical efficacy of 50 mg/day of vitamin E in a population suffering from coronary heart disease. This population showed no changes with respect to cardiovascular events during the follow-up.[42]

The Cambridge Heart Antioxidant Study (CHAOS) tested the hypothesis if treatment with a high dose of α-tocopherol would reduce subsequent risk of myocardial infarction and cardiovascular death in patients with established ischemic heart disease. The study included 2002 patients with angiographically proven coronary atherosclerosis, and they were assigned α-tocopherol (800 IU or 400 UI daily) or placebo. The patients had their progress followed for a median of 510 days. This trial showed that in patients with symptomatic coronary atherosclerosis, α-tocopherol treatment substantially reduced the rate of nonfatal myocardial infarction, with beneficial effects apparent after 1 year of treatment. However, no significant reduction in fatal myocardial infarction was recorded.[43,44]

The GISSI-Prevenzione trial[45] assessed the efficacy of vitamin E and n-3 polyunsaturated fatty acids (PUFAs) on cardiovascular death, nonfatal myocardial infarction, or stroke in patients with recent myocardial infarction. In this study, 11,324 patients were randomly assigned supplements of n-3 PUFAs (1 g daily), vitamin E (300 mg daily), both, or none for 3.5 years. The primary combined efficacy endpoint encompassed death, nonfatal myocardial infarction, and stroke outcomes. Intention-to-treat analyses were done according to a factorial design (two-way) and by treatment group (four-way). Treatment with n-3 PUFAs significantly lowered the risk of the primary endpoint in the two- and four-way analyses. By contrast with the results for n-3 PUFAs, the results for vitamin E did not provide evidence of efficacy, although it was possible to see a significant decrease of cardiovascular deaths in the four-way analysis. Moreover, 300 mg/day of synthetic vitamin E daily (which is equivalent to about 150 mg natural vitamin E[25]) is below the range in which clinical trials report positive results.

Similarly, the Heart Outcomes Prevention Evaluation (HOPE) Study was a double-blind, randomized trial, conducted to evaluate the effects of ramipril and vitamin E in 9,541 patients at high risk for cardiovascular events. Patients were randomly assigned to receive either 400 IU of vitamin E from natural sources or an equivalent placebo daily for 4 to 6 years. In this study, vitamin E did not reduce the incidence of cardiovascular events, as compared with the incidence among patients assigned to placebo, during the follow-up period.[46]

The Secondary Prevention with Antioxidants of Cardiovascular Disease in End-stage Renal Disease (SPACE) Trial[47] investigated the effect of high-dose vitamin E supplementation on CVD outcomes in hemodialysis patients with preexisting CVD. This population was chosen because it is well established that patients undergoing chronic hemodialysis are exposed to increased oxidative stress induced by the membranes used in dialysis.[48,49] In this study, 196 patients were randomized to receive 800 IU/day vitamin E or matching placebo and had their progress followed for a median 519 days. The primary endpoint was a composite variable consisting of myocardial infarction, ischemic stroke, peripheral vascular disease, and unstable angina. Among hemodialysis patients treated with high-dose vitamin E, a 54% reduction was attained in the primary endpoint, contributed to largely by the reduction in total myocardial infarction (70%). The study was small, but the results are suggestive. Antioxidant therapy would be expected to have a greater treatment effect on patients in greater oxidative stress, and hemodialysis patients are in greater oxidative stress than other patient groups.[47] The accelerated cardiovascular disease event rate observed in hemodialysis patients, contributed to by increased oxidative stress, was shown to be reduced by antioxidant therapy.

A negative result came from the Heart Protection Study (HPS) trial, which included 20,536 adults from the United Kingdom. These participants had coronary disease, other occlusive arterial disease, or diabetes and were randomly allocated to receive antioxidant vitamin supplementation (600 mg of vitamin E, 250 mg of vitamin C, and 20 mg of β-carotene daily) or matching placebo. This vitamin regimen approximately doubled the plasma concentration of α-tocopherol, increased that of vitamin C by one-third, and quadrupled that of β-carotene. After a 5-year treatment period, there were no significant differences in all-cause mortality or in myocardial infarction or coronary death or in stroke between the two groups of participants.[50]

In addition to secondary prevention studies (which included patients with documented or known vascular disease), the Primary Prevention Project (PPP) studied the efficacy of vitamin E among patients who had one or more cardiovascular risk factors (hypertension, diabetes, or early family history of coronary disease). In this study, 4,495 people were randomly allocated to receive aspirin (100 mg) or no aspirin, and vitamin E or no vitamin E. After a mean follow-up period of 3.6 years, the trial was prematurely stopped on ethical grounds when newly available evidence from other trials documented the benefit of aspirin in primary prevention. Vitamin E showed no effect on any pre-specified endpoint, even if the findings could be regarded as a false-negative result, because of the inadequate power of a prematurely interrupted trial.[51]

The effect of antioxidant vitamins was also investigated using surrogate endpoints such as carotid atherosclerotic progression. Fang and colleagues[52] tested the effect of vitamin E (400 UI × 2) plus vitamin C (500 mg × 2) in 40 patients 0–2 years after cardiac transplantation. The primary endpoint was the change in average intimal index (plaque area divided by vessel area) measured by intravascular ultrasonography. During 1 year of treatment, the intimal index increased in the placebo group by 8% (SE 2%) but did not change significantly in the treatment group. Despite the small sample size, which was due to the limited number of patients that undergo this procedure, the study was of particular interest because cardiac transplantation is associated with oxidative stress, which may contribute to the development of accelerated coronary arteriosclerosis.

The Antioxidant Supplementation in Atherosclerosis Prevention (ASAP) Study[53] demonstrated that a combination of 136 IU vitamin E plus 250 mg of slow-release vitamin C twice daily slows down atherosclerotic progression in hypercholesterolemic patients. The subjects included 520 smoking and nonsmoking men and postmenopausal women aged 45 to 69 years with serum cholesterol <5.0 mmol/L. The progression of common carotid artery (CCA) atherosclerosis was carried out by high-resolution ultrasonography. After 6 years of follow-up, covariance analysis revealed that in both sexes, supplementation reduced the main study outcome, the slope of mean CCA intima-media thickness, by 26%. It was of note that the treatment was more effective in patients with low baseline values of vitamin C.

Most trials with antioxidants used vitamin E likely because epidemiologic studies documented that regular consumption of this vitamin reduced the risk of cardiovascular events.[2] Patient selection of these trials was therefore based on the hypothesis that all patients at risk of CVD could have benefits from supplementation with this vitamin. Therefore, many primary and secondary interventional trials, such the GISSI-prevenzione, the HOPE, and the PPP studies, did not consider antioxidant status as entry criterion and did not report any data inherent to bioavailability of vitamin E.[45,46,51] The lack of information on antioxidant status and vitamin E availability complicates the interpretation of the results of these trials. We demonstrated, in fact, that about 30% of subjects did not have any increase of vitamin E plasma levels unless vitamin E was consumed after food intake.[31] This finding has been recently supported by Carroll and Schade,[54] who showed a significant increment of plasma vitamin E when supplement was given immediately before meals. Among antioxidant trials, six reported plasma values of vitamin E in control population.[42,43,47,50,52,53] Assuming that values of vitamin E <5 μmol/mmol cholesterol identify patients at risk for CVD,[25] we argue that only three studies included patients with low antioxidant status. Among these trials, the ATBC provided negative results, whereas the other two studies[47,52] demonstrated that vitamin E alone or in combination with vitamin C significantly reduced cardiovascular events.

CONCLUSION

On the basis of these considerations, we can conclude that there is compelling evidence that enhanced oxidative stress is detectable in patients with classic risk factors for atherosclerosis, but its impact in the context of atherosclerosis progression is still unclear. This uncertainty is due to the lack of a clear prospective study indicating that markers of oxidative stress, such as blood lipid peroxides or urinary F_2-isoprostanes, are of some value for predicting the progression of atherosclerosis, even if there some evidence suggesting that antibodies against oxidized LDL may be of some utility.[26] Conversely, epidemiologic studies seem to indicate that low antioxidant status increases the risk for CVD. Clinical characteristics of patients with low antioxidant status have not been defined and should be studied in the future. So far, clinical trials with antioxidants have included patients without evaluating either oxidative stress or antioxidant status. Such indiscriminate enrollment could account for the negative results of antioxidant trials recently emphasized by meta-analysis.[55]

Moreover, as Steinberg and Witztum recently discussed,[1] the antioxidants might be effective in inhibiting the initial stages of human atherosclerosis and yet be ineffective or much less effective in reducing plaque instability and rupture. If this were the case, it might be necessary to find some way to assess early stages of lesion development (perhaps by high-resolution ultrasound or magnetic resonance imaging) rather than relying on the usual late clinical endpoints. Of course, if the development of early lesions were successfully inhibited, there should eventually be a decrease in the frequency of clinical events, but in that case, the trials might need to extend beyond the conventional 5 years.

Another issue that deserves further attention is the choice of appropriate antioxidant treatment. So far, several mechanisms, including enzymatic and non-enzymatic oxidation of LDL, have been proposed, but the exact process leading to LDL accumulation within the vessel wall is still unclear. This fact creates uncertainty in the type of antioxidants that could be relevant for inhibiting atherosclerotic progress. Thus, future trials with antioxidants should not be discouraged; conversely, better identification of criteria identifying potential candidates for antioxidant treatment, together with the choice of an adequate daily regimen of antioxidants, should be studied.

REFERENCES

1. STEINBERG, D. & J.L. WITZTUM. 2002. Is the oxidative modification hypothesis relevant to human atherosclerosis? Do the antioxidant trials conducted to date refute the hypothesis? Circulation **105:** 2107–2111.
2. JHA, P. et al. 1995. The antioxidant vitamins and cardiovascular disease: a critical review of epidemiologic and clinical trial data. Ann. Intern. Med. **123:** 860–872.
3. VIOLI, F., F. MICHELETTA & L. IULIANO. 2002. How to select patient candidates for antioxidant treatment? Circulation **106:** e195 [author reply e195].
4. PEARSON, T.A. 2002. New tools for coronary risk assessment: what are their advantages and limitations? Circulation **105:** 886–892.
5. GRIENDLING, K.K. et al. 1994. Angiotensin II stimulates NADH and NADPH oxidase activity in cultured vascular smooth muscle cells. Circ. Res. **74:** 1141–1148.
6. TADDEI, S. et al. 1998. Vitamin C improves endothelium-dependent vasodilation by restoring nitric oxide activity in essential hypertension. Circulation **97:** 2222–2229.
7. MEZZETTI, A., F. CIPOLLONE & F. CUCCURULLO. 2000. Oxidative stress and cardiovascular complications in diabetes: isoprostanes as new markers on an old paradigm. Cardiovasc. Res. **47:** 475–488.
8. TIMIMI, F.K. et al. 1998. Vitamin C improves endothelium-dependent vasodilation in patients with insulin-dependent diabetes mellitus. J. Am. Coll. Cardiol. **31:** 552–557.
9. COSENTINO, F. et al. 1997. High glucose increases nitric oxide synthase expression and superoxide anion generation in human aortic endothelial cells. Circulation **96:** 25–28.
10. WOLIN, M.S. 2000. Interactions of oxidants with vascular signaling systems. Arterioscler. Thromb. Vasc. Biol. **20:** 1430–1442.
11. GUZIK, T.J. et al. 2002. Mechanisms of increased vascular superoxide production in human diabetes mellitus: role of NAD(P)H oxidase and endothelial nitric oxide synthase. Circulation **105:** 1656–1662.
12. OHARA, Y. et al. 1995. Dietary correction of hypercholesterolemia in the rabbit normalizes endothelial superoxide anion production. Circulation **92:** 898–903.
13. DAVI, G. et al. 1997. In vivo formation of 8-Epi-prostaglandin F2 alpha is increased in hypercholesterolemia. Arterioscler. Thromb. Vasc. Biol. **17:** 3230–3235.
14. SANGUIGNI, V. et al. 2002. Increased superoxide anion production by platelets in hypercholesterolemic patients. Thromb. Haemost. **87:** 796–801.
15. TAKEMOTO, M. & J.K. LIAO. 2001. Pleiotropic effects of 3-hydroxy-3-methylglutaryl coenzyme a reductase inhibitors. Arterioscler. Thromb. Vasc. Biol. **21:** 1712–1719.
16. FERRO, D. et al. 2000. Simvastatin inhibits the monocyte expression of proinflammatory cytokines in patients with hypercholesterolemia. J. Am. Coll. Cardiol. **36:** 427–431.
17. DE CATERINA, R. et al. 2002. Low-density lipoprotein level reduction by the 3-hydroxy-3-methylglutaryl coenzyme-A inhibitor simvastatin is accompanied by a related reduction of F_2-isoprostane formation in hypercholesterolemic subjects: no further effect of vitamin E. Circulation **106:** 2543–2549.

18. MORROW, J.D. et al. 1995. Increase in circulating products of lipid peroxidation (F_2-isoprostanes) in smokers. Smoking as a cause of oxidative damage. N. Engl. J. Med. **332:** 1198–1203.
19. WEN, Y. et al. 1996. Lipid peroxidation and antioxidant vitamins C and E in hypertensive patients. Ir. J. Med. Sci. **165:** 210–212.
20. PIERDOMENICO, S.D. et al. 1998. Low-density lipoprotein oxidation and vitamins E and C in sustained and white-coat hypertension. Hypertension **31:** 621–626.
21. TSUCHIYA, M. et al. 2002. Smoking a single cigarette rapidly reduces combined concentrations of nitrate and nitrite and concentrations of antioxidants in plasma. Circulation **105:** 1155–1157.
22. MAXWELL, S.R. et al. 1997. Antioxidant status in patients with uncomplicated insulin-dependent and non-insulin-dependent diabetes mellitus. Eur. J. Clin. Invest. **27:** 484–490.
23. LEONHARDT, W. et al. 1996. Impact of concentrations of glycated hemoglobin, alpha-tocopherol, copper, and manganese on oxidation of low-density lipoproteins in patients with type I diabetes, type II diabetes and control subjects. Clin. Chim. Acta **254:** 173–186.
24. NOUROOZ-ZADEH, J., C.C. SMITH & D.J. BETTERIDGE. 2001. Measures of oxidative stress in heterozygous familial hypercholesterolaemia. Atherosclerosis **156:** 435–441.
25. PRYOR, W.A. 2000. Vitamin E and heart disease: basic science to clinical intervention trials. Free Radic. Biol. Med. **28:** 141–164.
26. PRATICO, D. et al. 1998. Vitamin E suppresses isoprostane generation in vivo and reduces atherosclerosis in ApoE-deficient mice. Nat. Med. **4:** 1189–1192.
27. HELMERSSON, J. et al. 2004. Association of type 2 diabetes with cyclooxygenase-mediated inflammation and oxidative stress in an elderly population. Circulation **109:** 1729–1734.
28. VAN DER LOO, B. et al. 2002. Cardiovascular aging is associated with vitamin E increase. Circulation **105:** 1635–1638.
29. GEY, K.F. et al. 1991. Inverse correlation between plasma vitamin E and mortality from ischemic heart disease in cross-cultural epidemiology. Am. J. Clin. Nutr. **53:** 326S–334S.
30. GEY, K.F. 1994. Optimum plasma levels of antioxidant micronutrients: ten years of antioxidant hypothesis on arteriosclerosis. Bibl. Nutr. Diet. :84–99.
31. IULIANO, L. et al. 2001. Bioavailability of vitamin E as function of food intake in healthy subjects: effects on plasma peroxide-scavenging activity and cholesterol-oxidation products. Arterioscler. Thromb. Vasc. Biol. **21:** E34–E37.
32. RIEMERSMA, R.A. et al. 1991. Risk of angina pectoris and plasma concentrations of vitamins A, C, and E and carotene. Lancet **337:** 1–5.
33. SINGH, R.B. et al. 1995. Dietary intake, plasma levels of antioxidant vitamins, and oxidative stress in relation to coronary artery disease in elderly subjects. Am. J. Cardiol. **76:** 1233–1238.
34. FEKI, M. et al. 2000. Vitamin E and coronary heart disease in Tunisians. Clin. Chem. **46:** 1401–1405.
35. MEZZETTI, A. et al. 2001. Vitamin E and lipid peroxide plasma levels predict the risk of cardiovascular events in a group of healthy very old people. J. Am. Geriatr. Soc. **49:** 533–537.
36. GALE, C.R. et al. 2001. Antioxidant vitamin status and carotid atherosclerosis in the elderly. Am. J. Clin. Nutr. **74:** 402–408.
37. MCQUILLAN, B.M. et al. 2001. Antioxidant vitamins and the risk of carotid atherosclerosis: the Perth Carotid Ultrasound Disease Assessment Study (CUDAS). J. Am. Coll. Cardiol. **38:** 1788–1794.
38. SIMON, E. et al. 2001. Erythrocyte, but not plasma, vitamin E concentration is associated with carotid intima-media thickening in asymptomatic men at risk for cardiovascular disease. Atherosclerosis **159:** 193–200.
39. IANNUZZI, A. et al. 2002. Dietary and circulating antioxidant vitamins in relation to carotid plaques in middle-aged women. Am. J. Clin. Nutr. **76:** 582–587.
40. DWYER, J.H. et al. 2004. Progression of carotid intima-media thickness and plasma antioxidants: the Los Angeles Atherosclerosis Study. Arterioscler. Thromb. Vasc. Biol. **24:** 313–319.

41. The Alpha-Tocopherol, Beta-Carotene Cancer Prevention Study Group.1994. The effect of vitamin E and beta-carotene on the incidence of lung cancer and other cancers in male smokers. N. Engl. J. Med. **330:** 1029–1035.
42. RAPOLA, J.M. *et al.* 1997. Randomised trial of alpha-tocopherol and beta-carotene supplements on incidence of major coronary events in men with previous myocardial infarction. Lancet **349:** 1715–1720.
43. STEPHENS, N.G. *et al.* 1996. Randomised controlled trial of vitamin E in patients with coronary disease: Cambridge Heart Antioxidant Study (CHAOS). Lancet **347:** 781–786.
44. MITCHINSON, M.J. *et al.* 1999. Mortality in the CHAOS trial. Lancet **353:** 381–382.
45. GRUPPO ITALIANO PER LO STUDIO DELLA SOPRAVVIVENZA NELL'INFARTO MIOCARDIO. 1999. Dietary supplementation with n-3 polyunsaturated fatty acids and vitamin E after myocardial infarction: results of the GISSI-Prevenzione trial. Lancet **354:** 447–455.
46. YUSUF, S. *et al.* 2000. Vitamin E supplementation and cardiovascular events in high-risk patients: the Heart Outcomes Prevention Evaluation Study Investigators. N. Engl. J. Med. **342:** 154–160.
47. BOAZ, M. *et al.* 2000. Secondary prevention with antioxidants of cardiovascular disease in endstage renal disease (SPACE): randomised placebo-controlled trial. Lancet **356:** 1213–1218.
48. LOUGHREY, C.M. *et al.* 1994. Oxidation of low-density lipoprotein in patients on regular haemodialysis. Atherosclerosis **110:** 185–193.
49. BOAZ, M. *et al.* 1999. Serum malondialdehyde and prevalent cardiovascular disease in hemodialysis. Kidney Int. **56:** 1078–1083.
50. HEART PROTECTION STUDY COLLABORATIVE GROUP. 2002. MRC/BHF Heart Protection Study of antioxidant vitamin supplementation in 20,536 high-risk individuals: a randomised placebo-controlled trial. Lancet **360:** 23–33.
51. DE GAETANO, G. 2001. Low-dose aspirin and vitamin E in people at cardiovascular risk: a randomised trial in general practice. Collaborative Group of the Primary Prevention Project. Lancet **357:** 89–95.
52. FANG, J.C. *et al.* 2002. Effect of vitamins C and E on progression of transplant-associated arteriosclerosis: a randomised trial. Lancet **359:** 1108–1113.
53. SALONEN, R.M. *et al.* 2003. Six-year effect of combined vitamin C and E supplementation on atherosclerotic progression: the Antioxidant Supplementation in Atherosclerosis Prevention (ASAP) Study. Circulation **107:** 947–953.
54. CARROLL, M.F. & D.S. SCHADE. 2003. Timing of antioxidant vitamin ingestion alters postprandial proatherogenic serum markers. Circulation **108:** 24–31.
55. IULIANO, L. *et al.* 2000. Radiolabeled native low-density lipoprotein injected into patients with carotid stenosis accumulates in macrophages of atherosclerotic plaque: effect of vitamin E supplementation. Circulation **101:** 1249–1254.

Future Directions in Preclinical Vitamin E Research

Panel Discussion A

LESTER PACKER, *Moderator*
ANGELO AZZI, KLAUS KRAEMER, NESRIN OZER, HELMUT SIES, ETSUO NIKI, FRANCESCO VIOLI, AND GOVIND VATASSERY, *Panel*

LESTER PACKER: Welcome everyone to the first of two round table discussions. In this session we have asked the panel to focus on the future directions of *preclinical* vitamin E research. Each panel member is asked to identify a strategy, a disorder, or an area that has potential preclinical value with respect to vitamin E. A lot of different views will be represented that will, it is hoped, point to some valuable insights.

MARET TRABER: I'd like to suggest that vitamins A and D are really known to have nuclear effects. Regina Brigelius-Flohé has pointed the direction towards nuclear receptors with her findings that α-tocopherol, and some of the tocotrienols, bind to PXR. We also know that drug troglitazone binds to PPAR-γ, and I'd like to suggest that vitamin E may have hugely important nuclear receptor effects, possibly relating to PXR, that haven't been studied but that represent a really fruitful area for investigation.

ANGELO AZZI: Since we are working in this direction, I can say something more about it. Nuclear receptors are an intriguing possibility. In addition to their possible existence, we're also thinking in terms of possible alternatives such as binding of vitamin E to co-receptors responsible for modulating effector macromolecules. However, we should be aware of the fact that before the other nuclear receptors were discovered they were not there, and before the vitamin E receptor is discovered, we don't know what it is—it may be totally different from nuclear receptors. We also need to know how gene expression is regulated by α-tocopherol, because we know that not all tocopherols act in the same way. It is known that α-tocopherol has unique properties and that γ-tocopherol is different from it. The other tocopherols and tocotrienols might have therapeutic effects. In certain models they show, for instance, antitumoral activity. This is both my scientific vision and my personal research target.

COMMENT: It is curious. We recently demonstrated that metabolites can have a sort of biological effect that is similar to their precursors. So how can they do the same job? They are more hydrophilic, when you put them outside the cell, so how they can reach the same intracellular target or targets? This suggests that there are probably other proteins or mechanisms that can lead vitamin-E-like molecules to be involved in trafficking.

MARET TRABER: I'd like to respond to that because it's critical to recognize that the concentrations, at least in the plasma, are 10-fold lower for γ-CEHC than γ-tocopherol, and α-CEHC is a thousand times lower than α-tocopherol. People using trolox, a water-soluble form of vitamin E, say that it has the same effects, but, in point of fact, being water-soluble is exactly not what α-tocopherol is. So, I'm not sure that we can say yet what those metabolites are doing *in vivo*. Are they just forms to get rid of other than α-tocopherol form, or do they have some real biologic activity?

ANGELO AZZI: Maret, do you know the concentration of these metabolites near the P450 where they are produced, before they reach the plasma? Most probably, their concentration is very high locally, and therefore they might exert modulatory functions, which cannot be conceivable at the concentrations present in plasma.

MARET TRABER: Well, Angelo, do you know the level of oxidized lipids in the membrane near where PKC arrives, and does α-tocopherol prevent oxidation of membrane lipids in that vicinity?

ANGELO AZZI: These types of studies are not conceivable at the present time.

ETSUO NIKKI: One of the issues that has emerged recently is the role of reactive oxygen species and nitrogen species, even lipid peroxides and antioxidants including vitamin E, as signaling messengers. As a physiologically important signaling messenger, the formation, concentration, time, site, and quantity should be strictly controlled. This point is very important, and in that sense free radicals may not be good candidates as signaling messengers, because free radicals are difficult to control with respect to their formation and reaction. The concentrations of tocopherols and metabolites at the microenvironment are the critical point.

LESTER PACKER: So, here is point that might be worth considering: we know that tocopherols and tocotrienols can be metabolized and catabolized in a few cell types, but what about other tissues in the body? What kind of strategy can be devised to learn about these pathways in different tissues? Right now we are just looking at a couple of cells, in just a few places.

ANGELO AZZI: Since you mentioned possible differences in tissues, I'm wondering whether by looking at tocopherol we are looking at a right cellular effector of tocopherol functions. Is it possible that tocopherol is phosphorylated in cells and that tocopherol phosphate is the real effector molecule? Is a tocopherol phosphorylation state maintained by a kinase and a phosphatase? Can they be specifically regulated? Is tocopherol phosphate and not tocopherol the molecule that will reach the right targets and provide the right signaling function?

LESTER PACKER: I knew we would come to tocopherol phosphate at some point, although I didn't know when you would mention it. Now that you have, I think maybe we should elaborate a bit more on tocopherol phosphate. Where does it come from? What evidence do we have that it's something that we should take seriously? Do you want to comment on that?

ANGELO AZZI: My comment was only hypothetical, and I didn't want to provide any scientific information. However, after the discovery that this molecule exists in tissues, I think it would be important to ask the following question: is tocopherol phosphate an "accident" in tissues, or is it something that nature decided to have for some reason, such as a deposit form of tocopherol? Alternatively, α-tocopherol phosphate or other forms of tocopherol phosphates may have signaling functions.

LESTER PACKER: Is anything known about kinases and phosphatases that act on tocopherol phosphate?

ANGELO AZZI: We are studying that—it's our future direction.

MARET TRABER: What is the level of tocopherol phosphate—do we know? Is it 10 times more than tocopherol, or a tenth of tocopherol?

PANEL DISCUSSION A: FUTURE DIRECTIONS IN PRECLINICAL RESEARCH

ANGELO AZZI: I don't have any quantitative data. The only thing I know is that it exists in tissues.

MARET TRABER: So, then when we get to that argument of natural versus synthetic, if tocopherol has to be phosphorylated, one critical issue will be how important the 2S center is since it may radically alter the specificity of the tocopherol transfer protein.

ANGELO AZZI: Everybody's allowed to make hypotheses and to verify them experimentally; the field is open. I wanted to mention these ideas because I believe they are important, but I don't want to lead anybody in the wrong direction.

LESTER PACKER: So, does anybody in the audience know something about tocopherol phosphate that we haven't heard about from Angelo?

ESRA OGRU: Together with my colleague at Phosphagenics Australia, Bruce Butler, we're trying to currently optimize our method to quantitatively detect α-tocopherol phosphate in tissues. Our tissue studies currently range from liver to adipose tissue, and we're still struggling with our analytical method. Together with Dr. Azzi, we're trying to understand why this compound is better than α-tocopherol.

QUESTION: What you do mean by *better*?

ESRA OGRU: These are just very early studies, but we're trying to understand how it could be better in terms of gene modulation and in gene regulation relating to atherosclerosis.

ANGELO AZZI: The data suggest it is better because it is acting on the same reactions, but at lower concentrations.

QUESTIONER: So, it has a high potency then?

ANGELO AZZI: The efficacy of tocopherol phosphate at 10 times lower concentrations prompted us to try to understand why this is so. It may be that the ester enters the cells more efficiently than tocopherol, thus delivering a higher local concentration of the vitamin after hydrolysis; alternatively it may have special properties.

QUESTION: Dr. Azzi, you have suggested that there might be some information on its toxicity. Has sufficient information been gathered on the safety, tolerance, toxicity, etc. of α-tocopherol phosphate in living systems, especially in whole animals?

ANGELO AZZI: Yes, there are data that have been obtained on toxicity in rats; I don't have the figures in front of me, but you had to go to massive doses to show its toxicity.

NORMAN KRINSKY: Am I correct in assuming that the α-tocopherol acetate is not an antioxidant?

ANGELO AZZI: As such, α-tocopherol acetate, having the OH group, cannot be an antioxidant in the sense of α-tocopherol. Tocopherol phosphate is, as well, not an antioxidant. The question is whether they are hydrolyzed or not.

NORMAN KRINSKY: But, if it's functioning in its phosphorylated form, wouldn't that resolve the issue of whether vitamin E is functioning as an antioxidant or not.

ANGELO AZZI: That's exactly the point that we have been trying to face these days.

QUESTION: Angelo, have you done studies in which you've looked at feeding different levels of tocopherol to see whether this changes the level of the tocopherol phosphate?

ANGELO AZZI: This study has been planned and will be carried out in collaboration with Nesrin Kartal-Özer in Turkey.

WILLIE COHN: About 10 years ago it was shown that tocopherol phosphate can be cleaved by a number of esterases in the body, and in particular, in the small intestine.

I would like to remind you of something that quite important. Many, many molecules that show hormonal activity occur at very small doses. The doses of retinoic acid, for example, are much smaller than those of, say, γ-tocopherol. The active molecules of vitamin E could really occur at very, very minute amounts, and we should even take into consideration what Achim Stocker has said at this very meeting about the tocopherol quinone. This is a very important molecule that we should also not forget. But what is important is that on this basis, because probably the active forms occur at minute amounts, you cannot really discuss the isomeric forms because we also have also the RR form, and probably at sufficient amounts, that would form adequate amounts of active metabolites.

LESTER PACKER: Good comment.

HELMUT SIES: When the compound is not phosphorylated, it has a free hydroxyl group and that's the tocopherol we know. Mohsen said yesterday that 15 years ago the New York Academy of Sciences held a meeting entitled "Beyond Deficiency,"[a] and now maybe we should call this meeting "Beyond Antioxidant Function," or something like that. But we still should remember that there is the free hydroxyl group and it is of interest to try to pin down whether the hydroxyl group can provide an antioxidant function. Another point that came from Dr. Jens Thiele's group relates to a place where there are no living cells, where tocopherol is transported by the sebum to the skin. So, it would be of interest to show here, where there are no nuclei, where tocopherol can find its potential receptor; it is a good to look at an antioxidant function. Also, we had a deep discussion on the early atherosclerosis question, and Roland Stocker showed that the amount of vitamin E, or the amount of α-tocopherol, which is present in the oxidized form, or one of the oxidized forms, tocopherol quinone, is increased as compared to the concentration in plasma. Whether that reflects an antioxidant function or something else is not known. But we should not completely rule out the base from where vitamin E research is coming from, and we should continue in this line of activity as well. Of course, this doesn't have the same excitement found in studying tocopherol phosphate and possible receptors, but it is highly interesting as well. The breakthrough with PXR represents a new level of refinement in this field, as vitamin E is identified as a ligand to a nuclear receptor. Whether that's the most important function remains to be seen.

LESTER PACKER: No doubt this will be found in other systems where receptors are not present, wherein just the pure antioxidant activities can be researched.

COMMENT: So, pursuant to your suggestions, I'll wave the flag for the eye lens, where you have cells that are nucleated right next to cells that are denucleated, and in fact have "dumped" all their organelles. By ignoring the epidemiological data you have a tremendous opportunity to ask those questions and, in fact, you can even make lens explants denucleate, so that once again you may have a good system in which to work.

COMMENT: I would like to suggest that the occurrence of tocopherol phosphate in tissue should be replicated by more labs, in general, and that we should also look to see whether there would be potential for other derivatives of vitamin E to have the same function as tocopherol phosphate.

---

[a]Published as *Beyond Deficiency: New Views on the Function and Health Effects of Vitamins.* Edited by Lawrence J. Machlin and Howerde E. Sauberlich. Vol. 669 of the *Annals of the New York Academy of Sciences* (1992).

PANEL DISCUSSION A: FUTURE DIRECTIONS IN PRECLINICAL RESEARCH

ANGELO AZZI: I fully agree. The reason why I brought up this issue in public, and have not kept it in the drawer, was indeed to have the data replicated, especially the possibility that other tocopherols, such as γ-tocopherol, may be phosphorylated and might have different functions as well. This is also being studied in Australia.

COMMENT: I wanted to bring attention to an area that was discussed by Dr. Heller with regard to the regulation of eNOS with vitamin E, and the possibility that it would be mediated to association with carbolin 1 and lipid domains.This very interesting area of tocopherol function should be investigated. It fits well with some data we have in immune cells showing that vitamin E can increase immune synapse formation, which is an event that is very much dependent on lipid domains and some of the proteins that are associated with it. Again, this area needs further attention.

COMMENT: With regard to Regina Briselius-Flohé's talk, the disappointment about endothelial function and eNOS, with regards to forearm blood flow and other measures, is that if you look at the majority of studies in patients or in volunteers that they've been null. This is unlike the case with ascorbate intravenous infusion and even high-dose oral ascorbate. Why is it that with vitamin E, in all its forms, when given to humans and subject to meta-analysis of the effects on endothelial vasoreactivity, you arrive at a null result? So it's nice biochemistry, but I'm not sure why it doesn't translate to clinical benefit.

LESTER PACKER: I'd like to call upon Govind Vatassery to say something about that.

GOVIND VATASSERY: This is a good time for me to come in, because you were talking about nitric oxide synthase. I want to remind everybody, if you need reminding, that the deficiency symptom in humans is really ataxia, which is vitamin E deficiency and which can be cured by vitamin E administration. It's a real pure vitamin E deficiency syndrome that actually exhibits, as a phenotype, cerebral ataxia, as a symptom. Obviously, this gives rise to the importance of the cerebellum as well as the nervous system. Dr. Muller already had talked to you about some of the neuroconduction velocity studies. So, we do need a number of studies in this particular area. One of the things that we deal with when we are talking about preclinical studies is that the effectiveness of the particular compound to be used,and which compound to use, and how much to use is still up in the air, as far as many of the studies are concerned. More studies are needed, with regard to the nervous system per se, concerning the different forms of vitamin E, and the kind of effects they have in this tissue. The other point I wanted to make is in relation to nitric oxide, which is a transmitter in the nervous system. There might be a connection there, and we need more studies along those lines, as well.

LUCILLA POSTON: I will go back to the discussion about flow-mediated dilatation because unfortunately it is the only estimate that we have of endothelium-dependent relaxation *in vivo*. We can look at ACH ionophoresis and so on, but that's the one everybody uses. I would remind everybody that flow-mediated dilatation in conduit vessels, like the brachial artery and the carotid, is not actually physiologically relevant. Basal NOS is important in those vessels. If we really want to look at eNOS-mediated dilatation, which is physiologically relevant, in terms of peripheral vascular resistance, you need to look at much smaller vessels. The best thing to do there is to take small arteries from biopsies, as we've done many times, and look at flow-mediated dilatation in an isolated system. Flow-mediated dilatation in the brachial artery is a tiny change in the diameter of the vessel, and it's not entirely nitric oxide mediated—there is a prostacyclin-mediated component. We need to be very careful about extrapolation of what we see in the conduit vasculature to what we think might be happening in the peripheral circulation. There's great heterogeneity in the mechanisms of vasodilatation from large to small vessels.

DAVID MULLER: To continue Dr. Vatassery's point on the neurologic role of vitamin E, I think what ought to be pointed out is that it may provide a very good clue to potential function of α-tocopherol. Is it the pathology? The neuropathology is highly specific, and it's described as a primary axonopathy, so, it is affecting the axon first, and the demyelination effect is secondary. But, on top of that, it's described as a dying-back axonopathy. If you think of a neuron, which has got to provide all the "goodies" for this very long cell, the problem is at the end of the cell, and it's taking a long time to cause the problem. Studies on repletion suggest that it can be corrected very rapidly, so all this information together should provide clues as to its role. We've got to bear the neuropathology in mind.

KENNY JIALAL: Since I raised the issue of flow-mediated dilation, I agree with you totally. It's in a vessel that doesn't get atherosclerosis, but researchers like Scott Kinley have shown its correlation with coronary flow-mediated dilation. So, for what it's worth, it's a surrogate. The point I was really trying to make, and I think it'll come out later also, is that this field has been draped in controversy, it's been bloodied. It's not "down for the count" yet, or it might be down as far as the National Institutes of Health thinks about antioxidants and vitamin E specifically. So if we can't translate the basic science into an *in vivo* situation and confirm it, we have a major problem—from those lousy clinical trials the NIH has drawn the conclusion that antioxidants are useless. So all future studies with antioxidants that the NIH looks at, they look at very critically.

ANGELO AZZI: I agree with you, Kenny, but the problem is that you are calling them antioxidants when they are not *only* antioxidants. If they were simple antioxidants, every individual would respond equally. These compounds have special properties—they recognize polymorphisms, for example. If we treat them as site-directed molecules, specific for a certain subgroup of the population, and not as generic antioxidants, we could design better clinical trials as well.

LESTER PACKER: Maybe.

NESRIN OZER: This is a very important issue—what *should* be the future direction in preclinical research on vitamin E? We started with epidemiologic data, which showed us that vitamin E has an important role in cardiovascular disease and some other diseases. Then laboratory research focused on what exactly vitamin E is doing. First, vitamin E was described as an antioxidant. Now we know that it has many functions in cell signaling—inhibition of smooth muscle cell proliferation described by Angelo, anti-inflammatory effects as described by Jialal. Also, as Maret touched on, there are nuclear receptors and tocopherol binding proteins. I think that what is important and what we should focus on are biomarkers, which correlate with cellular changes in cellular function.

FRANCESCO VIOLI: I completely agree. I would like to remind everyone that about 20 years ago an observation was made that indicated that the lower the level of blood vitamin E, the higher the risk of mortality from cardiovascular disease. So, a way to approach this issue is to measure vitamin E, and look for the progression of atherosclerosis. This is just what Dr. Jialal is doing, and we will do in the near future. If you select patients in whom the plasma level of vitamin E may be low, and you follow them for a year or two, you can see whether the progression of atherosclerosis is correlated to plasma levels of tocopherol. This is a way to see whether vitamin E is working in a better way, at least in the atheroscleric disease.

NESRIN OZER: Actually, my point is not only to follow vitamin E levels, but also other markers. For example, atherosclerosis is related to scavenger receptor CD36 expression and, as Angelo mentioned before, vitamin E inhibits CD36 expression in smooth muscle cells. Moreover, it would be very interesting to follow CD36 expression in blood cells such as monocytes.

COMMENT: I think you agree that this would not be easy to do in a large clinical trial since it's tough to measure in the cell, so you must choose something easier to do.

MARET TRABER: I'd like to come back to what happens in vitamin E–deficient humans because perhaps vitamin E is really not beneficial in atherosclerosis. Those vitamin E–deficient humans are not described as having heart disease at an early age. In fact, I don't think anybody has reported that they have particularly elevated risk. Certainly there's no more than maybe a hundred patients in the world so, and they are young. But they do have severe neurologic disease so the target tissue of the artery wall may be the wrong one.

ANGELO AZZI: Maret, I fully agree with you. We have to identify the function of vitamin E in human subjects first, and then we can develop the models in animals or in tissue culture, where we can assess the effects of different forms of vitamin E.

COMMENT: Dr. Traber, if I remember clearly, had a paper in *PNAS* showing that the double knock-out of the TTP transfer protein—that is, classic vitamin E deficiency on the background of Apo E or LDL receptor knock-out—resulted in less atherosclerosis. Is that true now, Maret?

MARET TRABER: That was an antioxidant function, and so we're discounting it.

COMMENT: But maybe patients show neurological symptoms much earlier than symptoms of heart and arterial disease. That's possible.

FULVIO URSINI: Just to make a further contribution about the possible physiological function of vitamin E, I wanted to remind you about two sets of experiments at the very beginning of my own career. They appear to be overlooked in the last few years. First, why did somebody invent the antioxidant function for vitamin E? It's because there were three guys around the world—Rick Nagle at Cincinnati, Trevor Slater in London, and Mario Dianzanni in Italy—who were studying carbon tetrachloride toxicity. They carried out very simple experiments in which all the animals were treated and then died. Next time they gave vitamin E and all the animals survived. You're not talking about the increasing risk of something. You're talking clear-cut facts. The miracle was carried out by α-tocopherol because it was transported: it was inserted in the membranes and it was providing a one-electron transfer to the carbon tetrachloride radical. So, the story is complete. How can everyone forget about these things? This was a clear-cut story in pathology, no risk factors needed—100% dead, 100% alive. A second part of the story has been completely overlooked for 20 years: There is a tremendous interaction of various enzymes and vitamin E. This is in nutrition, in pathology, in experimental pathology, in chemistry. There are tissues where there is selenium and vitamin E and just vitamin E alone. Also, we must never forget scurvy, a severe deficiency syndrome that can be treated. So far, thank God, there is no evidence that vitamin E is phosphorylated; otherwise it would never protect against oxygen toxicity. So we have to differentiate the effect of vitamin E from all the other phenols, and there are plenty. If you study botanical compounds, you find they control protein kinases, they control gene expression, and so on. The reason for my comment is that we should not forget these two critical experiments in the 1960s: Interaction with selenium is clear cut, as is 100% protection against carbon tetrachloride toxicity. We need to be reminded of this.

LESTER PACKER: Very well said.

SIMIN MEYDANI: We should also not forget that giving fish oil, which is oxidizing, induces vitamin E deficiency. That's how vitamin E deficiency was originally produced, by giving cod liver oil. The other thing I found interesting was a range of experiments presented here concerning the effect of vitamin E on global gene expression. I find it quite fascinating that there is this distinction between the effect of vitamin E, as far as the type of genes that are induced, or are affected, between primary cells and tumor cells. We had presentations showing that vitamin E in tumor cells inhibits cell cycle–related gene expression, whereas in primary cells it actually increases the expression of these genes. Looking into why there's this differentiation not only might tell us something about how vitamin E works, but could also tell us something about why cells turn into tumor cells. This is an area that is certainly worthy of further investigation.

ANGELO AZZI: I want to comment on what Simin has just said concerning the depletion of α-tocopherol by rancid diets. This doesn't prove that α-tocopherol is an antioxidant. This is chemistry and tocopherol can be destroyed by oxidants. If we want to conserve tocopherol in the body, as a unique molecule, we must protect it in order to avoid its destruction. The antioxidant function of tocopherol is incompatible with a signaling function. Either tocopherol is signaling, and then we have to protect it, or it is an antioxidant, and then we are to use it. Given what we have learned about vitamin E over the last 15 years, I think it would be unwise to develop new projects that focus on discovering or testing new antioxidants to find a better one than tocopherol. Instead we should focus on the actual biological role of this important micronutrient.

LESTER PACKER: Thank you. We don't want to get into the argument we had the other day, though. Klaus, can I ask you to make some comments?

KLAUS KRAEMER: We should revisit the biopotency of vitamin E. The animal models we have need to be refined so that we can develop vitamin E deficiency in a shorter time. Then we can use these models to determine the specific functions of all different vitamin E forms. We have had an extensive discussion on the potency ratio of all-rac- and RRR-alpha-tocopherols, gamma-tocopherol, and all other siblings of this family. It is important to determine the individual functions of vitamin E forms so that we can define vitamin E according to its biopotency rather than bioavailability.

MARET TRABER: And, to add to that, it would be really nice if suppliers would make some 2S form for us to test, because we've got the deficient animals.

ETSUO NIKI: I would like to return to the basic antioxidant function. As many have pointed out, we have good markers for lipid peroxidation. Many people agree that vitamin E reduces the level of lipid peroxidation *in vivo*. But we do not know its significance, if lipid peroxidation or lipid peroxidation products are the cause or consequence of diseases or disorders. That's something we have to prove, and by doing so, we can get some answers regarding this function of vitamin E. I don't say it is the only function, but undoubtedly one of the important functions of vitamin E.

LESTER PACKER: Thank you all for your contributions to this discussion.

Future Directions in Clinical Vitamin E Research

Panel Discussion B

LESTER PACKER, *Moderator*
JEFFREY BLUMBERG, ISHWARLAL JIALAL, JOE LUNEC, SIMIN MEYDANI, FRANCESCO VIOLI, AND WALTER WILLETT, *Panel*

LESTER PACKER: We'll follow the same strategy that we used for the Panel A discussion.

JOE LUNEC: I'd like to address the subject of biomarkers and their relevance. It's important to remember that biomarkers can have different meanings for different people. For instance, one or two presenters have talked about the measurement of 8-oxo-dG, which certainly is a DNA-damaged product, but depending on where you measure it, it's a repair product as well. Now, depending on how you want to interpret the measure of 8-oxo-dG could determine whether you consider vitamin E an antioxidant or even a pro-oxidant. For instance, if you look for 8-oxo-dG in urine, as we have done in a vitamin C trial, it is elevated. The problem is, the immunoassay that measures 8-oxo-dG measures the free form of 8-oxo-dG, and measures it as a putative repair product. So, what you're actually measuring is an increase in repair, which of course is a protective effect. So, I'm afraid it's another question of the duck quacking, but not quite walking.

KENNY JIALAL: Yesterday I presented preliminary data from our study investigating the effects of *RRR*-alpha-tocopherol on biomarkers of oxidative stress and inflammation in patients with coronary artery disease. It is important with biomarkers of oxidative stress, since we are measuring footprints of what has already happened, that we follow the strategy that Jackson Roberts and Jason Morrow have employed with the isoprostanes; this is really the way to go because it's a measure of *in vivo* lipid peroxidation. There is no question that F2 isoprostane measured by chromotography–mass spectrometry is a measure of *in vivo* lipid peroxidation. By the same token, measuring nitrotyrosine reliably in urine or plasma also serves as a good footprint of oxidative/nitrative stress. However, with the DNA oxobases, some go up, and some go down and there has been disagreement concerning artifacts. We need to have stable markers of an *in vivo* process, and of all the markers of lipid peroxidation that are coming to fruition, the isoprostanes seem to fit the role, and they are also present in the atherosclerotic vessel.

MOHSEN MEYDANI: Joe, before you respond to that, I have a question for you. There are commercial ELISA kits available for F2 isoprostane measurement, and many investigators are using them because they're much easier than GC/MS. What is your view on GC/MS–determined markers versus the kit?

JOE LUNEC: Mohsen, it's almost as if you've read my mind. We've had a very proactive flag raised for the measurement of isoprostanes, but it's a question of how you measure them. Not everybody has GC/MS facilities, and if you haven't got them, don't try to measure F2-isoprostanes, because you won't be successful. If you use a kit, and you compare your findings with those obtained with GC/MS, you get totally different results. This is all related to how specific the antibodies are. The situation may get better, but unless you've got very good quality control, you have to be very careful about just picking a biomarker and not really thinking about the method for measuring it and how specific it is.

MOHSEN MEYDANI: Although you get different levels, is there a good correlation between the approaches that one can rely on?

JOE LUNEC: There is a correlation, yes.

SIMIN MEYDANI: Isoprostane measurement is also influenced by the type of fat in the diet, so it can be nonspecific.

WALTER WILLETT: Clearly, good biomarkers would help move this field forward. Of course, we would like to have evidence that the biomarker is related to the clinical event of interest, and eventually we might have that with F2 isoprostanes. Part of the current problem, however, is that the isoprostanes are fairly unstable as well as variable within a subject. We've tried looking at blood levels of isoprostanes in our epidemiologic studies, but haven't been able to use them due to instability and variability. It would be very helpful to have some biomarkers of oxidative stress that could be related to cardiovascular disease incidence, and then we could really examine the whole sequence of events.

SAMAR BASU: I'd like to comment about these biomarkers, oxidative stress and isoprostanes. We have been working for about 10 years with prostaglandins. Now you're saying that GC/MS is absolutely one of the best methods when you start measuring isoprostanes, because their levels are so low in normal plasma. But if you consider measuring isoprostanes in urine, their concentrations are much higher. Incidentally, within 30 seconds, prostaglandins metabolize in the serum. Isoprostanes have a much longer half-life, about 4 or 5 minutes. So when you get oxidative stress, you have a continuation of the production of isoprostanes, so you can always find F2 isoprostanes in the urine, but you need a method that can justify the experimental conditions, like CCl4–induced oxidative stress. If you do these studies and measure isoprostanes, you can see a 100-fold increase in F2 isoprostanes within an hour. Also, if you give these animals vitamin E you can get a reduction in the concentration of isoprostanes. Both Jason Morrow's group and our group agree on this approach. Oxidative stress models such as CCl4 always provide the same results. If this is the case, then you can use antibody-based assays, or GC/MS. With the antibody method you can examine thousands of samples in a short time period, but with the GC/MS, you are more limited. Both methods work well to measure oxidative stress.

QUESTION: There are other markers, C-reactive protein among them, which the American Heart Association accepts as a marker of atherosclerosis. How sensitive is CRP to vitamin E treatment?

KENNY JIALAL: We're now talking about two totally different measurements. We have great difficulty with oxidative stress. What is a free radical reaction? What is a footprint? I disagree with Simin—there are isoprostane assays that Jackson Roberts has used that can measure different isoprostanes. There is a whole array of various assays with which you can measure different isoprostanes. But CRP, as I said in my presentation, is a stable marker. It's a protein with a half-life of 19 hours. It's not specific, but it's downstream, a stable marker of the inflammatory process. At least three groups, as I reviewed in my presentation, have shown that CRP is significantly reduced with vitamin E therapy.

WALTER WILLETT: We should go back and look at our data. I'm not sure that we looked carefully at the relation between vitamin E and CRP and other inflammatory markers. One thing we have been looking at are fluorescent products in the plasma or serum, and this is an old measurement. Dr. Wu in our group has shown that these do predict coronary heart disease, which is interesting. This line has potential, and identifying the specific fluorescent products could be informative. These fluorescent products are very stable. If you measure subjects 6 months apart, the correlation is very high, and and that's what we need to do if we're going to be looking at clinical influence in human populations. Of all the markers we've looked at, these fluorescence products are amongst the most promising, even though they are nonspecific.

LESTER PACKER: With Marion Dietrich and Gladys Block, we've just reported (J. Am. Coll. Nutr. **23:** 141–147) that vitamin C can lower the CRP levels, so there's a lot of factors that are going to be affecting this level, and unless we have some better understanding of what these factors are and how important they are in determining the basic level of CRP, it's always going to be a bit difficult to use them as a marker.

COMMENT: We published a paper recently in *Circulation*. We have checked that there is no correlation on CRP, at least within type 2 diabetes. We do, however, have correlation with the prostaglandins that are mediated by cycloxygenases. In all our studies where we see inflammation, there is some oxidative stress.

MICHAEL GAZIANO: CRP is a good marker related to cardiovascular disease in our large studies, but it's also related to the risk factors of oxidative stress, like cigarette smoking and obesity, and is reversed by changes in those factors. Now, as an aside, I think that once you have all the risk factors in the model, CRP becomes a much less valuable marker. It's really a reflection of the atherosclerotic process. Once you adjust for all known risk factors, including smoking and obesity, you get very little contribution to the model. While CRP is interesting mechanistically. I'm not sure we have to have it to be able to predict disease in clinical studies.

JOE LUNEC: You have to be very careful, because markers like CRP, particularly related to an inflammatory response, rise, plateau, and then go down again, depending on whether there's reduction in inflammation. If you measure isoprostanes at any one point on that curve, you might get a positive correlation or you might not, and so you have to be very careful how you interpret these results. We can't talk about CRP's being related to lipid peroxidation, protein oxidation, or DNA oxidation directly.

COMMENT: But if there's constant inflammation of an artery in a patient, you have a constant production of CRP, so the value isn't going down or on a plateau—rather, the inflammation is growing and getting worse.

JOE LUNEC: Unfortunately, diseases aren't like that. They're not pure in terms of responses. For instance, we've looked at patients with rheumatoid arthritis. One of the classic ways of looking at disease activity in rheumatoid arthritis is to measure CRP response to therapy. If you give anti-inflammatory drugs, then you reduce the CRP, and you will reduce the lipid peroxidation products that you're measuring as part of rheumatoid arthritis. These are sometimes, but not always, related in time, and so you have to be very careful because sometimes patients are in remission. Rheumatoid arthritis isn't considered to be a "sexy" disease because you don't die from joint pains, but in fact, a lot of patients with rheumatoid arthritis have increased susceptibility to cardiovascular disease. It's pretty tricky to sort out the CRP that is related to the inflammation due to cardiovascular problems compared to the generalized inflammation from joint swelling.

COMMENT: I'm not clear why we're talking about biomarkers—biomarkers for *what*? Are we talking about biomarkers *of* stress or *for* stress? Is oxidative stress, in fact, now accepted as a risk factor? and if so, for what—for inflammation or for disease? Is the pathway Mohsen talked about a causative or a causal defect? Are we talking about biomarkers for disease or for markers of disease?

JEFFREY BLUMBERG: I'll try to answer that. We can use "biomarkers" for a number of different purposes—as indicators of mechanism of action, as risk factors for chronic disease, or as indices useful to measure biochemical responses to an intervention. The central problem with biomarkers of oxidative stress is the lack of evidence fully validating any of them as an integral part of disease etiology or pathogenesis. Thus, even when we demonstrate a reduction in the biomarker in response to an antioxidant intervention, we don't know whether we have actually slowed the onset or progression of the disease or, at least, that part of the process that the biomarker is supposed to reflect. Of course, we need to keep in mind that even if the biomarker were valid, other parallel pathogenic pathways may exist such that the clinical outcome would not be much affected.

Also, I've been really excited by the material presented at this meeting and the emphasis on the non-antioxidant mechanisms of vitamin E which may prove relevant to its physiological actions and putative health benefits. I was particularly struck by listening to the discussions about Eric Klein's SELECT study and Mike Gaziano's presentation on randomized clinical trials and the skepticism about the potential for success in demonstrating an unequivocal benefit on some disease outcome. Are we truly ready to receive good news on a positive outcome or will we merely be critical about the relevance of the dose, duration or form of vitamin E, the choice of population or biomarkers, or the risk of potential adverse effects? If the SELECT study indicates a 25% reduction in the risk of prostate cancer, will there be an agreement about the value of vitamin E and selenium supplementation in men? Or will there be a call for studies instead with gamma-tocopherol in a lower risk cohort and warnings about an uncertainty concerning adverse effects of the supplement on unstudied chronic diseases or nutrient–drug interactions? Indeed, the potential toxicity of vitamin E has been raised here several times. Mohsen Meydani declared E to be a very safe vitamin, while others have suggested doses of 1800 or 2000 mg posed potential risks, particularly in interacting with other antioxidants.

I am not always sure we have thoroughly considered the potential outcomes of benefit or toxicity before investing tens of millions of dollars in very large-scale, long-term trials. What would have happened had the ATBC study resulted in a significant reduction in lung cancer in smokers? Would we suggest that smokers take an antioxidant supplement rather than quit smoking? But before I sound too negative about clinical trials, I would like to wonder aloud whether we are here too narrowly considering the way in which strategies for preventive nutrition should be considered. We have been discussing vitamin E in detail, but most often without reference to the full antioxidant network. Although the SELECT study of prostate cancer is employing both vitamin E and selenium, why was lycopene not included? In the AREDS trial of cataract and macular degeneration with vitamins C and E, beta-carotene and zinc, why was lutein not included? Given the potential pro-oxidant actions of homocysteine, why are antioxidant interventions not combined with folic acid and vitamins B6 and B12? If we are interested looking for nutritional solutions to public health problems and not just mechanisms of action, we need less of a tunnel vision and more of a broad focus recognizing that while one nutrient, like vitamin E, may have many actions (and mechanisms) against many diseases, that many nutrients can benefit a single disease.

I want to second the opinion I've heard several times that we must look more carefully at the eligibility criteria employed in clinical trials—whether for primary or secondary prevention. We need to consider carefully whether we want to recruit subjects into an antioxidant study who have high intakes of dietary antioxidants and/or no evidence of oxidative stress. We also need now to include genomic measures, such as gene polymorphisms, into our study designs. In addition to Eric Klein's data on PON 1 and MRS 1, the recent results from the WAVE study suggest that vitamin E is beneficial in increasing luminal diameter in women with a haptoglobin 1 allele, but may decrease this parameter in those with the more common a haptoglobin 2 allele.

WALTER WILLETT: I wouldn't worry too much over Jeff's point about whether we are ready for a positive result. It would be nice if we had a positive result from some of these trials. We probably don't have the data to start additional primary prevention trials with vitamin E at this point in time. As Dr. Gaziano mentioned, there are a handful of trials under way, and we just need to let some of these play out. Some of these trials were started a number of years ago. The Women's Health Study, for example, will soon be providing some data, and it is more relevant because it has a population that's more similar to the epidemiologic populations in which we saw lower risks of coronary heart disease among women who took vitamin E supplements. Thus the Women's Health Study more closely replicates the epidemiologic studies than the randomized trials that have been published so far.

It is absolutely right that the population is very important because it can lead to very different results. We have a good example, I believe, with hormone replacement therapy and the Women's Health Initiative. In the epidemiologic studies, there have been consistently lower risks of coronary heart disease for women who take hormone replacement therapy. The Women's Health study seemed to say the opposite, but in fact, the Women's Health Study randomized women who were not at all like the women who typically use hormonal replacement. Women normally using hormone replacement therapy usually start at the time of menopause, but in the Women's Health Initiative women as old as 75 were randomized. A subgroup analysis recently published from the Women's Health Initiative showed protection from coronary heart disease among women who started hormone replacement therapy within a short time after menopause. But almost opposite answers can be obtained if you pick a different population.

In the case of vitamin E, as has been mentioned already, we shouldn't only be considering persons who already have coronary heart disease, as has been the case in most of the intervention trials that have been done so far. As Dr. Meydani described, for people who have coronary heart disease in these trials, the state of good practice is to give them antiplatelet drugs, statins, and ACE inhibitors. There's very heavy-duty polypharmacology going on in these patient groups. In our epidemiologic studies we routinely exclude sick people to begin with, and so populations that are being studied are extremely different. We will have new data from the ongoing trials, but it's not totally clear that there will be a crystal-clear answer. If we get a relative risk of 0.8, not quite statistically significant, there would be ambiguities. If we do get a positive result, it will raise more questions about the dose and type of vitamin E, and the mechanisms. This is the normal process of science. Whatever we find will be interesting, and we'll have to interpret the results, as we always do, in light of all the evidence regarding possible complications and other benefits.

JEFFREY BLUMBERG: I look forward to the outcomes of these studies, like the Women's Health Study and SU.VI.MAX. But Kenny makes an important point that some of these trials, even at 6 or 7 years' duration, may be too short to detect benefit of cardiovascular disease in women. This may be partly responsible for the results of the ASAP study, where the women showed no benefit, but the men were quite responsive. So we must keep gender and duration in mind when considering new trials as well as dosage form and amount and combinations of nutrients.

KENNY JIALAL: I made a similar point earlier. It's true that women get heart disease, but there's a 10-year lag between women and men for heart disease. If you choose a population of men and women, and include the same number of each at the beginning of the study, you're already diluting your endpoint. The ASAP study showed benefit in men with cholesterol over 200 mg/dL, but not women. Also, David Waters and his group showed increased cardiovascular mortality in women given synthetic E and C. However, this has not been shown in other studies, but the point we are discussing today is that a lot of these clinical trials didn't even measure antioxidant levels.

Antioxidants as supplements have been dismissed based on clinical trials, the majority of which have not measured antioxidant levels, let alone biomarkers of oxidative stress and inflammation. So, for those who are going to conduct clinical trials and investigation, the plea from now on is that, at the minimum, they measure reliable markers of oxidative stress and inflammation. This is why we've been getting into the nitty gritty of oxidative stress markers. Also we see from Angelo Azzi's PKC studies, our work on 5-lipoxygenase and on tyrosine kinase of CD36, and other work on COX 2 from Simin, that vitamin E is a biological-response modifier. Therefore in future studies of vitamin E it is imperative to look not only at oxidative stress and the so-called antioxidant effect, but also at the anti-inflammatory effects. There is no doubt about the usefulness of CRP. We heard about it in rheumatoid arthritis; it is one of the most stable markers we have of inflammation as long as you measure it properly: in the steady state, two samples a month apart using a high-sensitivity assay, and the value has got to be less than 10 mg per liter to exclude macro-inflammation, trauma, infection, etc. With these caveats, you have an excellent biomarker for research for looking at inflammation. You can go upstream in the cascade and look at inflammatory cytokines, chemokines, and soluble cell adhesion molecules. When you look at the whole thing properly, the CRP assay stands up as the best biomarker we have for inflammation at this point, and in more than 20 studies it has proven to be a good risk marker for cardiovascular disease. A recent study in the *New England Journal* by Danesh *et al.* suggests that the increase in risk is not 2-fold but 50%. But whichever way you look at it, CRP tells you more than what we know with the established risk factors. This is clearly shown in the Women's Health study, in which a high CRP predicted greater risk than LDL cholesterol or the Framingham risk score.

I think we could tolerate a positive finding. I think we could handle it from a large-scale trial. I'll second Walt's notion that the trials are an adjunct to our knowledge of the field, but in a very specific way. They don't answer all the questions. We have more flexibility to answer questions in observational epidemiology. We can pose subtly nuanced questions. The trials are designed to answer very specific questions, and perhaps sometimes these are misguided and perhaps other times not. At this point, it's very reasonable that the SELECT trial won't address all the questions about vitamin E. However, there's a question out there because the ATBC trial showed this lower rate of prostate cancer. Was that due to chance in people who took short-term vitamin E, synthetic vitamin E? If we give it to people, maybe for a little bit longer, will we reduce the risk of prostate cancer? This is a very legitimate question.

Maybe we picked the wrong population for cardiovascular disease, the wrong endpoints, even the wrong duration and the wrong dose. The question is still out there—should we be taking vitamin E to prevent prostate cancer? There's enormous utility in answering this one question, and understanding that we have the field of randomized trials targeted in a very focused way.

JEFF BLUMBERG: I agree. I admit to being deliberately provocative in my previous statements. After all the null results we've seen, I too would welcome a significant, positive study. I had been trying to comment on the discussions occurring over the last two days that suggested to me that if we do obtain a particular health benefit, would the people at this conference be able to agree about the value of supplementation for that condition or instead find only arguments for delaying application while searching for other doses and combinations and fearing potential adverse outcomes? If the intent of large-scale trials like the SELECT is to be able to make health recommendations to the general public, then we must find some way to agree on dealing with an apparent benefit of a dietary supplement.

MOHSEN MEYDANI: Now that you have already heard about Simin's positive results, what we are going to do about that?

SIMIN MEYDANI: When it comes to biological markers, we've talked about oxidative stress, and one marker that is sensitive to vitamin E, but maybe not related to cardiovascular disease, but certainly to infectious diseases and cancer, is T cell function. T cell function is sensitive to both deficiency and supplemental increases in vitamin E. We have data showing that there is a very nice correlation between the plasma level of vitamin E and *in vivo* measures of T cell function, that is, delayed-type hypersensitivity skin response and response to hepatitis B vaccine. I therefore think that this is a marker that could be utilized easily in some of the trials. It could also be useful if you're looking at biopotency of different types of tocopherols, or comparing synthetic versus natural vitamin E. The other point I wanted to make is that I know we are focused on cardiovascular diseases and cancer because those are the killing diseases in the developed countries, but let's not forget that the number one cause of mortality and morbidity around the world is infectious disease. There are new data indicating that vitamin E could be beneficial as far as protecting against some of these infectious diseases. Perhaps some of the focus needs to be shifted to diseases other than cardiovascular disease and cancer, if you're evaluating functions of vitamin E, or considering its benefits or adverse effects.

COMMENT: I have to support Jeff's opinion that we are not ready to accept a positive function of vitamins and antioxidants. As we have seen with the ATBC study, using relatively high levels of β-carotene, there's no recommendation possible for the general population on account of the ATBC's study on the effects of lung cancer. And maybe we need some softer endpoints that are modulated by vitamin E, like the effect on the immune function, so that we could make recommendations to the public.

JEFFREY BLUMBERG: I would point out there was a positive outcome in reducing the progress of age-related macular degeneration in the ARED Study. Although there was some initial excitement about the value of a high dose antioxidant supplement for eye health, many researchers then began to criticize the application of the results, arguing the dose of zinc was too high, the formula should have included lutein, the trial wasn't relevant to people at only moderate risk, and so on.

JOHN HATHCOCK: In terms of progressing, vitamin E is not a drug, thank God. It need not be a drug. We don't want it to be, but I've worked with more drugs than I have with nutrients, and I would suggest that in terms of developing protocols for clinical studies, it might be a good idea to involve people and organizations who have done drug studies, because those are the most rigorously conducted studies. This helps to focus, right up front, on such questions as what is the basis for the study? what is the evidence? and what are the expectations? It will help to put your thought processes in the right order, and then help with designing, implementing, and interpreting the study. People with that kind of experience can be very helpful, and by taking this approach it does not make vitamin E a drug, as some people have mistakenly thought it is. You can benefit a lot from involving people with the process that is involved in teasing answers out of data.

JEFFREY BLUMBERG: I agree. I would not like to define nutrients as drugs for many reasons, but I would point out that in virtually all the secondary prevention studies, such as HOPE and HPS, the question asked was: Is vitamin E an effective adjunctive agent to well-established polypharmacy regimens? That is, these trials actually investigated whether vitamin E, when added to antiplatelet therapy, beta blockers, calcium channel blockers, statins, ACE inhibitors, diuretics, anticoagulants, and/or other therapies, results in a further reduction in the risk of second cardiac events. The answer to this question now appears to a pretty firm *no*. But perhaps it was a bit optimistic, based on primary prevention studies, to expect vitamin E to add substantially to the overlapping mechanisms, like antiplatelet actions, endothelial responsiveness, antioxidation effects, etc., of these drugs with their other pharmacologic actions as well. I wonder whether it's feasible to readily design secondary prevention studies that carefully balance or account for all the standard drug therapies being given to these patients. This situation presents significant confounding elements to the basic question being posed for these studies.

COMMENT: I take slight exception to what you are saying, in the sense that, had the ARED study come through with a clear observation, particularly with early grades, for instance, of retinal disease or cataract, people would have been thrilled, and there would probably be a good reason to be thrilled. My second point is that as scientists, it's probably not our job yet to be overly enthusiastic and raise unrealistic expectations. A certain amount of healthy scepticism is probably the appropriate responses to these studies. Even if our study had shown that we could even cure cataracts, our response would still have to be guarded because, as Walter has reminded us, populations are different, studies are designed differently, and there should be more of a consensus of observations before we come out too strong and raise unrealistic expectations. But even with the ARED study there is an application: it was appropriate for people with fairly advanced AMD. That is where the positive results were, and I think most ophthalmologists are highly recommending it. Maybe this is before they should, because it's not been supported by as many other studies as they really need to make it a strong observation. But I think that clinicians are in fact doing the appropriate thing, at least in this case. Now maybe they should be looking at cardiovascular disease and finding out that beta-carotene is dangerous, but that's what we're here for. I would make one more plea, and that is that researchers look for new and additional biomarkers. One of the problems that most aging cells and aging tissues face is a lot of protein damage.

JEFFREY BLUMBERG: There certainly are some protein oxidation products that can be used as biomarkers. However, I feel we should also be taking greater advantage of physiological measures as they appear to be more integrative markers of clinical action, in contrast to the biomarkers of oxidative injury to DNA, lipids, and protein, that is, the specific footprints of free radical reactions. For example, Simin Meydani's point is well taken that we should be looking at T cell–mediated immune responses as a physiologic biomarker. This is a meaningful parameter, beyond merely demonstrating a physiological response to vitamin E, in that it directly addresses broad natural defense mechanisms against disease. Similarly, flow-mediated dilation of the vasculature presents another good redox-sensitive physiological marker, particularly for cardiovascular disease.

LESTER PACKER: So, Simin, if T cell function was used in a multi-center trial, what kinds of complications would you see? Do you think it would be easy to get comparable results?

SIMIN MEYDANI: It depends on the size of the study and what the clinical end point is. I don't know whether in a study with 30,000 participants you would want to use a marker like that unless it is directly related to the clinical outcome of interest. Or, for example, it might be premature to use T cell function, if the clinical endpoint is cardiovascular disease, although recent studies indicate that inappropriate T cell function contributes to development of cardiovascular disease. But for large clinical trials, where the endpoint is related to the function of the immune cells, that would be a very good marker. We've been discussing biopotency of different types of tocopherols, and a biological marker like T cell function is an excellent marker in this regard, whether it works through antioxidant or non-antioxidant function.

LESTER PACKER: I was also concerned about whether different centers would be able to carry out the assays in the correct manner so that the results could be comparable.

SIMIN MEYDANI: That should not be a problem because these assays can be standardized. It is more important to make sure that it is appropriate for the clinical endpoint of interest.

KENNY JIALAL: Simin, I believe that at the last meeting there was a South African group that showed with measles that vitamin supplementation led to a better outcome.

SIMIN MEYDANI: Right; I think there is more evidence now for the effectiveness of antioxidants against viral diseases, which is why I think investigating the relationship between antioxidants and infectious diseases will have important implications for global health. We are seeing a lot of new, emerging viral diseases worldwide, so that might be an area where the future focus should be.

MOHSEN MEYDANI: One thing we haven't touched on in this meeting is AIDS. Does anyone have any comment on vitamin E in relation to AIDS and HIV?

SIMIN MEYDANI: It would be purely speculative, because obviously nothing has been done in humans. Some animal studies were carried out looking at some of the markers of T cell function, and they found some beneficial effect, but no work has been done in humans. There are strong indications, as far as the mechanisms are concerned, that antioxidant supplementation could be beneficial because T cell functions, similar to the case in the elderly, are suppressed in patients with HIV. One can only speculate that it could be beneficial, but it's just speculation.

JEFFREY BLUMBERG: That is interesting as we have very preliminary data from HIV-positive subjects that they have significantly elevated isoprostanes compared to healthy controls. We know that patients with HIV and AIDS have very low glutathione levels and N-acetylcysteine has been used as a supplement in those patients. I don't know whether there is a clear clinical benefit to increasing these patients' glutathione status, but in terms of an approach to restore levels towards normal, this seems reasonable.

QUESTION: Do these patients also have a very high CRP level?

KENNY JIALAL: The big problem with AIDS is that the antiretroviral treatment is leading to this epidemic of metabolic syndrome, dyslipidemia, and coronary artery disease. We're come back to cardiovascular disease and how you treat that in patients with HIV is a big problem.

COMMENT: Some of my colleagues, including Frank Polk, who started this study, made a prospective evaluation of nutritional factors in relation to progression of HIV disease before it was actually known to be HIV disease. This was a MAC cohort and the results were published a number of years ago. There was a clear, inverse relationship, an apparent benefit, from high intake of niacin and other B vitamins. Bozi in Tanzania confirmed that finding in a randomized trial among HIV-positive women. There was also a strong adverse relation with high zinc intake, but as I remember, there was not much for vitamin E.

SIMIN MEYDANI: Marianna Bahm and colleagues have also performed similar studies, and they found an inverse association with selenium and progression of disease.They were not able to demonstrate any association with vitamin E, and I think they're now conducting a clinical trial with selenium.

SAMAR BASU: I have some comments in line with what Dr. Jialal is talking about, the selection of biomarkers. There was a concern in the NIH several years back as to which biomarkers could be used as oxidative stress biomarkers in relation to many of these diseases. So we have been participating in a biomarker study—Biomarkers of Oxidative Stress (BOSS). There are 14 different groups selected from the United-States. CCl4, a classical model for oxidative stress, was used and samples have been sent to various participating laboratories. These samples have been analyzed for various kinds of oxidative stress biomarkers, including isoprostanes, which at present seems to be a promising biomarker. There are two papers on this scheduled for publication. We have been seeing that isoprostanes are one of the best biomarkers, as measured by GC/MS or antibody-based methods, all of them have showing excellent correlations.

JEFFREY BLUMBERG: Isoprostanes are the best validated biomarker available for lipid peroxidation. But if we are talking about approaches to characterizing oxidative stress, it is critically important to recognize that no single biomarker will suffice to reflect all its facets. A wonderful biomarker for lipid peroxidation may not at all reflect DNA oxidation or protein oxidation. We are most often limited in human studies by ready access only to blood and urine, but we must be cautious about extrapolating findings in these matrices to other tissues or making inferences about the distribution and kinetics of these biomarkers. A prudent approach, whenever feasible, is to adopt a panel of biomarkers of oxidative stress. It is simply not reasonable, though not uncommon, to pick a single biomarker, like MDA or 8OHdG, in a single tissue and presume it to reflect accurately and fully oxidative stress in those cells or other tissues in the body.

LESTER PACKER: In closing this discussion, I would like to do is ask each panel member if they have any jewel or nugget they would like to leave with us.

SIMIN MEYDANI: In some of the intervention trials, we need to also pay attention to the status of some of the other nutrients. I have, for example, noticed that if you look at some of the European countries, they have a lower level of vitamin C, for example, in plasma compared to those in the United States. When you use a high level of supplementation, for example, with vitamin E, in the context of lower levels of vitamin C, you might find very different results than if you had an adequate level of vitamin C. The same could be true for other nutrients. I think the differences in nutritional status could explain some of the controversies observed in the literature.

WALTER WILLETT: Most important to me is continuing to talk to each other, because it's clear that we're getting very different pictures working in our own isolated areas. The challenge here is to put all of these pieces together and understand how vitamin E relates to human health.

KENNY JIALAL: I want to congratulate the organizers on putting on an excellent symposium. Joe Lunec, I just want to reiterate the fact that if you're going to measure a biomarker of lipid peroxidation, then it should relate to lipid peroxidation. If you're going to measure a marker of protein oxidation, then relate it to protein oxidation, and DNA oxidation also. There has to be a mechanistic point for its being measured if you're going to say something about effect. On a positive note, as I'm probably the last one to say something, I think we're getting better at measuring biomarkers, and I think we should progress further in the future to improve the robustness of these markers.

LESTER PACKER: Thank you all very much for your participation.

Fluorescent Tocopherols as Probes of Inter-Vesicular Transfer Catalyzed by the α-Tocopherol Transfer Protein

JEFFREY K. ATKINSON,[a] PHILLIP NAVA,[a] GRANT FRAHM,[a] VALERIE CURTIS,[b] AND DANNY MANOR[b]

[a]*Department of Chemistry and Centre for Biotechnology, Brock University, St. Catharines, Ontario, Canada*

[b]*Division of Nutritional Sciences, Cornell University, Ithaca, New York*

ABSTRACT: Novel fluorescent analogues of α-tocopherol have been prepared that incorporate the useful fluorophores nitrobenoxadiazyl (NBD) and anthroyloxy (AO). Both fluorescent tocopherol analogues bind specifically to recombinant human tocopherol transfer protein (hTTP). The NBD-α-tocopherol is particularly useful for protein-binding assays, whereas the AO-α-tocopherol was designed to be one of a pair of chromophores for a fluorescence resonance energy transfer (FRET) assay of intervesicular tocopherol transfer. It is now possible to follow AO-α-tocopherol transfer from donor lipid vesicles composed of predominantly phosphatidylcholine (PC) to acceptor lipid vesicles containing PC and a quenching lipid NBD-PE (2-dipalmitoyl-*sn*-glycero-3-phosphoethanolamine-*N*-[7-nitro-2-1,3-benzoxadiazol-4-yl]). The presence of hTTP substantially increases the rate of AO-α-tolcopherol transfer over the uncatalyzed spontaneous rate.

KEYWORDS: α-tocopherol transfer protein; fluorescent analogues; lipid transfer proteins

The α-tocopherol transfer protein (α-TTP) is now understood to be a key mediator in the selective retention of dietary α-tocopherol.[1] However, the molecular mechanism by which α-TTP selectively harvests *RRR*-α-tocopherol and mediates its transfer to circulating lipoproteins in plasma is not well described. The similarity of α-TTP to several other lipid-binding proteins of the CRAL-TRIO family (Pfam entry PF00650) and the recent publication of the three-dimensional structure of human α-TTP[2] hint that the mechanism of inter-membrane tocopherol transfer may involve direct association with membrane surfaces in a manner similar to that postulated for Sec14p, a yeast phosphatidylinositol transfer protein.

Despite this similarity in structure and possibly in function, little is known about intracellular tocopherol transfer from one lipid environment to another. To visualize

---

Address for correspondence: Jeffrey K. Atkinson, Department of Chemistry and Centre for Biotechnology, Brock University, St. Catharines, Ontario, Canada. Voice: 905-688-5550; fax: 905-682-9020.

jatkin@brocku.ca

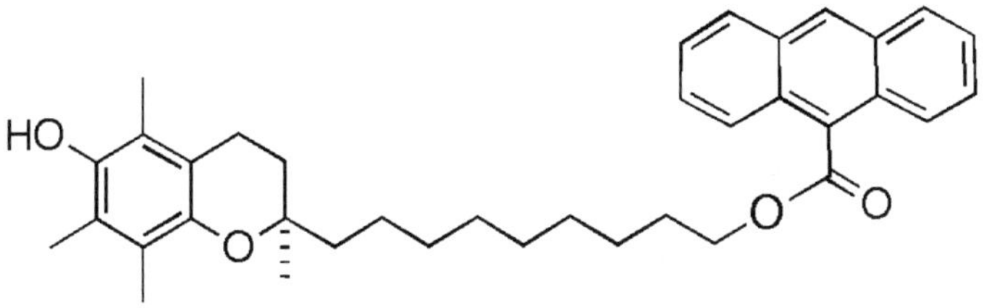

**C9-anthroyloxy-α-tocopherol
(C9-AO-α-Toc)**

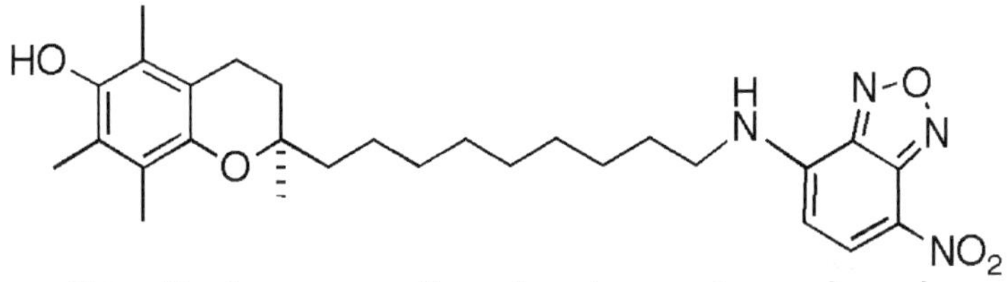

**C9-nitrobenzoxadiazolamino-α-tocopherol
(C9-NBD-α-Toc)**

FIGURE 1. Fluorescent analogues of α-tocopherol.

the catalysis of lipid transfer by α-TTP, we have prepared unique fluorescent tocopherol analogues to act as reporters of the location and amount of material in a specific environment. The tocopherol analogues that we have prepared are shown in FIGURE 1.

METHODS

Analogues with different side-chain lengths have been prepared, but only the nine-carbon (C9), straight-chain versions are reported here. Briefly, they were synthesized by addition of an ω-hydroxyalkylphosphonium salt to Trolox aldehyde as previously described.[3] The fluorophores were then attached to the terminal functional group (OH or NH_2) using well-known chemistries of the fluorophore derivatives.

Fluorescence resonance energy transfer (FRET) assays were performed by monitoring the spontaneous and α-TTP-catalyzed transfer of C9-AO-Toc between donor lipid vesicles and acceptors. Large unilamellar vesicles (approximate diameter: 100 nm) composed of 98% bovine liver phosphatidylcholine and 2% C9-AO-Toc, were prepared by extrusion through polycarbonate filters. Acceptor vesicles were composed of 90% phosphatidylcholine and 10% NBD-PE (2-dipalmitoyl-*sn*-glycero-3-phosphoethanolamine-*N*-[7-nitro-2-1,3-benzoxadiazol-4-yl]). Fluorescence intensity of the C9-AO-Toc (excitation at 366 nm; emission at 440 nm) was followed

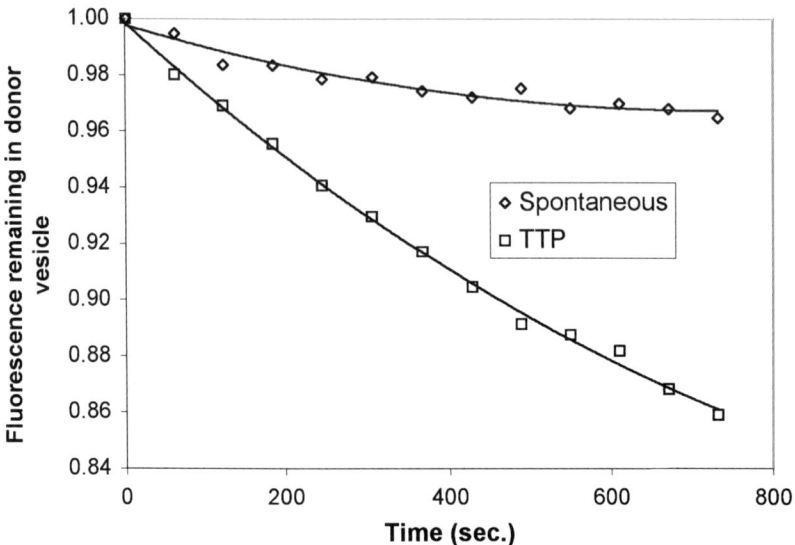

FIGURE 2. Assay of transfer of 9-AO-tocopherol between LUVs.

over time using a fluorometer (Quantamaster 2000, Photon Technologies International, London, Ontario). Transfer assays were begun by mixing a prepared solution of donor vesicles (158 μM total lipids, 3.2 μM C9-AO-Toc) with acceptor vesicles (315 μM), either containing 6.3 μM α-TTP or no protein for controls.

RESULTS

Both the C9-NBD-α-Toc and C9-AO-α-Toc specifically bound to recombinant human α-TTP with K_d values of approximately 30 nM and 70 nM, respectively, substantiating their use as specific labels for assessing binding to tocopherol transfer proteins. The AO-α-Toc labels were designed to act as one partner of a FRET pair, the other being a suitable partner such as NBD-labeled phosphatidylethanolamine. FIGURE 2 shows the time-dependent loss of fluorescence from donor vesicles loaded with C9-AO-Toc as they transfer either spontaneously or under the catalysis of α-TTP.

CONCLUSIONS

The rate of tocopherol transfer between unilamellar vesicles can be monitored using newly prepared fluorescent tocopherols in a FRET assay. α-TTP is shown to catalyze this transfer in a specific manner. This system will allow further investigations to be made regarding the effects of vesicle lipid composition, curvature, competing tocopherols, and other lipids that have been shown to have some affinity for α-TTP. Current studies include similar FRET assays performed between α-TTP loaded with

C9-AO-α-Toc and acceptor vesicles under stopped-flow conditions in a similar manner as has been done with fatty-acid-binding proteins.[4] Additionally, these fluorescent tocopherol analogues will allow for the investigation of intra-cellular vitamin E trafficking in cultured cells.

REFERENCES

1. TRABER, M.G. & H. ARAI. 1999. Molecular mechanisms of vitamin E transport. Annu. Rev. Nutr. **19:** 343–355.
2. MEIER, R. *et al.* 2003. The molecular basis of vitamin E retention: structure of human alpha-tocopherol transfer protein. J. Molec. Biol. **331:** 725–734.
3. LEI, H.S. & J. ATKINSON. 2000. Synthesis of phytyl- and chroman-derivatized photoaffinity labels based on alpha-tocopherol. J. Org. Chem. **65:** 2560–2567.
4. STORCH, J. & A.E. THUMSER. 2000. The fatty acid transport function of fatty acid-binding proteins. Biochim. Biophys. Acta **1486:** 28–44.

Gene–Nutrient Interactions Exemplified by the α-Tocopherol Content of Tissues from α-Tocopherol Transfer Protein–Null Mice Fed Different Dietary Vitamin E Concentrations

YUNSOOK LIM,[a] BETTINA C. SCHOCK,[a] KISHORCHANDRA GOHIL,[a] SCOTT W. LEONARD,[b] LESTER PACKER,[c] CARROLL E. CROSS,[a] AND MARET G. TRABER[a,b]

[a]*Center for Comparative Respiratory Biology and Medicine, Department of Internal Medicine, University of California, Davis, Davis, California, USA*

[b]*Department of Nutrition and Food Management, Linus Pauling Institute, Corvallis, Oregon, USA*

[c]*Department of Molecular Pharmacology and Toxicology, University of Southern California, Los Angeles, California, USA*

KEYWORDS: α-tocopherol; α-tocopherol transfer protein; vitamin E deficiency

Alpha-tocopherol transfer protein (α-TTP) is a liver cytosolic transport protein responsible for maintenance of plasma α-tocopherol (α-T) concentrations. Symptoms of vitamin E deficiency, including neurological disorders such as ataxia, in α-TTP–deficient (TTP$^{-/-}$) mice can be attenuated if dietary α-T is sufficiently augmented. We reviewed the current knowledge of the regulation of plasma and tissue α-T manipulated by dietary α-T in α-TTP $^{-/-}$ mice. These include all characteristics, gene profile, and plasma and tissue α-T levels in α-TTP $^{-/-}$ mice fed diets containing different α-T levels in all published and unpublished data on α-TTP $^{-/-}$ mice. In mice fed normal diets that contained 35–150 mg α-T/kg, cerebral cortex α-T concentrations in TTP$^{-/-}$ mice were 0.25 nmol/g, but were 100-times greater in TTP$^{+/+}$ mice. On α-T supplementation at 600 mg/kg diet, cerebral cortex and cerebellar levels of α-T in TTP$^{-/-}$ mice were only 1.8 and 2.6 nmol/g, respectively. Nonetheless, these increases were sufficient to prevent neurological symptoms and to suppress lipid peroxidation in TTP $^{-/-}$ mice. Furthermore, α-T supplementation can be sufficient to prevent abnormalities such as infertility in α-TTP $^{-/-}$ mice.

Liver α-T levels in TTP$^{-/-}$ mice are 34–47% of TTP$^{+/+}$ mice when fed normal α-T diets (35–150 mg α-T/kg). But plasma and other tissue α-T levels are very low in TTP$^{-/-}$ mice (1–14.2% of tissue α-T levels in TTP$^{+/+}$ mice). Plasma and other tissue

Address for correspondence: Maret G. Traber, Ph.D., Linus Pauling Institute, Oregon State University, 571 Weniger Hall, Corvallis, OR 97331. Voice: 541-737-7977.
maret.traber@orst.edu

levels of α-T in TTP$^{-/-}$ mice on the different diets showed considerable variability, suggesting tissue-specific mechanisms for regulating α-T.

This review suggests that liver α-T can be modulated by dietary α-T in TTP$^{-/-}$ mice. However, plasma and other tissue α-T levels in α-TTP$^{-/-}$ mice do not appear to be directly related to the amounts of dietary α-T. Therefore, α-TTP$^{-/-}$ mice will provide an ideal model for investigating the specific role of α-T in different tissues and genes associated with α-T in health and disease and for dissociating antioxidant functions of α-T from its non-antioxidant functions.

REFERENCES

1. JISHAGE, K. *et al.* 2001. α-tocopherol transfer protein is important for the normal development of placental labyrinthine tropoblasts in mice. JBC **276:** 1669–1672/
2. KAEMPF-ROTZOLL, D.E. *et al.* 2002. α-tocopheol transfer protein is specifically localized at the implantation site of pregnant mouse uterus. Biol. Reprod. **67:** 599–604
3. Leonard, S.W. *et al.* 2002. Incorporation of deuterated RRR- or all-rac-α-tocopherol in plasma and tissues of α-tocopherol transfer protein null mice. Am. J. Clin. Nutr. **75:** 555–560
4. SCHOCK, B.C. *et al.* 2004. Enhanced inflammatory responses in α-tocopherol transfer protein null mice. Arch. Biochem. Biophys. **423:** 162–169.
5. GOHIL, K. *et al.* 2003. Gene expression profile of oxidant stress and neurodegeneration in transgenic mice deficient in α-tocopherol transfer protein. Free. Rad. Biol. Med. **35:** 1343–1354.
6. TERASAWA, Y. *et al.* 2000. Increased atherosclerosis in hyperlipidemic mice deficient in α-tocopherol transfer protein and vitamin E. Proc. Natl. Acad. Sci. USA **97:** 13830–13834.
7. YOKOTA, T. *et al.* 2001. Delayed-onset ataxia in mice lacking a-tocopherol transfer protein: model for neuronal degeneration caused by chronic oxidative stress. Proc. Natl. Acad. Sci. **98:** 15185–15190.

Intracellular Localization of α-Tocopherol Transfer Protein and α-Tocopherol

JINGHUI QIAN,[a] KATHLEEN WILSON,[a] PHIL NAVA,[b] SAMANTHA MORLEY,[a] JEFFREY ATKINSON,[b] AND DANNY MANOR[a]

[a]*Division of Nutritional Sciences, Cornell University, Ithaca, New York, USA*
[b]*Department of Chemistry, Brock University, St. Catharines, Ontario, Canada*

ABSTRACT: The mechanism of action of tocopherol transfer protein (TTP) and its role in the intracellular processing of vitamin E were investigated using confocal fluorescence microscopy. The results from this work suggest that TTP functions by transporting vitamin E from endocytic organelles to other locations in the cell.

KEYWORDS: tocopherol transfer protein; vitamin E

The alpha tocopherol transfer protein (α-TTP) is a critical regulator of tocopherol status in mammals. It functions by facilitating the secretion of tocopherol from the liver to circulating lipoproteins. Humans carrying mutations in the TTP gene have low plasma tocopherol levels and develop the syndrome called ataxia with vitamin E deficiency (AVED). To gain insight into the mechanism by which α-TTP facilitates tocopherol secretion, we developed an inducible expression system for TTP in human and rat hepatocyte cell lines. We characterized these cell lines with respect to TTP-dependent tocopherol secretion, and to the intracellular localization of both α-TTP and fluorescently labeled α-tocopherol.

In the TetOn-TTP cell line, treatment with tetracycline leads to expression of the TTP protein, and to significant increase in secretion of tocopherol to the media. Under the same conditions, confocal immunofluorescent microscopy reveals that TTP exhibits a punctate cellular distribution pattern. Since TTP co-localizes with the EEA1 marker, we conclude that it associates with the endosomal compartment. To study the intracellular trafficking of tocopherol, we synthesized a fluorescent derivative of α-tocopherol, in which the 7-*nitro*-2,1,3-benzoxadiazole (NBD) fluorophore is attached to the phytyl chain of the tocopherol. Shortly (5 min) after incubation with the cells, we observe NBD-tocopherol to localize at the cell periphery, where it appears to associate with the plasma membrane. The tocopherol then progressively moves to the cell interior, with the ligand localizing at a perinuclear compartment within 30 minutes. The time-dependence of the internalization process suggests that the tocopherol is "traveling" in the endocytosis pathway. At longer times (30–

Address for correspondence: Danny Manor, Division of Nutritional Sciences, Cornell University, Ithaca, NY 14853. Voice: 607-255-6085; fax: 607-225-1033.
dm43@cornell.edu

40 min) we observe that NBD-tocopherol is co-localized with α-TTP in a vesicular perinuclear compartment.

CONCLUSION

Our results suggest that tocopherol is internalized by an endocytotic process. The localization of TTP to endosomal compartments suggests a way by which TTP can regulate tocopherol secretion in hepatocytes.

Structure–Function Relationship in the Tocopherol Transfer Protein

S. MORLEY,[a] C. PANAGABKO,[b] A. STOCKER,[c] J. ATKINSON,[b] AND D. MANOR[a]

[a]*Cornell University, Ithaca, New York, USA*
[b]*Brock University, St. Catharines, Ontario, Canada*
[c]*ETH, Zurich, Switzerland*

ABSTRACT: The role of specific amino acid residues in mediating the biochemical functions of tocopherol transfer protein (TTP) was investigated using site-directed mutagenesis and functional assays. These findings further current understanding of TTP mechanism of action and its role in human health.

KEYWORDS: tocopherol transfer protein; vitamin E

Tocopherol transfer protein (α-TTP) is soluble 32-kDa protein expressed in liver that selectively binds alpha tocopherol. That TTP plays a critical role in vitamin E transport is evident from the physiological impact of mutations in the TTP gene. Thus, humans harboring heritable mutations in the TTP gene display low plasma vitamin E levels and a neurodegenerative syndrome termed ataxia with vitamin E deficiency (AVED). Essentially identical symptoms arise in mouse models in which TTP expression is specifically disrupted. In cultured hepatocyte cell lines, overexpression of TTP leads to enhanced secretion of cellular tocopherol to the media. From these observations a model for TTP function was developed in which the protein somehow regulates a novel, alpha-tocopherol–specific secretion pathway. However, the molecular mechanisms underlying this activity are, at present, unknown. *In vitro* characterization of TTP relies on the protein's "signature" activity, namely, the facilitation of tocopherol transfer between lipid bilayers. Neither the molecular mechanism underlying tocopherol transfer, nor its relevance to TTP function *in vivo* are well understood. To arrive at a better-defined picture of TTP function, we used site-directed mutagenesis to generate a series of substitution mutations in the protein. In our choices of target residues for mutagenesis, we were guided by the naturally ocurring mutations in human AVED patients, and by the recently solved three-dimensional structure of TTP. To test the functionality of the TTP mutants, we purified them from overexpressing bacteria, and measured their tocopherol transfer activity *in vitro*. We have also utilized urea-induced denaturation experiments to assess

Address for correspondence: Danny Manor, Division of Nutritional Sciences, Cornell University, Ithaca, NY, 14853. Voice: 607-255-6085; fax: 607-255-1033.
dm43@cornell.edu

overall folding and stability of the mutated proteins in comparson to the wild-type TTP.

We find that all AVED TTP mutations retain significant tocopherol transfer activity. Mutations associated with the severe, early-onset form of the disease (namely, the R59W, E141K and R221W substitutions) exhibit a 2–3-fold kinetic impairment in the ability to catalyze tocopherol transfer). TTP variants possessing the mild, later-onset AVED substitutions (R192H, H101Q, and A120T) or a mutation in the protein's basic patch (R68A) exhibited tocopherol transfer activities that were virtually indistinguishable from the wild-type protein. These results show that TTP's activity in the tocopherol transfer assay *in vitro* does not fully capture its biochemical activities *in vivo*. Thus, we propose that for proper maintainance of tocopherol status *in vivo*, TTP is likely to have additional, as-yet unknown functions, such as interactions with other cellular components.

We also find that occupancy of the ligand-binding pocket significantly protects TTP against denaturant-induced unfolding. Possibly TTP's amphipathic helical "lid," which changes conformation upon tocopherol binding, contributes significantly to the overall stability of the protein.

α-Tocopherol Affects Androgen Metabolism in Male Rat

LUCA BARELLA,[a] CRISTINA ROTA,[b] ELISABETH STÖCKLIN,[a] AND GERALD RIMBACH[c]

[a]*DSM Nutritional Products, Research and Development, Human Nutrition and Health, CH-4303 Kaiseraugst, Switzerland*

[b]*Hugh Sinclair Human Nutrition Unit, School of Food Biosciences, University of Reading, Whiteknights, Reading RG6 6AP, United Kingdom*

[c]*Christian Albrechts University of Kiel, Institute of Food Science and Nutrition, D-24105 Kiel, Germany*

ABSTRACT: The Alpha-Tocopherol Beta-Carotene Cancer Prevention Study has provided the first evidence implicating vitamin E in hormone synthesis. The effect of vitamin E on stereoidogenesis in testes and adrenal glands was assessed in growing rats using Affymetrix gene-chip technology. Dietary supplementation of rats with vitamin E (60 mg/kg feed) for a period of 429 days caused a significant repression of genes encoding for proteins centrally involved in the uptake (low-density lipoprotein receptor) and *de novo* synthesis (for example, 7-dehydrocholesterol reductase, 3-hydroxy-3-methylglutaryl coenzyme A synthase, 3-hydroxy-3-methylglutaryl-coenzyme A reductase, isopentenyl-diphosphate delta-isomerase, and farnesyl pyrophosphate synthetase) of cholesterol, the precursor of all steroid hormones. The present investigation indicates that dietary vitamin E may induce changes in stereoidogenesis by affecting cholesterol homeostasis.

KEYWORDS: vitamin E; hormone; androgen; gene expression; testes; adrenal; cholesterol

INTRODUCTION

Vitamin E (VE), which is considered the most effective lipid-soluble, chain-breaking antioxidant, protects cellular membranes from lipid peroxidation. Many types of cancers are believed to be the result of oxidative damage to DNA by free radicals. Thus, several studies have addressed the question whether VE may prevent carcinogenesis. In 1995, a large intervention trial, the Alpha-Tocopherol Beta-Carotene Cancer Prevention (ATBC) Study, has shown that male smokers supplemented with VE experienced 32% lower incidence and 41% decreased mortality from prostate cancer than did those not taking the supplement.[1] Several mechanisms of action

Address for correspondence: Luca Barella, DSM Nutritional Products, Research and Development, Human Nutrition and Health, CH-4303 Kaiseraugst, Switzerland. Voice: +41 (0)61 688 5292; fax: +41 (0)61 688 96 84.

luca.barella@dsm.com

TABLE 1. Effect of dietary vitamin E supplementation on gene expression in rat testis and adrenal glands

Affymetrix Accession Number	Gene Description	Fold Change P value	Organ and Function
AB016800_at	7-dehydrocholesterol reductase	−4.61 $P<0.01$	Testes Cholesterol biosynthesis
rc_AI177004_s_at	3-hydroxy-3-methyl-glutaryl-coenzyme a synthase	−2.12 $P<0.05$	Adrenal gland Cholesterol biosynthesis
X55286_g_at	3-hydroxy-3-methyl-glutaryl-coenzyme a reductase	−2.0 $P<0.01$	Adrenal gland Cholesterol biosynthesis
AF003835_at	isopentenyl-diphosphate delta isomerase	−2.89 $P<0.01$	Adrenal gland Cholesterol biosynthesis
M89945mRNA_at	farnesyl diphosphate synthase	−1.06 $P<0.01$	Adrenal gland Cholesterol biosynthesis
X13722_at	low density lipoprotein receptor	−3.72 $P<0.01$	Adrenal gland Cholesterol uptake

have been proposed to explain the potential chemoprotective effect of VE. Potential mechanisms include protection of DNA integrity, modulation of immune function, and interference with hormone production. The latter hypothesis is supported by the ATBC Study, which indicated that men who received α-tocopherol had significantly lower serum levels of androstenedione and testosterone than did those who received a placebo.[2] The mechanism behind this inhibitory effect of VE on androgen production remains largely unknown. The objective of this study was the investigation of the molecular mechanisms of action of VE on the pituitary-gonadal axis in male rat.

METHODS

Two groups (five animals each) of male rats were randomly assigned to either a diet deficient in VE or to a control diet containing 60 mg RRR-α-tocopheryl acetate per kg feed for 429 days. Affymetrix U34A high-density oligonucleotide microarrays comprising more than 7,000 genes were used to assess the transcriptional response of the testis[3] and the adrenal glands.

RESULTS

This experimental strategy identified several genes that were chronically altered by dietary VE. Animals supplemented with VE showed a consistent down regulation of the enzyme 7-dehydrocholesterol reductase (7-DCH) in the testes when compared to the animals deficient in VE.[3] Furthermore, in the adrenal glands of VE-supplemented rats, the low-density lipoproteins receptor (LDL-R) as well as a number of enzymes involved in cholesterol biosynthesis—that is, 3-hydroxy-3-methylglutaryl coenzyme A synthase (HMG-CoA-S), 3-hydroxy-3-methylglutaryl-coenzyme A reductase (HMG-CoA-R), isopentenyl-diphosphate δ-isomerase (IP δ-I) and farnesyl pyrophosphate synthetase (FPP-S)—were found to be down-regulated (TABLE 1). Measurement of plasma androgens showed a moderate decrease in testosterone (data not shown) and a significant decrease in dehydrotestosterone[4] in animals supplemented with VE.

DISCUSSION

This study demonstrates that dietary VE intake has long-term effects on the pituitary-gonadal axis in male rat. VE was found to affect the transcriptional activation of a number of genes encoding for proteins centrally involved in the uptake and *de novo* synthesis of cholesterol, the precursor of all steroid molecules. In the testes, VE was found to decrease 7-DCH, which catalyzes the last steps in the synthesis of cholesterol. In the adrenal glands, cholesterol synthesis (see HMG-CoA-S, HMG-CoA-R, IP delta-I, and FPP-S) and cholesterol uptake (see LDL-R) were downregulated by VE. Adrenals are the primary source of dehydroepiandrosterone (DHEA), which is also synthesized from cholesterol as its precursor. Taken together, these data give new insights into the possible molecular mechanisms underlying the observed decrease in plasma DHEA and testosterone in men supplemented with vitamin E.[2]

REFERENCES

1. ALBANES, D., O.P. HEINONEN, J.K. HUTTUNEN, *et al.* 1995. Effects of alpha-tocopherol and beta-carotene supplements on cancer incidence in the Alpha-Tocopherol Beta-Carotene Cancer Prevention Study. Am. J. Clin. Nutr. **62**(Suppl.): 1427S–1430S.
2. HARTMAN, T.J., J.F. DORGAN, K. WOODSON, *et al.* 2001. Effects of long-term alpha-tocopherol supplementation on serum hormones in older men. Prostate **46**: 33–38.
3. ROTA, C., L. BARELLA, A.M. MINIHANE, *et al.* 2004. Alpha-tocopherol affects gene expression in rat testis. IUBMB Life **56**: 277–280.
4. BARELLA, L., P.Y. MULLER, M. SCHLACHTER, *et al.* 2004. Identification of the hepatic molecular mechanisms of action of alpha-tocopherol using global gene expression profile analysis in rats. Biochim. Biophys. Acta **1689**: 66–74.

The Transcriptional Signature of Vitamin E

AMY JOHNSON AND DANNY MANOR

Division of Nutritional Sciences, Cornell University, Ithaca, New York 14853, USA

ABSTRACT: To investigate the ability of RRR-α-tocopherol to regulate gene expression, we interrogated RNA samples from treated cultured cells with Affymetrix oligonucleutodie arrays. We find that vitamin E potently regulates the expression of ca. 230 genes, functioning in metabolism, cell-cycle progression, and transcriptional regulation.

KEYWORDS: tocopherol; vitamin E; transcription

Vitamin E, the principal lipid-soluble antioxidant in mammalian tissues, is a family of eight structurally related tocopherol and tocotrienol vitamers. In recent years α-tocopherol (α-TOH) was shown to exhibit several activities that appear to be independent of its antioxidant function and that have yet to be fully characterized. Among those activities are modulation of enzymatic activities, protein stability, and cell proliferation. In addition, several studies implicate a role for α-TOH as a transcriptional regulator that modulates the expression of multiple genes; however, the distinction between α-TOH's antioxidant and non-antioxidant transcriptional activities is unclear, and the ability of other tocopherol forms to regulate transcription remains largely unexplored. We set out to identify genes whose transcription is regulated by α-tocopherol in a specific manner, and to evaluate whether α-TOH's genomic effects stem from a specific transcriptional response or from a general response to redox/antioxidant status. Toward this end, we cultured HepG2 C3A cells with control media or with media supplemented with 100 µM α-TOH. After 48 hours, total RNA was isolated from triplicate plates, and used to synthesize fluorescently labeled cRNA. Triplicate human DNA oligonucleotide microarrays (Affymetrix) were then used to interrogate the different samples. Since β-TOH is similar to α-TOH in its structure and free-radical scavenging ability, it was included as an additional treatment group, in which we intended to assess transcriptional responses to changes in cellular oxidation/redox status. From this experiment we obtained a list of genes that are significantly regulated by vitamin E.

We observed that, in most cases, β-tocopherol exhibited similar or greater transcriptional activities to those seen upon α-tocopherol treatment. The genes that responded to vitamin E belong to several functional categories including lipid metabolism, signal transduction, and cell proliferation. We also observed changes in the transcription of a number of transcription factors that may be the primary responders to vitamin E. Of particular interest were genes that encode key regulatory

Address for correspondence: Danny Manor, Division of Nutritional Sciences, Cornell University, Ithaca, NY, 14853. Voice: 607-255-6085; fax: 607-255-1033.
dm43@cornell.edu

enzymes in the biosynthetic pathway of cholesterol. To confirm transcriptional regulation observed in the expression arrays, real-time and semi-quantitative RT-PCR was utilized in independent experiments to assess the transcriptional effects of tocopherols on four differentially expressed genes. In addition, dose–response and time course experiments were carried out to validate and further characterize the nature of the observed transcriptional regulation. Our results suggest that both α- and β- tocopherol can act as transcriptional regulators in cultured cells. The differences in the regulatory effects of the two vitamers provide further insight into tocopherol-dependent mechanisms that regulate gene expression in the body.

α- and γ-Tocopherol Plasma and Urinary Biokinetics following α-Tocopherol Supplementation

JUDITH C.P. EICHHORN,[a] ROSALIND LEE,[a] CHRISTINA DUNSTER,[a] SAMAR BASU,[b] AND FRANK J. KELLY[a]

[a]*School of Health & Life Sciences, King's College, London, UK*

[b]*Uppsala Medical School, Uppsala University, Sweden*

KEYWORDS: vitamin E; α-tocopherol; γ-tocopherol; carboxyethyl-hydroxy-chromans; CEHC; supplementation

BACKGROUND

Because of the potential beneficial effects of α-TOH on health, there is much interest in oral intake of α-TOH, especially in high doses. Although 35% of the adult population take α-TOH supplements, little research attention is paid to the actual biotransformation and metabolism of α- and γ-TOH *in vivo*, in particular with increased intake. Our aim was to investigate the impact of increased levels of α-TOH intake for 21 days on plasma α- and γ-TOH and urinary tocopherol metabolite concentrations.

STUDY DESIGN

Subjects ($n=38$) were given daily 15, 100, 200, and 400 mg α-TOH acetate for 21 days. Blood and urine samples were taken before supplementation (baseline) and weekly during supplementation and a 3-week washout period. Each subject underwent all four treatments. Plasma α- and γ-TOH were assayed with HPLC with UV detector and adjusted for cholesterol. Urinary α- and γ-2,5,7,8-tetramethyl-2(2′-carboxyethyl)-6-hydroxy-chroman (CEHC) and α-quinone lactone (QL) concentrations were analyzed by GC/MS and corrected for creatinine.

Address for correspondence: Judith Eichhorn, Department of Life Sciences, King's College London, 150 Stamford Street, London, SE1 9NN, UK. Voice: +44 20 7848 3893; fax +44 20 7848 3891.

judith.eichhorn@kcl.ac.uk

TABLE 1. Plasma tocopherols and urinary metabolite concentrations over the 21-day α-tocopherol supplementation period as percentage of baseline values

	Plasma Tocopherols		Urinary Metabolites		
	α-TOH	γ-TOH	α-QL	α-CEHC	γ-CEHC
Baseline	100	100	100	100	100
15 mg	105.1*	80.4**	89.9	107.1*	78.5
100 mg	140.2**	48.2**	168.0**	326.9**	113.4
200 mg	147.8**	40.4**	257.9**	551.6**	117.1
400 mg	151.0**	28.2**	325.5**	821.9**	132.5

NOTE: Values are geometric means over the 21-day supplementation period expressed as percentage of starting baseline values. *$P < 0.05$; **$P < 0.0001$.

RESULTS

Generally all doses of α-TOH acetate supplementation for 21 days resulted in increased plasma α-TOH and decreased γ-TOH concentration. Both urinary α-CEHC and α-QL concentrations increased in a dose-dependent manner to α-TOH, but γ-CEHC concentration did not change significantly throughout the different doses of supplementation. The concentration of the tocopherols and their metabolites went back to baseline within a week post supplementation.

CONCLUSION

Elevated plasma α-TOH and decreased γ-TOH concentrations by increased levels of oral α-TOH intake (≥15mg) suggest that α-TOH replaces plasma γ-TOH, which recently is found to have unique *in vivo* activities itself. The decrease of γ-TOH does not lead to an increase in γ-CEHC excretion, which may imply that other degradation and excretion routes are present for γ-TOH. In contrast, the excretion of urinary α-CEHC is positive correlated to plasma α-TOH concentration and therefore might reflect the amount of α-TOH exceeding the requirement of the body or capacity of involved factors.

ACKNOWLEDGMENT

This work was funded by the UK Food Standards Agency.

Oxidized Vitamin E and Ubiquinone

Competition for Binding Sites of the Mitochondrial Cytochrome bc_1 Complex?

LARS GILLE, WOLFGANG GREGOR, KATRIN STANIEK, AND HANS NOHL

Research Institute of Pharmacology and Toxicology of Oxygen Radicals, University of Veterinary Medicine Vienna, Vienna, Austria

KEYWORDS: mitochondrial bc_1 complex; tocopheryl quinone; ubiquinone; vitamin E; oxygen radicals

One of the most remarkable properties of vitamin E is its radical scavenging activity, which protects biomembranes from oxidative damage.[1] During its antioxidative activity both *in vitro* and *in vivo* small amounts of oxidized vitamin E (α-tocopheryl quinone, TQ) are continuously formed and accumulated in membranes.[2] In contrast to vitamin E, the bioactivity of the metabolite TQ in those membranes had not yet been extensively studied.

In view of TQ's structural similarity to the mitochondrial electron carrier ubiquinone (UQ) (FIG. 1), we developed the hypothesis that TQ could possibly interfere with the functions of ubiquinone in the mitochondrial respiratory chain. UQ is reduced by mitochondrial complexes I and II and in turn oxidized by complex III (electron bifurcation at the cytochrome bc_1 complex). In particular, the latter process was considered to be a source of mitochondrial $O_2^{\cdot-}$ formation modulated by various inhibitors and mitochondrial membrane constituents.[3,4] This high susceptibility towards oxygen radical formation prompted us to study the influence of substoichiometric amounts of TQ on the substrate properties of reduced UQ in isolated bc_1 complex, which was essentially free from both quinones.

Therefore we were able to study the activity of TQ and/or UQ as substrates and their binding to the isolated mitochondrial bc_1 complex independently, using low molecular weight analogues. Redox changes of either *b* cytochromes or cytochrome *c* were assessed by photometric detection in the presence and in the absence of inhibitors for the ubiquinone binding sites at the bc_1 complex.

In a first step the suitability of reduced UQ (UQH_2) and reduced TQ (TQH_2) as substrates for the bc_1 complex using cytochrome *c* as acceptor was compared. Experimental data revealed that TQH_2 shows a quinol:cytochrome *c* oxidoreductase activity about 500 times lower than UQH_2. This clearly demonstrates that TQ cannot replace UQ as an electron carrier in the respiratory chain. However, the apparent K_M values for both compounds were in a similar range (UQH_2: 398 µM; TQH_2: 85 µM),

---

Address for correspondence: Lars Gille, Research Institute of Pharmacology and Toxicology of Oxygen Radicals, University of Veterinary Medicine Vienna, Veterinärplatz 1, A-1210 Vienna, Austria. Voice: +43-1-25077-4407; fax: +43-1-25077-4490.

lars.gille@vu-wien.ac.at

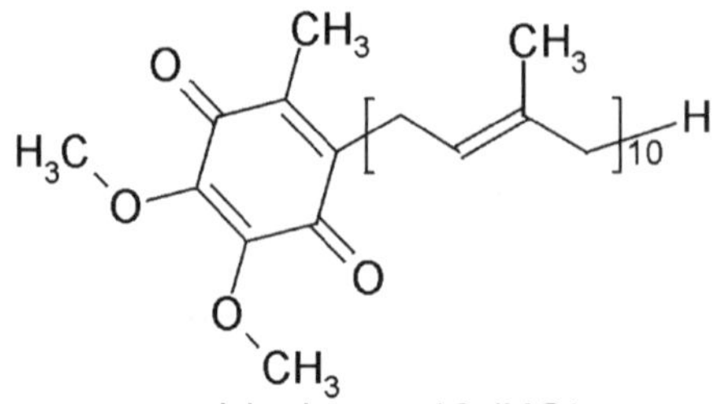

ubiquinone-10 (UQ)

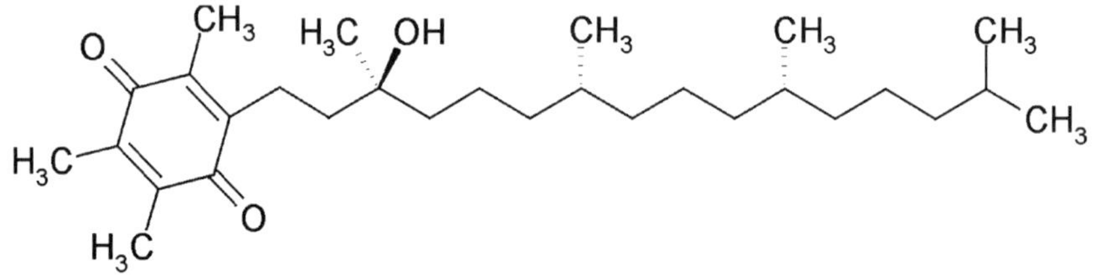

RRR-α-tocopheryl quinone (TQ)

FIGURE 1. Structure of ubiquinone-10 (UQ) and RRR-α-tocopheryl quinone (TQ).

indicating even a slightly stronger binding of TQ than of UQ to the bc_1 complex. In freshly isolated rat liver mitochondria about 3% of vitamin E is present in its oxidized form TQ. The physiological ratio of TQ to UQ in these mitochondria was about 1:20. Therefore, we tested the influence of substoichiometric amounts of TQ with respect to UQ on the quinol:cytochrome *c* oxidoreductase activity of UQH_2. In order to maintain a defined redox state of the substrate quinone/quinol pool, the sum of TQ and UQ was kept constant at 50%, and the remaining 50 % was UQH_2. While a turnover rate of 73 nmol reduced cytochrome *c*/min was observed without TQ under such experimental conditions, already at 10% TQ it declined to 65, and at 50% TQ to about 40. This continuous decrease of turnover rates at the bc_1 complex with increasing TQ concentrations suggested binding properties of this quinone which are different from the native substrate UQ. In order to elucidate TQ-specific binding properties we studied the ability of TQ/TQH_2 to oxidize/reduce *b*-cytochromes of the bc_1 complex in the presence of the Q_i site-specific inhibitor antimycin A, and the Q_o site-specific inhibitor myxothiazol. The potency of both quinones as oxidants at the Q_i pocket was similar.

In contrast, at the Q_o pocket TQH_2 proved to be an inefficient reductant of *b* cytochromes, leading to a slower and incomplete reduction under double block conditions (antimycin A plus myxothiazol).[5] Only after addition of oxidized UQ reduction levels typically achieved with UQH_2 were observed (FIG. 2A).

Kinetic measurements confirmed that TQ preferably exchanges reducing equivalents with the Q_i pocket of the complex, while UQ, the native substrate, binds equally

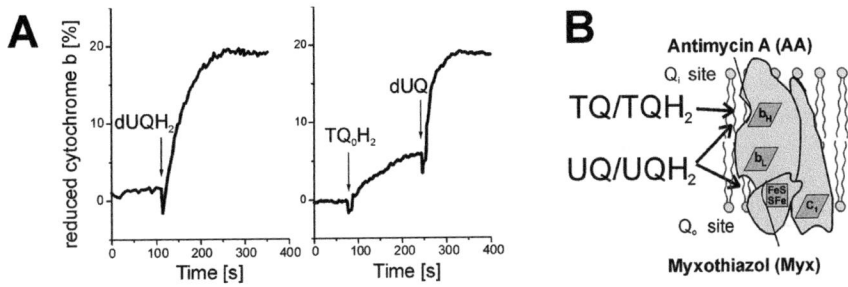

FIGURE 2. Comparison of TQH_2 and UQH_2 as substrate for the bc_1 complex. (**A**) Reduction state of b cytochromes in the bc_1 complex in the presence of myxothiazol and antimycin A after addition of either $dUQH_2$ or TQ_0H_2 plus dUQ. (**B**) Scheme of the bc_1 complex with preferred interaction sites for TQ/TQH_2 and UQ/UQH_2.

effectively to both the Q_i and Q_o pocket of the complex. These asymmetric binding properties of TQ are the rationale for its poor substrate properties and its rather inhibiting effect at the bc_1 complex (FIG. 2B). Experiments to quantify the amount of $O_2^{\bullet-}$ released by UQH_2-oxidizing bc_1 complex demonstrated an inhibiting influence of TQ as well.

The findings of this study suggest a function of the couple vitamin E/TQ as redox sensor in the respiratory chain, which is able to slow down respiration in peroxidizing mitochondrial membranes with increasing amounts of oxidized vitamin E.

ACKNOWLEDGMENTS

This work was supported by Grant P16244-B08 from the Austrian Science Fund (FWF).

REFERENCES

1. BRIGELIUS-FLOHÉ, R. & M.G. TRABER. 1999. Vitamin E: function and metabolism. FASEB J. **13:** 1145–1155.
2. HAM, A.J. & D.C. LIEBLER. 1995. Vitamin E oxidation in rat liver mitochondria. Biochemistry **34:** 5754–5761.
3. GILLE, L. & H. NOHL. 2001. The ubiquinol/bc_1 redox couple regulates mitochondrial oxygen radical formation. Arch. Biochem. Biophys **388:** 34–38.
4. GILLE, L., K. STANIEK & H. NOHL. 2001. Effects of tocopheryl quinone on the heart: model experiments with xanthine oxidase, heart mitochondria, and isolated perfused rat hearts. Free Radic. Biol. Med. **30:** 865–876.
5. VON JAGOW, G. & W.D. ENGEL. 1981. Complete inhibition of electron transfer from ubiquinol to cytochrome b by the combined action of antimycin and myxothiazol. FEBS Lett. **136:** 19–24.

Antioxidant Properties of Chromanols Derived from Vitamin E and Ubiquinone

WOLFGANG GREGOR,[a] CHRISTIAN ADELWÖHRER,[b] THOMAS ROSENAU,[b] GOTTFRIED GRABNER,[c] AND LARS GILLE[a]

[a]*Research Institute for Pharmacology and Toxicology of Oxygen Radicals, University of Veterinary Medicine Vienna, Vienna, Austria*

[b]*Institute of Chemistry, Agricultural University of Vienna, Vienna, Austria*

[c]*Institute of Theoretical Chemistry and Structural Biology, University of Vienna, Vienna, Austria*

> KEYWORDS: EPR; laser flash photolysis; oxachromanol; ubichromanol; ubichromenol; chromanoxyl; chromenoxyl

To be efficient antioxidants, new chromanol derivatives must have a number of chemical and biological properties: (i) fast and irreversible reduction of lipid-derived oxygen radicals; (ii) long lifetime of the resulting chromanoxyl radicals; (iii) fast recycling of the chromanols by endogenous reductants; (iv) low toxicity; and (v) eventual degradation to endogenous metabolites. A complete set of kinetic parameters describing reactions (i)–(iii), obtained under comparable conditions, is therefore desirable, although rarely reported in the literature. We newly synthesized the 2,4-*cis*- and 2,4-*trans*-oxachromanol[1] (Cis, Trans) as well as the dimeric twin chromanol[2] (Twin). In addition, we synthesized ubichromenol[3] (UCe) from ubiquinone-10, and ubichromanol (UCa) from UCe (see FIGURE 1 for all structures).

To investigate the influence of the second ring oxygen in Cis and Trans, the rigid pyran fusion of Twin and the methoxy substituents of UCa and UCe on the electronic properties of these compounds, we collected kinetic data for reactions (i)-(iii) in simple chemical systems, including α-tocopherol (Toc) and pentamethyl chromanol (Penta) as a reference. The primary antioxidant reactivity (i) was quantified in terms of the rate constants (k_1) of the reaction with the blue stable radical diphenyl picryl hydrazyl (DPPH) as a routinously used model for lipid peroxyl radicals. Stopped-flow spectrophotometry in the msec to min timescale yielded second-order k_1 values (in $M^{-1}\ s^{-1}$) for the decay of the 517-nm DPPH absorption in ethanol: 380 ± 10 (Twin), 250 ± 10 (Toc, Penta), 140 ± 50 (UCe), 120 ± 20 (UCa), 110 ± 10 (Cis) and 70 ± 10 (Trans). In addition, we found that Twin can donate 4 electrons (in contrast to 2 for the other compounds) to excess DPPH in aqueous acetonitrile, as anticipated from its dimeric structure. To address the chromanoxyl stability (ii), we first char-

---

Address for correspondence: Lars Gille, Research Institute of Pharmacology and Toxicology of Oxygen Radicals, University of Veterinary Medicine Vienna, Veterinärplatz 1, A-1210 Vienna, Austria. Voice: +43-1-25077-4407; fax: +43-1-25077-4490.
  lars.gille@vu-wien.ac.at

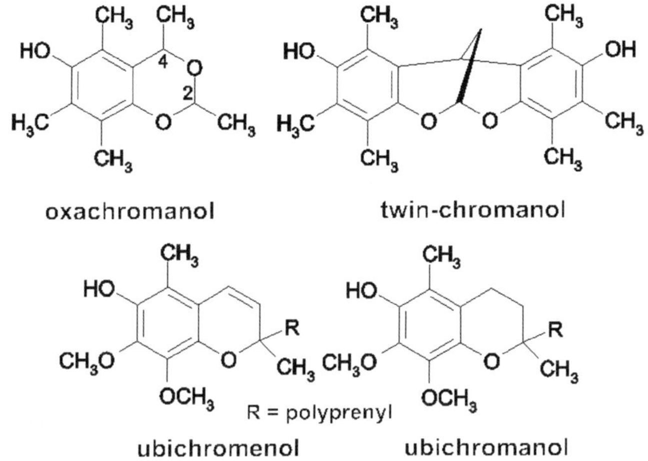

FIGURE 1. Structures of the antioxidants used in this work.

acterized these radicals by UV/VIS (FIG. 2) and electron paramagnetic resonance (EPR) spectroscopy. One-electron oxidation of the chromanols in acetonitrile with UV light (FIG. 2A, Cis, Trans and Twin) or with DPPH (UCa and UCe) yielded radicals which showed optical transitions peaking at ca. 410–425 nm, similar to Toc/Penta (except a shift to 475 nm for UCe) and EPR spectra with similar but distinct hyperfine patterns compared to Toc/Penta; especially Twin showed a more complex pattern, indicating a more delocalized unpaired electron. UCa and UCe yielded broader EPR transitions; however, the larger hyperfine splittings fit published spectra from short-chain analogues.[4] Fast recording of optical chromanoxyl spectra with a diode array detector (FIG. 2B), after reaction of the chromanols with known concentrations of DPPH, yielded absorption coefficients ($\varepsilon/M^{-1}cm^{-1}$) of the radicals in ethanol: ca. 5000 (Penta), 4000 (Toc and Cis), 3000 (UCa), 2000 (Twin and Trans), and 1000 (UCe). These values were used to calculate rate constants (k_2) for the second-order decay (predominantly disproportionation) of the chromanoxyl absorption, again measured by stopped-flow photometry after generating the radicals with DPPH in ethanol. We obtained k_2 values (in $M^{-1} s^{-1}$) of ca. 3200 ± 200 (Cis), 1100 ± 300 (UCa), 630 ± 60 (Penta), 580 ± 50 (Toc), 390 ± 40 (Trans), 180 ± 5 (Twin) and 30 ± 5 (UCe), indicating that Trans, Twin, and UCe are converted to more stable radicals than Toc/Penta. We attribute the exceptional stability of the chromenoxyl radical of UCe to its additional double bond in the pyran ring. Radicals generated by PbO_2 oxidation of the chromanols decayed with similar kinetics. As an additional control, the analysis of time-dependent EPR spectra resulted in similar k_2 values as well. Finally we measured rate constants (k_3) for the chromanol recycling reaction (iii) using ascorbate as reductant. Laser photolysis (at 266 nm) of the chromanols, incorporated in cationic tetradecyl trimethyl ammoniumbromide micelles, in the presence of ascorbate, yielded k_3 values of 1.10^7–1.10^8 $M^{-1} s^{-1}$ with Toc/UCa and Trans ranging at the low and high limit, respectively, except for UCe,

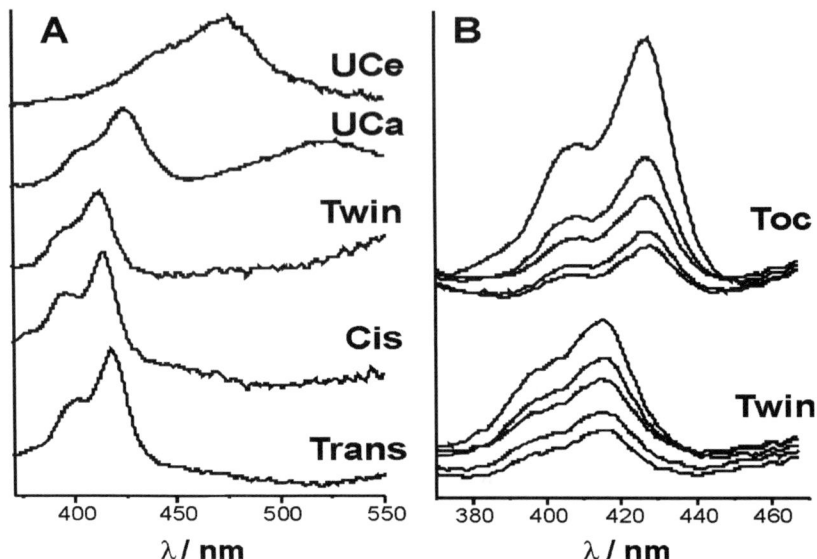

FIGURE 2. (A) Transient UV/VIS spectra of chromanoxyl radicals in acetonitrile. (B) Chromanoxyl spectra at 15-sec intervals in ethanol, showing a slower decay of Twin versus Toc.

which failed to produce the radical photochemically. The value for Toc is close to the published one.[5] Preliminary experiments in homogenous solution (ethanol) with decylubiquinol instead of ascorbate as reductant yielded rate constants in the range of 10^4–10^5 M^{-1} s^{-1}.

Of all antioxidants tested, Twin is a promising candidate for biological studies: in ethanol its antioxidant activity is 50% greater than that of Toc, and its higher radical stability and fast ascorbate reaction should make antioxidant recycling efficient. On the other hand, in addition to an antioxidant activity of ca. 50 % compared to Toc, the ubiquinone derivatives might be interesting in terms of the aforementioned criterion (v).

ACKNOWLEDGMENTS

This work was supported by the Grant P16244-B08 from the Austrian Science Fund (FWF). Technical assistance by Werner Stammberg and helpful advice for the synthesis of UCa by Dr. Thomas Netscher (DSM Nutritional Products) is gratefully acknowledged.

REFERENCES

1. ROSENAU T. *et al.* 2002. Synthesis and oxidation behavior of 2,4,5,7,8-pentamethyl-4H-1,3-benzodioxin-6-ol, a multifunctional oxatocopherol-type antioxidant. J. Org. Chem. **67:** 3607–3614.

2. ROSENAU T. et al. 2002. Calixarene-type macrocycles by oxidation of phenols related to vitamin E. Angew. Chem. Int. Ed. **41:** 1171–1173.
3. IMADA I. & H. MORIMOTO. 1964. Photochemical reaction of ubiquinone (35). Chem. Pharm. Bull. **12:** 1047–1051.
4. MUKAI K. et al. 1984. ESR studies of coenzyme Q_1 chromanoxyl and chromenoxyl radicals. Tetrahedron Lett. **25:** 1929–1932.
5. BISBY R.H. & A.W. PARKER. 1991. Reactions of the α-tocopheroxyl radical in micellar solutions studied by nanosecond laser flash photolysis. FEBS Lett. **290:** 205–208.

Vitamin E in Uremia and Dialysis Patients

FRANCESCO GALLI, UMBERTO BUONCRISTIANI, CARMELA CONTE, CRISTINA AISA, AND ARDESIO FLORIDI

Department of Internal Medicine, Section of Applied Biochemistry and Nutritional Sciences, University of Perugia, Perugia, Italy

ABSTRACT: Vitamin E therapy (based either on oral supplements or new dialysis methods such as vitamin E-coated hemodialysers) has been suggested to yield a better clinical outcome in hemodialysis (HD) patients than in other populations of patients. Among other factors, the presence of a modified vitamin E status might help to explain this apparently paradoxical response to vitamin E. In this study we investigated 104 regular HD patients. The results indicate that, besides having a low dietary intake, these subjects show some abnormalities in the levels and metabolism of vitamin E, such as a disproportion between plasma tocopherols and lipids, low levels of γ-T, and CEHC accumulation. Although further studies are needed to confirm the clinical relevance of vitamin E therapy in HD, these findings might lead to recommending a higher vitamin E intake in these patients.

KEYWORDS: vitamin E; tocopherol; CEHCs; uremia; hemodialysis; end-stage renal disease; oxidative stress; lipid oxidation; antioxidants

INTRODUCTION

It is now believed that in maintenance hemodialysis (HD) the administration of vitamin E may provide clinical advantages greater than in other populations of patients. In fact, several reports showed abnormalities of the antioxidant defense network and accumulation of indices of oxidative stress in plasma and blood cells in patients undergoing HD. These aspects may contribute to sustain the entire comorbidity in these patients, and particularly atherosclerotic cardiovascular disease (CVD), anemia, and chronic inflammation (reviewed in Himmelfarb *et al.*[1] and Galli *et al.*[2]).

The controlled intervention trial SPACE[3] demonstrated that vitamin E supplementation can lower the incidence of some major CVD events associated with HD and particularly myocardial infarction. Other small studies have provided positive results as regards the role of vitamin E in preventing plasma lipid peroxidation, anemia, and some events associated with chronic inflammation and immune dysfunction (see references in Refs. 1 and 2).

Address for correspondence: Francesco Galli, Ph.D., University of Perugia, Department of Internal Medicine, Section of Applied Biochemistry and Nutritional Sciences, Via del Giochetto, 06126 Perugia, Italy. Fax: +39 075 585 7441.
  f.galli@unipg.it

This study evaluates some aspects that may give reason for the therapeutic role of vitamin E in patients with end-stage renal disease (ESRD). In a cross-sectional evaluation we investigated whether vitamin E levels and metabolism are modified in ESRD, and whether and to which extent these changes may lead to a recommendation to implement the intake of vitamin E in these patients in order to prevent or delay ESRD co-morbidity. Our findings are in agreement with other studies in the literature and they suggest that HD patients might benefit from vitamin E therapy.

METHODS

In the past 5 years this laboratory has measured vitamin E levels of 104 ESRD patients from five different dialysis centers in Italy and one in Hungary, and 111 healthy controls.

Subject Characteristics

All the patients were on regular HD with low- or high-flux hemodialysers used in standard bicarbonate HD or hemodiafiltration. There were 61 males and 43 females aged 61±11 years and on dialysis for 27±29 months (mean±SD). Exclusion criteria were severe malnutrition, liver dysfunction, overt infectious disease, interfering therapies and antioxidant supplementation, problems with the arteriovenous fistula, and malignancy. Co-morbidity included CVD (hypertension, left ventricular hypertrophy often associated with coronaropathy and angina, instrumental evidence of carotid plaques, and aortic calcifications), anemia, diabetes, dyslipidemia (hypertriglyceridemia and lowered HDL/LDL ratio), leukopenia, and amyloidosis-related bone disease. The most common drugs were i.v. iron and erythropoietin, different combinations of anti-hypertensive drugs, folates, and calcium and phosphorus binders. Healthy controls were matched for sex and age: there were 68 males and and 43 females whose age was 58±19 years (mean ± SD); exclusion criteria in the controls were severe malnutrition, liver dysfunction, overt infectious disease, interfering therapies and antioxidant supplementation, diabetes, anemia, CVD, and malignancy.

Vitamin E Intake

All the subjects maintained their usual dietary regimen. The vitamin E intake was assessed in 16 HD patients and 10 healthy controls in the area of Perugia by means of a food-frequency questionnaire consisting of four 24-hr dietary recalls, two carried out weekdays and two on the weekend.

Lipids, Vitamin E, and CEHC Analysis in Plasma

Blood samplings and analyses were performed as described in Galli et al.[4]

RESULTS AND DISCUSSION

The present data (TABLE 1) are in agreement with the majority of the reports in literature (see Galli[5] and Himmelfarb et al.[6] and references therein), showing that

TABLE 1. Plasma levels of lipids, vitamin E, and CEHC metabolites in 111 healthy control subjects and 104 ESRD patients on regular hemodialysis

	Healthy Controls	HD Patients	Statistics[a]
Total cholesterol (mmol/L)	5.38 ± 0.61	6.16 ± 1.55	$P < 0.05$
Ttriglycerides (mmol/L)	1.22 ± 0.39	2.71 ± 1.19	$P < 0.01$
α-Tocopherol (mmol/L)	28.4 ± 3.5	28.9 ± 6.7	NS
γ-Tocopherol (mmol/L)	2.44 ± 0.36 ($n = 28$)	1.38 ± 0.49 ($n = 39$)	$P < 0.01$
α-Tocopherol (mmoL/mmol TL)	4.30 ± 0.52	3.26 ± 0.75	$P < 0.01$
γ-Tocopherol (mmoL/ mmol TL)	0.37 ± 0.05 ($n = 2$)	0.16 ± 0.06 ($n = 39$)	$P < 0.01$
α-CEHC (nmol/L)	16.8 ± 7.5 ($n = 10$)	79.2 ± 28.3 ($n = 14$)	$P < 0.01$
γ-CEHC (nmol/L)	190.7 ± 61.0 ($n = 10$)	688.6 ± 180.3 ($n = 14$)	$P < 0.01$

The results are mean ± SD.
ABBREVIATIONS: NS, not significant; CEHCs, carboxyethyl-hydroxychroman metabolites; TL, total lipids (total cholesterol + triglycerides).
[a]The Student-Newman-Keuls test for multiple comparisons was applied to evaluate differences between the two groups.

the absolute levels of α-T in HD patients are often normal or slightly increased. On the contrary, γ-T was significantly decreased. To our knowledge only three studies have measured plasma γ-tocopherol (γ-T) levels in patients undergoing HD. The data from our laboratory[4] and that of Traber[7] suggested that plasma γ-T before HD may be lower than normal. Himmelfarb et al.[6] reported a mean concentration of γ-T three times higher in HD patients than in healthy controls. Therefore, these data need to be confirmed by further studies.

Patient stratification for co-morbidity, dialysis membranes and methods, and pharmacological therapy does not seem to influence vitamin E levels, except in the case of dyslipidemia. In fact, there is a positive correlation between total lipid and α-T (but not γ-T) levels in plasma (r = 0.429; $P < 0.05$). It is of note that both α-T and γ-T levels in plasma decreased when corrected for total lipids. According to the literature,[8] in the presence of hyperlipidemia, the practice of showing both the uncorrected and lipid-corrected vitamin E levels should be recommended to provide more complete clinical and nutritional information.

The analysis of carboxyethyl-hydroxychroman metabolites (CEHCs) shows a marked accumulation of these metabolites in ESRD (more than 3-fold the mean control value). Previously, we demonstrated that this event follows the degree of loss of renal function[4] and vitamin E supplementation strongly exacerbates this accumulation in ESRD.[6,7]

The intake of vitamin E was lower than the RDA in all the patients and controls (7 ± 4 vs. 10 ± 4 mg/d; P = NS).

CONCLUSIONS

In apparent contrast with the findings in the general patient population, the SPACE study[3] and several smaller studies showed that the administration of vitamin E to HD patients very often may result in positive clinical outcomes.[5] This has lead to the hypothesis that HD patients may have a particularly high beneficial effect from vitamin E administration. Possible reasons for this particular responsiveness could be a marked incidence of oxidative stress and CVD that are often combined with hyperlipidemia and a defective antioxidant protection. Moreover, the potency of vitamin E administration might be significantly enhanced in HD by the accumulation of CEHCs that have been proposed to possess some biological functions helpful in preventing CVD and inflammation (reviewed in Hensley et al.[9]).

The results in this study show that, in the presence of a low dietary intake, HD patients show some abnormalities in the levels and metabolism of vitamin E, such as a disproportion between tocopherols and circulating lipids, a defect in the levels of γ-T and the accumulation of CEHCs in plasma. These findings may provide further support to the aforementioned hypothesis leading to the recommendation of a higher intake of vitamin E in patients undergoing HD with the ultimate goal of restoring (or likely surpassing) the vitamin E/lipid ratio found in healthy subjects. In the case of oral supplementation protocols, particular care should be paid to avoid depletion of non-alpha homologues by sustained metabolization.[6,7] Actually, non-alpha homologues, and particularly γ-T, may play a role in preventing oxidative stress, inflammation and CVD.[9]

In any case, appropriate biomarkers that would confirm the individual compliance to and the clinical outcome of vitamin E therapy should be assessed. Large-population intervention trials on HD patients are needed to confirm the therapeutic role of vitamin E in ESRD.

REFERENCES

1. HIMMELFARB, J., P. STENVINKEL, T.A. IKIZLER & R.M. HAKIM. 2002. The elephant in uremia: oxidant stress as a unifying concept of cardiovascular disease in uremia. Kidney Int. **62:** 1524–1538.
2. GALLI, F., A. FLORIDI & U. BUONCRISTIANI. 2002. Oxidant stress in hemodialysis patients. Contrib. Nephrol. **137:** 371–378.
3. BOAZ, M., S. SMETANA, T. WEINSTEIN, et al. 2000. Secondary prevention with antioxidants of cardiovascular disease in endstage renal disease (SPACE): randomised placebo-controlled trial. Lancet **356:** 1213–1218.
4. GALLI, F., A.G. FLORIDI, A. FLORIDI & U. BUONCRISTIANI. 2004. Accumulation of vitamin E metabolites in the blood of renal failure patients. Clin. Nutr. **23:** 205–212.
5. GALLI, F. 2002. Vitamin E-modified dialyzers. Contrib. Nephrol. **137:** 95-105.
6. HIMMELFARB, J., J. KANE, E. MCMONAGLE, et al. 2003. Alpha and gamma tocopherol metabolism in healthy subjects and patients with end-stage renal disease. Kidney Int. **64:** 978–991.
7. SMITH, K.S., C.L. LEE, J.W. RIDLINGTON, et al. 2003. Vitamin E supplementation increases circulating vitamin E metabolites tenfold in end-stage renal disease patients. Lipids **38:** 813–819.
8. TRABER, M.G. & I. JIALAL. 2000. Measurement of lipid-soluble vitamins: further adjustment needed? Lancet **355:** 2013–2014.
9. HENSLEY, K., E.J. BENAKSAS, R. BOLLI, et al. 2004. New perspectives on vitamin E: gamma-tocopherol and carboxyethylhydroxychroman metabolites in biology and medicine. Free Radic. Biol. Med. **36:** 1–15.

Oxidative Stress and Changes in α- and γ-Tocopherol Levels during Coronary Artery Bypass Grafting

A.T. ULUS,[a] A. AKSOYEK,[a] M. OZKAN,[a] S.F. KATIRCIOGLU,[a]
B. VESSBY,[b] AND S. BASU[b]

[a]*Cardiovasculer Surgery Clinic, Ozel Yasam Hospital, Ankara, Turkey*

[b]*Sections of Geriatrics and Clinical Nutrition Research, Faculty of Medicine, Uppsala University, Uppsala, Sweden*

ABSTRACT: We studied whether cardiopulmonary bypass (CPB) has any immediate impact on the initiation of antioxidative defenses in the body by measuring F$_2$-isoprostanes and α- and γ-tocopherol, respectively. 8-iso-PGF$_{2\alpha}$ levels increased significantly within 3 minutes and until the end of CPB. α-Tocopherol levels increased gradually at 20 min during CPB and continued until 6 hours after CPB. γ-Tocopherol levels followed a similar fashion at the end of CPB. 8-iso-PGF$_{2\alpha}$ and tocopherol levels kept at basal level 12 and 24 hours post CPB. These findings suggest that an increased free radical–induced oxidative stress together with a gradual appearance of antioxidative defense system during and after CPB.

KEYWORDS: antioxidants; isoprostanes; ischemia–reperfusion; oxidative stress; cardiopulmonary bypass; humans

INTRODUCTION

Cardiopulmonary bypass (CPB) is associated with oxidative injury and inflammatory response involving oxygen free radicals.[1] This possibly causes through the peroxidation of lipid molecules. α-Tocopherol, an endogenous lipid-soluble chain-breaking antioxidant, is known to protect cells from the diverse actions of oxygen free radicals by donating its hydrogen atom.[2] Vitamin E is shown to be beneficial in the injury caused by free radicals during CPB.[3] However, reports on plasma α-tocopherol levels during CPB are conflicting.[4,5] Thus, the goal of this study was to investigate the involvement of oxidative stress and vitamin E response during and following coronary bypass surgery, after protamin infusion, and at 24 hours after CPB in patients undergoing open-heart surgery.

Address for correspondence: Dr. S. Basu, Sections of Geriatrics and Clinical Nutrition Research, Faculty of Medicine, Uppsala University, Uppsala, Sweden. Voice: +46 18 6117958; fax: +46 18 6117976.
  samar.basu@pubcare.uu.se

TABLE 1. Clinical characteristics of patients

Characteristics	Group ($n = 20$)
Mean age (years)	60.5 ± 9.8 (40–76)
Women / men	4/16 (25 %)
Unstable angina	4 (20 %)
Previous MI	8 (40 %)
Single-vessel disease	5
Bivascular disease	9
Trivascular disease	6
Number of distal anastomoses	41
Mean cross-clamp time (min)	24.6 ± 8.4
Mean CPB time (min)	59.2 ± 26.6

MI: myocardial infarction; CPB: cardiopulmonary bypass.

SUBJECTS AND METHODS

A total of 20 patients with elective, isolated, first-time coronary artery bypass grafting was included in the study (TABLE 1). After the standard intravenous anesthetic management CPB was established by cannulation of the ascending aorta and the right atrium, with moderate hypothermia. Myocardium was preserved with topical hypothermia and antegrade-retrograde cardioplegia administration. Myocardial revascularization was done by grafting the internal mammary artery and when necessary by saphenous vein grafting. The mean aortic cross-clamp time was 24.6 ± 8.4 minutes and cardiopulmonary perfusion time was 59.2 ± 26.6.

Blood samples were collected from the radial artery: (i) baseline; pre-operatively, T0); (ii) after endotracheal intubation (T1); (iii) 3 min after the starting the CPB (T2); (iv) 10, 20, and 30 min during the CPB (T3, T4, T5); (v) at the end of CPB (T6); (vi) after the protamin infusion (T7); and (vii) 6, 12, and 24 hours after the end of operation from the radial artery (T8, T9, T10). The plasma samples were analysed for 8-iso-PGF$_{2\alpha}$, a major F$_2$-isoprostane, as described by Basu.[6] Plasma α- and γ-tocopherol levels were assayed by using HPLC with fluorescence detection. The results were expressed as mean ± SEM. A P value <0.05 was considered to be significant. Differences between the two groups were calculated by an analysis of variance model (ANOVA) with factors of time point.

RESULTS

Oxidative Injury as Measured by Plasma 8-iso-PGF$_{2\alpha}$

The levels of 8-iso-PGF$_{2\alpha}$ in plasma increased after the pre-induction (T0) and remained high during the whole CPB period (TABLE 2). Although the levels of 8-iso-PGF$_{2\alpha}$ increased after induction and intubation, this was not statistically significant ($P>0.05$). This difference became significant and reached at its height 3 minutes

TABLE 2. The mean levels of free-8-iso-PGF$_2$ in peripheral plasma at various times before, during, and after cardiopulmonary bypass

Time	8-iso-PGF$_2$ (pmol/L)
T0 (baseline; pre-induction)	110.69 ± 15.88
T1 (post intubation)	145.15 ± 20.41
T2 (3 min after CPB)	266.85 ± 26.71*γ
T3 (10 min after CPB)	253.59 ± 26.12 γ
T4 (20 min after CPB)	209.85 ± 20.63γ
T5 (30 min after CPB)	198.76 ± 23.45γ
T6 (at the end of CPB)	155.73 ± 26.38*
T7 (after the protamin infusion)	141.26 ± 13.39
T8 (6 hr after the operation)	99.70 ± 13.05*
T9 (12 hr after the operation)	93.03 ± 18.10
T10 (24 hr after the operation)	105.5 ± 213.43

γ $P<0.05$ according to baseline (T0)
* $P<0.05$ between the two consecutive periods.

after the beginning of the CPB and cross-clamping of the aorta ($P<0.05$). The difference was still observed until 30 minutes of CPB compared to the baseline values ($P<0.05$). It began to decrease at the end of the CPB (T6) according to CPB state ($P<0.05$). It reached approximately baseline levels 6 hr after CPB (T8), and this was statistically significant when compared to the levels at the previous period ($P<0.05$). There was no difference in the levels of 8-iso-PGF$_{2\alpha}$ in plasma observed at the subsequent period until the last blood sample taken 24 hr after the start of bypass surgery. Neither was there any difference in the levels of 8-iso-PGF$_{2\alpha}$ in plasma before or after anaesthesia induction or protamin infusion ($P<0.05$).

Antioxidant Levels as Measured by Plasma alpha- and gamma-Tocopherol

Lipid-corrected α-tocopherol levels were gradually increased after the pre-induction period (T0) (TABLE 3). It became significant at 20 min of CPB (T4) when compared to the previous measurement ($P<0.05$). α-Tocopherol levels increased significantly at the end of the CPB (T6) and after protamin infusion (T7) ($P<0.05$). These increments returned to the baseline levels at 6 hours after the CPB (T8). γ-Tocopherol levels were also gradually increased after the induction and intubation (T0). It become statistically significant ($P<0.05$) at the end of the CPB when compared with the previous level (T6), and after the protamin infusion (T7) compared to the baseline levels ($P<0.05$). Thereafter, it returned to baseline level 6 hours after the CPB (T8), and remained at the same levels 24 hr after CPB. There was no difference in the levels of tocopherols in plasma before and after anesthesia induction.

TABLE 3. The mean levels of tocopherols (adjusted to lipids) in peripheral plasma at various times before, during, and after cardiopulmonary bypass

Time	α-tocopherol (mg/mmol)	γ-tocopherol (mg/mmol)
T0 (baseline; pre-induction)	1.86 ± 0.14	0.072 ± 0.017
T1 (post intubation)	1.91 ± 0.13	0.078 ± 0.019
T2 (3 min after CPB)	1.90 ± 0.23	0.085 ± 0.018
T3 (10 min after CPB)	1.93 ± 0.17	0.083 ± 0.022
T4 (20 min after CPB)	2.01 ± 0.16*	0.091 ± 0.027
T5 (30 min after CPB)	1.94 ± 0.16	0.084 ± 0.021
T6 (at the end of CPB)	2.03 ± 0.12*	0.103 ± 0.016*
T7 (after the protamin infusion)	2.16 ± 0.25*	0.120 ± 0.025*γ
T8 (6 hr after operation)	1.80 ± 0.11*	0.069 ± 0.013*
T9 (12 hr after operation)	1.79 ± 0.14	0.071 ± 0.016
T10 (24 h after operation)	1.79 ± 0.13	0.070 ± 0.015

γ $P<0.05$ according to baseline (T0)
* $P<0.05$ between the two consecutive periods.

DISCUSSION

In this study we have analyzed two different important biochemical pathways: isoprostanes, a non-enzymatic free radical–mediated oxidation product of arachidonic acid, in order to assess oxidative injury; and tocopherol levels during and following 24 hr after CPB. The results demonstrate that 8-iso-PGF$_{2\alpha}$ is increased significantly in the plasma during bypass, and continued until the end of CPB, indicating a rapid involvement of oxidative injury, which corroborated our earlier findings.[1] However, after a successful end of the CPB operation, free radical–derived oxidative products returned to basal levels, indicating acute involvement of free radicals, possibly by the disruption of ischemia–reperfusion.

The α- and γ-tocopherol levels were gradually increased after the pre-induction period and during CPB; they returned to baseline levels 6 hr after CPB. These results, together with the increase in circulatory isoprostane during CPB, provide further evidence that upregulation of free radical reactions during CPB is compensated by the successive appearance of antioxidants, namely, α- and γ-tocopherols. The latter finding corroborates an earlier study with CPB.[7] A higher production of circulatory γ-tocopherol during CPB is of current interest. The role of γ-tocopherol was mostly ignored because of its relatively low concentration *in vivo*.[8] Evidence indicates that γ-tocopherol may be important in the defense against lipid oxidation. α– and γ-Tocopherol levels were significantly increased after protamin infusion, and returned to baseline level 6 hours after coronary bypass. In conclusion, oxidative stress and antioxidants during CPB might play a major role in postoperative complications. An upregulation of tocopherols during and after CPB evidences an imbalance between oxidants and antioxidative defense system. This argues for an early counter-regulation of free radical reactions by potential therapeutic means that might have a significant impact on CPB–related complications.

REFERENCES

1. ULUS, A.T., A. AKSOVEK, M. OZKAN, *et al.* 2003. Cardiopulmonary bypass as a cause of free radical induced-oxidative stress and enhanced circulatory isoprostanes in humans. Free Radic. Biol. Med. **34:** 911–917.
2. COGHLAN, J.G., W.D. FLITTER, S.M. CLUTTON, *et al.* 1993. Lipids peroxidation and changes in vitamin E levels during coronary artery bypass grafting. J. Thorac. Cardiovasc. Surg. **106:** 268–274.
3. YAU, T.M., R.D. WEISEL, D.A. MICKLE, *et al.* 1994. Vitamin E for coronary bypass operations. J. Thorac. Cardiovasc. Surg. **108:** 302–310.
4. WEISEL, R.D., D.A.G. MICKLE, C.D. FINKLE, *et al.* 1989. Myocardial free-radical injury after cardioplegia. Circulation **80** (Suppl.) III: 14–18.
5. BALLMER, P.E., W.H. REINHART, P. JORDAN, *et al.* 1994. Depletion of plasma vitamin C but not of vitamin E in response to cardiac operations. J. Thorac. Cardiovasc. Surg. **108:** 311–320.
6. BASU, S. 1998. Radioimmunoassay of 8-iso-prostaglandin F2 alpha: an index for oxidative injury via free radical catalysed lipid peroxidation. Prostagl. Leukot. Essent. Fatty Acids **58:** 319–325.
7. TANGNEY, C.C., J.S. HANKINS, M.A. MURTAUGH & W. PICCIONE. 1998. Plasma vitamins E and C concentrations of adult patients during cardiopulmonary bypass. J. Am. Coll. Nutr. **1:** 162–170.
8. BEHRENS, W.A. & R. MADERE. 1996. Alpha- and gamma tocopherol concentrations in human serum. J. Am. Coll. Nutr. **5:** 91–96.

Cigarette Smoking Increases Human Vitamin E Requirements as Estimated by Plasma Deuterium-Labeled CEHC

SCOTT W. LEONARD,[a] RICHARD S. BRUNO,[a] RAJASEKHAR RAMAKRISHNAN,[b] TAMMY BRAY,[a] AND MARET G. TRABER[a]

[a]*Linus Pauling Institute, Corvallis, Oregon 97331, USA*

[b]*Columbia University, College of Physicians and Surgeons, New York, New York 10027, USA*

ABSTRACT: Cigarette smoking (CS) is a well-described oxidant burden in humans. We hypothesized that CS would accelerate α-tocopherol (α-T) utilization leaving less for metabolite (CEHC) production. After labeled α-T consumption (75 mg each of d_3-*RRR*-α-TAc and d_6-*all-rac*-α-TAc) by smokers and nonsmokers ($n = 10$/group), CS increased α-T disappearance and decreased plasma and urinary CEHCs. Plasma d_3/d_6-α-T ratios were approximately 1.4 during supplementation and approximately 2 from days 5 to 17. d_3/d_6-α-CEHC ratios were on average 0.29 ± 0.05, confirming that *all-rac*-α-tocopherol is metabolized more efficiently. CEHC may be a good marker of vitamin E status, and smokers may have an increased vitamin E requirement.

KEYWORDS: cigarette smoking; α-tocopherol; vitamin E; CEHC

MATERIALS AND METHODS

Healthy, normolipidemic volunteers (nonsmokers, $n = 10$; smokers, $n = 10$) were selected for this study on the basis of age (18–35 years), nonnutritional supplement use (> 6 months), and exercise status (< 5 h/w of aerobic activity). Nonsmokers ($n = 6$ men, 4 women) were selected on the basis of never having smoked or resided with a smoker. Smokers ($n = 6$ men, 4 women) were selected if they smoked > 10 cigarettes/day. To confirm smoking status, we measured urinary cotinine (metabolite of nicotine) using a radioimmunoassay (Diagnostics Products Corp, Los Angeles, CA).

On six consecutive evenings, participants ingested a deuterated α-T supplement (75 mg each of d_3-*RRR*-α-TAc and d_6-*all-rac*-α-TAc) immediately after a standard meal. On average, this meal contained 1,143 kcal (43% carbohydrate, 17% protein, 41% fat), 35 mg ascorbic acid, and 2.7 mg α-T.

Blood samples were obtained after an overnight fast (10–12 h) on days −6, −5, −4, −3, −2, −1, 0, 1, 2, 3, 4, 5, 6, 8, 10, 13, 15, 17 (negative days denote supplementation

Address for correspondence: Maret G. Traber, Ph.D., Linus Pauling Institute, 571 Weniger Hall, Oregon State University, Corvallis, OR 97331, USA. Voice: 541-737-7977; fax: 541-737-5077.

maret.traber@oregonstate.edu

period). Blood was obtained from the antecubital vein into blood collection tubes (Vacutainer; Becton Dickinson, Franklin Lakes, NJ) containing 0.05 mL 15% K_3 EDTA or sodium heparin. Smokers were asked to refrain from smoking for 1 h before blood collection to alleviate the transient oxidative stress effects. Urine was collected for 24 h on three occasions: before supplementation (day –6), day 0, and day 17.

Plasma-labeled and unlabeled tocopherols were extracted according to procedures outlined by Podda et al.[1] and were analyzed using a liquid chromatography/ mass spectrometry (LC/MS) method.[2] Plasma and urinary labeled and unlabeled tocopherol metabolites (α- and γ-CEHCs) were extracted[3] and measured by LC/MS[4] and gas chromatography/mass spectrometry (GC/MS),[5] respectively. Ascorbic and uric acid were measured by HPLC with amperometric detection as previously described.[6] Plasma $F_{2\alpha}$-isoprostanes were measured on selected days throughout the study by GC/MS as previously described.[7] Total cholesterol and triglycerides were measured using kits obtained from Sigma Diagnostics (procedure No. 343 and 401, respectively) and performed in accordance with the manufacturer's instructions.

There were no differences at baseline between smokers and nonsmokers for age, sex, height, weight, body mass index, plasma lipids (total cholesterol and triglycerides), α-tocopherol, γ-tocopherol, uric acid, or ascorbic acid concentrations. Smokers were found to have increased lipid peroxidation, as measured by plasma $F_{2\alpha}$-isoprostanes.

The percentage of d_3-α-T $\{\%d_3\text{-}\alpha\text{-}T = [d_3\text{-}\alpha\text{-}T/(d_0\text{-}\alpha\text{-}T + d_3\text{-}\alpha\text{-}T + d_6\text{-}\alpha\text{-}T)] \times 100\}$ was calculated from the plasma α-tocopherol concentrations for each subject, at each time point, and was fitted by a two-compartment model, as described previously.[8] The two compartments were assumed to have reached the same concentration at the end of 6 days of deuterated α-tocopherol supplementation. Fitting was by nonlinear least squares, assuming measurement error to have a constant coefficient of variation. Labeled α-tocopherol half-lives were calculated as $t_{1/2} = \ln(2)/$disappearance rate constant.

Plasma % α-CEHC $\{\%d_x\text{-}\alpha\text{-CEHC} = [\%d_x\text{-}\alpha\text{-CEHC}/(d_0\text{-}\alpha\text{-CEHC} + d_3\text{-}\alpha\text{-CEHC} + d_6\text{-}\alpha\text{-CEHC})] \times 100\}$ was calculated from the plasma α-CEHC concentrations for each subject, at each time point up to 5 days after dosing, at which time the labeled α-CEHC concentrations became undetectable. The areas under the plasma α-CEHC concentration curves (AUCs) were calculated, according to the trapezoidal rule for day –5 through day 5. Results were considered to be statistically significant at the 95% confidence level ($P < 0.05$).

RESULTS AND DISCUSSION

After 6 days of supplementation, plasma total α-T (sum of d_0-, d_3- and d_6-α-T) more than doubled ($P < 0.0001$) in nonsmokers (from 15.3 ± 2.8 µM at baseline to 35.5 ± 5.8 µM on day 0) and in smokers (from 14.6 ± 3.8 µM at baseline to 32.1 ± 10.2 on day 0).

Mathematical modeling was performed using plasma%d_3-α-T from days 0 through 17. The α-T fractional disappearance rates in cigarette smokers (0.215 ± 0.001) were approximately 13% greater than that in nonsmokers (0.191 ± 0.001 pools/day; $P < 0.05$). Corresponding α-tocopherol half-lives were 10 h shorter in cigarette smokers (79 ± 4) compared with nonsmokers (89 ± 4 h; $P < 0.05$).

Given the limited data on α-tocopherol metabolism, we hypothesized that plasma or urinary vitamin E metabolite (CEHC) concentrations might serve as good biomarkers for vitamin E status. Plasma d_3- and d_6-α-CEHC concentrations were detectable only during supplementation and for the subsequent 5 days. Plasma d_3- and d_6-α-CEHC AUCs were lower in smokers compared with nonsmokers ($P < 0.05$). For urinary α-CEHC excretion, there were no differences between smokers and nonsmokers in urinary unlabeled and labeled α-CEHCs at baseline or on day 0. However, by day 17, urinary total α-CEHC was lower in smokers compared with nonsmokers. These latter data suggest that less α-tocopherol metabolism occurred in smokers because less "excess" α-tocopherol was available for degradation.

To evaluate whether natural and synthetic vitamin E (administered as 1:1 d_3-RRR-α- and d_6-all-rac-α-Tacs) were equally well utilized, we calculated the plasma d_3/d_6-α-T ratios in the subjects. During supplementation (days –6 to 0), the plasma d_3/d_6-α-T ratios were 1.48 ± 0.01. Upon cessation of supplementation, the ratio increased, reaching a ratio of 1.81 ± 0.24 at day 5 and increased to approximately 2. Previously, the half-life of SRR-α-T was calculated to be 15 h,[9] which suggests that, theoretically if all $2S$-α-Ts behave similarly to SRR-α-T, 12–15 h after the dose the d_3/d_6-α-T ratio should be 1.5. The observed values during supplementation are consistent with this prediction. Upon cessation of dosing, theoretically it should take approximately four half-lives for 95% of the $2S$-α-T to disappear from the plasma. This prediction was also met; the plasma d_3/d_6-α-T ratio = 2 after 5 days suggests that only $2R$-α-Ts are retained in the plasma and serve as vitamin E, as suggested by the Food and Nutrition Board in the 2000 Dietary Reference Intakes.[10]

The plasma d_3/d_6-α-CEHC ratios in the subjects documented the increased synthesis of α-CEHC from synthetic vitamin E. These ratios were on average 0.29 ± 0.05 (FIG. 1), confirming our previous work[11] that all-rac-α-tocopherol is metabolized three times more efficiently than is RRR-α-tocopherol. Plasma labeled α-CE-

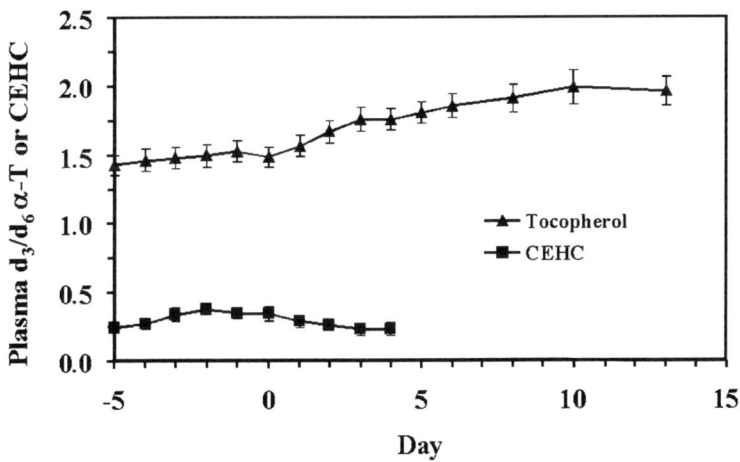

FIGURE 1. Plasma ratios (mean ± SE) of d_3/d_6-α-Ts and d_3/d_6-α-CEHCs in subjects receiving supplement from day –5 to day 0 with 1:1 ratio of approximately 75 mg each d_3-RRR- and d_6-all-rac-α-TAcs.

HCs were no longer detectable after day 5, suggesting that once the 2S-α-Ts have been removed from the fast-turning-over pool of α-Ts, there is little 2S-α-T available for metabolism.

In conclusion, cigarette smoking resulted in increased α-tocopherol utilization as shown by a faster α-T fractional disappearance rate. Accordingly, there was less α-T available for metabolism, and, as predicted, a corresponding decrease in the plasma and urinary α-CEHC was observed. Thus, smokers have an increased vitamin E requirement, and CEHC may be a good biomarker of vitamin E status. This statement is supported by lower plasma deuterium-labeled T concentrations, which corresponded to lower plasma CEHC concentrations in smokers compared with nonsmokers.

REFERENCES

1. PODDA, M. et al. 1996. Simultaneous determination of tissue tocopherols, tocotrienols, ubiquinols, and ubiquinones. J. Lipid Res. **37:** 893–901.
2. VAULE, H., S.W. LEONARD & M.G. TRABER. 2004. Vitamin E delivery to human skin; studies using deuterated α-tocopherol measured By APCI LC-MS. Free Radic. Biol. Med. **36:** 456–463.
3. LODGE, J.K. et al. 2000. A rapid method for the extraction and determination of vitamin E metabolites in human urine. J. Lipid Res. **41:** 148–154.
4. HIMMELFARB, J. et al. 2003. Alpha and gamma tocopherol metabolism in healthy subjects and patients with end-stage renal disease. Kidney Int. **64:** 978–991.
5. GALLI, F. et al. 2002. Gas chromatography mass spectrometry analysis of carboxyethyl-hydroxychroman metabolites of alpha- and gamma-tocopherol in human plasma. Free Radic. Biol. Med. **32:** 333–340.
6. FREI, B., L. ENGLAND & B.N. AMES. 1989. Ascorbate is an outstanding antioxidant in human blood plasma. Proc. Natl. Acad. Sci. USA **86:** 6377–6381.
7. MORROW, J.D. & L.J. ROBERTS II. 1994. Mass spectrometry of prostanoids: F2-isoprostanes produced by non-cyclooxygenase free radical-catalyzed mechanism. Methods Enzymol. **233:** 163–174.
8. TRABER, M.G. et al. 2001. Vitamin E kinetics in smokers and nonsmokers. Free Radic. Biol. Med. **31:** 1368–1374.
9. TRABER, M.G., R. RAMAKRISHNAN & H.J. KAYDEN. 1994. Human plasma vitamin E kinetics demonstrate rapid recycling of plasma *RRR*-α-tocopherol. Proc. Natl. Acad. Sci. USA **91:** 10005–10008.
10. FOOD AND NUTRITION BOARD & INSTITUTE OF MEDICINE. 2000. Dietary Reference Intakes for Vitamin C, Vitamin E, Selenium, and Carotenoids. National Academy Press. Washington.
11. TRABER, M.G., A. ELSNER & R. BRIGELIUS-FLOHE. 1998. Synthetic as compared with natural vitamin E is preferentially excreted as alpha-CEHC in human urine: studies using deuterated alpha-tocopheryl acetates. FEBS Lett **437:** 145–148.

Effects of Vitamin E Depletion/Repletion on Biomarkers of Oxidative Stress in Healthy Aging

BRIGITTE M. WINKLHOFER-ROOB,[a] ANDREAS MEINITZER,[a,b] MICHAELA MARITSCHNEGG,[a] JOHANNES M. ROOB,[c] GHOLAMALI KHOSCHSORUR,[b] JOSEP RIBALTA,[d] ISABELLA SUNDL,[a] SANDRA WUGA,[a] WILLIBALD WONISCH,[b] BEATE TIRAN,[b] AND EDMOND ROCK[e] FOR THE VITAGE STUDY GROUP

[a]*Human Nutrition & Metabolism Research and Training Center, Institute of Molecular Biosciences, Karl-Franzens University, A-8010 Graz, Austria*

[b]*Clinical Institute of Medical and Chemical Laboratory Diagnostics, Medical University, 8036 Graz, Austria*

[c]*Division of Clinical Nephrology, Department of Internal Medicine, Medical University, A-8036 Graz, Austria*

[d]*Lipid Research Unit, University Rovira i Virgili, 43201 Reus, Spain*

[e]*UMMM INRA-Theix, 63122 St. Genes Champanelle, France*

ABSTRACT: The effects on *ex vivo* LDL resistance to oxidation and biomarkers of *in vivo* oxidative stress in response to 3-month dietary vitamin E restriction to 25% of recommended intake and 2-month unrestricted dietary intake and supplementation with 800 IU/d were studied in 100 healthy, nonsmoking 20–75-year-old volunteers. Significant changes in vitamin E status were associated with decreases and increases, respectively, in LDL resistance to oxidation in the depletion and supplementation period and with decreases in lipid peroxidation and oxidative DNA modification in the supplementation period. Healthy aging was not associated with enhanced susceptibility to oxidation in the depletion period.

KEYWORDS: vitamin E; dietary restriction; supplementation; aging; nonsmokers; oxidative stress; malondialdehyde; 8-isoprostanes; 8-hydroxydeoxyguanosine; peroxides; LDL oxidation; vitamin C; lycopene; β-carotene; glutathione peroxidase.

Address for correspondence: Brigitte M. Winklhofer-Roob, M.D., Associate Professor of Pediatrics, Human Nutrition & Metabolism Research and Training Center, Institute of Molecular Biosciences, Karl-Franzens University, Schubertstrasse 1, A-8010 Graz, Austria. Voice: +43-316-380-5490; fax: +43-316-380-9857.
brigitte.winklhoferroob@uni-graz.at

BACKGROUND

Although the effects of vitamin E supplementation on individual biomarkers of oxidative stress have been studied previously, data are lacking on the effects of dietary vitamin E depletion and on the simultaneous effects on a panel of biomarkers of oxidative stress.

STUDY AIMS

The aim of this part of the European Commission–funded project VITAGE was to investigate the effects of low dietary vitamin E intake of approximately 25% of the recommended intake and subsequent vitamin E supplementation on biomarkers of oxidative stress in healthy, nonsmoking 20–75-year-old volunteers.

SUBJECTS AND METHODS

One hundred healthy, male nonsmoking Austrian volunteers 20–75 years of age and not taking supplements were enrolled in the study. For the depletion period, a special diet was created to be cooked on-site for restricting vitamin E intake to approximately 25% of the recommended intake. Depletion was followed by unrestricted dietary intake and a daily supplement of 800 IU/d of RRR α-tocopherol (Etocovit; Richter Pharma AG, Wels, Austria) for 2 months. The study protocol was approved by the Ethics Committee of the Medical University of Graz and informed consent was obtained from the volunteers. Vitamin E[1] and C[2] and carotenoid[1] status were determined by HPLC, as were plasma malondialdehyde[3] and urinary 8-hydroxydeoxyguanosine[4] concentrations. In addition, 8-isoprostanes[5] (Cayman EIA kit) and total peroxides[6] (Dr. Tatzber KEG kit) were determined in plasma and glutathione peroxidase[7] in erythrocytes, along with *ex vivo* LDL resistance to oxidation[8] and oxidative protein modifications using monoclonal antibodies against 8-hydroxynonenal-modified proteins[9] and Western blot analysis.

RESULTS

Effects on Antioxidant Status in Plasma and Erythrocytes

Plasma α-tocopherol concentrations decreased significantly in the depletion period and roughly doubled in the supplementation period, whereas γ-tocopherol concentrations decreased in both periods to final concentrations of less than 30% of baseline values. Plasma ascorbate concentrations did not change, plasma carotenoids decreased, and selenium-dependent glutathione peroxidase activity increased during depletion.

Effects on LDL Antioxidants and Resistance to Oxidation

Changes in LDL α-tocopherol concentrations were comparable to those in plasma and were associated with a significant ($P < 0.001$) decrease in LDL resistance to oxidation in the depletion period and increase in LDL resistance in the supplementation period. Changes in LDL resistance were dependent on changes in LDL α-tocopherol content ($P < 0.001$) both in the depletion and supplementation period. They were also dependent on age such that decreases in LDL resistance to oxidation in the depletion period decreased with age.

Effects on Biomarkers of Oxidative Stress

Although none of the biomarkers of oxidative stress changed in the depletion period, there was a significant ($P < 0.001$) decrease in lipid peroxidation (plasma 8-isoprostanes and plasma total peroxides) and oxidative DNA modification (urinary 8-hydroxydeoxyguanosine) in the supplementation period.

SUMMARY AND CONCLUSIONS

Taken together, these results demonstrate that short-term dietary vitamin E intake of approximately 25% of recommended intake enhances *ex vivo* LDL susceptibility to oxidative stress but does not significantly increase biomarkers of *in vivo* oxidative stress. Supplementation with vitamin E to above average levels in healthy, male non-smoking volunteers significantly enhances antioxidant protection, as evidenced by decreased LDL susceptibility to oxidation and decreased biomarkers of lipid peroxidation and oxidative DNA modification.

ACKNOWLEDGMENTS

This study was conducted with financial support from the Commission of the European Communities, specific RTD programme "Quality of Life and Management of Living Resources," QLK1-CT-1999-00830, VITAGE. It does not necessarily reflect its views and in no way anticipates the Commission's future policy in this area. Additional support by the Government of Austria (bm:bwk), and Roche Vitamins Europe, Basel, Switzerland is gratefully acknowledged.

REFERENCES

1. AEBISCHER, C.P., J. SCHIERLE & W. SCHÜEP. 1999. Simultaneous determination of retinol, tocopherols, carotene, lycopene, and xanthophylls in plasma by means of reversed-phase high-performance liquid chromatography. Method. Enzymol. **299:** 348–362.
2. LYKKESFELDT, J., S. LOFT & H.E. POULSEN. 1995. Determination of ascorbic acid and dehydroascorbic acid in plasma by high-performance liquid chromatography with coulometric detection—are they reliable markers of oxidative stress? Anal. Biochem. **299:** 329–335.
3. KOSCHSORUR, G.A., B.M. WINKLHOFER-ROOB, H. RABL, *et al.* 2000. Evaluation of a sensitive HPLC method for the determination of malondialdehyde, and application of the method to different biological materials. Chromatographia **52:** 181–184.
4. LENGGER, C., G. SCHÖCH & H. TOPP. 2000. A high-performance liquid chromatographic method for the determination of 8-oxo-7,8-dihydro-2′-deoxyguanosine in urine from man and rat. Anal. Biochem. **287:** 65–72.

5. ROBERTS, L.J. II & J.D. MORROW. 1994. Isoprostanes. Novel markers of endogenous lipid peroxidation and potential mediators of oxidant injury. Ann. N.Y. Acad. Sci. **15:** 237–242.
6. TATZBER, F., S. GRIEBENOW, W. WONISCH & R. WINKLER. 2003. Dual method for the determination of peroxidase activity and total peroxide-iodide leads to a significant increase of peroxidase activity in human sera. Anal. Biochem. **316:** 147–153.
7. PAGLIA, D.E. & W.N. VALENTINE. 1967. Studies on the quantitative and qualitative characterization of erythrocyte glutathione peroxidase. J. Lab. Clin. Med. **70:** 158–169.
8. BERGMANN, A.R., P. RAMOS, H. ESTERBAUER & B.M. WINKLHOFER-ROOB. 1997. RRR-α-tocopherol can be substituted for by trolox in determination of kinetic parameters of LDL oxidizability by copper. J. Lipid Res. **38:** 2580–2588.
9. WAEG, G., G. DIMSITY & H. ESTERBAUER. 1996. Monoclonal antibodies for detection of 4-hydroxynonenal modified proteins. Free Radic. Res. **25:** 149–159.

Consumption of Sesame Oil Muffins Decreases the Urinary Excretion of γ-Tocopherol Metabolites in Humans

JAN FRANK,[a] AFAF KAMAL-ELDIN,[a] AND MARET G. TRABER[b]

[a]*Department of Food Science, Swedish University of Agricultural Sciences, Uppsala, Sweden*

[b]*Linus Pauling Institute, Oregon State University, Corvallis, Oregon, USA*

ABSTRACT: Sesame seed and oil consumption previously increased human plasma γ-tocopherol (γ-T) concentrations. This was attributed to the sesame lignans sesamin and sesamolin. Here, we studied the inhibition of vitamin E metabolism by a single dose of sesame oil lignans coingested with deuterated α- and γ-tocopherols in human volunteers. The urinary excretion of γ-T metabolites was significantly lower in sesame oil treated than in control subjects. Concentrations of tocopherols in blood were not affected by the treatment. In conclusion, a single dose of sesame oil, containing 136 mg sesame lignans (sesamin and sesamolin), reduces the urinary excretion of co-administered γ-T in humans.

KEYWORDS: carboxyethyl hydroxychromans; CEHC; lignans; sesame; sesamin; sesamolin; tocopherol; vitamin E

INTRODUCTION

The consumption of sesame seeds[1] or sesame oil[2] previously increased plasma γ-tocopherol (γ-T) concentrations in humans. This effect was attributed to sesame lignans such as sesamin and sesamolin, which, in rats, decreased the excretion of urinary γ-T metabolites (γ-carboxyethyl hydroxychromans [γ-CEHC]).[3] In a human hepatoblastoma cell line, sesamin inhibited the enzymatic degradation of γ-T to γ-CEHC.[4] Despite this clear evidence, both *in vivo* and *in vitro*, for an inhibition of γ-tocopherol metabolism by dietary sesame lignans, this has not been directly examined in humans. We hypothesized that the simultaneous consumption of sesame oil lignans and α- and γ-tocopherol would inhibit the side-chain degradation of γ-T and reduce its urinary excretion as γ-CEHC in humans.

Address for correspondence: Jan Frank, Department of Food Science, Swedish University of Agricultural Sciences, Box 7051, 750 07 Uppsala, Sweden. Voice: +46-18-672063; fax: +46-18-672995.

jan.frank@lmv.slu.se

TABLE 1. Intake of vitamin E (mg) from muffins (d0) and supplements (d2 and d6, respectively) upon treatment

Treatment	Intake of Vitamin E upon Treatment (mg)					
	d-0 α-T	d-6 α-T	Sum α-T	d-0-γ-T	d-2 γ-T	Sum γ-T
Corn oil muffins	2.8	50.0	52.8	13.2	50.0	63.2
Sesame oil muffins	2.4	50.0	52.4	13.0	50.0	63.0

METHODS

Volunteers ($n = 10$) consumed a breakfast with muffins containing either corn oil or sesame oil (94 mg sesamin, 42 mg sesamolin) with a capsule containing deuterium-labeled α-tocopherol (d6-α-T) and γ-tocopherol (d2-γ-T) in a crossover design with 4 weeks' washout. The vitamin E contents of the muffins and capsules are given in TABLE 1. Blood and urine samples were collected over 72 hours and analyzed for labeled (d6 and d2, respectively) and unlabeled (d0) tocopherols and their metabolites (CEHCs).

RESULTS

Concentrations of tocopherols in blood did not differ between treatments. Urinary d0-α-CEHC concentrations were not significantly affected by the treatment and d6-α-CEHC was not detectable. Excretion of d0-γ-CEHC in urine was lower, although not significantly, in subjects eating sesame oil muffins and peaked 6–12 hours after supplementation (sesame oil muffin [SOM], 1.1 ± 0.7; corn oil muffin [COM] 1.6 ± 0.7 µmol/g creatinine) and returned to baseline after 48 hours (SOM, 0.9 ± 0.4; COM, 0.7 ± 0.4 µmol/g creatinine). Urinary excretion of d2-γ-CEHC was significantly lower in sesame oil than in corn oil–treated subjects between 6–12 hours (SOM, 0.3 ± 0.2; COM, 1.0 ± 0.7 µmol/g creatinine; $P < 0.01$) and at peak excretion between 12 and 24 hours after treatment (SOM, 0.6 ± 0.4; COM, 1.1 ± 0.7 µmol/g creatinine; $P < 0.05$).

DISCUSSION

In support of our hypothesis, consumption of sesame oil lignans did reduce the urinary excretion of total γ-CEHC (FIG. 1) and d2-γ-CEHC. The inhibition of γ-T metabolism was more pronounced for the coadministered d2-γ-T than for d0-γ-T. This may hint of a direct effect of sesame lignans on first-pass metabolism of vitamin E. However, the singular ingestion of sesame oil lignans in this trial did not change blood concentrations of γ-T. Previous studies reporting an increase in blood γ-T made use of repeated doses of sesame lignans,[1,2] which appear to be a prerequisite to achieve an increase in γ-T concentrations.

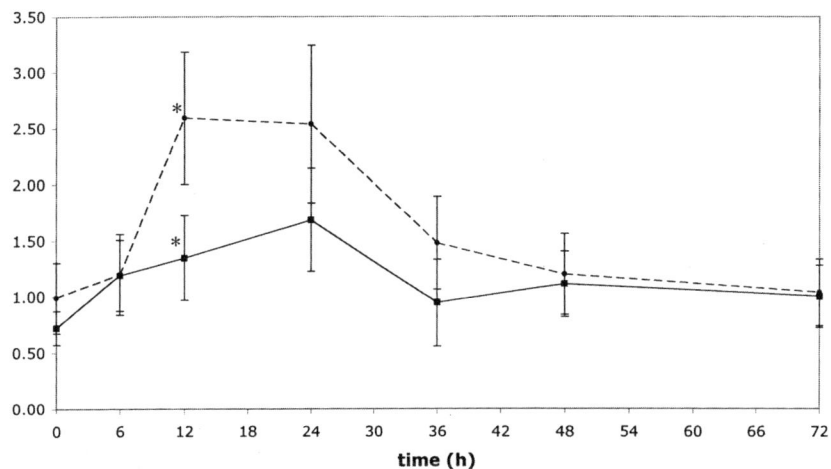

FIGURE 1. Urinary excretion of γ-tocopherol metabolites (d0- + d2-γ-CEHC; μmol/g creatinine) in subjects ($n = 10$) eating sesame oil (*solid line*) or corn oil (*dashed line*) muffins with comparable α-T and γ-T contents. Significantly different at $P < 0.02$.

CONCLUSIONS

A single dose of sesame oil, containing 136 mg sesame lignans (sesamin and sesamolin), inhibits the metabolism of co-administered γ-tocopherol in humans and leads to a reduced excretion of its urinary metabolites.

REFERENCES

1. COONEY, R.V. *et al.* 2001. Effects of dietary sesame seeds on plasma tocopherol levels. Nutr. Cancer **39:** 66–71.
2. LEMCKE-NOROJÄRVI, M. *et al.* 2001. Corn and sesame oils increase serum γ-tocopherol concentrations in healthy Swedish women. J. Nutr. **131:** 1195–1201.
3. IKEDA, S., T. TOHYAMA & K. YAMASHITA. 2002. Dietary sesame seed and its lignans inhibit 2,7,8-trimethyl- 2(2'-carboxyethyl)-6-hydroxychroman excretion into urine of rats fed γ-tocopherol. J. Nutr. **132:** 961–966.
4. PARKER, R.S., T.J. SONTAG & J.E. SWANSON. 2000. Cytochrome P4503A-dependent metabolism of tocopherols and inhibition by sesamin. Biochem. Biophys. Res. Commun. **277:** 531–534.

Characterization of Cellular Uptake and Distribution of Vitamin E

YOSHIRO SAITO, YASUKAZU YOSHIDA, KEIKO NISHIO, MIEKO HAYAKAWA, AND ETSUO NIKI

Human Stress Signal Research Center, National Institute of Advanced Industrial Science and Technology, Ikeda, Osaka 563-8577, Japan

ABSTRACT: We previously reported that tocotrienols acted as more potent inhibitors against selenium deficiency–induced cell death than the corresponding tocopherol isoforms (*J. Biol. Chem.* 2003;278:39428–39434). In the present study, we first compared the differences in the cellular uptake between α-tocopherol (α-Toc) and α-tocotrienol (α-Toc-3). The initial rate of cellular uptake of α-Toc-3 was 70-fold higher than that of α-Toc. Subcellular fractionation analysis of α-Toc-3 and α-Toc–fortified cells showed similar cellular distribution of these antioxidants, which was directly proportional to the lipid distribution. The cells containing similar amounts of α-Toc-3 and α-Toc showed similar resistance against the oxidative stress caused by peroxides. These results suggest that the apparent higher cytoprotective effect of α-Toc-3 than α-Toc is primarily ascribed to its higher cellular uptake.

KEYWORDS: vitamin E; tocotrienol; cellular uptake; oxidative stress; antioxidant

INTRODUCTION

Tocotrienol (Toc-3) differs from the corresponding tocopherol (Toc) only in the aliphatic tail. Chemically, Toc and Toc-3 are closely related[1]; however, it has been observed that they have widely varying degrees of biological activity.[1-3] Additionally, there are some reports on the beneficial effects of Toc-3 compared with Toc.[4-6] We have recently reported that Toc-3 acted as more potent inhibitors than the corresponding Toc isoforms against selenium deficiency–induced cell death, in which the causative role of oxidative stress was also demonstrated.[7] α-Tocotrienol (α-Toc-3) was the most potent inhibitor against cell death caused by selenium deficiency among the isoforms of vitamin E. In the present study, we characterized the accelerated cellular uptake of α-Toc-3 compared with α-Toc. We also demonstrated the cellular distribution of α-Toc-3 and the resistance of α-Toc-3–fortified cells against oxidative stress.

Address for correspondence: Yoshiro Saito, Ph.D., Human Stress Signal Research Center, National Institute of Advanced Industrial Science and Technology, 1-8-31 Midorigaoka, Ikeda, Osaka 563-8577 Japan. Voice: +81-72-751-8293; fax: +81-72-751-9964
yoshiro-saito@aist.go.jp

MATERIALS AND METHODS

Cell Culture

Jurkat E6-1 cells, human T-leukemia (American Tissue Type Collection, Rockville, MD), were maintained in RPMI-1640 medium containing 10% heat-inactivated fetal calf serum (serum medium). For studies on the uptake of vitamin E, the cells (3×10^5 cells/mL) were cultured in serum-free RPMI-1640 medium containing 5 µg/mL human insulin, 5 µg/mL human transferrin, 92 nM $FeCl_3$, 100 nM sodium selenite, and 2.5 mg/mL bovine serum albumin (ITSA-RPMI), as described previously.[8]

Determination of Intracellular Vitamin E

Intracellular vitamin E was detected using HPLC systems with electrochemical detection as described previously.[9] Cell samples in PBS were mixed with chloroform/methanol (2:1), and then cellular vitamin E in the lower chloroform layer was analyzed with an HPLC using a postcolumn amperometric electrochemical detector.

Subcellular Fractionation of Cells

α-Toc-3 and α-Toc–fortified cells were fractionated by the previously described method[10] with slight modification. The cells were homogenized by nitrogen decompression using Parr Cell Disruption Bombs. The nuclear fractions were prepared by centrifugation at 500g for 10 min and suspended in a homogenizing buffer. Mitochondrial fraction was obtained from postnuclear fractions by centrifugation at 5,000g for 10 min, and the microsomal and cytosolic fractions were obtained by centrifugation at 105,000g for 60 min. The distribution of each subcellular fraction was judged by standard enzymatic measurements, cytochrome c oxidase (mitochondrial marker), NADPH-cytochrome c reductase (microsomal marker), and lactate dehydrogenase (cytosolic marker) as reported previously.[11] The cell constituents were extracted with chloroform and methanol (2:1 by volume), and lipids in the chloroform layer were analyzed by using a thin-layer chromatography equipped with a flame ionization detection system.[12] The total molar lipid content of each cell fraction was determined using these authentic samples and average molecular weight as follows: for phosphatidylcholine, 1,2-dimyristoyl-rac-glycero-3-phosphocholine (Sigma, St. Louis, MO) and 677.9; for phosphatidylethanolamine, L-α-phosphatidylethanolamine from egg yolk (Sigma) and 746.1; for triacylglycerol, triolein (Nacalai, Kyoto, Japan) and 885.4; for cholesterol, cholesterol (Sigma) and 386.7.

Determination of Cell Viability

For the determination of cell viability, MTT assay was conducted for the indicated times. The treated cells were incubated with 0.5 mg/mL MTT at 37 °C for 2 h. Isopropyl alcohol containing 0.04 N HCl was added to the culture medium (3:2, by volume), and they were mixed using a pipette until the formazan was completely dissolved. The optical density of formazan was measured at 570 nm.

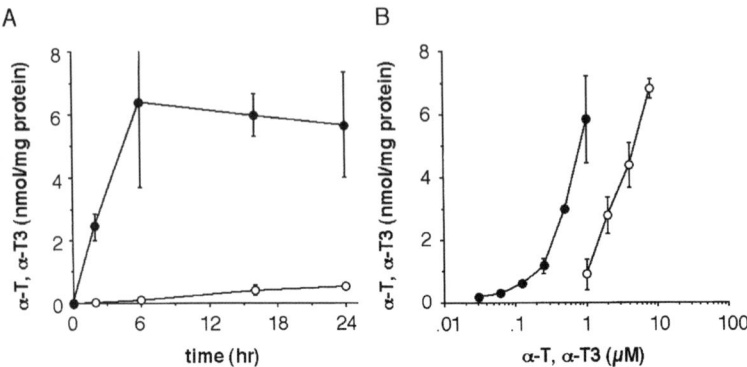

FIGURE 1. Cellular uptake of α-tocotrienol and α-tocopherol into Jurkat cells. The cells (3× 10⁵ cells/mL) were cultured in serum-free RPMI-1640 medium (ITSA-RPMI) with α-tocotrienol (α–Toc-3) or α-tocopherol (α-Toc) for the indicated times, and the cellular vitamin E content was measured using an HPLC system with an electrochemical detector. (**A**) 1 μM α-Toc-3 (*closed circle*) or 1 μM α-Toc (*open circle*) for the indicated times. (**B**) Variable amounts of α-Toc-3 (*closed circle*) or α-Toc (*open circle*) for 24 h. Mean values of cellular vitamin E content are shown with standard error ($n = 3$).

RESULTS

Characterization of Accelerated Cellular Uptake of α-Toc-3

To investigate the biological effectiveness of α-Toc-3, we first determined the cellular uptake of this antioxidant. When Jurkat cells were cultured in a serum-free RPMI-1640 medium (ITSA-RPMI) containing 1 μM α-Toc-3, the cellular content of α-Toc-3 increased with incubation time and reached a plateau after 6 h of incubation time (FIG. 1A). In the case of α-Toc, cellular content increased linearly with incubation time up to 72 h. Most strikingly, the initial rate of cellular uptake of α-Toc-3 was found to be 70-fold higher than that of α-Toc. A dose-dependent study of cellular uptake of vitamin E revealed accelerated incorporation of α-Toc-3, which was found to be 6.5- and 2.2-fold higher than that of α-Toc after incubation for 24 h (FIG. 1B) and 72 h (data not shown), respectively. The cellular contents of vitamin E in selenium-deficient and sufficient media were not significantly different after 72 h of incubation time (data not shown).

Cellular Distribution of α-Toc-3

To investigate the distribution of α-Toc-3 in cellular organelles, we fractionated cells preincubated with 1 μM α-Toc-3 for 24 h into their organelles by centrifugation, and the contents of α-Toc-3 were quantified. α-Toc-3 was mainly enriched in the microsomal fraction of the cells (FIG. 2A). In the α-Toc–treated cells, a distribution similar to that of α-Toc-3 was observed (FIG. 2B). Of interest, the subcellular contents of both α-Toc-3 and α-Toc were directly proportional to the lipid distribution in a similar manner (FIG. 2C). The same subcellular fractionation study was also

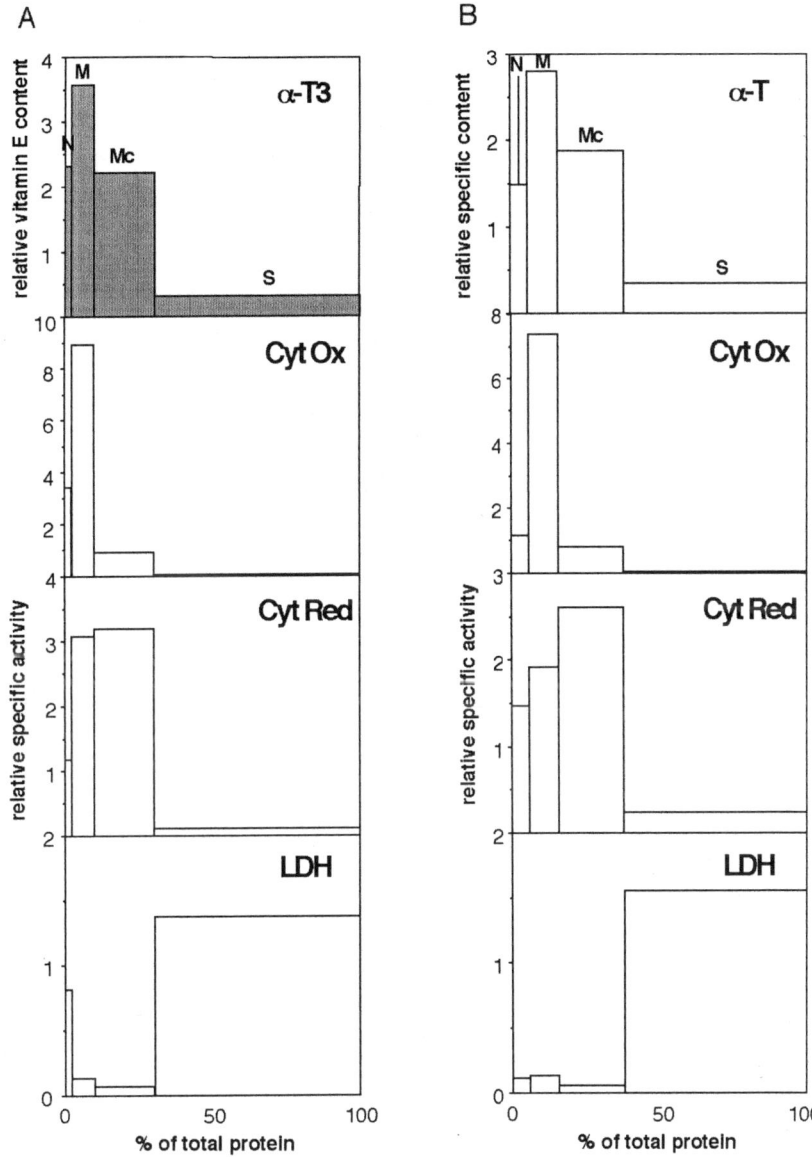

FIGURE 2. Subcellular localization of α-tocotrienol and α-tocopherol. Cells were cultured in ITSA-RPMI containing 1 μM α-Toc-3 (**A**) or α-Toc (**B**) for 24 h. These cells were fractioned by differential centrifugation into nuclear fraction (N), mitochondrial fraction (M), microsomal fraction (Mc), and cytosolic fraction (S), and the contents of vitamin E and protein were measured. The distribution of marker proteins was determined by enzymatic activity. Cytochrome c oxidase (Cyt Ox), NADPH–cytochrome c reductase (Cyt Red), and lactate dehydrogenase (LDH) were measured as marker enzymes of mitochondria, microsome, and cytosol, respectively.

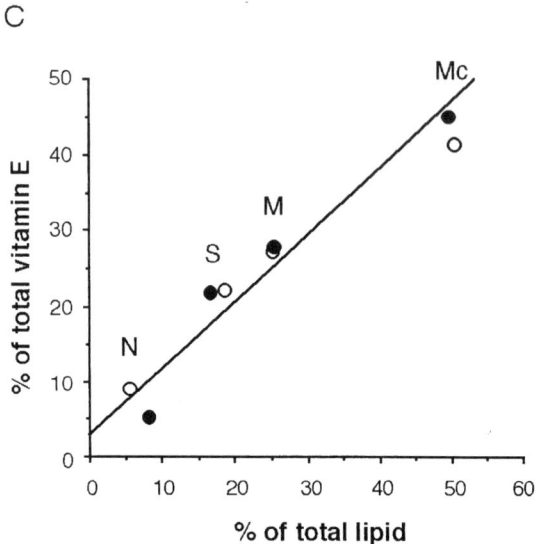

FIGURE 2 — *continued*. (C) Correlation between vitamin E (α-Toc-3, *closed circle*; α-Toc, *open circle*) and lipid contents in subcellular fractions.

conducted on cells treated for 3 h, and the similar cellular distribution was observed between α-Toc-3 and α-Toc (data not shown).

Antioxidative Function of a-Toc-3

We determined the effects of α-Toc-3 against the oxidative stress caused by several peroxides. According to the observation shown in FIGURE 1B, the cells were treated with either 1 μM α-Toc-3 or 6 μM α-Toc for 24 h to obtain the cells containing the same amounts of antioxidants. It was found in fact that the cells thus obtained contained 6.2 ± 2.6 and 5.9 ± 3.6 nmol/mg protein of α-Toc-3 and α-Toc, respectively. They exerted similar protective effects against the peroxide-induced cell death (FIG. 3). The effects against lipophilic cumene hydroperoxide were more significant than those against hydrophilic hydrogen peroxide (FIG. 3A and B).

DISCUSSION

α-Toc is the major vitamin E *in vivo* and exerts the highest biological activity. Additionally, there are some reports on the beneficial effects of Toc-3 compared with Toc. We also reported the potent preventive effect of α-Toc-3 against cell death caused by selenium deficiency.[7] In the present study, we observed an accelerated cellular uptake of α-Toc-3 compared with α-Toc, and the maximum difference between these was 70-fold at 6 h of incubation time (FIG. 1A). The difference in the cellular uptake after 72 h of incubation was 2.2-fold, which corresponded well with the dif-

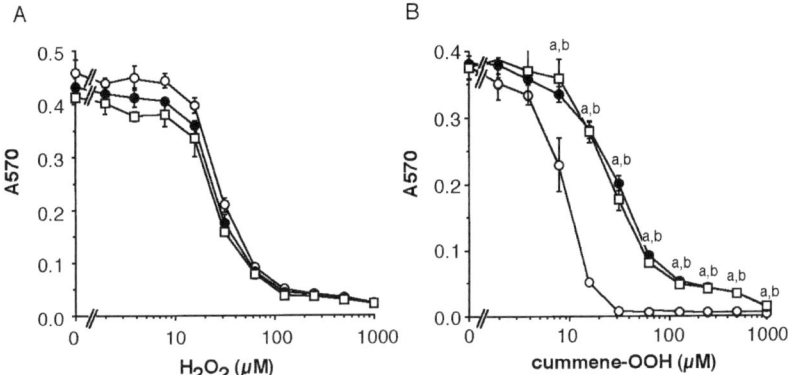

FIGURE 3. Effect of α-tocotrienol on the cell death caused by variable hydroperoxides. Cells were cultured in ITSA-RPMI without (*open circle*) and with 1 μM α-Toc-3 (*open square*) or 6 μM α-Toc (*closed circle*) for 24 h, and then cells were washed and treated with variable amounts of hydrogen peroxide (**A**) and cumene hydroperoxide (**B**) for 6 h. The cell viability was measured by MTT assay, and the means ± SE of the three experiments are shown. In (**B**) a = $P < 0.05$ when compared with α-Toc-3–fortified cells and control cells; b = $P < 0.05$ when compared with α-Toc–fortified cells and control cells.

ference in their ED_{50} value of the inhibitory effect on the cell death caused by selenium deficiency in 72 h of incubation time,[7] the ratio being 2.8-fold. Therefore, it was suggested that the more potent inhibitory effect of α-Toc-3 compared with α-Toc on cell death may be ascribed mainly to the accelerated cellular uptake. Noguchi et al. also found that α-Toc-3 inhibited the endothelial expression of adhesion molecules more strongly than α–Toc and that this inhibitory effect of vitamin E analogues correlated well with its intracellular concentrations.[5] It has been reported that tocotrienols are more readily transferred between membranes than are tocopherols.[13] In this report, using 14:0 PC unilamelar liposomal membranes, we found the maximum differences between α-Toc-3 and α-Toc on the incorporation into membranes was under two-fold as estimated by ESR spin probe technique. Although there are differences in the experimental conditions between culture cells and liposome membranes, it seems that higher intermembrane mobility of α-Toc-3 contributes to the accelerated cellular uptake of this antioxidant. Further work on the mechanism of accelerated cellular uptake of α-Toc-3, especially the feasibility of the existence of specific transfer system, is necessary in the future.

It is noteworthy that the content of vitamin E in the cultured cells is quite low. In the case of Jurkat cells cultured with RPMI-1640 medium containing 10% fetal bovine serum, the cellular content of α-Toc was 0.83 nmol/10^9 cells, which was approximately only 1% of the lymphocytes in human blood. Brigelius-Flohé previously reported that the conventional cell culture media do not adequately supply cells with vitamin E[14] because of the low content of this antioxidant in bovine serum as compared with that of human serum. A standardized supplementation with vitamin E seems to be important to yield reproducible results in investigations related to the function of antioxidants, oxidative stress, and redox-modulated signaling pathway.

Note that the subcellular distribution was similar between α-Toc-3 and α-Toc and that the contents were linearly correlated with lipid contents (FIG. 2). These results suggest that the cellular distribution of vitamin E is determined primarily by the lipid distribution. Although some articles have reported the existence of vitamin E-regulatory proteins such as α-tocopherol transfer protein (α-TTP), cytosolic tocopherol-associated protein (TAP), and tocopherol binding protein (TBP) (reviewed in Brigelius-Flohe and Traber[2] and Blatt et al.[3]), relatively small amounts of cellular vitamin E should bind to these proteins. The mechanism by which vitamin E is redistributed within the cell and reaches mitochondria and the nucleus has not been elucidated. Currently, vitamin E-regulatory proteins such as α-TTP, TAP, and TBP are regarded as candidates for cellular transporter of vitamin E.

It was found that α-Toc-3– and α-Toc–fortified cells exerted similar protective effects against lipophilic cumene hydroperoxide-induced cell death. It is known that the potency of radical-scavenging antioxidants in the cell is determined not only by the chemical reactivity toward radicals, but also by other factors including localization, concentration, and mobility at the microenviroment.[13,15] It has been reported that the reactivities of tocotrienols against peroxyl radical in homogeneous solution is substantially the same with the corresponding tocopherols.[13,16] It is also known that tocotrienols and tocopherols have similar mobilities within the membranes.[13] Taken together with our results such as resistance against oxidative stress and cellular distribution and these reports, it is thought that cellular α-Toc-3 functions as antioxidant equal to α-Toc.

In conclusion, the present study shows the accelerated uptake of α-Toc-3 compared with α-Toc in cultured cells, and the similarities of cellular distribution and antioxidative function between α-Toc-3 and α-Toc. These results indicate that the higher cytoprotective effect of α-Toc-3 over α-Toc observed in certain cases may be ascribed to its higher cellular uptake. Why α-Toc-3 uptake is so much faster than that for α-Toc is a subject for future study.

REFERENCES

1. PACKER, L., S.U. WEBER & G. RIMBACH. 2001. Molecular aspects of alpha-tocotrienol antioxidant action and cell signalling. J. Nutr. **131**: 369S–373S.
2. BRIGELIUS-FLOHE, R. & M.G. TRABER. 1999. Vitamin E: function and metabolism. FASEB J. *13:* 1145–1155.
3. BLATT, D.H., S.W. LEONARD & M.G. TRABER. 2001. Vitamin E kinetics and the function of tocopherol regulatory proteins. Nutrition *17:* 799–805.
4. CHAO, J.T., A. GAPOR & A. THERIAULT. 2002. Inhibitory effect of delta-tocotrienol, a HMG CoA reductase inhibitor, on monocyte-endothelial cell adhesion. J. Nutr. Sci. Vitaminol. (Tokyo) **48**: 332–337.
5. NOGUCHI, N., R. HANYU, A. NONAKA, et al. 2003. Inhibition of THP-1 cell adhesion to endothelial cells by alpha-tocopherol and alpha-tocotrienol is dependent on intracellular concentration of the antioxidants. Free Radic. Biol. Med. **34**: 1614–1620.
6. KHANNA, S., S. ROY, H. RYU, et al. 2003. Molecular basis of vitamin E action: tocotrienol modulates 12-lipoxygenase, a key mediator of glutamate-induced neurodegeneration. J. Biol. Chem. **278**: 43508–43515.
7. SAITO, Y., Y. YOSHIDA, T. AKAZAWA, et al. 2003. Cell death caused by selenium deficiency and protective effect of antioxidants. J. Biol. Chem. **278**: 39428–39434.

8. SAITO, Y. & K. TAKAHASHI. 2002. Characterization of selenoprotein P as a selenium supply protein. Eur. J. Biochem. **269:** 5746–5751.
9. YOSHIDA, Y., N. ITO, S. SHIMAKAWA, *et al.* 2003. Susceptibility of plasma lipids to peroxidation. Biochem. Biophys. Res. Commun. **305:** 747–753.
10. DE DUVE, C., B.C. PRESSMAN, R. GIANETTO, *et al.* 1955. Tissue fractionation studies. 6. Intracellular distribution patterns of enzymes in rat-liver tissue. Biochem. J. **60:** 604–617.
11. IMAI, H., K. NARASHIMA, M. ARAI, *et al.* 1998. Suppression of leukotriene formation in RBL-2H3 cells that overexpressed phospholipid hydroperoxide glutathione peroxidase. J. Biol. Chem. **273:** 1990–1997.
12. OGASAWARA, M., K. TSURUTA & S. ARAO. 2002. Flame photometric detector for thin-layer chromatography. J. Chromatogr. A **973:** 151–158.
13. YOSHIDA, Y., E. NIKI & N. NOGUCHI. 2003. Comparative study on the action of tocopherols and tocotrienols as antioxidant: chemical and physical effects. Chem. Phys. Lipids **123:** 63–75.
14. LEIST, M., B. RAAB, S. MAURER, *et al.* 1996. Conventional cell culture media do not adequately supply cells with antioxidants and thus facilitate peroxide-induced genotoxicity. Free Radic. Biol. Med. **21:** 297–306.
15. YOSHIDA, Y., N. NOGUCHI, A. WATANABE, *et al.* 2002. Antioxidant action of 2,2,4,6-tetra-substituted 2,3-dihydro-5-hydroxybenzofuran against lipid peroxidation: effects of substituents and side chain. Free Radic. Res. **36:** 1171–1178.
16. SUARNA, C., R.L. HOOD, R.T. DEAN, *et al.* 1993. Comparative antioxidant activity of tocotrienols and other natural lipid-soluble antioxidants in a homogeneous system, and in rat and human lipoproteins. Biochim. Biophys. Acta. **1166:** 163–170.

Vitamin E Exhibits Concentration- and Vitamer-Dependent Impairment of Microsomal Enzyme Activities

T.J. SONTAG AND R.S. PARKER

Division of Nutritional Sciences, Cornell University, Ithaca, New York 14853, USA

KEYWORDS: vitamin E; tocotrienols; tocopherols; liver; microsomes; enzyme activity; inhibition; kinetics

INTRODUCTION

Vitamin E is a generic term for a structurally related group of lipophilic molecules that reside in the lipid bilayer of cell membranes. The various vitamers differ in their methylation around the chromanol head group and the saturation of the phytyl tail, with the tocopherols possessing a saturated phytyl tail and the tocotrienols an unsaturated tail containing 3 double bonds. The tocopherols and tocotrienols have been reported to differ in their physiological functions, including their antioxidant and apoptotic activity.[1,2] The tocotrienols are known to affect organizational properties of lipid bilayers to a greater extent than the tocopherols, such as the order of the liquid crystalline phase at the C10-13 region of the membrane phospholipid chain, and increased anisotrophic motion within the membrane.[3]

We previously reported the ω-oxidation pathway of vitamin E initiated by the tocopherol-omega-hydroxylase cytchrome P450 enzyme (CYP4F2)[4] and have observed the inhibitory effects of the tocotrienols on their own metabolism at high concentrations. We here compare the effects of tocopherols and tocotrienols on microsomal membrane enzymatic activity.

METHODS

Rat liver microsomes were prepared by differential centrifugation (100,000 × g pellet). Insect cell microsomes selectively expressing recombinant human cytochrome P450, cytochrome c reductase, and +/− recombinant cytochrome $b5$, were purchased from BD Gentest. Tocopherols and tocotrienols (alpha- and gamma-) were incorporated into microsomes in the presence of NADPH. The activities of several microsomal enzymes including the tocopherol-omega-hydroxylase were evalu-

---

Address for correspondence: R.S. Parker, Cornell University, Ithaca 14853, NY. Voice: 607-255-2661; fax: 607-255-1033.
rsp3@cornell.edu

ated at varying membrane vitamer concentrations with variations in membrane environment considered.

RESULTS

Studies of the CYP450 tocopherol-omega-hydroxylase activity toward vitamin E reveals self-inhibition of metabolism by the tocotrienols, but not by tocopherols. The tocotrienol-specific inhibitory effect is observed for activity of P450s which do not metabolize vitamin E, including testosterone-6-beta- and -16-alpha-hydroxylation reactions, 7-ethoxycoumarin-O-deethylation, and lauric acid omega-1-hydroxylation, but not for other P450s tested, indicating that the observed effects are not generalizable to all P450 activities.

Kinetic analysis of inhibition of testosterone metabolism by tocotrienol indicates a noncompetitive mechanism of inhibition, with variation in V_{max}, but similar K_m values in the presence or absence of tocotrienol. Kinetics similar to tocotrienol's were observed for CYP450 arachidonic acid 20-hydroxylation.[5] These effects were suggested to be caused by several possible mechanisms: substrate/product inhibition, micellar aggregation of substrate, physical effects of the substrate on membrane/enzyme, or detergent activity rearrangement of electron transfer system. We found that, in a manner similar to that of vitamin E, unsaturated fatty acids inhibit P450 activity to a much greater extent than their saturated counterparts.

The addition of recombinant CYP450 reductase (CPR) to the rat liver microsomal system did not reverse the inhibitory effect of tocotrienols. Likewise, no effect of the tocotrienols was observed on CYP450 reductase activity toward cytochrome c. Insect microsomes expressing CYP3A4 +/− cytochrome b5 were compared for sensitivity to membrane tocotrienols. In the absence of cytochrome b5, the addition of tocotrienols to the microsomal membrane was not as inhibitory toward P450 activity.

CONCLUSIONS

We observed that tocotrienols exhibited effects on membrane enzymes that were not shared by tocopherols. These effects were not due to the competitive action of tocotrienols on enzyme binding sites. The P450 inhibition appears to be a general phenomenon of lipids possessing an unsaturated carbon chain. The effect may be due in part to disruption of the electron-transfer system of P450 activity as removal of cytochrome b5 from the microsomal system reduces the effects of the tocotrienols on cytochrome P450 activity.

REFERENCES

1. SERBINOVA, E., V.E. KAGAN, D. HAN & L. PACKER. 1991. Free Rad. Biol. Med. **10:** 263–275.
2. YU, W., M. SIMMONS-MENCHACA, A. GAPOR, *et al.* 1999. Nutr. Cancer **33:** 26-32.
3. SUZUKI, Y.J., M. TSUCHIYA, S.R. WASSALL, *et al.* 1993. Biochemistry **32:** 10692–10699.
4. SONTAG, T.J. & R.S. PARKER. 2002. J. Biol. Chem. **277:** 25290–25296.
5. XU, F., J.R. FALCK, P.R. ORTIZ DE MONTELLANO & D.L. KROETZ. 2004. J. Pharmacol. Exp. Ther. **308:** 887–895.

The Decrease in γ-Tocopherol in Plasma and Lipoprotein Fractions Levels Off within Two Days of Vitamin E Supplementation

ISABELLA SUNDL,[a] ULRIKE RESCH,[a] ANDREAS R. BERGMANN, JOHANNES M. ROOB,[b] AND BRIGITTE M. WINKLHOFER-ROOB[a]

[a]*Human Nutrition & Metabolism Research and Training Center, Institute of Molecular Biosciences, Karl-Franzens University, A-8010 Graz, Austria*

[b]*Division of Clinical Nephrology, Department of Internal Medicine, Medical University, 8036 Graz, Austria*

ABSTRACT: The effects of vitamin E supplementation on α- and γ-tocopherol concentrations were studied in plasma and lipoprotein fractions of five healthy volunteers taking 1000 IU/day of RRR α-tocopherol for 4 days. Although plasma α-tocopherol increased, γ-tocopherol decreased. Compared with baseline, γ-/α-tocopherol ratios decreased from 48 h onward ($P < 0.001$). They all leveled off within 48 h. From 12 h onward, γ-/α-tocopherol ratios were higher in VLDL and IDL than in LDL and HDL, indicating that γ-tocopherol is better maintained in triglyceride-rich lipoprotein fractions. These data suggest that vitamin E supplementation exceeding 2 days does not further decrease γ-tocopherol concentrations.

KEYWORDS: vitamin E; supplementation; α-tocopherol; γ-tocopherol; α-/γ-tocopherol ratio; plasma; lipoproteins; VLDL; IDL; LDL; HDL

INTRODUCTION

Several studies have demonstrated that vitamin E supplements consisting exclusively of α-tocopherol not only increase α-tocopherol concentrations, but also decrease γ-tocopherol concentrations both in plasma and in low-density lipoproteins (LDL).[1,2]

STUDY AIMS

The aim of the present study was to further explore the effects of vitamin E supplementation by studying the kinetics of α- and γ-tocopherol concentrations and γ-/α-tocopherol ratios in plasma and in the different lipoprotein fractions.

SUBJECTS AND METHODS

Five healthy volunteers aged 24 to 29 years, three females, two males, received a daily supplement of 1,000 IU of RRR α-tocopherol for 4 days. Blood was drawn before and 3, 6, 9, 12, 24, 48, 72, and 96 h after the initial vitamin E dose. At 24, 48, 72, and 96 h, blood was drawn after an overnight fast, while subjects were consuming a free diet from baseline to 12 h. VLDL, IDL, LDL, and HDL fractions were isolated by discontinuous density gradient ultracentrifugation. In brief, plasma density was adjusted to 1.41 g/mL with KBr and 3 mL plasma was overlayered by three EDTA buffer solutions prepared with KBr of decreasing density (solution A: d = 1.080 g/mL, solution B: d = 1.050 g/mL, solution C: d = 1 g/mL) and the lipoprotein fractions were separated by ultracentrifugation at 40,000 rpm at 10°C for 22–24 h according to Chapman *et al.*[3] Concentrations of α- and γ-tocopherol were determined in plasma and in the lipoprotein fractions as described.[4] Changes over 96 h were analyzed by Friedman Repeated Measures ANOVA on Ranks.

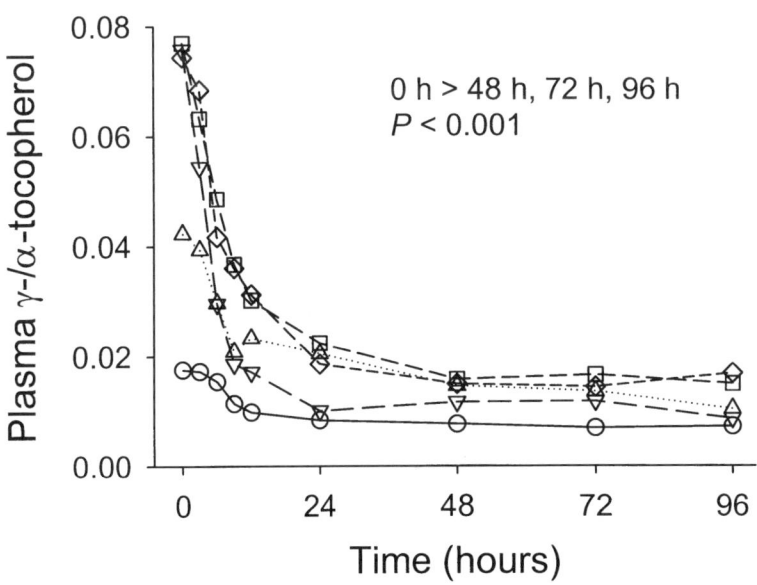

FIGURE 1. Kinetics of plasma γ-/α-tocopherol ratios in five volunteers taking 1,000 IU/day of RRR α-tocopherol for 4 days. Blood was drawn before and 3, 6, 9, 12, 24, 48, 72, and 96 h after the initial supplement.

RESULTS

Plasma

Plasma α-tocopherol concentrations increased significantly, as expected. They leveled off within 48 h. In contrast, γ-tocopherol concentrations decreased from 6 h onward and leveled off at 24 h. The ratios of plasma γ-/α-tocopherol decreased and leveled off within 48 h; the decrease from baseline was significant at 48 h, 72 h, and 96 h ($P < 0.05$, All Pairwise Multiple Comparison Procedure, Dunn's Method).

Lipoprotein Fractions

γ-Tocopherol concentrations in the lipoprotein fractions VLDL, IDL, LDL, and HDL showed the same trend as γ-tocopherol concentrations in plasma and leveled off between 24 and 48 h. In VLDL, the decrease from baseline in ratios of γ-/α-tocopherol was significant at 24, 48, and 72 h and in IDL, LDL and HDL at 48, 72, and 96 h ($P < 0.05$). γ-/α-Tocopherol ratios in the different lipoprotein fractions did not differ between the fractions up to 9 h. From 12 to 96 h, γ-/α-tocopherol ratios were significantly higher in VLDL compared with LDL, from 12 to 72 h in VLDL compared with HDL and from 12 to 72 h in IDL compared with LDL.

While between-subject variability was high at baseline, it decreased substantially during vitamin E supplementation, both in plasma and in the lipoprotein fractions.

SUMMARY AND CONCLUSIONS

The decrease in γ-tocopherol concentrations and in the ratios of γ-/α-tocopherol leveled off within 48 h of vitamin E supplementation, suggesting that long-term vitamin E supplementation exceeding 2 days does not further decrease γ-tocopherol concentrations. The ratios of γ-/α-tocopherol were lower in LDL and HDL than in VLDL and IDL from 12 h onward, indicating that γ-tocopherol is better maintained in triglyceride-rich lipoprotein fractions.

REFERENCES

1. WINKLHOFER-ROOB, B.M., O. ZIOUZENKOVA, H. PUHL, et al. 1995. Impaired resistance to oxidation of low density lipoprotein in cystic fibrosis: Improvement during vitamin E supplementation. Free Radic. Biol. Med. **19:** 725–733.
2. HUANG, H.Y. & J.A. LAWRENCE. 2003. Supplementation of diets with α-tocopherol reduces serum concentrations of γ- and δ-tocopherol in humans. J. Nutr. **133:** 3137–3140.
3. CHAPMAN, M.J., S. GOLDSTEIN, D. LAGRANGE & P.M. LAPLAUD. 1981. A density gradient ultracentrifugal procedure for the isolation of the major lipoprotein classes from human serum. J. Lipid Res. **22:** 339–358.
4. ZIOUZENKOVA, O., B.M. WINKLHOFER-ROOB, H. PUHL, et al. 1996. Lack of correlation between the α-tocopherol content of plasma and LDL, but high correlations for γ-tocopherol and carotenoids. J. Lipid Res. **37:** 1936–1946.

Does Aging Affect the Response of Vitamin E Status to Vitamin E Depletion and Supplementation?

BRIGITTE M. WINKLHOFER-ROOB,[a] JOHANNES M. ROOB,[b] MICHAELA MARITSCHNEGG,[a] GRETE SPRINZ,[c] DORIS HILLER,[a] ELISABETH MARKTFELDER,[a] MELANIE PREINSBERGER,[a] SANDRA WUGA,[a] ISABELLA SUNDL,[a] BEATE TIRAN,[d] NICOLAS CARDINAULT,[e] JOSEP RIBALTA,[f] EDMOND ROCK[e] AND THE VITAGE STUDY GROUP

[a]*Human Nutrition & Metabolism Research and Training Center, Institute of Molecular Biosciences (IMB), Karl-Franzens University, A-8010 Graz, Austria*

[b]*Division of Clinical Nephrology, Department of Internal Medicine, Medical University, A-8036 Graz, Austria*

[c]*Academy of Dietetics, A-8010 Graz, Austria*

[d]*Clinical Institute of Medical and Chemical Laboratory Diagnostics, Medical University, 8036 Graz, Austria*

[e]*UMMM INRA-Theix, St. Genes Champanelle, France*

[f]*Lipid Research Unit, University Rovira i Virgili, 43201 Reus, Spain*

ABSTRACT: A vitamin E depletion/supplementation study was conducted in 100 healthy 20–75-year-old volunteers. The responses of vitamin E status to 3-week dietary vitamin E restriction to approximately 25% of recommended intake and 2-month unrestricted dietary intake plus 800 IU/d of RRR-α-tocopherol were studied as a function of age. Plasma α-tocopherol concentrations were closely related to cholesterol concentrations, which increased with age ($P < 0.001$). Upon dietary restriction, plasma α-tocopherol concentrations decreased significantly ($P < 0.001$) but independently of age. Plasma α-tocopherol responses to supplementation increased significantly with age, but this effect disappeared after standardization for cholesterol. γ-Tocopherol concentrations decreased to less than 30% of baseline.

KEYWORDS: vitamin E; status; dietary restriction; supplementation; aging; α-tocopherol; γ-tocopherol; healthy men; nonsmokers

Address for correspondence: Brigitte M. Winklhofer-Roob, M.D., Associate Professor of Pediatrics, Human Nutrition & Metabolism Research Training Center, Institute of Molecular Biosciences, Karl-Franzens University, Schubertstrasse 1, A-8010 Graz, Austria. Voice: +43-316-380-5490; fax: +43-316-380-9857.
brigitte.winklhoferroob@uni-graz.at

Ann. N.Y. Acad. Sci. 1031: 381–384 (2004). © 2004 New York Academy of Sciences.
doi: 10.1196/annals.1331.050

BACKGROUND

Although numerous studies have demonstrated the effects of vitamin E supplementation on vitamin E status, data on the effects of low vitamin E intake in healthy subjects are confined to a single report.[1] Given that vitamin E is extremely widespread in the human diet, vitamin E deficiency is hardly achieved under nonpathological conditions. However, dietary restriction due to low-fat diets may well be associated with low vitamin E intake and as yet poorly characterized consequences.

STUDY AIMS

The aims of this part of the European Commission-funded project VITAGE were to study (1) the responses of vitamin E status to restricted dietary vitamin E intake for 3 weeks, followed by unrestricted dietary intake and vitamin E supplementation for 2 months and (2) the effects that age might have on the changes observed as a result of these interventions.

SUBJECTS AND METHODS

One hundred healthy male nonsmoking Austrian volunteers 20–75 years of age and not taking supplements were enrolled in the study. For the depletion period, a special diet was created to be cooked on-site that restricted vitamin E intake to approximately 25% of recommended intake. Depletion was followed by unrestricted dietary intake and a daily supplement of 800 IU/d of RRR α-tocopherol (Etocovit; Richter Pharma AG, Wels, Austria) for 2 months. The study protocol (FIG. 1) was approved by the ethics committee, and informed consent was obtained from the volunteers. Vitamin E status was assessed by α- and γ-tocopherol concentrations in plasma and LDL[2] and total vitamin E in buccal mucosal cells (BMCs).[3]

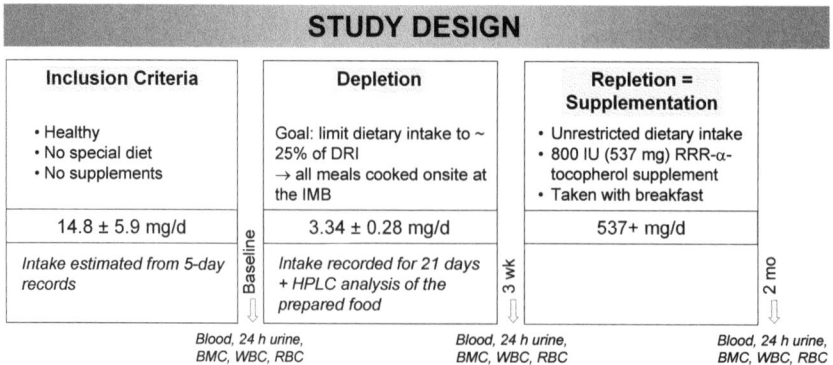

FIGURE 1. Study design of the vitamin E depletion/repletion (supplementation) study completed by 100 healthy nonsmoking 20–75-year-old male volunteers.

RESULTS

Vitamin E–Reduced Diet

The diet used was composed such that dietary vitamin E intake could be restricted to 3.35 ± 0.28 mg/day. This amount was equivalent to 28% of the recommended dietary allowances of 12 mg/day[4] and 22% of the more recent dietary reference intakes (DRI) of 15 mg/day.[5]

Effects of Depletion and Supplementation

Vitamin E restriction for 3 weeks significantly reduced ($P < 0.001$) α-tocopherol concentrations in plasma and LDL and total vitamin E in BMCs. Supplementation increased plasma α-tocopherol concentrations from 25.0 ± 6.56 to 53.6 ± 14.2 μmol/L. In contrast, both vitamin E restriction and supplementation decreased γ-tocopherol concentrations in plasma and LDL to final concentrations of less than 30% of baseline values.

Effects of Age

Plasma α-tocopherol concentrations were closely related to cholesterol concentrations ($r = 0.77$, $P < 0.001$), which showed a significant increase with age ($P < 0.001$). Changes in α-tocopherol concentrations during the depletion period were not dependent on age. In contrast, the response of plasma α-tocopherol concentrations to supplementation increased significantly with age ($P = 0.002$). However, this age effect disappeared when plasma α-tocopherol concentrations were standardized for cholesterol concentrations.

DISCUSSION AND CONCLUSIONS

When given for a duration of 3 weeks, a diet restricting vitamin E intake to approximately 25% of the recommended intake is associated with a significant decrease in vitamin E status, affecting both α- and γ-tocopherol concentrations in plasma, LDL, and BMCs. It is expected that continuing vitamin E restriction at that level over a longer period of time will have an even more pronounced effect, as demonstrated by long-term reduced dietary vitamin E intake with data available not before 3 months of depletion.[1] Vitamin E supplementation almost doubled plasma α-tocopherol concentrations, and concentrations achieved matched those previously reported.[6–8]

Of interest, healthy aging does not have a negative impact on vitamin E status. Vitamin E status was well maintained in healthy nonsmoking aging men and linked to an increase in cholesterol concentrations with age. Increases in cholesterol concentrations with age in healthy subjects have been reported,[9] and close relations between plasma α-tocopherol and cholesterol concentrations have been shown to be major determinants of vitamin E status.[10,11]

A 3-week period of low vitamin E intake reduced vitamin E status independently of age, indicating that healthy, elderly nonsmoking men are not more susceptible to dietary restriction than their younger counterparts. In contrast, the effects of supplementation were even more pronounced in the elderly, most likely as a result of higher plasma lipid concentrations.

ACKNOWLEDGMENTS

This study was conducted with financial support from the Commission of the European Communities, specifically the RTD program "Quality of Life and Management of Living Resources," QLK1-CT-1999-00830, VITAGE. The study does not necessarily reflect the views of the Commission and in no way anticipates the Commission's future policy in this area. Additional support of the Government of Austria (bm:bwk) and Roche Vitamins Europe, Basel, Switzerland is gratefully acknowledged.

REFERENCES

1. HORWITT, M.K. 1960. Vitamin E and lipid metabolism in man. Am. J. Clin. Nutr. **8:** 451–461.
2. AEBISCHER, C.P., J. SCHIERLE & W. SCHÜEP. 1999. Simultaneous determination of retinol, tocopherols, carotene, lycopene, and xanthophylls in plasma by means of reversed-phase high-performance liquid chromatography. Methods Enzymol. **299:** 348–362.
3. LYAN, B., V. AZAIS-BRAESCO, N. CARDINAULT, et al. 2001. Simple method for clinical determination of 13 carotenoids in human plasma using an isocratic high-performance liquid chromatographic method. J. Chromatogr. B Biomed. Sci. Appl. **751:** 297–303.
4. FOOD AND NUTRITION BOARD, NATIONAL RESEARCH COUNCIL. 1989. Recommended dietary allowances, 10th ed. National Academy Press. Washington, DC.
5. FOOD AND NUTRITION BOARD, INSTITUTE OF MEDICINE. 2000. Dietary reference intakes for vitamin C, vitamin E, selenium and carotenoids. National Academy Press. Washington, DC.
6. ROOB, J.M., G. KHOSCHSORUR, A. TIRAN, et al. 2000. Vitamin E attenuates oxidative stress induced by intravenous iron in patients on hemodialysis. J. Am. Soc. Nephrol. **11:** 539–549.
7. TOUSOULIS, D., C. ANTONIADES, C. TENTOLOURIS, et al. 2003. Effects of combined administration of vitamins C and E on reactive hyperemia and inflammatory process in chronic smokers. Atherosclerosis **170:** 261–267.
8. DESIDERI, G., M.C. MARINUCCI, G. TOMASSONI, et al. 2002. Vitamin E supplementation reduces plasma vascular cell adhesion molecule-1 and von Willebrand factor levels and increases nitric oxide concentrations in hypercholesterolemic patients. J. Clin. Endocrinol. Metab. **87:** 2940–2945.
9. WINKLHOFER-ROOB, B.M., M.A. VAN'T HOF & D.H. SHMERLING. 1997. Reference values for plasma concentrations of vitamin E and A and carotenoids in a Swiss population from infancy to adulthood, adjusted for seasonal influences. Clin. Chem. **43:** 146–153.
10. THURNHAM, D.I., J.A. DAVIES, B.J. CRUMP, et al. 1986. The use of different lipids to express serum tocopherol:lipid ratios for the measurement of vitamin E status. Ann. Clin. Biochem. **23:** 514–520.
11. WINKLHOFER-ROOB, B.M., P.E. TUCHSCHMID, L. MOLINARI & D.H. SHMERLING. 1996. Response to a single oral dose of all-rac-α-tocopheryl acetate in patients with cystic fibrosis and in healthy individuals. Am. J. Clin. Nutr. **63:** 717–721.

The Maximal Amount of α-Tocopherol Intake from Foods Alone in U.S. Adults (1994–1996 CSFII)

An Analysis by Linear Programming

XIANG GAO, PARKE E. WILDE, JANICE E. MARAS, ODILIA I. BERMUDEZ, AND KATHERINE L. TUCKER

The Jean Mayer USDA Human Nutrition Research Center on Aging at Tufts University, Boston, Massachusetts 02111, USA

KEYWORDS: α-tocopherol; linear programming; DRI

The 2000 Dietary Reference Intakes (DRIs) for vitamin E increased the Recommended Daily Allowance (RDA) from 10 and 8 mg of α-tocopherol (α-TC) equivalents per day for adult men and women, respectively, to 15 mg α-tocopherol for both men and women.[1] Only 8.0% of men and 2.4% of women in the United States were shown to meet this new Estimated Average Requirement (EAR) for vitamin E (12 mg) from foods alone.[2] This raises the question of whether the new EAR for vitamin E is a reasonable goal within the context of achievable dietary patterns.

OBJECTIVES

The current study was designed to determine the maximal amount of α-TC intake that may be obtained from food within the general U.S. diet and to examine the effect of different food group intakes on this amount.

METHODS

Data from 4,852 men and 4,656 women aged older than 18 years were obtained from the 1994–1996 Continuing Survey of Food Intakes by Individuals (CSFII). Subjects were stratified into four subgroups by age (19–50 or >50 yr) and sex. Two 24-hour recalls were used to collect dietary intake data. Fifty-eight food subgroups were collapsed based on similar nutrient components. Linear programming was used

---

Address for correspondence: Katherine L. Tucker, Ph.D., The Jean Mayer USDA Human Nutrition Research Center on Aging at Tufts University, 711 Washington Street, Boston, MA 02111. Voice: 617-556-3351; fax: 617-556-3344.

katherine.tucker@tufts.edu

to generate diets with maximal α-TC intake, while meeting a set of constraints (TABLE 1), including palatability, DRI, energy, and fat intake limits.

RESULTS

When saturated fat (SFAT) was limited to ≤10% of total energy, the maximal α-TC intakes were 25.5, 21.3, 18.5, and 15.0 mg for male young (aged 19–50 yr) and older adults (>50 yr) and female young and older adults, respectively. However, these amounts decreased to 20.6, 16.3, 16.0, and 11.5 mg, respectively, when a total fat (TFAT) constraint (≤30% of total energy) was added. With the SFAT constraint, the maximal α-TC intakes increased with increased intake of fruit and vegetables, nuts, and oils and fats. An umbrella relationship was observed between maximal α-TC and bread and cereal intake. When the TFAT constraint was added, associations between maximal α-TC with intake of fruit and vegetables, nuts, and bread and cereals remained the same, but became negative for intake of fats and oils. When we set total energy intake at 2,000 kcal and used the SFAT constraint, the maximal α-TC diet, generated by linear programming, contained three servings of breads and cereals, eight servings of fruit and vegetables, two servings of meat, one serving of milk and dairy products, eight servings of fats and oils, and two servings of nuts and seeds. When the TFAT constraint was added, consumption of breads and cereals, fruit and vegetables, and fats and oils changed to 6, 11, and 0 servings, whereas the other food groups remained the same.

CONCLUSIONS

The current DRI for vitamin E can be met from foods for all age–sex groups, except for women older than 50 yr with total fat restricted to ≤30% of energy. However, with fat intake ≤30% of energy, food group choices that can provide adequate α-TC intake are limited and always contain nuts and seeds, a food group not regularly consumed by many Americans.

ACKNOWLEDGMENTS

This work was supported by NIA Grant AG10425-05 and by the U.S. Department of Agriculture, under agreement no. 581950-9-001.

REFERENCES

1. INSTITUTE OF MEDICINE, NATIONAL ACADEMY OF SCIENCE. 2000. Dietary Reference Intakes for Vitamin C, Vitamin E, Selenium, and Carotenoids. National Academy Press. Washington, DC.
2. MARAS, J.E. *et al.* 2004. Intake of alpha-tocopherol is limited among US adults. J. Am. Diet Assoc. **104:** 567–575.

Current Status of Vitamin E Nutriture

JASPREET K.C. AHUJA, JOSEPH D. GOLDMAN, AND ALANNA J. MOSHFEGH

Food Surveys Research Group, Beltsville Human Nutrition Research Center, Agricultural Research Service, Beltsville, Maryland 20705, USA

ABSTRACT: Vitamin E intake status requires reassessment because the recommended levels have been increased and take into account only the α-tocopherol form of vitamin E. A database of α-tocopherol values for more than 7,000 foods was developed and applied to dietary data from the National Health and Nutrition Examination Survey 1999–2000. Usual intake distributions were determined and evaluated for adequacy. Ninety percent or more of the adults studied had their usual intakes below the current Estimated Average Requirement. Several observations—the prevalence of inadequate intakes of vitamin E, absence of signs of deficiency in the U.S. population, and increasing evidence that vitamin E helps reduce chronic disease risk—point to a need for further research.

KEYWORDS: vitamin E; α-tocopherol; Food and Nutrient Database for Dietary Studies (FNDDS); National Health and Nutrition Examination Survey (NHANES) 1999–2000; dietary intakes; food sources

INTRODUCTION

Vitamin E intake status requires reassessment. The recommended average daily intake levels for adult men and women have been increased by the Food and Nutrition Board (FNB) of the National Academy of Sciences[1] and take into account only the α-tocopherol (AT) form of vitamin E. In the past, vitamin E activity in foods was expressed as α-tocopherol equivalents (ATEs) because other naturally occurring forms (β-, γ-, δ-tocopherol and tocotrienols) were thought to contribute towards it. The Food and Nutrition Board has also recommended new approaches for assessing nutrient intakes of groups—adjusting the distribution of intakes for day-to-day variations and then determining the adequacy of intakes by using the probability approach or the Estimated Average Requirement (EAR) cut-point method.[2]

The purpose of this study was to assess vitamin E intakes from foods (expressed as mg AT) for different age/gender groups in the U.S. population. To accomplish this assessment, this study used a new database of α-tocopherol values, current dietary intake data, and the new approach to determine adequacy. Major food sources of α-tocopherol were also determined.

Address for correspondence: Jaspreet K.C. Ahuja, Food Surveys Research Group, Beltsville Human Nutrition Research Center, 10300 Baltimore Avenue, Building 005, BARC-W, Beltsville, MD 20705. Voice: 301-504-0178; fax: 301-504-0377.
jahuja@rbhnrc.usda.gov

Ann. N.Y. Acad. Sci. 1031: 387–390 (2004). © 2004 New York Academy of Sciences.
doi: 10.1196/annals.1331.052

METHODS

Data presented are based on dietary intake information obtained from 8,244 individuals, aged 1 year and over, in the National Health and Nutrition Examination Survey (NHANES) 1999–2000. Details of the survey design and data collection methods are detailed elsewhere.[3] The dietary intake information was coded according to values provided by the United States Department of Agriculture's Food and Nutrient Database for Dietary Studies (FNDDS), release 1.0,[4] which includes values for vitamin E as mg AT. For intakes to be evaluated according to the EAR cut-point method, 2 days of dietary data were needed. Hence, measures of within-person variation for α-tocopherol were estimated with 2-day data from the Continuing Survey of Food Intakes by Individuals (CSFII) 1994–96, 1998.[5] These variation measures were applied to the NHANES data to develop usual intake distributions for 16 age/gender groups. These distributions were developed according to the Iowa State University method and the software C-Side, version 1.02.[6] To determine food sources of α-tocopherol, foods were grouped into 71 predefined food groups used in reporting of CSFII 1994–96, 1998 data,[5] and the contribution of each food group to α-tocopherol intake was estimated using SAS, version 8.02.

TABLE 1. Usual intakes of α-tocopherol by age and sex, NHANES 1999–2000

Group	Sample Size	Usual Mean (mg)	Percentiles			EAR	Percent under EAR
			10	50	90		
Children 1–3	571	4.1	2.6	3.8	5.8	5	80.5
Children 4–8	772	5.2	3.5	4.9	7.1	6	74.8
Male							
9–13 y	536	6.0	3.7	5.6	8.8	9	90.9
14–18 y	680	7.5	4.2	7.0	11.4	12	92.1
19–30 y	451	7.3	4.5	6.9	10.4	12	96.0
31–50 y	648	8.5	4.7	7.7	12.9	12	87.0
51–70 y	630	7.7	4.2	7.1	11.9	12	90.5
70+ y	354	6.7	3.3	5.8	11.2	12	92.1
19 and over	2,083	7.8	4.3	7.2	12.1	12	89.8
Females							
9–13 y	561	5.3	3.5	5.0	7.5	9	96.6
14–18 y	666	5.7	3.6	5.5	8.0	12	99.6
19–30 y	618	5.7	3.7	5.5	7.9	12	99.7
31–50 y	740	6.7	3.8	6.3	10.2	12	95.5
51–70 y	654	6.3	3.4	5.6	9.9	12	95.7
70+ y	363	5.4	2.7	4.8	8.9	12	97.3
19 and over	2,375	6.3	3.5	5.7	9.6	12	96.3

TABLE 2. Main food contributors of α-tocopherol for adult men and women

Food Group	Examples of Top Contributors in the Group	Percent Contribution
Mixtures	Spaghetti sauce,[a] pizza,[a] chili,[a]	19.0
Fried potatoes	Potato chips, french fries	7.1
Salad dressings	Ranch, Italian, mayonnaise	6.0
Cakes, cookies, pastries, pies	Doughnuts, apple pie	5.7
Tomatoes	Raw tomatoes, tomato-vegetable juice, tomato catsup	4.3
Eggs	Fried eggs, omelets, boiled eggs	4.1
Nuts and seeds	Peanut butter, peanuts, almonds	3.9
Crackers, popcorn, pretzels, corn chips	Tortilla chips, popcorn popped in oil, corn-cheese puffs and twists	3.9

[a]Mainly from tomato products.

RESULTS

Mean dietary AT intake and the 10th, 50th, and 90th percentiles of usual dietary AT intake are shown in TABLE 1. Also included are the EAR and the percentage of the population with intakes below the EAR. The mean intake of AT is low across all groups, and the majority of the U.S. population has intakes lower than the EAR. The proportion of children below the EAR ranges from 75% for 4–8 year olds to almost 100% for 14–18 year old girls. Ninety percent or more of adults have intakes below the EAR. Inadequate intakes are more prevalent in females than males. TABLE 2 lists the food groups, along with examples of individual foods, ranked by percent contribution to total dietary intake of AT in the diets of adults. Top food sources are mixture foods (including spaghetti with sauce, pizza, and chili) and fried potatoes (including potato chips and french fries).

CONCLUSIONS

The majority of the U.S. population does not meet the current dietary recommendations of 15 mg AT/day. As expected, dietary vitamin E intakes reported as mg AT are lower than those reported as mg ATEs. The mean intake of 8.8 mg ATEs was reported with the use of NHANES 1999–2000 data,[7] and 9.9 mg ATEs for males and 7.1 mg ATEs for females, 20 and older, were reported with the use of CSFII 1994–1996 data.[6] Maras and colleagues reported intakes of 6.7 mg AT and 4.7 mg AT with the use of CSFII data.[8] Our analysis shows slightly higher intakes, a result that may be attributed to the use of a different sample, a different methodology, or the new database of AT values.

Vitamin E is mainly obtained in the diet through foods low in AT but high in frequency of consumption. Given the prevalence of inadequate intakes, vitamin E nutriture could be improved by increasing intake of foods high in AT. Further research is needed because there is an absence of evidence of deficiency in the U.S. population, and increasing evidence of benefits of vitamin E in reducing the risk of certain chronic diseases.

REFERENCES

1. INSTITUTE OF MEDICINE. 2000. Dietary Reference Intakes for Vitamin C, Vitamin E, Selenium, and Carotenoids. Food and Nutrition Board. National Academy Press. Washington, DC.
2. MURPHY, S.P., S.I. BARR & M.I. POOS. 2002. Using the new Dietary Reference Intakes to assess diets: a map to the maze. Nutr. Rev. **60(9):** 267–275.
3. U.S. DEPARTMENT OF HEALTH AND HUMAN SERVICES. 2003. NHANES 1999–2000 Data Files. Available at <www.cdc.gov/nchs/about/major/nhanes/NHANES99_00.htm>.
4. U.S. DEPARTMENT OF AGRICULTURE, AGRICULTURAL RESEARCH SERVICE. 2004. USDA Food and Nutrient Database for Dietary Studies, Release 1.0. Available at <http://www.barc.usda.gov/bhnrc/foodsurvey/home.htm>.
5. U.S. DEPARTMENT OF AGRICULTURE. AGRICULTURE RESEARCH SERVICE. 2000. Continuing Survey of Food Intake by Individuals 1994–96, 1998. National Technical Information Service. CD-Rom. NTIS Accession no. PB2000-500027.
6. INSTITUTE OF MEDICINE. 2000. Dietary Reference Intakes: Applications in Dietary Assessment. Food and Nutrition Board. National Academy Press. Washington, DC.
7. ERVIN, R.B. *et al.* 2004. Dietary intake of selected vitamins for the United States Population: 1999–2000. Advance data. Mar. 12, 339:1–4. National Center for Health Statistics. Hyattsville, MD.
8. MARAS, J.E. *et al.* 2004. Intake of α-tocopherol is limited among U.S. adults. J. Am. Diet. Assoc. **104(4):** 567-575.

γ-Tocotrienol Metabolism and Antiproliferative Effect in Prostate Cancer Cells

CARMELA CONTE, ALESSANDRO FLORIDI, CRISTINA AISA, MARTA PIRODDI, ARDESIO FLORIDI, AND FRANCESCO GALLI

Department of Internal Medicine, Section of Applied Biochemistry and Nutritional Sciences, University of Perugia, Perugia, Italy

ABSTRACT: In this study, we evaluated the antiproliferative effect of tocotrienols (T3) and the presence of a specific vitamin E metabolism in PC3 and LNCaP prostate cancer cells. These cell lines are able to transform tocopherols (T) and T3 in the corresponding carboxyethyl-hydroxychromans metabolites (CEHCs). The extent of this metabolism and the inhibitory effect on cell growth followed the order of magnitude α-T<α-T3<γ-T<γ-T3. The partial inhibition of γ-T3 metabolism by ketoconazole did not influence cell proliferation. These early findings may suggest that the transformation of vitamin E to CEHC is mostly a detoxification mechanism useful to maintain the malignant properties of prostate cancer cells.

KEYWORDS: vitamin E; tocotrienol; tocopherol: carboxyethyl-hydroxychroman; CEHC; prostate cancer cells; hepatocarcinoma cells; cytochrome P-450

We recently demonstrated that γ-tocopherol (γ-T) and γ-carboxyethyl-hydroxychroman (γ-CEHC), when compared with their alpha homologues, show a much stronger inhibitory effect on prostate cancer cell growth.[1] This effect is mediated by cyclin D1 pathway downregulation with consequent arrest of the cell cycle in the G1 phase. The antiproliferative effect of tocotrienols (T3) and the presence of a specific vitamin E metabolism on prostate cancer cells remain thus far uninvestigated. As a suggestive hypothesis, CEHC formation might represent an underlying event of the antiproliferative effect that the different vitamin E homologues exert on prostate cancer cells. Therefore, we compared in PC3 and LNCaP prostate cancer cells the uptake and transformation of different vitamers, and particularly γ-T and T3, and their effect on cell growth.

Address for correspondence: Francesco Galli, Ph.D., University of Perugia, Department of Internal Medicine, Section of Applied Biochemistry and Nutritional Sciences, Via del Giochetto, 06126 Perugia, Italy. fax: +39-075-585-7441.
  f.galli@unipg.it

TABLE 1. Concentrations of α-CEHCs and γ-CEHCs in the culture media of PC3 prostate cancer cells (1.5×10^6 cells) supplemented for 72 h with 50 μM of α-T, γ-T, and their T3 homologues

Sample	α-CEHCs μmol/L (% of the control)	γ-CEHCs μmol/L (% of the control)
Control	0.06 ± 0.02 (–)	0.53 ± 0.13 (–)
α-T	0.11 ± 0.05 (200)	0.46 ± 0.11 (88)
α-T3	0.16 ± 0.07 (285)	0.65 ± 0.46 (123)
γ-T	0.03 ± 0.11 (83)	2.62 ± 0.65 (496)
γ-T3	0.26 ± 0.12 (470)	4.01 ± 0.99 (756)

METHODS

Cell culture conditions and proliferation assay for the two prostate cancer cell lines PC-3 and LNCaP were the same as in Galli et al.[1] The cells were cultured in the presence of alpha and gamma homologues of tocopherols and T3 in the concentration range 0–100 μM. Metabolic processing of the test compounds was investigated in these two cell lines and in the hepatoblastoma cell line Hep-G2 supplemented for 72 h with the test compounds. In some experiments, before the supplementation step with T3, the cells were preincubated for 4 h in the presence of the CYP3A inhibitor ketoconazole (1 μM).[2] The supernatants and cells were processed for the analysis of metabolite and vitamin homologues as described in Galli et al.[3] with some changes. In brief, 100 μL of a 0.23 M solution of ascorbic acid and δ-CEHCs or Trolox as internal standards for the HPLC or GCMS analysis was added to 5 mL of culture medium. After acidification with 60 μL of 6N HCl, the metabolites were extracted once with 20 mL diethyl ether containing 1% w/v BHT. The analysis was performed with HPLC-ECD or GCMS as described in Galli et al.[3,4] To measure cell vitamin E, the cell pellet was suspended in 1 mL of PBS. After sonication, Tocol was added as internal standard and the liposoluble vitamins were extracted with 5 mL hexane containing 1% w/v BHT. The organic phase was collected and dried down under a stream of nitrogen gas and resuspended in 200 μL of the mobile phase used for the HPLC analysis.

RESULTS AND DISCUSSION

The supplementation of PC3 cells with γ-T, γ-T3, and their alpha homologues lead to a significant transformation to the corresponding CEHCs. This metabolism is particularly marked in the case of γ-T3 (TABLE 1). The alpha homologues showed the lowest response of transformation to α-CEHC. In all the test compounds, the concentration of CEHCs released in the culture media was linearly dependent on the quantity of vitamer precursors taken up by the cells. FIGURE 1 shows in detail the direct correlation existing between uptake and transformation of either γ-T or γ-T3 as a function of the amount of vitamer added to the culture medium in the concentration range 0–100 μM. Of importance, γ-T3 showed a higher uptake and transformation rate than γ-T. Similar results were obtained with the cell line LNCaP (not shown).

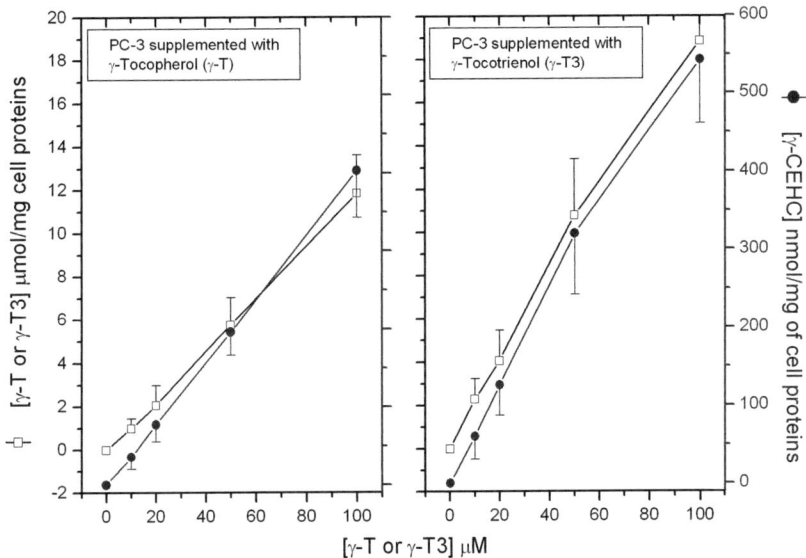

FIGURE 1. Dose-dependence of the uptake and transformation of γ-T and γ-T3 in PC3 cells (1.5×10^6) supplemented for 72 h with the two compounds in the concentration range 0–100 μM.

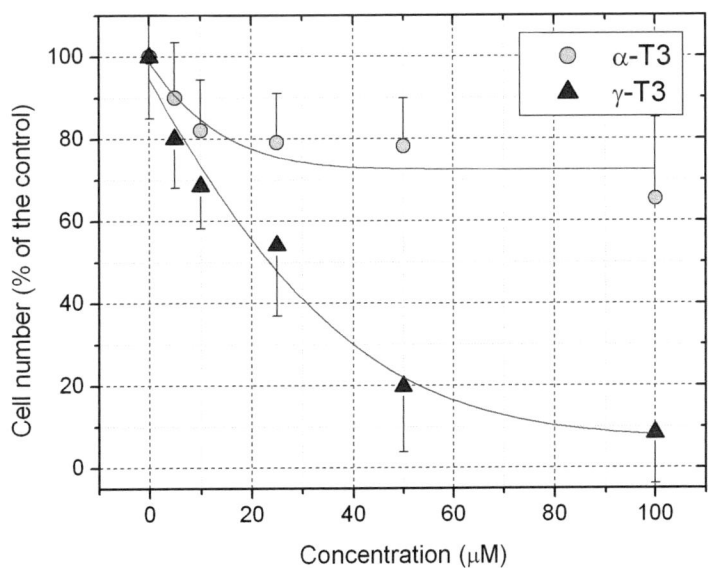

FIGURE 2. Concentration-dependent effect of α-T3 or γ-T3 on PC3 cancer cell growth. The cells were cultured under the same conditions summarized in TABLE 1.

For comparison, we also evaluated the transformation response in Hep-G2 cells under the same experimental conditions. This cell line produced from three- to six-fold higher concentrations of CEHCs as compared with prostate cancer cells. The supplementation of PC3 or LNCaP cells with γ-T3 inhibits the cell growth in a concentration-dependent manner (FIG. 2), and this effect was superior to that in the case of γ-T. Consistent with previous findings on tocopherol homologues,[1] this effect was specific for γ-T3, whereas α-T3 was much less effective. The supplementation of PC3 cells with γ-T3 in the presence of 1 μM ketoconazole, an inhibitor of the CytP-450–mediated transformation of vitamin E in Hep-G2 cells,[2] does not seem to affect the decrease of the cell growth induced by γ-T3 (not shown).

CONCLUSIONS

In conclusion, PC3 and LNCaP show a specific vitamin E metabolism that is influenced by the uptake rate and type of homologue tested with the order of magnitude α-T<α-T3<γ-T<γ-T3. The same order of magnitude was observed for the antiproliferative effect exerted by these compounds. These findings weaken the hypothesis that CEHCs might be the biological effectors of the antiproliferative activity of vitamin E in prostate cancer cells. In this respect, it seems probable that prostate cancer cells transform vitamin E homologues to CEHCs exclusively as a detoxification mechanism useful to maintain their malignant properties. Further studies are required to verify this aspect.

REFERENCES

1. GALLI, F., A.M. STABILE, M. BETTI, et al. 2004. The effect of alpha- and gamma-tocopherol and their carboxyethyl hydroxychroman metabolites on prostate cancer cell proliferation. Arch. Biochem. Biophys. **423:** 97–102.
2. PARKER, R.S. & J.E. SWANSON. 2000. A novel 5′-carboxychroman metabolite of gamma-tocopherol secreted by HepG2 cells and excreted in human urine. Biochem. Biophys. Res. Commun. **269:** 580–583.
3. GALLI, F., R. LEE, C. DUNSTER & F.J. KELLY. 2002. Gas chromatography mass spectrometry analysis of carboxyethyl-hydroxychroman metabolites of alpha- and gamma-tocopherol in human plasma. Free Radic. Biol. Med. **32:** 333–340.
4. GALLI, F., A.G. FLORIDI, A. FLORIDI & U. BUONCRISTIANI. 2004. Accumulation of vitamin E metabolites in the blood of renal failure patients. Clin. Nutr. **23:** 205–212.

In Utero Origins of Cancer

Maternal Dietary Vitamin E, Fetal Oxidative DNA Damage, and Postnatal Carcinogenesis in p53 Knockout Mice

CONNIE SHIHSIN CHEN[a] AND PETER G. WELLS[a,b]

[a]*Faculty of Pharmacy, University of Toronto, Toronto, Ontario, Canada M5S 2S2*

[b]*Department of Pharmacology, University of Toronto, Toronto, Ontario, Canada M5S 2S2*

KEYWORDS: fetal redox status; reactive oxygen species (ROS); p53-deficient mice; vitamin E; cancer

Reactive oxygen species (ROS) can oxidatively damage cellular macromolecules such as DNA, and ROS-mediated oxidative stress has been implicated in cancer initiation and promotion (FIG. 1).[1,2] The developing conceptus (embryo and fetus) generally has less than 5% of the antioxidative capacity of adults,[3–6] potentially leaving it at greater risk from endogenous oxidative stress.[6] Previously, we found that dietary supplementation with the antioxidant vitamin E (*all-rac-α*–tocopherol-acetate) reduced embryonic DNA oxidation and embryopathies in outbred CD-1 mice.[7,8] Also, *in utero* exposure of cancer-prone p53 knockout mouse[9] conceptuses to dietary vitamin E in high doses (10% [w/w]) altered conceptal DNA oxidation and enhanced postnatal cancer in the offspring, providing evidence for redox-dependent *in utero* origins of cancer (FIG. 2).[10] Here, we investigated the effect of conceptal exposure to low-dose dietary vitamin E on postnatal carcinogenesis.

METHODS

Virgin +/– p53 knockout females were placed on either a normal or 0.1% [w/w] vitamin E–supplemented diet for 4 weeks and mated with +/– p53 knockout males. Vitamin E supplementation was stopped on the day of birth. The offspring were *p53*-genotyped and observed for spontaneous tumor development. Fetal DNA oxidation (8-oxo-7,8-dihydro-2′-deoxyguanosine) was analyzed in tissues taken on gestational days 13 and 19 using high-performance liquid chromatography with electrochemical detection.

Address for correspondence: Peter G. Wells, Faculty of Pharmacy, University of Toronto, 19 Russell Street, Toronto, ON, Canada M5S 2S2. Voice: 416-978-3221; fax: 416-267-7797.
pg.wells@utoronto.ca

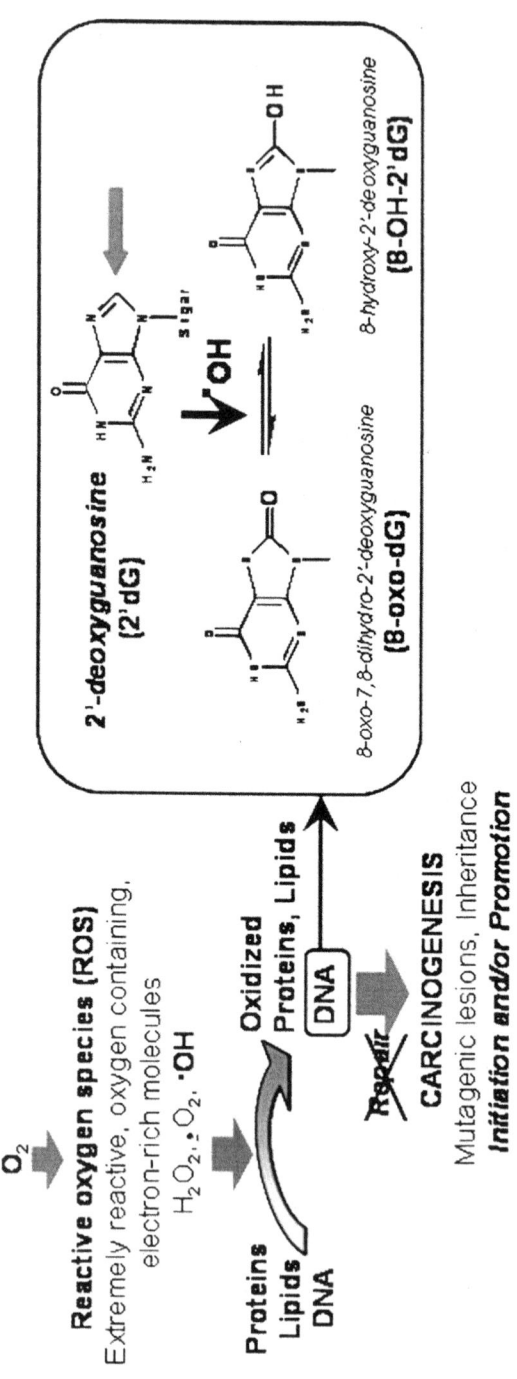

FIGURE 1. Role of ROS in carcinogenesis. Highly reactive ROS can damage critical cellular macromolecules, including DNA, which, in turn, if unrepaired, can be mutagenic, teratogenic, and carcinogenic.

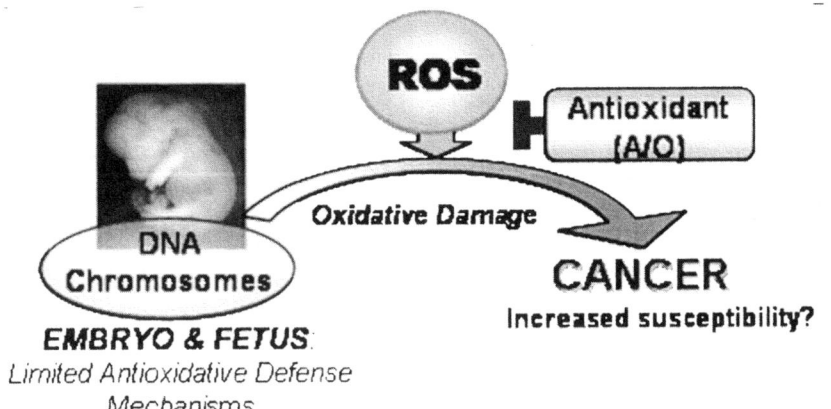

FIGURE 2. Higher risk of the fetus to ROS-mediated carciogenesis? Measurable oxidative stress occurs normally in embryos and fetuses (conceptuses). However, the conceptus has very low protective antioxidative capacity, constituting less than 5% of adult levels, and may be more susceptible to ROS-initiated damage and consequences. The teratological importance of DNA damage is illustrated in p53 knockout mice, which have deficient DNA repair and exhibit enhanced susceptibility to ROS-initiating teratogens.[11] Similarly, we hypothesized that the conceptus is more susceptible to ROS-initiated cancer, and that *in utero* exposure to the antioxidant vitamin E may alter the risk for postnatal carcinogenesis.

RESULTS

Compared with offspring from dams supplemented with control diet, *in utero* exposure to low-dose vitamin E delayed postnatal tumorigenesis in +/− p53 knockout offspring ($P < 0.05$) and increased their median survival age by 5% ($P < 0.05$). p53-*null* offspring were not protected. Low-dose vitamin E did not appear to alter the tumor spectrum. Embryonic DNA oxidation was 84% and 58% higher in untreated null p53-deficient embryos compared to heterozygous and wild-type littermates, respectively ($P < 0.05$). High-dose, but not low-dose, vitamin E reduced DNA oxidation in null p53-deficient embryos by 36% ($P < 0.05$) but not heterozygous or wild-type littermates. In the fetus, the effects of vitamin E varied substantially by dose and by fetal tissue type. Both high-dose and low-dose vitamin E reduced DNA oxidation in the fetal brain by 42% and 33% in −/− and +/− p53-deficient offspring, respectively ($P < 0.01$). This effect was not seen in wild-type brains. Low-dose vitamin E did not afford significant protection in other tissues. In contrast, high-dose vitamin E enhanced fetal skin DNA oxidation by 42–91% in both −/− and +/− p53-deficient offspring, respectively ($P < 0.05$), but not in wild-type skin. These effects were not observed in other tissues.

CONCLUSIONS

The delay in postnatal carcinogenesis effected by *in utero* low-dose vitamin E exposure provides new evidence for *in utero* origins of cancer and raises the possibility of new therapeutic strategies. The reduction in fetal brain DNA oxidation by low-dose vitamin E in both −/− and +/− p53-deficient fetuses suggests a ROS-dependent mechanism for *in utero* carcinogenesis and the protective effect of low-dose vitamin E. The elevation of fetal skin DNA oxidation by high-dose vitamin E in −/− and +/− p53-deficient fetuses is consistent with the potential for a related but contrasting pro-oxidant mechanism. These highly variable effects of vitamin E on DNA oxidation in different tissues reveal the difficulty in anticipating its effects in different cell types. The reduction in embryonic DNA oxidation by both high- and low-dose vitamin E in null p53-deficient offspring on gestational day 13 suggests that cancer is not originating during the embryonic period, and that high-dose vitamin E may be protective for developmental processes other than cancer. The protective effects of low-dose vitamin E appear to be insufficient if both p53 alleles are lost. In contrast, the tumor-enhancing effects of high-dose vitamin E were evident in both −/− and +/− p53-deficient offspring.[10] These results show that carcinogenesis in some cases can be modified by altering fetal redox status, suggesting novel carcinogenic mechanisms and potential therapeutic strategies.

ACKNOWLEDGMENTS

This work was supported by the National Cancer Institute of Canada and the Canadian Institutes of Health Research.

REFERENCES

1. HALLIWELL, B. & J. GUTTERIDGE. 1999. Free Radicals in Biology and Medicine, 3rd ed. Oxford University Press. New York.
2. FLOYD, R.A. 1999. The role of 8-hydroxyguanine in carcinogenesis. Carcinogenesis **11:** 1447–1450.
3. EL-HAGE, S. & S.M. SINGH. 1990. Temporal expression of genes with higher mRNA levels during in utero development in mice. Dev. Genet. **11:** 149–159.
4. LIU, L. & P.G. WELLS. 1995. DNA oxidation as a potential molecular mechanism mediated drug-induced birth defects: phenytoin and structurally related teratogens initiated the formation of 6-hydroxy-2-deoxyguanosine *in vitro* and *in vivo* in murine maternal hepatic and embryonic tissues. Free Radic. Biol. Med. **19:** 639–648.
5. WINN, L.M. & P.G. WELLS. 1999. Maternal administration of superoxide dismutase and catalase in phenytoin teratogenicity. Free Radic. Biol. Med. **26:** 266–274.
6. NICOL, C.J., J. ZIELENSKI, L.C. TSUI & P.G. WELLS. 2000. An embryoprotective role for glucose-6-phosphate dehyrodgenase in developmental oxidative stress and chemical teratogenesis. FASEB J. **14:** 111–127.
7. CHEN, C.S. & P.G. WELLS. 2001. Effect of dietary vitamin E on endogenous and phenytoin-initiated embryonic DNA oxidation. Toxicol. Sci. [Suppl.: The Toxicologist] **60:** 48 [abstract 234].
8. MARICIC, J., C.S. CHEN & P.G. WELLS. 2002. Effects os maternal dietary vitamin E supplementation on developmental biology and phenytoin embryopathies. Toxico. Sci. [Suppl.: The Toxicologist] **66:** 23 [abstract 109].
9. DONEHOWER, L.A., M. HARVEY, B.L. SLAGLE, *et al.* 1992. Mice deficient for p53 are developmentally normal but susceptible to spontaneous tumors. Nature **35:** 215–221.
10. CHEN, C.S. & P.G. WELLS. 2002. In utero origins of cancer in p53 knockout mice: maternal dietary vitamin E, fetal oxidative DNA damage and postnatal carcinogenesis. Toxicologist **61:** 1502.
11. NICOL, C.J., M.L. HARRISON, R.R. LAPOSA, I.L. GIMELSHTEIN & P.G. WELLS. 1995. A teratoligc sppressor role for p53 in benzo[a]pyrene-treated transgenic p53-deficient mice. Nature Genetics **10:** 181–187.

γ-Tocopherol Induces Apoptosis in Androgen-Responsive LNCaP Prostate Cancer Cells via Caspase-Dependent and Independent Mechanisms

QING JIANG,[a,b] JEFF WONG,[b] AND BRUCE N. AMES[a,b]

[a]*Children's Hospital–Oakland Research Institute, 5700 Martin Luther King Jr. Way, Oakland, California 94609, USA*

[b]*Division of Biochemistry and Molecular Biology, University of California at Berkeley, Berkeley, California 94720, USA*

ABSTRACT: We found that γ-tocopherol, the predominant vitamin E form in diets, but not α-tocopherol, which is the exclusive form of vitamin E in most supplements, exhibited antiproliferation effect on prostate (PC-3, LNCaP) and lung (A549) cancer cells. γ-Tocopherol induced apoptosis in androgen-sensitive LNCaP but not androgen-resistant PC-3 cells. Consequently, γ-tocopherol treatment caused cytochrome *c* release and caspase-9, -3 and -7 activation. However, the apoptosis could not be completely reversed by an irreversible pancaspase inhibitor, indicating that an alternative caspase-independent pathway may also be involved. Our study suggests that γ-tocopherol may be valuable in the prevention and therapy for certain types of cancer.

KEYWORDS: γ-tocopherol; vitamin E; apoptosis; caspase; prostate cancer

BACKGROUND AND HYPOTHESIS

Eicosanoids derived from arachidonic acid through cyclooxygenase (COX)– and lipoxygenase (LOX)–mediated reactions play important roles in progression of certain types of cancer. It has been shown that inhibitors of COX and LOX can inhibit cancer cell proliferation in cell cultures and reduce the risk of human cancer.[1–3] Our recent studies indicate that γ-tocopherol (γ-T), the major form of vitamin E in U.S. diets, but not α-tocopherol (α-T), the predominant form of vitamin E in tissues and plasma, exhibits anti-inflammatory activities by inhibiting COX- and possibly LOX-catalyzed formation of prostaglandin E and leukotriene B, respectively.[4–6] These observations led to the current hypothesis that γ-tocopherol may be useful as an anticancer agent.

Address for correspondence: Qing Jiang, Ph.D., Department of Foods and Nutrition, Purdue University, West Lafayette, IN 47907. Voice: 765-494-2483; fax: 765-494-0674.
Qjiang@purdue.edu

RESULTS

In the current study, we report that γ-T, but not α-T, dose-dependently inhibited cancer cell proliferation in androgen-sensitive (LNCaP) and androgen-resistant (PC-3) prostate cells, as well as lung adenocarcinoma (A549), as indicated in the MTT assays. Of importance, γ-T, at 50 μM, had no effects on normal human prostate epithelial cells after 4 days of treatment. The antiproliferation effect of γ-T was partially reversed by the addition of arachidonic acid or linoleic acid, the substrates for cyclooxygenase and lipoxygenase. Further studies showed that γ-T treatment induced apoptosis in LNCaP but not PC-3 cells, as indicated by DNA fragmentation using gel electrophoresis. γ-T treatment led to the release of cytochrome c from mitochondria to cytosolic compartments. Consequently, an activation of caspase-9, -3, and -7 and the cleavage of PARP were observed. These results indicate that γ-T treatment led to the activation of the caspase pathway. In addition to the caspase-dependent pathway, apoptosis also appears to be mediated by caspase-independent mechanisms because the pan-caspase inhibitor, Z-VAD-fmk, did not completely reverse γ-T-induced apoptosis as indicated by MTT assay and DNA fragmentation. Although z-VAD-fmk inhibited the formation of active caspase-3, it did not completely prevent PARP cleavage. In search of the upstream event, we found that γ-T treatment did not appear to significantly affect BCl-2 and BCl-xL protein expression or the phosphorylation of Akt.

CONCLUSIONS

Our findings, in line with the potentially beneficial effect implicated in the recent epidemiologic studies,[7] suggest that γ-T may be useful in the prevention and therapy of prostate and possibly other types of cancer.

REFERENCES

1. AVIS, I. *et al.* 2001. Five-lipoxygenase inhibitors can mediate apoptosis in human breast cancer cell lines through complex eicosanoid interactions. FASEB J. **15:** 2007–2009.
2. DING, X.Z., W.G. TONG & T.E. ADRIAN. 2001. Cyclooxygenases and lipoxygenases as potential targets for treatment of pancreatic cancer. Pancreatology **1:** 291–299.
3. MARNETT, L.J. 1992. Aspirin and the potential role of prostaglandins in colon cancer. Cancer Res. **52:** 5575–5589.
4. JIANG, Q. *et al.* 2000. Gamma-tocopherol and its major metabolite, in contrast to alpha-tocopherol, inhibit cyclooxygenase activity in macrophages and epithelial cells. Proc Natl Acad Sci USA **97:** 11494–11499.
5. JIANG, Q. & B.N. AMES. 2003. Gamma-tocopherol, but not alpha-tocopherol, decreases proinflammatory eicosanoids and inflammation damage in rats. FASEB J. **17:** 816–822.
6. JIANG, Q. *et al.* 2001. Gamma-Tocopherol, the major form of vitamin E in the US diet, deserves more attention. Am. J. Clin. Nutr. **74:** 714–722.
7. HELZLSOUER, K.J. *et al.* 2000. Association between alpha-tocopherol, gamma-tocopherol, selenium, and subsequent prostate cancer. J. Natl. Cancer Inst. **92:** 2018–2023.

Antiangiogenic Potency of Vitamin E

TERUO MIYAZAWA, TSUYOSHI TSUZUKI, KIYOTAKA NAKAGAWA, AND MIKI IGARASHI

Food and Biodynamic Chemistry Laboratory, Graduate School of Agricultural Science, Tohoku University, Sendai 981-8555, Japan

ABSTRACT: We investigated the antiangiogenic property and mechanism of vitamin E compounds, with particular emphasis on tocotrienol (T3), a natural analogue of tocopherol (Toc). T3 inhibited both the proliferation and tube formation of bovine aortic endothelial cells, with δ-T3 appearing to have the highest activity. δ-T3 also reduced the vascular endothelial growth factor (VEGF)–stimulated tube formation by human umbilical vein endothelial cells. Moreover, δ-T3 inhibited the new blood vessel formation on the growing chick embryo chorioallantoic membrane (assay for *in vivo* angiogenesis). Orally administered T3 suppressed the tumor cell–induced angiogenesis in the mouse dorsal air sac assay. In contrast with T3, Toc showed very weak inhibition. Based on DNA microarray analysis, antiangiogenic effect of T3 was attributable in part to regulation of intracellular VEGF signaling (phospholipase C-γ and protein kinase C). Our findings suggest that T3 has potential as a therapeutic dietary supplement for preventing angiogenic disorders.

KEYWORDS: angiogenesis inhibitor; vitamin E; tocotrienol; tocopherol

INTRODUCTION

Angiogenesis, the formation of new blood vessels from a preexisting vascular bed, is of fundamental importance in several pathological states such as tumor growth, diabetic retinopathy, and rheumatic arthritis.[1] Angiogenesis normally involves a series of steps including endothelial cell activation and breakdown of the basement membrane, followed by proliferation, migration, and tube formation of the endothelial cells. If the progression of these abnormal processes can be minimized, the responsible food constituents might be used as therapeutic agents for the prevention of various angiogenesis-mediated disorders. Therefore, we previously have investigated food ingredients bearing antiangiogenic property by *in vitro* culture experiments.[2,3] As a result, vitamin E was screened out as an attractive angiogenesis inhibitor.

Vitamin E occurs in nature as at least eight different isoforms that include α-, β-, γ-, and δ-isomers of both tocopherol (Toc) and tocotrienol (T3). T3 is a minor plant constituent, especially abundant in palm oil and rice bran. T3 has an isoprenoid

---

Address for correspondence: Teruo Miyazawa, Food and Biodynamic Chemistry Lab, Graduate School of Agricultural Science, Tohoku University, Sendai 981-8555, Japan. Voice: +81-22-717-8904; fax: +81-22-717-8905.
miyazawa@biochem.tohoku.ac.jp

structure that differs from Toc bearing saturated phytyl side chain. Interestingly, in our previous studies,[2,3] T3 showed a higher antiangiogenic effect than Toc. Hence, in this study, the antiangiogenic property of T3 was investigated in detail by using well-characterized *in vitro* and *in vivo* systems. Moreover, the antiangiogenic mechanism of T3 was evaluated by DNA microarray analysis.

METHODS

For proliferation assay, bovine aortic endothelial cells (BAECs; Dainippon Pharmaceutical Co. Ltd., Osaka, Japan) were seeded at densities of 2×10^3 cells/well in a 100-μL minimum essential Eagle's medium (MEM; Sigma, St. Louis, MO) containing 10% fetal bovine serum (FBS) on 96-well collagen-coated culture plates (Asahi Techno Glass Co. Ltd., Tokyo, Japan). After incubation at 37°C in a 5% CO_2 incubator for 24 h, the cells were replaced in 100 μL fresh MEM containing 2% FBS and various concentrations of T3 or Toc. Twenty-four hours later, cell proliferation was evaluated by the WST-1 method.[4]

Tube formation was assessed using the three-dimensional culture method.[5] BAECs (1×10^5 cells/well) were preincubated for 24 h in a 1.5-mL MEM containing 10% FBS on 12-well collagen-coated culture plates. After removal of the medium, 0.5 mL of collagen gel solution (consisting of a mixture of 8 volumes of Vitrogen collagen, 1 volume of 10 times concentrated MEM, and 1 volume of 0.1 M NaOH) was overlaid. Fresh MEM (1.5 μL) containing 2% FBS and various concentrations of sample were added to each well. After incubation for 72 h, the length of the tube was measured. The effect of vitamin E on the vascular endothelial growth factor (VEGF)–stimulated tube formation of human umbilical vein endothelial cells (HUVECs) was evaluated by Angiogenesis kit (Kurabo Industries, Ltd., Osaka, Japan).

For DNA microarray analysis, total RNA was isolated from both T3-treated and untreated HUVECs by RNeasy Mini Kit (Qiagen, Valencia, CA). Reverse transcription to cDNA, hybridization with the DNA chip (CodeLink UniSet Human 1 Bioarray; Amersham, Tokyo, Japan), and signal analysis were conducted.

The *in vivo* antiangiogenic effect of vitamin E was evaluated by using chick embryo chorioallantoic membrane (CAM) assay[6] and mouse dorsal air sac (DAS) assay.[7] In the CAM assay, the fertilized chick eggs were preincubated at 37°C for 5 days. After that, the pellet containing sample at various concentrations was placed on the CAM. After incubation for 2 days, angiogenic response was evaluated by measuring the avascular zone in the CAM. In the DAS assay, DLD-1 human colon carcinoma cells (from the Cell Resource Center for Biomedical Research at Tohoku University, Sendai, Japan) were suspended in phosphate buffered saline (PBS) at a concentration of 1×10^8 cells/mL, and 0.1 mL of this suspension was injected into a chamber ring (Millipore Co., Billerica, MA). This chamber was implanted into a dorsal air sac prepared in a 5-week-old male ICR mouse (CLEA Japan, Inc., Tokyo, Japan). A food-grade T3 mixture (Tocomin 50; Carotech, Malaysia) or Toc (Eisai Co., Tokyo, Japan) was administrated orally to the mouse once a day at a dose of 0.5–4 mg/day for 5 days. After that, the implanted chamber was removed, and angiogenic response was assessed by counting newly formed capillary vessels within the area attached to the chamber.

RESULTS AND DISCUSSION

T3 at low micromolar range inhibited BAEC proliferation that was assessed by WST-1 method. The inhibitory potency of each T3 isomer varied markedly in the following order; δ- > β- > γ- > α-T3. Subjecting T3 (1–30 μM) to the BAEC tube formation assay, we confirmed that all the isomers significantly reduced the width and the length of endothelial tubes of BAECs. The ranked order of this inhibitory effect was δ- > β- > γ- > α-T3. On the other hand, Toc did not affect BAEC proliferation and tube formation even though increasing their Toc concentration at 100 μM. These results suggested that T3 may be a bioactive compound and that T3 has a potential for acting as an angiogenesis inhibitor, as previously reported by us.[2,3] Because, in the present study, δ-T3 would be a most potent antiangiogenic compound among vitamin E, we then investigated an effect of the compound on VEGF-stimulated tube formation of HUVECs. When HUVECs were co-cultivated with fibroblasts cultured in the presence of 10 ng/mL of VEGF for 11 days, the increases of tube-like structure were confirmed. Simultaneously adding δ-T3 (1 and 10 μM) with VEGF to the medium significantly reduced the VEGF-stimulated tube formation in HUVECs. VEGF is an endothelial cell–specific mitogen and an angiogenesis-inducer released by a variety of tumor cells and is known to play an important role in several pathological events such as tumor angiogenesis.[1] Hence, δ-T3 revealed potent antiangiogenic effect, presumably caused by the regulation of VEGF signaling. Indeed, based on DNA microarray analysis, δ-T3 downregulated the expression of VEGF receptor in HUVECs and blocked intracellular VEGF signaling (phospholipase C-γ and protein kinase C), which resulted in the inhibition of angiogenesis. On the other hand, in an *in vivo* model of angiogenesis, δ-T3 (125–1,000 μg) exhibited a dose-dependent inhibition in angiogenesis as assessed by CAM assay. Moreover, in the DAS assay, orally administered food-grade T3 mixture (4 mg/day) suppressed the tumor cell–induced angiogenesis. In contrast with T3, Toc showed very weak inhibition. These results suggest that T3 represents a member of a new class of dietary-derived antiangiogenic compounds. Angiogenic inhibitors derived from natural products have an advantage in that they are nontoxic at physiological doses, can be given orally, and can be easily obtained or manufactured.

In conclusion, vitamin E, especially of T3, exhibits the antiangiogenic property *in vitro* and *in vivo*. The results indicate that T3 has potential as a therapeutic dietary supplement for preventing angiogenic disorders.

REFERENCES

1. KIM, K.J., B. LI, J. WINER, *et al.* 1993. Inhibition of vascular endothelial growth factor-induced angiogenesis suppresses tumor growth *in vivo*. Nature **362:** 841–844.
2. INOKUCHI, H., H. HIROKANE, T. TSUZUKI, *et al.* 2003. Anti-angiogenic activity of tocotrienol. Biosci. Biotechnol. Biochem. **67:** 1623–1627.
3. MIYAZAWA, T., H. INOKUCHI, H. HIROKANE, *et al.* 2004. Anti-angiogenic potential of tocotrienol *in vitro*. Biochemistry (Moscow) **69:** 67–69.
4. ISHIYAMA, M., H. TOMINAGA, M. SHIGA, *et al.* 1996. A combined assay of cell viability and *in vitro* cytotoxicity with a highly water-soluble tetrazolium salt, neutral red and crystal violet. Biol. Pharm. Bull. **19:** 1518–1520.

5. MONTESANO, R., L. ORCI & P. VASSALLI. 1983. *In vitro* rapid organization of endothelial cells into capillary-like networks is promoted by collagen matrices. J. Cell Biol. **97:** 1648–1652.
6. OIKAWA, T., K. HIROTANI, O. NAKAMURA, *et al.* 1989. A highly potent anti-angiogenic activity of retinoids. Cancer Lett. **48:** 157–162.
7. KIUE, A., T. ABE, A. MORIMOTO, *et al.* 1992. Anti-angiogenic effect of 15-deoxyspergualin in angiogenesis model system involving human microvascular endothelial cells. Cancer J. **5:** 267–271.

Modulation of Cell Proliferation and Gene Expression by α-Tocopheryl Phosphates

Relevance to Atherosclerosis and Inflammation

ESRA OGRU,[a] ROKSAN LIBINAKI,[b] ROBERT GIANELLO,[b] SIMON WEST,[a] ADELINA MUNTEANU,[c] JEAN-MARC ZINGG,[c] AND ANGELO AZZI[c]

[a]*Phosphagenics Ltd., Melbourne 3000, Australia*

[b]*Department of Biochemistry and Molecular Biology, Monash University, Clayton, 3800, Australia*

[c]*Institute of Biochemistry and Molecular Biology, University of Bern, 3012 Bern, Switzerland*

> ABSTRACT: The effect of a mixture of α-tocopheryl phosphate plus di-α-tocopheryl phosphate (TPm) was studied *in vitro* on two cell lines, RASMC (from rat aortic smooth muscle) and human THP-1 monocytic leukemia cells. Inhibition of cell proliferation by TPm was shown in both lines and occurred with TPm at concentrations lower than those at which α-tocopherol was equally inhibitory. TPm led in nonstimulated THP-1 cells to inhibition of CD36 mRNA and protein expression, to inhibition of oxidized low-density lipoprotein surface binding and oxLDL uptake. In nonstimulated THP-1 cells, α-tocopherol had only very weak effects on these events.
>
> KEYWORDS: α-tocopheryl; di-α-tocopheryl phosphate; THP-1 cells

INTRODUCTION

A series of studies have drawn attention to the regulatory aspects of α-tocopherol on macrophages and smooth muscle cells. Modulation of signaling cascades and gene expression in these cells is at the basis of the preventive effect of α-tocopherol in atherosclerosis and inflammatory disease. A specific receptor for oxidized LDL (oxLDL) (the CD36 scavenger receptor) is expressed in endothelial cells, monocytes/macrophages, and cultured human aortic smooth muscle cells. Several studies have indicated that CD36 can transport oxLDL into the cytosol of these cells and that α-tocopherol inhibits oxLDL uptake by a mechanism involving downregulation of CD36 mRNA and protein expression.

Address for correspondence: Angelo Azzi, M.D., Department of Biochemistry and Molecular Biology, University of Bern, Buhlstrasse 28, Bern 3012, Switzerland. Voice413-16314131; fax: 413-16313737.
angelo.azzi@mci.unibe.ch

Recently, novel tocopherol derivatives have been described: the tocopheryl phosphate ester and the bis-tocopheryl phosphate ester, or di-α-tocopheryl phosphate (T_2P). The former compound is the ester derivative of phosphate with the hydroxyl group of tocopherol, whereas the latter is obtained by esterification of two tocopherol moieties with one phosphate molecule.[1]

Interest in tocopheryl phosphate derivatives has increased after the discovery that α-tocopheryl phosphate is present in plant and animal tissues as well as in food stuffs.[1] Furthermore, supplementation of the diet of rats with α-tocopheryl phosphate resulted in an increase deposition of tocopheryl phosphate in liver and adipose tissue and in an increase of α-tocopherol.[1] These findings prompt several questions, ranging from the possibility that α-tocopheryl phosphate is a reserve form of α-tocopherol to the hypothesis that it may represent an active compound capable of regulatory effects at the cellular level.

EXPERIMENTAL PROCEDURES

Materials

The mixture of α-tocopheryl phosphates, TPm (Phosphagenics Ltd.), was synthesized as follows. α-Tocopherol (51 g, 0.1 mol; RRR-α-tocopherol [Henkel, LaGrange, IL]) was reacted with P_4O_{10} (8.5 g, 30 mmol) under high shear conditions at 80–90°C to hydrolyze the residual polyphosphate bonds. Analysis of the resultant product using ^{31}P NMR indicated a mixture of α-tocopheryl phosphate, di-α-tocopheryl phosphate, and some residual inorganic phosphate. The TPm had the following composition: TP: 55.3%, T2P: 30.6%, α-tocopherol: 5%, inorganic phosphate: 2.6%, water: 1.9%, oleic acid: 1.0%, impurities (i.e., sterols): 3.57%. Stock solutions of TPm were prepared in ethanol with sonication. The tocopherol equivalents in the TPm is approximately 0.8 (i.e., 1 g TPm is equivalent to 0.8 g α-tocopherol). Stock solutions of α-tocopherol were prepared in ethanol.

The product also was used in some experiments (FIG. 1B) after conversion to the sodium form from the free acid form, as follows. The TPm was dissolved in ethanol and NaOH (in ethanol) was added at a 2:1 molar ratio of sodium to phosphorus. Removal of the ethanol was under reduced pressure. Stock solutions of the sodium form were prepared in 0.1% ethanol with sonication.

Cell Culture

Rat aortic smooth muscle cells (RASMCs; Cell Applications) were seeded in growth medium (DMEM/F12 + 10% serum) into six-well plates (25,000 cells/well). After 24 h, cells were washed twice with Hank's Buffered Salt Solution, and DMEM/F12 + 0.2% serum was added to each well. Cells were serum-starved for 48 h before treatments.

Human THP-1 monocytic leukemia cells (ATCC #TIB-202) were cultured in RPMI/10% FCS, 2 mM L-glutamine, 1.0 mM sodium pyruvate, and 4.5 g/L glucose. THP-1 cells (10^6 per plate) were plated 24 hours before treatments with α-tocopherol or tocopheryl phosphate mix at the concentrations indicated.

Proliferation Assay

RASMCs were grown and serum-starved as above. Treatment solutions containing drugs then were prepared in growth medium and added to each well (3 mL/well). The effect of α-tocopherol and TPm on smooth muscle cell proliferation was tested at three concentrations: 20, 50, and 100 μM. Control treatments included growth medium and growth medium + vehicles (ethanol did not exceed 0.1%). The experiment was performed in triplicate, and the mean and standard deviation were calculated for each treatment.

THP-1 cells were plated into six-well plates at 2×10^5 cells per well and treated with 0.1% ethanol (control), α-tocopherol (50 μM), or TPm at the indicated concentrations. The cells were counted in duplicate with a hemocytometer at 0, 24, and 48 h. The experiment was performed in triplicate, and the mean and the standard deviation were calculated for each treatment.

RT-PCR

Total RNA was isolated using a RNA extraction kit from Qiagen. Semiquantitative assays for CD36 mRNA expression were performed with a RT-PCR kit (Perkin-Elmer).

Western Blots

Western blots were done according to standard methods with monoclonal mouse anti-human CD36 primary antibody (Ancell) and sheep anti-mouse IgG secondary antibody coupled to horseradish peroxidase (AmershamPharmaciaBiotech).

FACS Analysis

For FACS, the cells were pretreated for 24 hours with 50 μM tocopherol, TPm, or 0.1% ethanol solvent (control).

Uptake and Binding of oxLDL-DiO

Labeling of oxLDL with DiO (Intracell Corporation) was done basically as previously described.[2,3] Uptake and binding of oxLDL-DiO was studied by FACS.

RESULTS

Inhibition of Cell Proliferation by TP

The effect of TPm on cell growth was checked in RASMCs and human monocytes (THP-1). The growth of RASMC was significantly inhibited by TPm at concentrations of 20 μM (Fig. 1A). Similarly, treatment of THP-1 cells with TPm for 24 hours led to growth inhibition only with higher TPm concentrations (60 μM). However, for the 48-hour treatments TPm at 30 μM inhibited proliferation strongly (Fig. 1B).

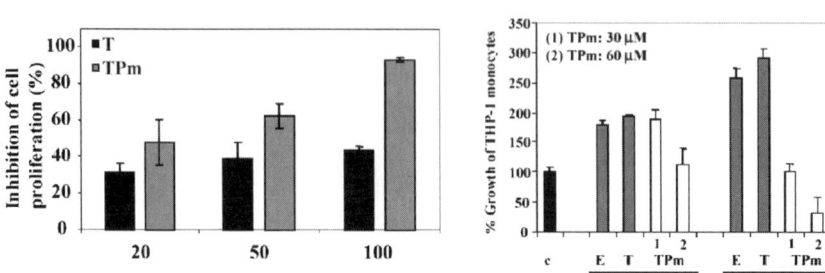

FIGURE 1. (A, B) Effect of TPm (sodium form) and tocopherol on proliferation of rat aortic smooth muscle cells (RASMCs) and THP-1 monocytes. (From Munteanu, Zingg, Ogru et al.[9] Reproduced by permission.)

Effect of TPm and α-Tocopheryl Phosphate on Apoptosis

High concentrations of TPm were cytotoxic to THP-1 cells determined by trypan blue exclusion (data not shown). To assess whether THP-1 cells underwent apoptosis, DNA laddering was monitored (FIG. 2). THP-1 cells were incubated with increasing TPm concentrations, genomic DNA was extracted and separated on a 1% agarose gel. Low concentrations (5–46 μM) of TPm had no effect on DNA laddering, whereas high concentrations (46–184 μM) induced significant DNA degradation. These results indicated that growth inhibition with low concentrations of TPm is not the result of apoptosis.

Inhibition of CD36 Protein Expression by TPm

The expression of the CD36 scavenger receptor on smooth muscle cells and activated monocytes/macrophages recently was shown to be decreased by treatment with α-tocopherol, in what may represent one of the mechanisms of how vitamin E prevents development of atherosclerosis.[3,4] Therefore, it was interesting to measure whether and how strongly TPm was able to inhibit CD36 expression. THP-1 monocytes were treated for 24 hours with increasing concentrations of TPm (9–46 μM) and CD36 surface expression assayed by FACS. TPm strongly decreased CD36 expression, whereas α-tocopherol (50 μM) had no effect on nonstimulated THP-1 cells (FIG. 3 and FIG. 4).

Inhibition of CD36 mRNA Transcription by TPm

Vitamin E was shown to modulate the expression of several genes, including the CD36 scavenger receptor.[5] To assess whether TPm had similar effects, we assayed the expression of CD36 in nonstimulated THP-1 monocytes by semiquantitative RT-PCR. THP-1 cells were incubated for 24 hours with increasing concentrations of TP (5–46 μM), total RNA was isolated, and the expression of CD36 mRNA was quantified by RT-PCR. The expression of CD36 decreased with increasing concentrations of TPm (FIG. 5).

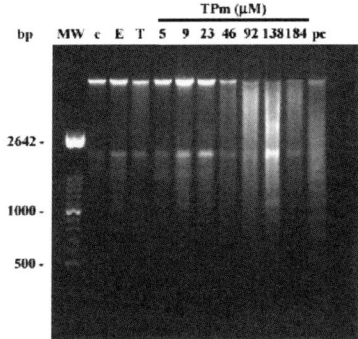

FIGURE 2. Effect of TPm and α-tocopherol on THP-1 cells apoptosis monitored by nuclear DNA laddering. THP-1 cells were incubated with control ethanol (E, 0.1%), α-tocopherol (T, 50 μM), or increasing concentrations of TPm for 24 hours. C, untreated control; pc, positive control. The experiment was repeated three times with similar results. (From Munteanu, Zingg, Ogru et al.[9] Reproduced by permission.)

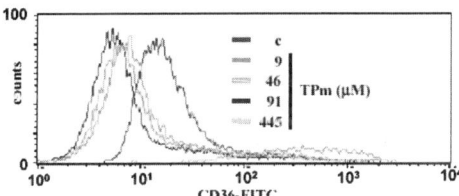

FIGURE 3. Inhibition of CD36 protein expression by TPm. THP-1 cells were incubated with increasing concentrations of TPm for 24 hours and CD36 expression quantified by FACS using an anti-human CD36-FITC antibody. The experiment was repeated three times with similar results. (From Munteanu, Zingg, Ogru et al.[9] Reproduced by permission.)

Inhibition of oxLDL-DiO Uptake and Binding by TPm

To assess whether decreased expression of CD36 leads also to decreased binding and uptake of oxLDL, we incubated nonstimulated THP-1 monocytes with increasing concentrations of TPm (9–46 μM), and uptake or binding of fluorescence-labeled oxLDL-DiO was analyzed by FACS. Parallel to the results of CD36 protein expression, TPm led to decreased binding and uptake of oxLDL-DiO (FIG. 6).

DISCUSSION

Recently, using a novel isolation method, we showed one of the synthetic analogues of tocopherol, the α-tocopheryl phosphate, to occur naturally in food and tissues.[1] Moreover, it was shown that low amounts of tocopherol can become phosphorylated and dephosphorylated, suggesting that the interconversion may

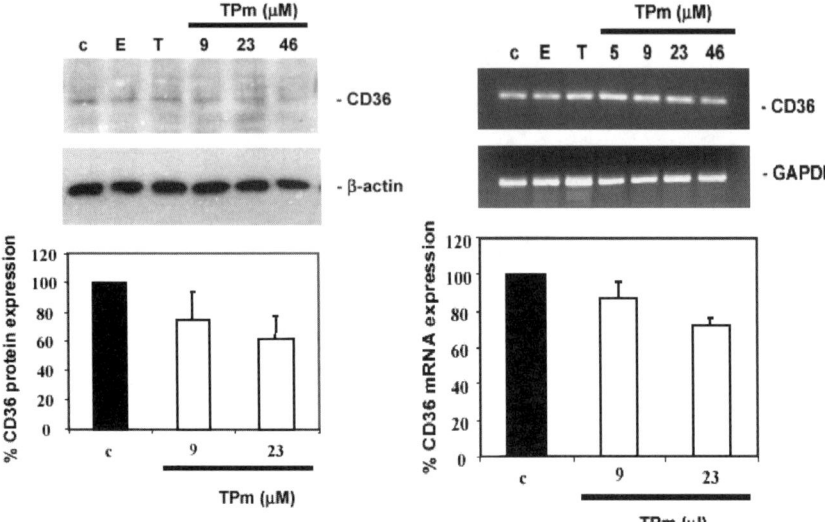

FIGURE 4. Inhibition of CD36 protein expression by TPm. THP-1 cells were incubated with solvent control ethanol (E, 0.1%), α-tocopherol (T, 50 μM), or increasing concentrations of TPm for 24 hours, and CD36 expression was quantified by Western blot analysis. As internal control, α-actin was used. The graph shows the mean and standard deviation from three experiments. (From Munteanu, Zingg, Ogru et al.[9] Reproduced by permission.)

FIGURE 5. Inhibition of CD36 mRNA transcription by TPm. THP-1 cells were incubated with solvent control ethanol (E, 0.1%), α-tocopherol (T, 50 μM), or increasing concentrations of TPm for 24 hours, and CD36 expression was quantified by RT-PCR. As internal control GAPDH was used. The graph shows the mean and standard deviation from two experiments.

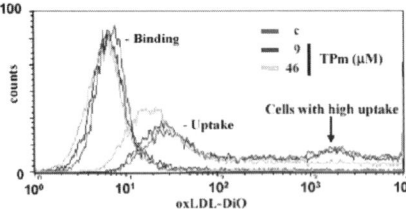

FIGURE 6. Inhibition of oxLDL-DiO uptake and binding by TPm. THP-1 cells were incubated with increasing concentrations of TPm for 24 hours. The uptake of oxLDL was measured after incubation with oxLDL-DiO (200 mg/mL) at 37°C for the last 6 hours.

serve some cellular functions. Several functions and activities have been suggested for tocopheryl phosphate: induction of hippocampal long-term potentiation, protection of mouse skin against ultraviolet-induced damage, activation of cAMP phophodiesterase, and activation of rat liver phenylalanine hydroxylase.

We have found that TPm reduces growth of rat aortic smooth muscle cells and human THP-1 monocytes more efficiently than α-tocopherol, even when using much lower concentrations of TPm compared to α-tocopherol. At these concentrations, no evidence of apoptosis was detected, suggesting that growth inhibition is the result of modulation of cellular signaling. Moreover, the expression of total CD36 protein in nonactivated THP-1 monocytes and on their surface is decreased by TPm treatment, whereas α-tocopherol had no effect. Decreased expression of CD36 protein led to decreased binding and uptake of oxLDL, suggesting that TPm could reduce the formation of foam cells.

Taken together, TPm shows activities like growth inhibition, CD36 mRNA, and protein expression that are similar to α-tocopherol, albeit at a much lower concentrations. It is conceivable that TPm acts at a cellular level in a way which is unrelated to that of α-tocopherol, similarly to what has been shown with the succinate ester. It might have direct effects at the level of signal transduction intermediate steps or in gene regulation. However, it may also be possible that the phosphorylated forms of tocopherol can be transported to the sites of action more efficiently than the non-phosphorylated one and that the effects observed with TPm at lower concentrations relative to α-tocopherol may be caused by higher local concentration than the latter. At lower concentrations, TPm usage may result in protection against atherosclerosis, in anti-inflammatory actions and in the defense of skin against ultraviolet light damage. More studies on the activities of TPm on gene expression and cellular signaling are required to solve these issues.

REFERENCES

1. OGRU, E., R. GIANELLO, R. LIBINAKI, et al., Eds. 2003. Vitamin E Phosphate: An Endogenous Form of Vitamin E. Medimond S.r.l. Bologna, Italy.
2. INNERARITY, T.L., R.E. PITAS & R.W. MAHLEY. 1986. Lipoprotein-receptor interactions. Methods Enzymol. **129:** 542–565.
3. RICCIARELLI, R., J.M. ZINGG & A. AZZI. 2000. Vitamin E reduces the uptake of oxidized LDL by inhibiting CD36 scavenger receptor expression in cultured aortic smooth muscle cells. Circulation **102:** 82–87.
4. DEVARAJ, S., I. HUGOU & I. JIALAL. 2001. Alpha-tocopherol decreases CD36 expression in human monocyte-derived macrophages. J. Lipid Res. **42:** 521–527.
5. AZZI, A., R. GYSIN, P. KEMPNA, et al. 2002. Regulation of gene and protein expression by vitamin E. Free Radic. Res. **36:** 30–35.
6. MULLER, D.P., J.A. MANNING, P.M. MATHIAS & J.T. HARRIES. 1976. Studies on the intestinal hydrolysis of tocopheryl esters. Int. J. Vitam. Nutr. Res. **46:** 207–210.
7. MATHIAS, P.M., J.T. HARRIES, T.J. PETERS & D.P. MULLER. 1981. Studies on the in vivo absorption of micellar solutions of tocopherol and tocopheryl acetate in the rat: demonstration and partial characterization of a mucosal esterase localized to the endoplasmic reticulum of the enterocyte. J. Lipid Res. **22:** 829–837.
8. LAURIDSEN, C., M.S. HEDEMANN & S.K. JENSEN. 2001. Hydrolysis of tocopheryl and retinyl esters by porcine carboxyl ester hydrolase is affected by their carboxylate moiety and bile acids. J. Nutr. Biochem. **12:** 219–224.
9. MUNTEANU, A., J.-M. ZINGG, E. OGRU, et al. 2004. Modulation of cell proliferation and gene expression by a-tocopheryl phosphates: relevance to atherosclerosis and inflammation. Biochem. Biophys. Res. Commun. **318:** 311–316.

Vitamin E Supplementation Reverses the Age-Associated Decrease in Effective Immune Synapse Formation in CD4+ T Cells

TANVIR AHMED,[a] MELISSA MARKO,[a] DAYONG WU,[a] HEEKYUNG CHUNG,[a] BRIGITTE HUBER,[b] AND SIMIN NIKBIN MEYDANI[a,b]

[a]*Nutritional Immunology Laboratory, Jean Mayer USDA Human Nutrition Research Center on Aging at Tufts University, Boston, Massachusetts 02111, USA*

[b]*Department of Pathology, Tufts School of Medicine, Boston, Massachusetts, USA*

ABSTRACT: Aging is associated with impairment of T cell function. We demonstrate here that age-associated declines in T cell signaling are due to the inability to form effective immune synapses at the site of the T cell receptor and antigen interaction. On the basis of our previous research with vitamin E (VE), we hypothesized that VE supplementation of old CD4+ T cells enhances effective immune synapse formation through increased translocation of signaling proteins. Using confocal microscopy, we found that when exposed to antigen-presenting cells, CD4+ T cells from old mice have a lower percentage of effective immune synapses compared to those from young mice. Furthermore, we show that *in vitro* and *in vivo* VE supplementation increases the percentage of old CD4+ T cells capable of forming a functional immune synapse. Further studies are under way to determine the mechanisms of age and VE-induced enhancement of effective immune synapse formation.

KEYWORDS: aging; vitamin E; T cell; immune synapse; signal transduction

BACKGROUND

Aging is associated with reduced interleukin (IL)-2 production and T cell proliferation, resulting in hyporesponsive cells. In turn, decreased IL-2 production has been shown to be due to the reduced ability of aging T cells to form effective immune synapses at the site of the T cell receptor and antigen interaction,[1] a required step in T cell signaling. Previously, we demonstrated that *in vitro* and *in vivo* vitamin E (VE) supplementation improves the immune response of old mice by enabling their T cells to produce more IL-2 and progress through the cell cycle.[2]

Address for correspondence: Simin Nikbin Meydani, Nutritional Immunology Laboratory, Jean Mayer U.S. Department of Agriculture Human Nutrition Research Center on Aging at Tufts University, 711 Washington Street, Boston, MA 02111. Voice: 617-556-3129; fax: 617-556-3224.
simin.meydani@tufts.edu

Ann. N.Y. Acad. Sci. 1031: 412–414 (2004). © 2004 New York Academy of Sciences.
doi: 10.1196/annals.1331.059

The objective of this study was to test the hypothesis that VE supplementation of old CD4+ T cells enhances effective immune synapse formation through increased translocation of signaling proteins to the site of the T cell and antigen interaction.

STUDY DESIGN

VE was administered *in vivo* by providing diets containing 30 ppm (control) or 500 ppm (supplemented)[3] to young and old mice for 4 weeks. VE was administered *in vitro* by isolating CD4+ T cells from young and old mice that had been fed laboratory chow, and supplementing these cells with 20 µg/mL[4] *dl*-α-tocopheryl acetate. Immune synapses formed between CD4+ T cells and antigen presenting cells, at single-cell level, were immunostained with antibodies against the signaling molecules LAT, Vav, and Zap70, followed by staining with fluorescent-tagged secondary antibodies and analyzed by confocal microscopy.[1]

RESULTS

CD4+ T cells from old mice had a lower percentage of effective immune synapses compared to those from young mice, as indicated by less redistribution of key signaling molecules to the site of the T cell/antigen-presenting cell interaction (see FIG-

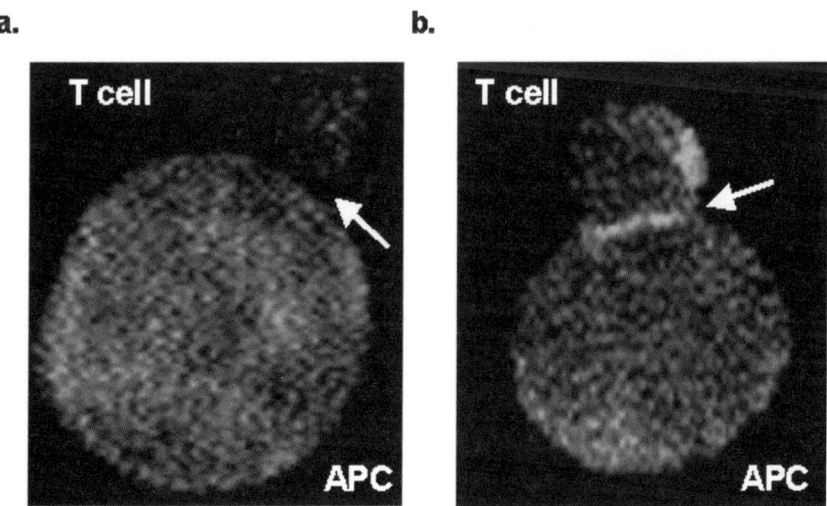

FIGURE 1. Confocal microscopy images of immune synapses. (**a**) Negative redistribution of signaling molecules causing ineffective immune synapses and potential defects in IL-2 transcription. (**b**) An increase in green fluorescence between the two cells (marked by the *arrow*) indicates an increase in redistribution of the signaling molecule that causes effective immune synapse formation and IL-2 transcription. In each image, the small cells are the CD4+ T cells from young or old mice, and the larger cells are the antigen-presenting cells.

URE 1 for examples of effective vs. ineffective immune synapses) (Vav 18 ± 1.8% vs. 36 ± 4.4%, LAT 12 ± 0.9% vs. 27 ± 2.6%, and Zap70 14 ± 2.0% vs. 28 ± 2.8%, respectively). *In vitro* and *in vivo* VE supplementation increased the percentage of old $CD4^+$ T cells capable of forming effective immune synapses (*in vitro:* Vav 18 ± 1.8% vs. 38 ± 5.5%, LAT 12 ± 0.9% vs. 40 ± 5.8%, and Zap70 14 ± 2.0% vs. 26 ± 2.8%, in control and VE groups, respectively; *in vivo:* Vav 19 ± 1.6% vs. 38 ± 2.5%; LAT 18 ± 1.4% vs. 31 ± 2.4%, and Zap70 16 ± 1.3% vs. 30 ± 4.8% in control and VE groups, respectively).

CONCLUSIONS

Immune synapse formation, a key early event in IL-2 production, and T cell proliferation are impaired in aged mice. We have shown, for the first time, that VE supplementation reverses this age-related event, leading to improved immune synapse formation and, ultimately, improved T cell function in aged mice.

ACKNOWLEDGMENTS

This work was supported by the NIA (R01 AG009140-10A1), the Office of Dietary Supplement (USDA contract 58-1950-9-001), a fellowship from the Unilever Health Institute, and a fellowship from the Ellison Medical Foundation–International Nutrition Foundation.

REFERENCES

1. TAMIR, A., M.D. EISENBRAUN, G.G. GARCIA & R.A. MILLER. 2000. Age-dependent alterations in the assembly of signal transduction complexes at the site of T cell/APC interaction. J. Immunol. **165:** 1243–1251.
2. ADOLFSSON, O., B. HUBER & S.N. MEYDANI. 2001. Vitamin E-enhanced IL-2 production in old mice: naïve but not memory T cells show increased cell division cycling and IL-2-producing capacity. J. Immunol. **167:** 3809–3817.
3. MEYDANI, S.N., M. MEYDANI, C.P. VERDON, *et al.* 1986. Vitamin E supplementation suppresses prostaglandin E1(2) synthesis and enhances the immune response of aged mice. Mech. Ageing Dev. **34:** 191–201.
4. MEYDANI, S.N., M. MEYDANI, J.B. BLUMBERG, *et al.* 1998. Assessment of the safety of supplementation with different amounts of vitamin E in healthy older adults. Am. J. Clin. Nutr. **68:** 311–318.

Synergistic Effect of Vitamin E and β-Carotene on the Suppression of Ovalbumin-Specific Immunoglobulin E Production in Mice

NORIKO BANDO, MASAMI YAMAMOTO, RINTARO YAMANISHI, AND JUNJI TERAO

Department of Food Science, Graduate School of Nutrition and Biosciences, University of Tokushima, Tokushima, 770-8503, Japan

KEYWORDS: immunoglobulin E (IgE) antibody; vitamin E; β-carotene; type I allergy

Vitamin E and other antioxidants such as carotenoids and flavonoids are suggested to be responsible for the anti-allergic effect of fruits and vegetables in epidemiologic studies.[1] Therefore, the effect of vitamin E on immunoglobulin E (IgE) production *in vivo* seems to be of much interest, as IgE antibody is well known to participate in the type I allergic reaction. We sought to determine whether or not supplementation with vitamin E and β-carotene, a typical carotenoid from plant foods, affects IgE production in the allergic model mice. The results strongly suggest that the combination of both antioxidants suppresses allergen-specific IgE production and total IgE production.

METHODS

BALB/c mice (female; 6 weeks of age) were given a diet supplemented with vitamin E and/or β-carotene for 3 weeks. These mice were then subcutaneously immunized twice with ovalbumin (OVA) without adjuvant. After 6 weeks, antiserum was obtained by decapitation with the mice under anesthesia. OVA-specific IgE production was evaluated with passive cutaneous anaphylaxis analysis. Total IgE and antigen-specific-IgG$_1$ concentrations in the serum were measured by the sandwich ELISA method.

Address for correspondence: Dr. Junji Terao, Department of Food Science, Graduate School of Nutrition and Biosciences, University of Tokushima, Kuramoto-cho 3-18-15, Tokushima, 770-8503, Japan. Voice: +81-88-633-7087; fax: +81-88-633-7089.
terao@nutr.med.tokushima-u.ac.jp

RESULTS

Diets with Vitamin E

Some mice were fed diets containing different amounts of vitamin E (α-tocopherol). The amounts included 0.5, 5, 10, and 50 mg of vitamin E per 100-g diet. The diet containing 5 mg of vitamin E was usually given to mice as a control diet. Passive cutaneous anaphylaxis analysis demonstrated that the mice fed the diet containing 5 mg of vitamin E produced OVA-specific IgE antibody. The lower level of antigen-specific IgE antibody was found in the mice fed the diet supplemented with 0.5, 10, and 50 mg of vitamin E. Lower IgE production in the case of the low vitamin E diet (0.5 mg per 100-g diet) may be explained by impairment of the immunological function due to vitamin E deficiency.

Diets with Basal Vitamin E Plus β-Carotene

Some mice received the basal diet (containing 5 mg of α-tocopherol acetate as vitamin E) with different amounts of β-carotene. The amounts included 2, 10, 50, and 250 mg of β-carotene. IgE production increased in the mice with 10 mg of β-carotene supplementation and decreased in the mice with 250 mg of β-carotene supplementation. Fifty milligrams of β-carotene supplementation had little effect on the

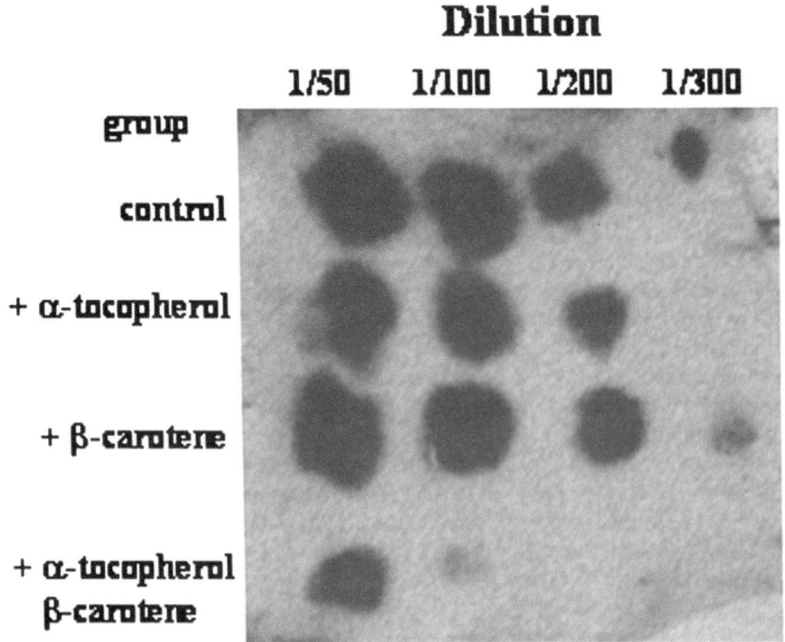

FIGURE 1. Passive cutaneous anaphylaxis analysis of allergen-specific IgE production in experimental amimals. (From Bando et al.[3] Reproduced by permission.)

IgE elevation. β-Carotene added to the diet might have been oxidized through the feeding period at 25°C, and this process might have resulted in the enhancement of IgE production by a pro-oxidant function of β-carotene oxidation products.

Combination Diets

The basal diet contained 5 mg of α-tocopherol acetate. In the combination diet, 5 mg of vitamin E and/or 50 mg of β-carotene were added to the basal diet in order to evaluate the effect of their combination. Vitamin E plus β-carotene effectively suppressed the allergen-specific IgE antibody as compared with either the case of vitamin E alone or the case of β-carotene alone (FIG. 1).[2] A similar effect was observed by addition of vitamin E and β-carotene on the level of total IgE and allergen-specific IgG_1, both Th2 immunoglobulins. Vitamin E and β-carotene were accumulated in the serum by supplementation with the respective compounds.

This phenomenon may reflect the synergistic antioxidative activity of vitamin E and β-carotene. It has been reported that vitamin E protects β-carotene from free radical-induced oxidation when the both compounds coexist. The provitamin A activity of β-carotene, as well as its antioxidative action, may be related to the combined effect of vitamin E and β-carotene on IgE production. Nevertheless, the literature shows that retinoic acid affects IgE production *in vitro* and *in vivo* through different functions.[3,4]

It is still unclear whether or not dietary β-carotene acts as a provitamin A for inhibiting IgE production. A high intake of β-carotene may induce a harmful effect by acting as a pro-oxidant through an unknown mechanism. It is unlikely, however, that a high dose of vitamin E and/or β-carotene exerts any undesirable effect, because the growth curve was not affected by a higher administration in this study. Therefore, intake of vitamin E together with β-carotene is helpful in the prevention of allergic IgE production.

CONCLUSION

The combination of dietary vitamin E and β-carotene suppresses IgE production dramatically in allergic model mice and would therefore help to attenuate the type I allergy syndrome.

REFERENCES

1. BUTLAND, B.K., D.P. STRACHAN & H.R. ANDERSON. 1999. Fresh fruit intake and asthma symptoms in young British adults: confounding or effect modification by smoking? Eur. Respir. **13:** 744–750.
2. BANDO, N., R. YAMANISHI & J. TERAO. 2003. Inhibition of immunoglobulin E production in allergic model mice by supplementation with vitamin E and β-carotene. Biosci. Biotechnol. Biochem. **67:** 2176–2182.
3. WORM, M., U. HERZ, J.M. KRAH, H. RENZ & B.M. HENZ. 2001. Effects of retinoids on *in vivo* and *in vitro* IgE production. Int. Arch. Allergy Immunol. **124:** 233–236.
4. STEPHANSEN, C.B., R. RASOOLY, X. JIANG, M.A. CEDDIA, C.T. WEAVER, R.A. CHANDRARATHA & R.P. BUCY. 2002. Vitamin A enhances in vivo Th2 development *via* retinoid X receptor pathway. J. Immunol. **168:** 4495–4503.

The Effect of Vitamin E on Secondary Bacterial Infection after Influenza Infection in Young and Old Mice

RAINA GAY,[a] SUNG NIM HAN,[a] MELISSA MARKO,[a] SARAH BELISLE,[a] RODERICK BRONSON,[b] AND SIMIN NIKBIN MEYDANI[a]

[a]*Nutritional Immunology Laboratory, Jean Mayer USDA Human Nutrition Research Center on Aging at Tufts University, Boston, Massachusetts 02111, USA*

[b]*Tufts University School of Veterinary Medicine, North Grafton, Massachusetts 01536, USA*

ABSTRACT: Mortality from influenza is high in the elderly. Deaths are mainly due to secondary complications, including *Staphylococcus aureus* (SA) infections. Vitamin E (E) supplementation reduces influenza in aged mice. This study determined the efficacy of E supplementation on secondary bacterial infections after influenza in young and old mice. C57BL/6 mice were fed diets containing 30 or 500 ppm E for 4 weeks. Priming with influenza significantly increased SA in the lungs of infected mice fed control diet. Age did not have a significant effect on SA infection alone or SA infection after influenza infection. E supplementation did not have a significant effect on SA infection alone. However, E supplementation abolished the priming effect of influenza on SA.

KEYWORDS: influenza; *Staphylococcus aureus*; pneumonia; vitamin E; aging; coinfection

BACKGROUND

Respiratory infections, of all infectious diseases, are the leading cause of death in the United States.[1,2] In the United States alone, influenza accounts for more than 10,000 deaths annually and more than 40,000 deaths during epidemic years.[3,4] These deaths are not typically due to influenza infection alone, but from the development of complications due to influenza infection.[5] Secondary bacterial infection is the most common life-threatening complication of influenza virus infection. *Staphylococcus aureus* (*S. aureus*) is one of the most common pathogens involved in influenza-associated bacterial pneumonia.[6] *S. aureus* is a particularly deadly bacteria in the elderly, and is most often observed in individuals, commonly found in nursing homes and hospitals, who have influenza infection.[7] For patients over 70 years of age, the mortality rate can climb to 75%.[8] Alternative strategies are needed to pre-

---

Address for correspondence: Simin Nikbin Meydani, Nutritional Immunology Laboratory, Jean Mayer USDA Human Nutrition Research Center on Aging at Tufts University, 711 Washington Street, Boston, MA 02111. Voice: 617-556-3129; fax: 617-556-3224.
Simin.Meydani@tufts.edu

vent severe disease in a population with elevated risk and compromised defenses. Viral infections in humans or mice can result in increased sensitivity to challenges with bacteria, bacterial products, or cytokine administration.[9] The changes observed with viral infection are all exacerbated with age. Factors such as improving antioxidant status may modulate the immune function, reduce tissue damage and bacterial colonization, and improve pulmonary resistance to secondary bacterial infection.[10] Previously we have shown that vitamin E supplementation significantly improves the immune response in aged mice and humans.[11] Furthermore, we showed that vitamin E supplementation reduces influenza viral infection in aged mice. In the present study we tested the hypothesis that vitamin E supplementation of mice will reduce the magnitude of, and subsequent mortality and morbidity from, secondary bacterial infection after influenza virus infection in mice.

STUDY DESIGN

Vitamin E was administered *in vivo* by feeding young and old mice diets containing 30 ppm (control) or 500 ppm (supplemented) for 4 weeks. Mice were infected intranasally with either influenza or PBS. At 7 days post infection, mice were intranasally infected with *S. aureus* or PBS. At 24 hours post bacterial infection, mice were euthanized and lungs were processed for viral and bacterial quantification. Pulmonary influenza viral titer was determined using MDCK cells, as previously described.[12] Quantitative bacterial cultures of lung homogenates were made using aliquots of homogenate spread on nutrient agar plates. Data were expressed as cfu/g lung (log 10) as previously described by LeVine *et al.*[13] Hematoxylin-eosin (H&E) staining was performed on lungs from mice for histologic analysis. Data were analyzed by a four by four ANOVA for overall effect of age, infections, and diet followed by Tukey's HSD for individual comparisons using SYSTAT 10 statistical package.

RESULTS

We performed a 2 (age; young, old) × 2 (diet; control, vitamin E) × 3 (pathogen; influenza, *S. aureus*, influenza + *S. aureus*) analysis of variance on change in weight over the course of the infection period, as well as on bacterial count. The result of the ANOVA indicated a significant effect of age, influenza, and a diet-by-age interaction on weight loss ($P<0.001$). There was no significant effect of age, diet, or influenza on bacterial infection alone. However a significant diet × influenza infection interaction on *S. aureus* counts was observed, indicating that vitamin E had influenced the effect of influenza on secondary bacterial infection ($P < 0.04$). Thus, a second 2 (age) × 3 (pathogen) ANOVA was performed within each diet group.

We did not observe a significant effect of age on bacterial counts. However, in mice fed the control diet (30 ppm vitamin E) we observed a significant effect of influenza infection on bacterial counts ($P = 0.03$).

Mice fed the control diet and infected with *S. aureus* alone exhibited a moderate level of bacterial infection. But, mice first infected with influenza, had significantly higher levels of *S. aureus* in the lungs ($P < 0.05$). In mice supplemented with vitamin

E, the priming effect of influenza on *S. aureus* infection was abolished such that the level of *S. aureus* was not significantly different than that observed in mice infected with *S. aureus* alone.

The priming effect of influenza infection on bacterial count was confirmed by pathologic evaluation. In control mice or mice infected with *S. aureus* alone, there was no evidence of any infection. Mice infected with influenza alone demonstrated focal lesions of infiltrating lymphocytes. However, in mice that had been coinfected with both influenza and *S. aureus*, we observed not only focal lesions of infiltrating lymphocytes, but bacterial bronchopneumonia due to an established *S. aureus* infection. Interestingly, we only observed the bronchopneumonia in animals first primed with influenza, and the bronchopneumonia was always within close proximity of the influenza-associated lesions. We did not observe a significant effect of age and vitamin E intervention on lung pathology.

CONCLUSIONS

In this animal model, age did not have a significant effect on *S. aureus* infection alone or *S. aureus* infection after influenza infection. Supplementation with vitamin E did not have a significant effect on *S. aureus* infection alone. Priming with influenza infection significantly increased *S. aureus* counts in the lungs of infected mice. Vitamin E supplementation abolished the priming effect of influenza infection on *S. aureus*. Vitamin E may exert its effect by a number of mechanisms, including reducing ROS, decreasing proinflammatory cytokines and adhesion molecule expression and production, and increasing surfactant antioxidant and antimicrobial activity. In future studies, we will investigate these mechanisms by the appropriate *in vitro* and *in vivo* experiments.

ACKNOWLEDGMENTS

This work was supported by USDA Contract # 58 1950 9 001, and a 2002 Glenn Foundation/AFAR Scholarship for Research in the Biology of Aging.

REFERENCES

1. RUBEN, F.L. *et al.* 1995. Clinical infections in the noninstitutionalized geriatric age group: methods utilized and incidence of infections. The Pittsburgh Good Health Study. Am. J. Epidemiol. **141:** 145–157.
2. PINNER, R.W. *et al.* 1996. Trends in infectious diseases mortality in the United States. JAMA 275: 189–193.
3. BENDER, B.S. & P.A. SMALL, JR. 1993. Heterotypic immune mice lose protection against influenza virus infection with senescence. J. Infect. Dis. **168:** p. 873–880.
4. SEATON, A., D. SEATON & A.G. LEITCH, Eds. 2000. Acute Upper Respiratory Tract Infection. *In* Crofton & Douglas's Respiratory Diseases, 5th ed. Blackwell Science. Malden, MA.
5. CENTERS FOR DISEASE CONTROL AND PREVENTION. 1995. Pneumonia and influenza death rates: United States, 1979–1994. MMWR **44:** 535–537.
6. HAN, S.N. & S.N. MEYDANI. 1999. Vitamin E and infectious diseases in the aged. Proc. Nutr. Soc. **58:** 697–705.

7. MARRIE, T.J., Pneumonia. Clin. Geriatr. Med., 1992. **8**(4): p. 721–34.
8. _____. 2000. Pneumonia. *In* Crofton & Douglas's Respiratory Diseases, 5th ed., op. cit., p. 402.
9. NGUYEN, K.B. & C.A. BIRON. 1999. Synergism for cytokine-mediated disease during concurrent endotoxin and viral challenges: roles for NK and T cell IFN-gamma production. J. Immunol. **162:** 5238–5246.
10. MEYER, K.C. 2001. The role of immunity in susceptibility to respiratory infection in the aging lung. Resp. Physiol. **128:** 23–31.
11. HAN, S.N. *et al.* 2000. Vitamin E supplementation increases T helper 1 cytokine production in old mice infected with influenza virus. Immunology **100:** 487–493.
12. BENDER, B.S., *et al.* 1992. Transgenic mice lacking class I major histocompatibility complex-restricted T cells have delayed viral clearance and increased mortality after influenza virus challenge. J. Exp. Med. **175:** 1143–1145.
13. LEVINE, A.M., V. KOENINGSKNECHT & J.M. STARK. 2001. Decreased pulmonary clearance of *S. pneumoniae* following influenza A infection in mice. J. Virol. Methods **94:** 173–186.

Effect of Concomitant Consumption of Fish Oil and Vitamin E on Production of Inflammatory Cytokines in Healthy Elderly Humans

DAYONG WU, SUNG NIM HAN, MOHSEN MEYDANI, AND SIMIN NIKBIN MEYDANI

Jean Mayer USDA Human Nutrition Research Center on Aging at Tufts University, Boston, Massachusetts 02111, USA

ABSTRACT: A beneficial effect of fish oil in reducing inflammatory and cardiovascular diseases has been suggested. This effect occurs in part through fish oil's inhibition of synthesis of pro-inflammatory cytokines. Epidemiologic studies have shown a link between increased intake of vitamin E in diet and reduced risk of cardiovascular disease. Since pro-inflammatory cytokines have been indicated in pathogenesis of cardiovascular diseases, the current study was designed to determine the effect of concomitant consumption of fish oil and vitamin E on interleukin (IL)-1β, IL-6, and tumor necrosis factor (TNF)-α production by peripheral blood mononuclear cells (PBMCs). Healthy elderly subjects consumed fish oil plus different doses of vitamin E for 3 months. The results indicated that, in general, fish oil inhibited production of pro-inflammatory cytokines and vitamin E did not interfere with this effect of fish oil; rather its supplementation might further contribute to the fish oil–induced inhibition of these cytokines, in particular at the 200 mg/d dose.

KEYWORDS: vitamin E; fish oil; inflammatory cytokines; aging

INTRODUCTION

Epidemiologic data, clinical trials, and experimental studies have suggested that consumption of fish oil might suppress inflammatory response and thus reduce the risk of inflammatory and cardiovascular diseases. The anti-inflammatory effect of fish oil is believed to occur, at least in part, through its reduction of pro-inflammatory cytokines. Epidemiological studies have shown a link between an increased dietary intake of vitamin E and a reduced risk of cardiovascular disease. Thus, combined consumption of fish oil and vitamin E is expected to further promote fish oil's beneficial effect on the cardiovascular system. Since pro-inflammatory cytokines have been indicated in the pathogenesis of cardiovascular diseases, the current study was designed to determine the effect of concomitant consumption of fish oil

Address for correspondence: Simin Nikbin Meydani, D.V.M., Ph.D., Nutritional Immunology Laboratory, Jean Mayer USDA Human Nutrition Research Center on Aging at Tufts University, 711 Washington Street, Boston, MA 02111. Voice: 617-556-3129; fax: 617-556-3224.
simin.meydani@tufts.edu

and vitamin E on production of interleukin (IL)-1β, IL-6, and tumor necrosis factor (TNF)-α by peripheral blood mononuclear cells.

METHODS

This randomized, double-blind, placebo-controlled study was conducted with 40 healthy male and female elderly subjects (>65 years) who were randomly assigned to four groups ($n=10$/group). All subjects received daily fish oil supplement in the form of 5 capsules of Omega-500™ fish oil containing 300 mg eicosapentaenoic acid (EPA) and 200 mg docosahexaenoic acid (DHA)/capsule together with the placebo (soybean oil), 100, 200, or 400 mg of vitamin E (*dl*-α-tocopherol in soybean oil) for 3 months. The subjects consumed the capsules daily for 3 months while continuing their typical food intake, dietary habits, and lifestyle. Blood samples were collected at baseline and 3 months after supplementation. Plasma fatty acids were analyzed by gas chromatography and plasma vitamin E was assessed by measuring α- and γ-tocopherol levels using a modified HPLC method. Peripheral blood mononuclear cells (PBMCs) were isolated from whole blood using Ficoll-Paque (Pharmacia Biotech, Piscataway, NJ) density gradient centrifugation. PBMCs in complete RPMI 1640 medium with 1% autologous plasma were cultured in the presence or absence of 1 µg/L lipopolysaccharide (LPS) for 24 hours. To measure total IL-1β (cell-associated and secreted), the samples were exposed to three freeze–thaw cycles before IL-1β concentration was determined by radioimmunoassay (RIA). The supernatants from PBMCs stimulated with Con A or PHA (50 mg/L) for 48 hours were collected to determine IL-6 and TNF-α production using a sandwich ELISA method.

RESULTS AND DISCUSSION

There was no difference in fatty acid profile among the groups at baseline. Both EPA and DHA, the n-3 PUFA, were significantly elevated after supplementation with fish oil. While arachidonic acid (AA, 20:4, n-6) levels decreased in all groups, a statistically significant change was observed in AA levels when all the groups were pooled for the fish oil effect ($7.30 \pm 0.29\%$ at baseline compared to $6.36 \pm 0.23\%$ after 3 months' supplementation, $P<0.01$).

There was no significant difference in plasma α-tocopherol levels among the groups at baseline. While no significant change in α-tocopherol level was found in the placebo group after 3 months of supplementation, plasma α-tocopherol levels were increased in all three vitamin E groups (31.9%, 25.1%, and 35.6% in 100 mg/d, 200 mg/d, and 400 mg/d groups, respectively). However, increased plasma vitamin E levels did not show a clear dose-dependent pattern and the increases were smaller compared to our previous studies in which vitamin E supplement was used alone, suggesting that fish oil interfered with absorption and/or metabolism of vitamin E. When plasma tocopherol levels were adjusted for plasma lipid levels, similar results were observed.

Compared to the baseline, LPS-stimulated IL-1β production was significantly reduced in the vitamin E 200 group by 42% but not in the other groups. Con A–stimulated IL-6 production did not change significantly in each group; however, when all groups were pooled, a significant decrease in IL-6 production was observed, suggesting a fish oil effect on IL-6 production. PHA-stimulated IL-6 production was not changed by supplementation in any group and an insignificant decrease was observed when all groups were pooled. While Con A–stimulated TNF-α production was not significantly changed in any of the groups, when all the groups were pooled for the effect of fish oil, a 20% reduction ($P=0.06$) was observed. PHA-stimulated TNFα production was significantly reduced in the vitamin E 200 group and no significant change was observed in any other groups or when all the groups were pooled.

In summary, vitamin E does not seem to interfere with the effect of fish oil on the inflammatory cytokines; rather its supplementation might further contribute to the fish oil–induced inhibition of these cytokines, in particular at the 200 mg/d dose.

ACKNOWLEDGMENTS

This work was supported by the NIH Grant RO1 AG11020, a USDA-NRICGP grant, and the U.S. Department of Agriculture, Agriculture Research Service, under contract number 53-K06-01.

Effect of Vitamin E on Prostacyclin (PGI$_2$) and Prostaglandin (PG) E$_2$ Production by Human Aorta Endothelial Cells

Mechanism of Action

DAYONG WU, LIPING LIU, MOHSEN MEYDANI, AND SIMIN NIKBIN MEYDANI

Jean Mayer USDA Human Nutrition Research Center on Aging at Tufts University, Boston, Massachusetts 02111, USA

ABSTRACT: Vitamin E has been suggested to reduce the risk of cardiovascular diseases. Prostanoids are vasoactive molecules, the change in whose production contributes to homeostasis and pathophysiology of the cardiovascular system. In the current study, we determined the effect of vitamin E on production of vasodilative PGI$_2$ and PGE$_2$ by human aorta endothelial cells (HAECs) and its underlying mechanism. Results showed that vitamin E increased production of both prostanoids by HAECs. This effect of vitamin E is due to increased release of substrate arachidonic acid, which in turn results from increased expression of phospholipase A$_2$ (PLA$_2$).

KEYWORDS: vitamin E; prostanoids; phospholipase A$_2$; endothelial cells

INTRODUCTION

Cardiovascular disease (CVD) is among the leading causes of death globally. Atherosclerosis is identified as a major factor in the pathogenesis of the majority of cases of CVD. Vascular dysfunction has been shown to contribute to the development of atherosclerosis. The endothelium plays a critical role in maintaining homeostasis of vasomotor function by producing vasoactive molecules. Vasodilator molecules such as nitric oxide and certain prostanoids constitute a protective mechanism in vasomotor function, which is viewed as one of the indicators of CVD risk. PGI$_2$ and PGE$_2$, both vasodilator prostanoids, are shown to counteract the function and/or inhibit secretion of vasoconstrictors such as thromboxane B$_2$ and endothelin-1 and thus have been indicated to play a role in prevention of CVD.

Epidemiologic and experimental studies have suggested that increased vitamin E intake may be linked to a reduced risk of developing CVD. Previously we showed that *in vitro* supplementation with vitamin E inhibited monocyte adhesion to human aorta endothelial cells (HAECs), endothelial expression of adhesion molecules, and

---

Address for correspondence: Dayong Wu, M.D., Ph.D., Nutritional Immunology Laboratory, Jean Mayer USDA Human Nutrition Research Center on Aging at Tufts University, 711 Washington Street, Boston, MA 02111. Voice: 617-556-3368; fax: 617-556-3224.

dayong.wu@tufts.edu

production of chemokines and inflammatory cytokines, all of which are involved in the initiation and development of atherosclerosis. To further determine the mechanism of preventive effect of vitamin E in CVD, in this study we sought to investigate whether vitamin E modulates the production of vasodilator prostanoid production and, if so, further determine its underlying mechanism.

METHODS

HAECs at passages 4 to 7 and 80% confluency were incubated with vitamin E (d-α-tocopherol) at 10, 20, 40, or 60 μM, or a vehicle control, for 24 hours, after which the medium was replaced by that containing IL-1β (10 ng/mL) to stimulate the cells for 20 hours. The culture supernatants were then collected to determine prostanoid concentrations using radioimmunoassay (RIA). PGI_2 was measured as its stable hydrolytic product 6-keto-$PGF_{1\alpha}$. To determine COX activity, cells were incubated in the presence of exogenous AA (30 μM) for 10 min. Aspirin (2 mM) was then added to stop COX activity and the supernatants were collected to determine the conversion of AA to 6-keto-$PGF_{1\alpha}$ or PGE_2 using RIA. To measure AA release, HAECs were incubated in the presence of [^{3}H]-AA (0.05 μCi/well) and different concentrations of vitamin E for 24 hours. The cells were then washed five times and were stimulated by IL-1β (10 ng/mL) for 5 hours. The supernatants were collected to determine released [^{3}H]AA. The cells were solubilized with 1N NaOH for measurement of cell-associated [^{3}H]AA. The radioactivity in the samples was measured by scintillation counting. AA release was calculated as released AA/(released AA + cell-associated AA) × 100%.

RESULTS AND DISCUSSION

Vitamin E dose-dependently increased PGI_2 production by 31, 90, 136, and 139% in unstimulated and by 34, 75, 102, and 50% in IL-1-stimulated HAECs for 10, 20, 40, and 60 μM vitamin E, respectively. Similarly, vitamin E increased PGE_2 production (40, 173, 279, and 342% in unstimulated and 48, 101, 99, and 77% in IL-1-stimulated HAECs for 10, 20, 40, and 60 μM vitamin E, respectively).

Biosynthesis of prostanoids is accomplished in a metabolic cascade starting from its precursor fatty acid, arachidonic acid (AA). AA is present in membrane phospholipids and released by the hydrolytic action of PLA_2. Released AA is metabolized to the unstable intermediate prostanoids by cyclooxygenase (COX), also called PGH_2 synthase. COX has bifunctional catalytic properties. It oxygenates and cyclizes AA to form PGG_2 via its cyclooxygenase function, and this is followed by the reduction of PGG_2 to PGH_2 via its peroxidase function. The intermediate product PGH_2 is then converted to different terminal prostanoids by the corresponding isomerases. Thus, to determine the mechanism of vitamin E–induced effect, we further assessed the effect of vitamin E on COX activity. The results showed that despite its enhancement of PGI_2 and PGE_2 production, vitamin E dose-dependently inhibited COX activity when determined as the synthesis of either 6-keto-$PGF_{1\alpha}$ or PGE_2 from the exogenous AA. When vitamin E was added at 10, 20, 40, and 60 μM, AA activity, determined as conversion to 6-keto-$PGF_{1\alpha}$, was reduced to 85, 59, 44, and 33% of control level in unstimulated HAECs and to 72, 44, 42, and 25% of control level in IL-1-stimulated HAECs, respectively. Similar results were observed when AA was determined as conversion of AA to PGE_2. We further determined the COX-1 (constitutive form) and COX-2 (inducible form) expression using Western blot and found that neither COX-1 nor COX-2 expression was affected by vitamin E supplementation.

Thus, we next determined the effect of vitamin E on AA release and PLA_2 expression. The results showed that vitamin E increased AA release by 95, 168, 208, and 222 in unstimulated and by 34, 89, 116, and 117% in IL-1-stimulated HAECs for 10, 20, 40, and 60 µM vitamin E, respectively. Western blot analysis showed that vitamin E increased expression of $cPLA_2$ in both unstimulated and IL-1–stimulated cells.

In conclusion, vitamin E has an opposite effect on two rate-limiting steps in biosynthesis of vasodilator prostanoid PGI_2 and PGE_2 in HAECs: increasing substrate AA release and inhibiting COX activity. The net effect is an increased production of both prostanoids, indicating that the substrate availability is the predominant factor through which vitamin E increases prostanoid production under these experimental conditions. Further, vitamin E–induced AA release is due to an increased $cPLA_2$ activity, which is, in turn, due to a higher a $cPLA_2$ expression. The vitamin E-induced increase in PGI_2 and PGE_2 production might contribute to its suggested beneficial effect in preventing CVD. In contrast to its effect on $cPLA_2$, vitamin E inhibited COX activity. This effect of vitamin E was not mediated through inhibiting COX-1 or COX-2 expression. The mechanism for inhibited COX catalytic activity in HAECs by vitamin E needs further investigation. It is speculated that vitamin E may suppress COX activity through reducing the generation of peroxide radicals, such as peroxynitrite, which are important co-factors for COX activity.

ACKNOWLEDGMENTS

This work was supported by the U.S. Department of Agriculture, Agriculture Research Service under contract number 53-K06-01.

Long-Term Vitamin E Deficiency in Mice Decreases Superoxide Radical Production in Brain

SARAH L. CUDDIHY,[a] ERIK S. MUSIEK,[b] JASON D. MORROW,[b] AND LAURA L. DUGAN[a]

[a]*Department of Neurology, Washington University School of Medicine, St. Louis, Missouri 63112, USA*

[b]*Department of Medicine and Pharmacology, Vanderbilt University School of Medicine, Nashville, Tennessee 37232, USA*

ABSTRACT: We investigated the effect of long-term vitamin E deficiency (38 weeks) on free radical (superoxide) production and free radical products (neuroprostanes and isoprostanes) and on mitochondrial function (oxygraph and electron transport chain activities) in C57B6J mice. We found that after 38 weeks, while liver was approximately 95% deficient, the brain had retained approximately 50% of its α-tocopherol. We also found that superoxide production was lowered in multiple brain regions of male vitamin E–deficient mice, as were neuroprostanes. Oxygraph studies showed higher respiratory control ratios (RCRs) in liver and lower RCRs in brain, which did not appear to be due to changes in electron transport chain activities. We conclude that vitamin E can function *in vivo* in both its traditional role as a lipid-soluble antioxidant as well as in non-traditional roles in the mitochondria.

KEYWORDS: α-tocopherol; vitamin E–deficient diet; superoxide; mitochondria

INTRODUCTION

Alpha-tocopherol is the major lipid-soluble chain-breaking antioxidant. It has also been shown to have a number of non-antioxidant roles. It is capable of inhibiting protein kinase C (PKC) activity and can also interact with phospholipase A2 and cyclooxygenase.[1–3] Upregulation of α-tropomycin and downregulation of vascular cellular adhesion molecule 1 (VCAM1) and the oxidized LDL scavenger receptor CD36 have also been shown.[4] The effect of vitamin E deficiency is less well understood. Thomas *et al.* found a significant decrease in mitochondrial complex I and IV activity in the skeletal muscle of α-tocopherol–deficient rats.[5] In addition, polarographic studies showed a reduction in the respiratory control ratio (RCR) of vitamin E–deficient isolated muscle mitochondria.[5] Another study showed that after

Address for correspondence: Laura L. Dugan, Department of Neurology, Campus Box 8111, Washington University School of Medicine, 660 South Euclid Avenue, St. Louis, MO 63110. Voice: 314-747-0467; fax: 314-362-9462.

duganl@neuro.wustl.edu

48 weeks of deficiency skeletal muscle mitochondria had decreased respiratory chain activities, whereas liver mitochondria had increased activities.[6] Suprisingly, previous studies on vitamin E deficiency have shown no significant difference in isoprostane or neuroprostane production in the cerebellum of C57B6J male mice on a vitamin E–deficient diet for 39 weeks.[7] In our study we analyzed the effect of vitamin E deficiency on multiple parameters of reactive oxygen species production in male C57B6 mice.

METHODS

Male C57B6 mice were placed on a vitamin E–deficient diet for 38 weeks. After determination of α-tocopherol, ROS production and products were analyzed in brain through *in vivo* dihydroethidium (DHE) oxidation (a measure of superoxide, $O_2^{-\bullet}$ radical production), neuroprostane production, and mitochondrial function (through oxygraph and electron transport chain activity).[8,7]

RESULTS

Tissues showed three categories of deficiency: (1) highly susceptible (liver >95% deficient); (2) moderately susceptible (non-nervous tissues such as heart ~80% deficient); and (3) resistant (nervous tissue such as cortex ~ 50–60% deficient). The state of mitochondrial coupling can regulate $O_2^{-\bullet}$ production, and we showed that by using *in vivo* DHE oxidation, $O_2^{-\bullet}$ was significantly lower in the CA1 region of brain, with multiple other regions showing a similar trend (FIG. 1). F4 neuroprostanes, an index of lipid peroxidation, were also significantly lower in cortex and basal ganglia of VED mice (FIG. 1b). Intact mitochondrial respiration by oxygraph showed that vitamin E–deficient (VED) mitochondria in brain had a lower control ratio (RCR), while mitochondria in liver had an increased RCR, indicating increased coupling of mitochondria (FIG. 2).

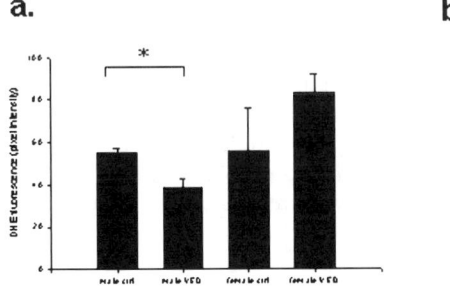
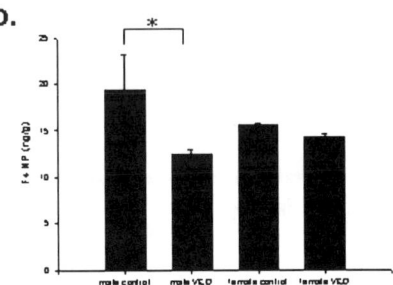

FIGURE 1. (**a**) Male vitamin E–deficient mice have less superoxide production in several regions of the brain: DHE oxidation in CA1 region of the hippocampus ($P=0.02$). (**b**) Male vitamin E–deficient mice have less F4 neuroprostanes in cortex ($P<0.05$) (control $n=3$; VED $n=3$).

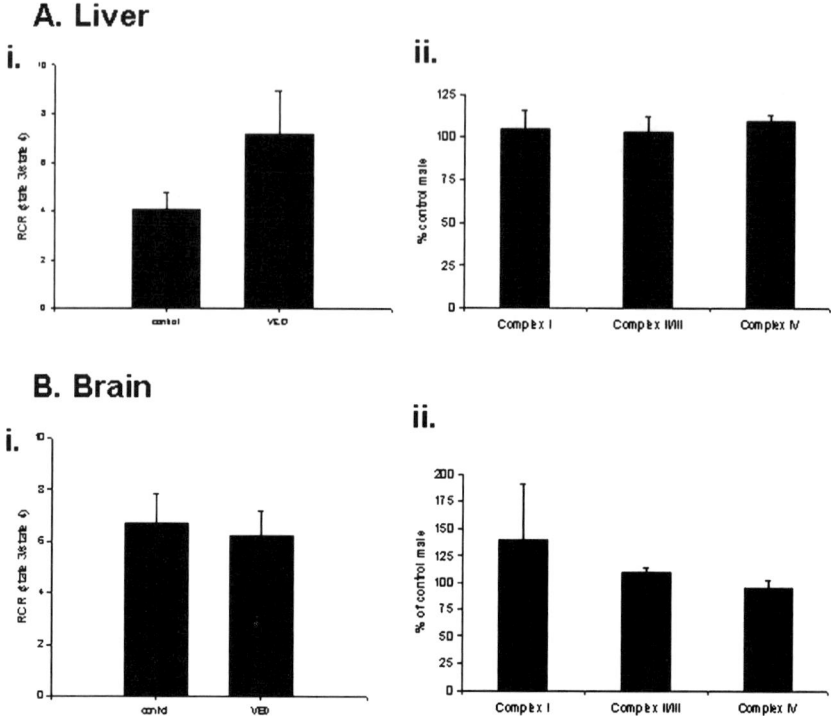

FIGURE 2. Vitamin E–deficient mice have more uncoupling in liver and less uncoupling in brain that is not due to changes in the electron transport chain: (**A**) liver; (**B**) brain. (**i**) respiratory control ratio (RCR) of week-38 male control and VED mice (RCR = state 3/state 4 respiration). (**ii**) Specific activity of electron transport chain complexes in VED mice as a % of controls ($n=3$).

DISCUSSION

Our results lend support to the idea that vitamin E plays a critical role in ROS production and neuronal function that is independent of its classic role as a chain-breaking antioxidant. As we see that vitamin E deficiency resulted in increased coupling of mitochondria in the liver, and decreased superoxide production and products of free radical attack (neuroprostanes), we theorize that α-tocopherol can act as a nonclassical uncoupler, and that deficiency leads to lower free radical $O_2^{-\bullet}$) production.

REFERENCES

1. KOYA, D., I.K. LEE, H. ISHII, et al. 1997. Prevention of glomerular dysfunction in diabetic rats by treatment with d-alpha-tocopherol. Am. Soc. Nephrol. **8:** 426–435.
2. RICCIARELLI, R., A. TASINATO, S. CLEMENT, et al. 1998. Alpha-tocopherol specifically inactivates cellular protein kinase C alpha by changing its phosphorylation state. Biochem. J. **334:** 243–249.

3. CHANDRA, V., J. JASTI, P. KAUR, et al. 2002. First structural evidence of a specific inhibition of phospholipase A2 by alpha-tocopherol (vitamin E) and its implications in inflammation: crystal structure of the complex formed between phospholipase A2 and alpha-tocopherol at 1.8 A resolution. J. Mol. Biol. **320:** 215–222.
4. AZZI, A., I. BREYER, M. FEHER, et al. 2000. Specific cellular responses to alpha-tocopherol. J. Nutr. **130:** 1649–1652.
5. THOMAS, P.K., J.M. COOPER, R.H. KING, et al. 1993. Myopathy in vitamin E deficient rats: muscle fibre necrosis associated with disturbances of mitochondrial function. J. Anat. **183:** 451–461.
6. RAFIQUE, R., A.H.V. SHAPIRA & J.M. COOPER. 2001. Sensitivity of respiratory chain activities to lipid peroxidation: effect of vitamin E deficiency. Biochem. J. **357:** 887–892.
7. REICH, E.E., K.S. MONTINE, M.D. GROSS, et al. 2001 Interactions between apolipoprotein E gene and dietary alpha-tocopherol influence cerebral oxidative damage in aged mice. J. Neurosci. **21:** 5993–5999.
8. QUICK, K.L. & L.L. DUGAN. 2001. Superoxide stress identifies neurons at risk in a model of ataxia-telangiectasia. Ann. Neurol. **49:** 627–635.

Tocopherol in Lipoproteins and Blood Cells after Cardiac Surgery

M. HACQUEBARD,[a] A. DUCART,[b] D. SCHMARTZ,[b] N. TEMBO,[a] AND Y.A. CARPENTIER[a]

[a]*L. Deloyers Laboratory for Experimental Surgery, Université Libre de Bruxelles, Brussels, Belgium*

[b]*Department of Anaesthesia, Erasme Hospital, Université Libre de Bruxelles, Brussels, Belgium*

ABSTRACT: Cardiac surgery was associated with a marked reduction in circulating LDL and HDL particles, which in turn largely affectd α-toc transport. α-toc was decreased in WBCs but not in PLTs and RBCs. An increased hydroperoxide content was observed in LDL and possibly in HDL after cardiac surgery.

KEYWORDS: vitamin E; alpha-tocopherol; acute phase; cardiac surgery; lipoproteins; blood cells

INTRODUCTION

The acute phase response (APR) is a systemic reaction to infectious and noninfectious injury in which multiple metabolic adaptations are induced by hormonal changes and inflammatory cytokines. This host response includes changes in hepatic synthesis of several plasma proteins (e.g., stimulated production of acute phase reactants), but also profound alterations in plasma lipids and lipoproteins.[1,2]

LDL and HDL are major alpha-tocopherol (α-toc) carriers in plasma and deliver it to cells and tissues. Plasma α-toc, as well as LDL- and HDL cholesterol levels are markedly reduced post surgery.[3,4] Whether the α-toc content per lipoprotein particle is changed after surgery is not clear.

The aim of this study was to determine the effect of cardiac surgery on the α-toc content in LDL and HDL lipoproteins as well as in blood cells.

METHODS

The study group included 20 patients undergoing coronary artery bypass graft or valve replacement. Blood samples were drawn at the time of induction of anesthesia

Address for correspondence: Mirjam Hacquebard, Laboratory for Experimental Surgery L. Deloyers. Université Libre de Bruxelles, Avenue J. Wybran 40, 1070 Brussels, Belgium. Voice: 00 32 2 520 09 19; fax: 00 32 2 520 82 81.

Mirjam.Hacquebard@ulb.ac.be

and again on day 2 post cardiac surgery. LDL and HDL were separated from the plasma of 15 patients. Total cholesterol (TC), α-toc^5 and hydroperoxides^6 were analyzed in LDL and HDL. Apo B-100 was measured in LDL and apo A-I and serum amyloid A (SAA) in HDL. Platelets (PLTs), white blood cells (WBCs) and red blood cells (RBCs) were isolated from blood samples of 5 patients. α-toc in PLTs, WBCs, and RBCs was expressed as a α-toc/phospholipid ratio. Statistical analyses were made with the paired Student's t test.

RESULTS

A similar decrease of TC (-41%; $P < 0.0001$) and of apoB (-40%; $P < 0.0001$) was observed in LDL post cardiac surgery, indicating a reduction in the number of circulating particles. The α-toc level in the LDL fraction was decreased by 40% ($P < 0.0001$). α-toc/TC and α-toc/apoB ratios remained unchanged. In HDL, α-toc and TC were reduced by 25% ($P < 0.001$) and 20% ($P < 0.01$), respectively, with a slightly reduced α-toc/TC ratio (-8%; $P = 0.04$); apo A-I decreased (-24%; $P = 0.002$) and SAA increased (50–1000-fold; $P = 0.04$). Hydroperoxide content was increased in LDL ($P = 0.017$) and possibly in HDL ($P=0.08$).

α-toc decreased by 22% ($P=0.026$) in WBCs, but remained unchanged in PLTs and RBCs.

CONCLUSIONS

These results indicate that the reduced α-toc level observed in the LDL fraction after cardiac surgery is entirely due to the reduced number of circulating LDL particles. In contrast a decreased α-toc content per HDL particle may possibly contribute to the reduced α-toc level observed post surgery in the HDL fraction.

The hydroperoxide content was increased in LDL and possibly in HDL after cardiac surgery. The reduced α-toc content observed in WBCs post surgery may result from α-toc consumption or from an increased release in the circulation of WBCs with a lower α-toc content.

REFERENCES

1. KHOVIDHUNKIT, W., R.A. MEMON, K.R. FEINGOLD & C. GRUNFELD. 2000. Infection and inflammation-induced proatherogenic changes of lipoproteins. J. Infect. Dis. (Suppl. 3) **181:** S462–S472.
2. KHOVIDHUNKIT, W., M.S. KIM, R.A. MEMON, et al. 2004. Effects of infection and inflammation on lipid and lipoprotein metabolism: mechanisms and consequences to the host. J. Lipid Res. **45:** 1169–1196.
3. COGHLAN, J.G., W.D. FLITTER, S.M. CLUTTON, et al. 1993. Lipid peroxidation and changes in vitamin E levels during coronary artery bypass grafting. J. Thorac. Cardiovasc. Surg. **106:** 268–274.
4. AKGÜN, S., N.H. ERTEL, A. MOSENTHAL & W. OSER. 1998. Postsurgical reduction of serum lipoproteins: interleukin-6 and the acute phase response. J. Lab. Clin. Med. **131:** 103–108.

5. TRABER, M.G. & H.J. KAYDEN. 1989. Preferential incorporation of α-tocopherol vs γ-tocopherol in human lipoproteins. Am. J. Clin. Nutr. **49:** 517–526.
6. JIANG, Z.Y., J.V. HUNT. & S.P. WOLFF. 1992. Ferrous ion oxidation in the presence of xylenol orange for detection of lipid hydroperoxides in low density lipoprotein. Anal. Biochem. **202:** 384–389.

Is *All-Rac*-α-Tocopherol Different from RRR-α-Tocopherol Regarding Cardiovascular Efficacy?

A Meta-Analysis of Clinical Trials

K. KRAEMER, W. KOCH, AND P.P. HOPPE

BASF Aktiengesellschaft, Ludwigshafen, Germany

ABSTRACT: A meta-analysis of 14 clinical studies with RRR- or *all-rac*-α-tocopherol (83,800 subjects) was performed to evaluate whether RRR and *all-rac* differ in cardiovascular efficacy based on those clinical endpoints that are most consistently documented in the publications of the studies. Odds ratios of treatment versus control for individual studies and for studies pooled by form were centered around unity, with no significant differences between vitamin E forms. The results corroborate the present opinion that vitamin E supplements up to 800 mg/d for up to 6.5 years are safe.

KEYWORDS: *all-rac*-α-tocopherol; RRR-α-tocopherol; vitamin E; meta-analysis; cardiovascular system

INTRODUCTION

A recent review of 11 clinical studies with RRR- (CHAOS, HOPE, SPACE, TAA, HATS, and ASAP) and *all-rac*-α-tocopherol (ATBC, GISSI, PPP, HPS, VEAPS) summarized benefits on primary endpoints for four studies with RRR (CHAOS, SPACE, TAA, ASAP), but none for studies with *all-rac*. The authors hypothesized that the form of vitamin E may be important for efficacy.[1] However, in the RRR studies showing benefits, two of the four primary endpoints were biomarker-type endpoints, and three large-scale studies with *all-rac* (GISSI, ATBC, PPP) showed benefits on secondary, but clinically important cardiovascular endpoints.

METHODS

We carried out a meta-analysis of 14 studies (TABLE 1) including the studies reviewed recently[1] and three further studies with *all-rac* (ADCS, AREDS, WAVE).[3–5] Patient numbers and endpoints were collected during a systematic review of publications and entered into a data table. Odds ratios (OR) of treatment vs. control and 95%

Address for correspondence: Klaus Kraemer, Ph.D., BASF Aktiengesellschaft, Human Nutrition, Scientific & Regulatory Affairs, ME/QR ? Li 725, Limburgerhof, 67117, Germany. Voice: +49-621-60-28712; fax: +49-621-60-6628712.
klaus.kraemer@basf-ag.de

TABLE 1. Overview of studies included in the meta-analysis

Trial	Patients' characteristics	Type of prevention[a]	Unit dose of AT	Dose of AT	Form of vitamin E	Follow-up (yr)	No. of subjects
ADCS	Alzheimer's disease	S	IU/d	2000	*all-rac*	2	341
AREDS	Age-related eye disease	P	IU/d	400	*all-rac*	6.6	4,757
ASAP	Hypercholesterolemia	P	IU/d	272	RRR	3	520
ATBC	Male smokers	P+S	IU/d	50	*all-rac*	5–8	29,133
CHAOS	Coronary atherosclerosis	S	IU/d	600	RRR	1.4	2,002
GISSI	Recent myocardial infarction	S	mg/d	300	*all-rac*	3–5	11,324
HATS	Coronary disease, low HDL	S	IU/d	800	RRR	3	160
HOPE	CVD, diabetes	P+S	IU/d	400	RRR	4–6	9,541
HPS	Coronary and occlusive arterial diseases, diabetes	P+S	mg/d	600	*all-rac*	5	20,536
PPP	Attendees to GP	P	mg/d	300	*all-rac*	3.6	4,495
SPACE	Chronic hemodialysis and CVD	S	IU/d	800	RRR	1.42	196
TAA	0 to 2 yr post cardiac transplant	S	IU/d	800	RRR	1	40
VEAPS	LDL cholesterol < 130 mg/dL	P	IU/d	400	*all-rac*	3	332
WAVE	Postmenopausal women with coronary stenosis	S	IU/d	800	*all-rac*	3.8	423
All studies							83,800

[a]P = primary prevention; S = secondary prevention.

confidence limits (CL) were estimated for individual studies and for studies pooled by form and overall. Estimations based on the random effects model were performed too; their results did not differ to a relevant extent from the simple formulas applied on pooled studies and therefore only the results of the latter are presented in this document.[2]

RESULTS

Odds ratios (RRR:control and *all-rac:*control) for endpoints are presented in FIGURE 1. For both RRR and *all-rac*, OR and CL limits were centered around unity,

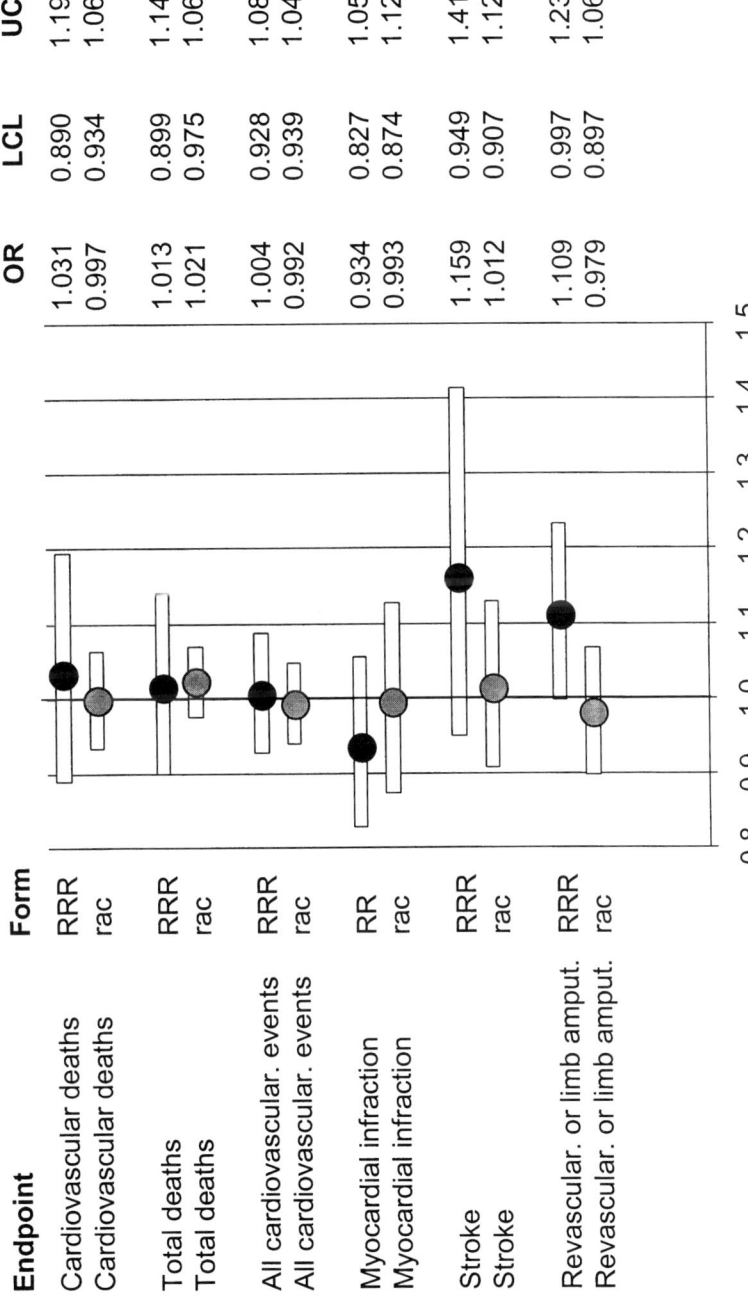

FIGURE 1. OR and 95% confidence limits (CL) for consistently documented cardiovascular endpoints; all studies pooled.

Endpoint	Form	OR	LCL	UCL
Cardiovascular deaths	RRR	1.031	0.890	1.195
Cardiovascular deaths	rac	0.997	0.934	1.063
Total deaths	RRR	1.013	0.899	1.141
Total deaths	rac	1.021	0.975	1.069
All cardiovascular. events	RRR	1.004	0.928	1.088
All cardiovascular. events	rac	0.992	0.939	1.047
Myocardial infraction	RR	0.934	0.827	1.055
Myocardial infraction	rac	0.993	0.874	1.127
Stroke	RRR	1.159	0.949	1.415
Stroke	rac	1.012	0.907	1.129
Revascular. or limb amput.	RRR	1.109	0.997	1.233
Revascular. or limb amput.	rac	0.979	0.897	1.068

indicating no significant effects of vitamin E on endpoints and no significant difference between vitamin E sources. The results also indicate, on the basis of 14 studies totaling 83,800 patients, that supplemental doses of RRR and *all-rac* for periods up to 6.6 years are safe. This is particularly evident for *all-rac,* for which we summarized the results of 8 studies with a total of 71,341 subjects.

DISCUSSION

Observational and experimental studies have suggested an important role of vitamin E in the prevention of cardiovascular disease. Results from clinical trials, however, are inconclusive regarding efficacy, suitability of the chosen endpoints, and form(s) and dosages of vitamin E required. This meta-analysis, by including all large clinical studies with RRR and *all-rac* and by using all relevant endpoints consistently documented in the publications, provides a more balanced view on cardiovascular efficacy of vitamin E compared with individual studies. The results do not support the hypothesis that the form of vitamin E may be important for efficacy. The possible reason for the low efficacy may be that only 4 of the 14 studies addressed primary prevention. The latter is more likely responsive to vitamin E than studies aiming at secondary prevention or primary and secondary prevention because vitamin E has shown to be effective mainly in early atherosclerosis, viz., in preventing LDL oxidation and fatty streak formation.

CONCLUSION

This meta-analysis of vitamin E effects on cardiovascular endpoints across 14 studies indicates no difference in efficacy between RRR and *all-rac*. The results also corroborate the present view that vitamin E supplements of either form at intakes from 50 to 800 mg/d are safe.

REFERENCES

1. JIALAL, I. & S. DEVARAJ. 2003. Antioxidants and atherosclerosis: don't throw out the baby with the bath water. Circulation **107:** 926–928.
2. BROCKWELL, S. & I. GORDON. 2001. A comparison of statistical methods for meta-analysis. Statistics in Medicine **20:** 825–840
3. SANO, M. *et al.* 1997. A controlled trial of selegiline, alpha-tocopherol, or both as treatment for Alzheimer's disease. The Alzheimer's Disease Cooperative Study. N. Engl. J. Med. **336:** 1216–1222.
4. AGE-RELATED EYE DISEASE STUDY RESEARCH GROUP. 2001. A randomized, placebo-controlled, clinical trial of high-dose supplementation with vitamins C and E and beta carotene for age-related cataract and vision loss: AREDS Report No. 9. Arch. Ophthalmol. **119:** 1439–1452.
5. WATERS, D.D. *et al.* 2002. Effects of hormone replacement therapy and antioxidant vitamin supplements on coronary atherosclerosis in postmenopausal women: a randomized controlled trial. JAMA **288:** 2432–2440.

Evolution of Serum α-Tocopherol in the Postprandial and Postabsorptive Phases in Type 1 Diabetes Mellitus

BEGOÑA MANUEL-Y-KEENOY,[a] ANN VAN CAMPENHOUT,[a] JAN VERTOMMEN,[a] LUC VAN GAAL,[b] AND IVO DE LEEUW[a]

[a]*Metabolic Research Unit, and* [b]*University Hospital, University of Antwerp, Belgium*

ABSTRACT: Blood glucose, lipids, α-tocopherol, and malondialdehyde were monitored in type 1 diabetes mellitus patients for 8 hours after a standard fat-rich breakfast and lunch. Although glucose and triglycerides increased, α-tocopherol decreased and malondialdehyde increased in the postprandial phase. In the postabsorptive phase values returned to fasting levels. These results point to the possible relevance of postprandial α-tocopherol depletion and lipid peroxidation to an increased cardiovascular risk in these patients.

KEYWORDS: type 1 diabetes mellitus; α-tocopherol; postprandial; postabsorptive; lipid peroxidation

INTRODUCTION

The 2- to 4-fold higher risk and mortality from cardiovascular disease in patients with diabetes mellitus (DM) has been independently associated with abnormalities of plasma lipid and lipoprotein metabolism[1] as well as with several pathologic effects of hyperglycemia. Studies on type 2 DM patients demonstrate that postprandial changes of both lipids and glucose can predict cardiovascular risk more strongly than fasting values[3,4] and that one of the underlying pathobiochemical links is oxidative stress. Less is known about the postprandial changes in type 1 DM and their role in the cardiovascular risk of these patients. Therefore we aimed in this study to describe the time course of postprandial and postabsorptive changes in lipids, α-tocopherol (α-T) and lipid peroxidation in type 1 DM.

METHODS

Patients on intensive insulin treatment (11 female/12 male; aged 42 ± 9 yr; duration of diabetes 17 ± 8 yr; HbA_{1c} 7.7 ± 0.8% and with no cardiovascular or irreversible microvascular complications) were hospitalized in the metabolic ward of the

Address for correspondence: B. Manuel-y-Keenoy, M.D., Ph.D., University of Antwerp (UA) campus Drie Eiken, Metabolic Research Unit (AMRU) T4.37, Universiteitsplein 1, B-2610 Wilrijk-Antwerp, Belgium. Voice: 32 3 8202573; fax: 32 3 8202574.
begona.manuelykeenoy@ua.ac.be

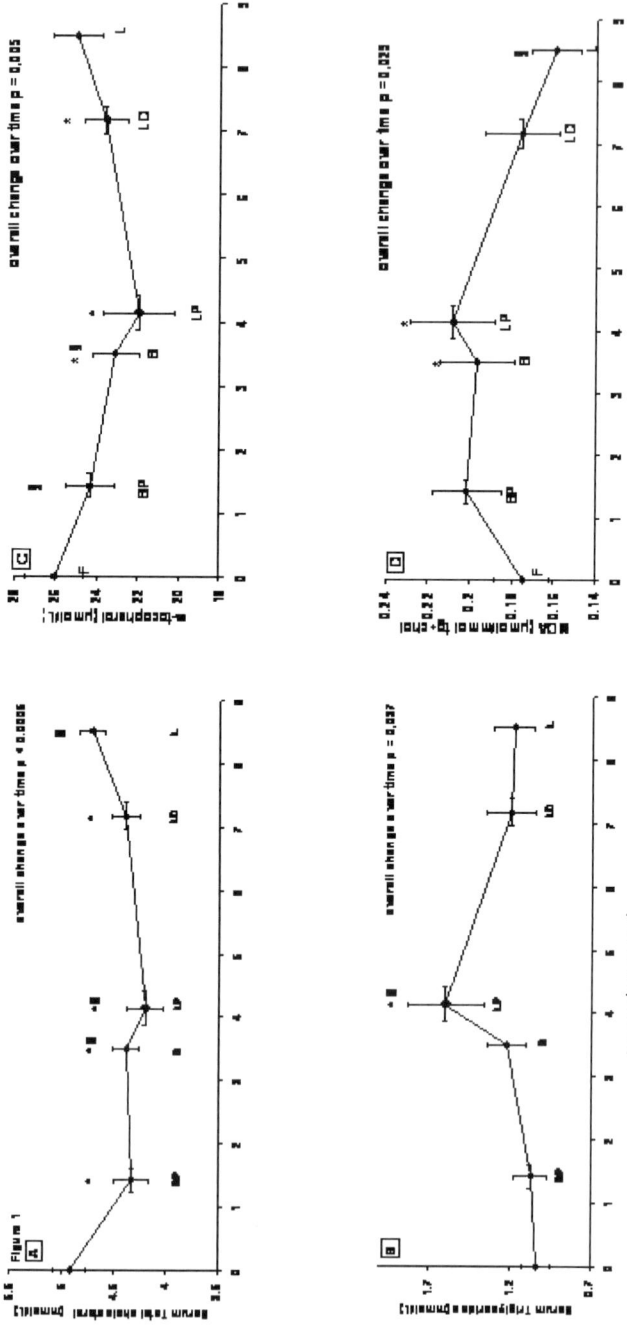

FIGURE 1. Time course of changes in serum cholesterol (A), triglycerides (B), plasma α-tocopherol (C) and malondialdehyde (D). Values were monitored at fasting F, just after the post-breakfast glucose peak BP, just before lunch B, just after the post-lunch glucose peak LP, just after the post-lunch glucose dale LD and 5 hours after lunch L. Shown are means ± SEM of 23 patients. P value denotes the significance of the overall change over time, calculated by repeated measures analysis of variance. * denotes $P < 0.05$ when contrasted to the value at fasting. § denotes $P < 0.05$ when contrasted to the preceding value.

Antwerp University Hospital; glycemia was monitored continuously via a subcutaneous device. The patients received a standard breakfast (883 kcal, 59% energy as fat, 4 mg tocopherol) and lunch (698 kcal, 50% energy as fat, 2 mg tocopherol). Blood samples were extracted at fasting (F), just after the post-breakfast glycemia peak (BP), 3.5 hours after breakfast and just before lunch (B), just after the post-lunch peak (LP), just after the post-lunch "dale" (LD), and 5 hours after lunch (L). Serum lipids were measured in the routine laboratory and α-T and malondialdehyde (MDA) by reverse-phase HPLC with detection at 292 and 532 nm, respectively.[6,7] Nine lipoprotein subfractions were separated by sequential gradient ultracentrifugation and their lipid composition (triglyceride, phospholipid and cholesterol) was determined using commercial kits. *In vitro* peroxidability was monitored by adding 5 μmol/L copper sulphate to each fraction containing 240 μg/mL protein and monitoring fluorescence at 360/440 nm excitation/emission.[8]

RESULTS

There were two clear hyperglycemic peaks (>300 mg/dL) after breakfast and lunch and a postprandial increase in serum triglycerides (by 55%), but a 12% decrease in both LDL and HDL cholesterol (FIG. 1). This was manifested as an increase of all the lipid components of the chylomicron fraction and of triglycerides in the VLDL fractions in contrast to decreases of all lipids in the LDL fractions and of triglycerides and phospholipids in the HDL fractions. Serum α-T (FIG. 1) decreased from 26.0 ± 6.7 μmol/L (4.43 ± 0.76 μmol/mmol lipid) at F to 24.3 ± 5.0 at BP ($P = 0.010$) and further to 23.1 ± 5.5 μmol/L (4.12 ± 0.82 μmol/ mmol lipid) 3 hours after breakfast B. Plasma MDA increased gradually from 1.02 ± 0.36 μmol/L at F to a maximum of 1.14 ± 0.40 at LP ($P = 0.028$). The postabsorptive phase (L, 5 hours after lunch) was characterized by a fall in glycemia to 85 mg/dL and a return of serum parameters to values similar to those at fasting. *In vitro* copper-induced peroxidation was unchanged in the LDL and HDL subfractions, but the lagtime of the VLDL fractions decreased from 91 ± 7 at F to 79 ± 6 minutes at L ($P < 0.05$).

CONCLUSIONS

In this group of patients we observe postprandial α-T depletion which is accompanied by increased *in vivo* lipid peroxidation (plasma MDA). However, the susceptibility to *in vitro* copper-induced peroxidation is not increased except for the VLDL and only in the postabsorptive phase. Alternatively, the time course of the various postprandial changes suggests that increased free radical production (originating from the increases in glucose and triglycerides) together with an increased clearance of LDL and α-T from the plasma, led to an oxidant-antioxidant imbalance which results in accumulation of MDA. Although further investigations are needed to elucidate the role played by meal composition and the insulin injections, we suggest that these postprandial changes are relevant to the increased cardiovascular risk in these patients. The recommendation to increase α-T intake during fat-rich meals is open for discussion.

REFERENCES

1. SYVANNE, M. & M.R. TASKINEN. 1997. Lipids and lipoproteins as coronary risk factors in non-insulin-dependent diabetes mellitus. Lancet (Suppl 1) **350:** SI20–SI23.
2. BROWNLEE, M. 2001. Biochemistry and molecular cell biology of diabetic complications. Nature **414:** 813–820.
3. TEMELKOVA-KURKTSCHIEV, T.S., C. KOEHLER, E. HENKEL, et al. 2000. Postchallenge plasma glucose and glycemic spikes are more strongly associated with atherosclerosis than fasting glucose or HbA1c level. Diabetes Care **23:** 1830–1834.
4. TENO, S., Y. UTO, H. NAGASHIMA, et al. 2000. Association of postprandial hypertriglyceridemia and carotid intima-media thickness in patients with type 2 diabetes. Diabetes Care **23:** 1401–1406.
5. CERIELLO, A. 2000. The post-prandial state and cardiovascular disease: relevance to diabetes mellitus. Diabetes Metab. Res. Rev. **16:** 125–132.
6. CAYE-VAUGIEN, C., M. KREMPF, P. LAMARCHE, et al. 1990. Determination of α-tocopherol in plasma, platelets and erythrocytes of type I and type II diabetic patients by HPLC. Int. J. Vitam. Nutr. Res. **60:** 324–330.
7. NIELSEN, F., B.B. MIKKELSEN, J.B. NIELSEN, et al. 1997. Plasma malondialdehyde as biomarker for oxidative stress: reference interval and effects of life-style factors Clin. Chem. **43:** 1209–1214.
8. ZHANG, A., J. VERTOMMEN, L. VAN GAAL & I. DE LEEUW. 1994. A rapid and simple method for measuring the susceptibility of low-density-lipoprotein and very-low-density lipoprotein to copper-catalysed oxidation. Clin. Chim. Acta. **227:** 159–173.

Topical α-Tocopherol Acetate in the Bulk Phase

Eight Years of Experience in Skin Treatment

GIORGIO PANIN,[a] RENATA STRUMIA,[b] AND FULVIO URSINI[c]

[a]*Hulka s.r.l. Rovigo, Italy*
[b]*Unit of Dermatology, University Hospital S. Anna, Ferrara, Italy*
[c]*Department of Biological Chemistry, University of Padova, Padova, Italy*

ABSTRACT: Clinical practice in dermatology indicates that α-tocopherol acetate is beneficial in xerosis, hyperkeratosis, asteatotic eczema, atopic dermatitis, superficial burns, cutaneous ulcers, onychoschizia and, in general, skin diseases in which an inflammatory process is activated. The positive effect results from the combination of biological activity, the absence of adverse reactions, and the physical effect of the α-tocopherol acetate oil. The viscosity of this oil in bulk phase accounts for a remarkable moisturizing effect and minimization of transepidermal water loss. This effect combines well with the antioxidant capacity of α-tocopherol released from the ester, and the recently emerging effect on reprogramming of gene expression.

KEYWORDS: α-tocopherol acetate (bulk phase); skin diseases; topical vitamin E; skin

INTRODUCTION

The first reports, indexed in Medline, about the use of vitamin E in dermatology appeared in the early 1950s, approximately 30 years after the discovery of this nutrient, the deficiency syndrome of which produced alterations of reproductive function. A topical or systemic treatment with vitamin E has been reported as beneficial in wound healing, X-ray injuries of the skin, senile skin, and a heterogeneous series of different dermatoses.

Later on, the elucidation of the redox properties of tocopherol[1,2] and the related "antioxidant theory" drove a large series of studies to unravel the relationships between free radical scavenging and skin protection.[3]

A large part of *in vitro* or *ex vivo* studies has been aimed at demonstrating that the protective effect of vitamin E on the skin is accounted for by its antioxidant properties.[4–6] Skin is, indeed, exposed to environmental oxidants (including oxygen itself) and inflammation is a major biological source of oxidants, and thus a protective ef-

---

Address for correspondence: Giorgio Panin, M.D., Ph.D., Hulka s.r.l., Via della Scienza 17, I-45100; Rovigo, Italy. Voice: +39 0425 471457; fax: +39 0425 988121.
g.panin@hulka.it

fect of vitamin E on skin aging, sunburn, and inflammatory diseases was first expected and than observed and rationalized on the basis of the efficient quenching of free radicals.[7]

Nevertheless, in 1993 in a exhaustive review of clinical data, K. Pehr and R. Forsey[8] reached the conclusion that "...there is still scant proof of vitamin E's effectiveness in treating certain dermatologic conditions..." and that "...research in well-designed controlled trials is needed to clarify vitamin E's role...."

To our knowledge fully controlled and evidence-based studies are still extremely scant. Nonetheless, the cosmeceutical use of vitamin E at different concentrations in different vehicles has became progressively more and more popular.

On the other hand, basic knowledge about the physiological function of vitamin E is today much more precise and new functions are emerging, not always nor necessarily related to the antioxidant effect.[9]

With the aim of suggesting possible insights, hopefully helping in bridging the gap between clinical experience and basic science, and looking forward for an evidence-based clinical validation for an use of vitamin E in dermatology, we would like to present examples of the practical clinical experience acquired by the company that first introduced, in Italy, the use of α-tocopherol acetate in bulk phase for the complementary treatment of different forms of skin disease.

TOPICAL VITAMIN E IN DERMATOLOGY

The idea of using the oily α-tocopherol acetate for topical skin treatment rests on the following evidence: (*a*) the redox chemistry of the vitamin, compatible with an antioxidant effect *in vivo*[10]; (*b*) the hydrolysis of the ester in the skin[11] and thus the pro-drug nature of the acetate; (*c*) the prospect of a physiological extracellular function of vitamin E, which is indeed secreted and readsorbed in the skin[12]; and (*d*) the virtual absence of adverse reactions.[13]

A further peculiar feature of the use of α-tocopherol acetate oil as a bulk phase is the absence of a vehicle in which the active species is dissolved. This results in a gain of chemical and microbiological stability and in the prevention of adverse reactions due to excipients. Furthermore, this viscous oil (TABLE 1) accounts for another, possibly relevant, effect. The use of treating the skin with oils[14] is, indeed, as old as our civilization, when our ancestors learned how to protect the skin by overspreading it with oils, most frequently the edible, and thus apparently safe, olive oil.

TABLE 1. Viscosity of different compounds used in cosmetic preparations

Compound	milliPascal per second
α-tocopherol acetate	5000
Glycerol	1270
Vaseline oil	180
Olive oil	70
Octyl-palmitate	50
Propylenic glycol	46
Jojoba oil	45

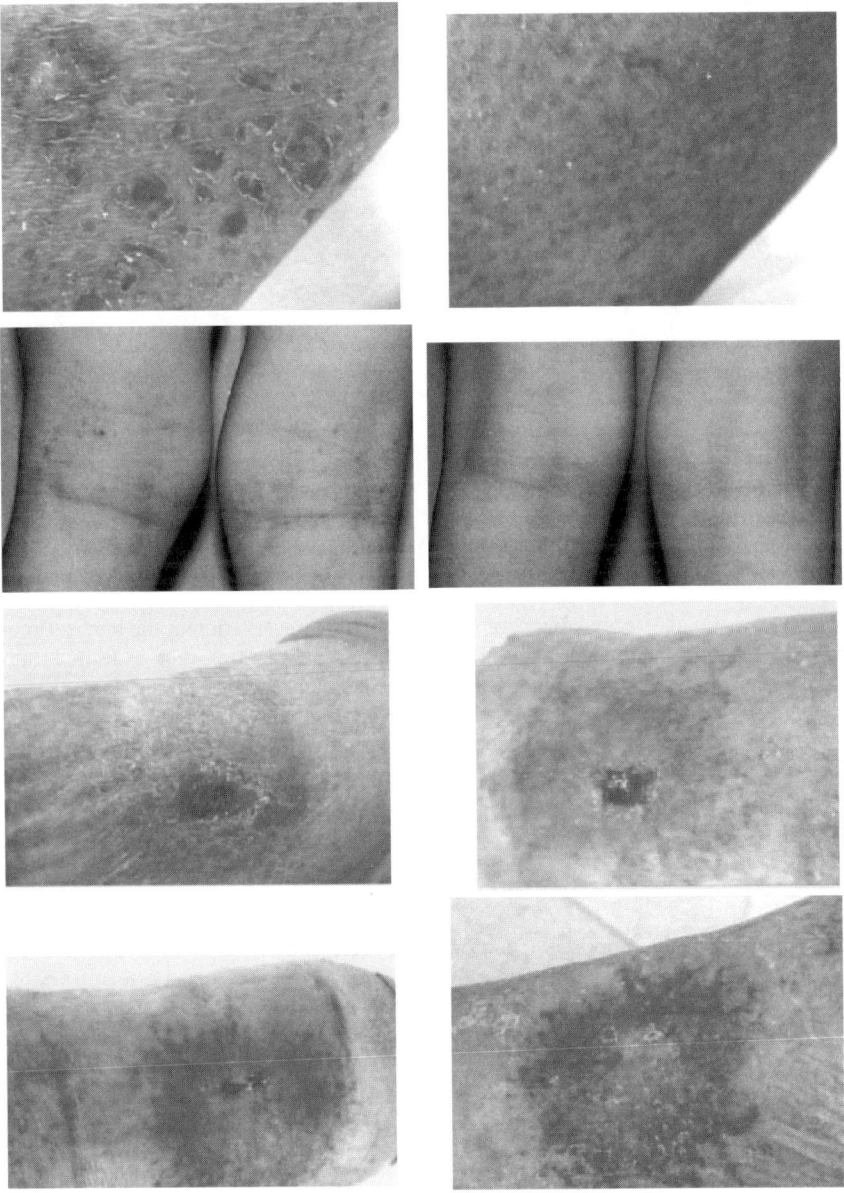

FIGURE 1. Effect of α-tocopherol acetate treatment in different skin diseases. *Top row*: asteatotic eczema. (*left*) dry and cracked skin; (*right*) disappearance of scales and dryness after 10 days of twice-a-day treatment. *Second row*: atopic dermatitis. (*left*) erythema, lichenification, and excoriation of knee flexures; (*right*) disappearance of symptoms after 7 days of treatment 2× daily. *Third row*: cutaneous ulcer. (*left*) venous long-standing ulcer in leg of old woman; (*right*) erythematous halo and blackish crust after 2 weeks of treatment 1× daily. *Fourth row*: cutaneous ulcer. (*left*) healing; reforming epithelium spreads over

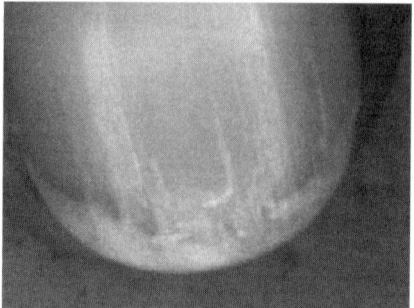 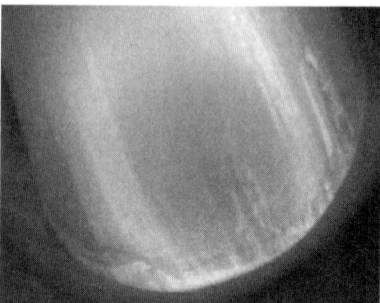

FIGURE 1. — *continued.*

granulation tissue after 4 weeks of treament 1× daily; (*right*) complete healing with brown halo after 6 weeks of treatment 1× daily. *Fifth row*: onychoschizia. (*left*) transverse splitting into layers near free edge; (*right*) good response to topical therapy after 3 months of treatment 2× daily.

The beneficial effect is now seen in relation to the preservation of the barrier function of the skin. In agreement with this notion, a minimization of the abnormal transepidermal water loss by topical vitamin E has been observed in atopic dermatitis.[15]

The oily α-tocopherol acetate can be seen, therefore, as a medical device capable of moisturizing the skin and preventing transepidermal water loss.

Examples of the efficiency of the treatment in some common skin disorders are shown in FIGURE 1.

CONCLUSIONS

Clinical practice supports the notion that treatment of the skin with vitamin E oil is beneficial in the vast majority of cases of xerosis, hyperkeratosis, asteatotic eczema, atopic dermatitis, superficial burns, cutaneous ulcers, and onychoschizia. However, only minimal beneficial effect, if any, has been observed in psoriasis, lichen ruber planus, seborrhoeic dermatitis, vitiligo, dyshidrotic eczema, and infectious diseases in general.

A remarkable effect of topical vitamin E oil is an amelioration of pruritus or pain associated with different diseases, independent of the efficiency on the peculiar features of the specific disease.

The common elements, shared by diseases where a clinical effect has been observed, could be tentatively recognized as an abnormal or inappropriate response to an injury associated with an inefficient repair system and to a more or less severe loss of the barrier function of the skin.

It is proposed that the observed clinical effect likely results from the combination of the redox chemistry of α-tocopherol, its biological activity as regulator of cellular response, and eventually the physical effect of the oil.

REFERENCES

1. BURTON, G.W., A. JOICE & K.U. INGOLD. 1982. First proof that vitamin E is major lipid-soluble, chain-breaking antioxidant in human blood plasma. Lancet **2**: 327.
2. SCARPA, M. et al. 1984. Formation of alpha-tocopherol radical and recycling of alpha-tocopherol by ascorbate during peroxidation of phosphatidylcholine liposomes: an electron paramagnetic resonance study. Biochim. Biophys. Acta **801**: 215–219.
3. FUCHS, J., R.J. MEHLLHORN & L. PACKER. 1989. Free radical reduction mechanisms in mouse epidermis skin homogenates. J. Invest. Dermatol. **93**: 633–640.
4. PACKER, L. & G. VALACCHI. 2002. Antioxidants and the response of skin to oxidative stress: vitamin E as a key indicator. Skin Pharmacol. Appl. Skin Physiol. **15**: 282–290.
5. THIELE, J.J. & L. PACKER. 1999. Noninvasive measurement of alpha-tocopherol gradients in human stratum corneum by high-performance liquid chromatography analysis of sequential tape strippings. Meth. Enzymol. **300**: 413–419.
6. KITAZAWA, M. et al. 1997. Interactions between vitamin E homologues and ascorbate free radicals in murine skin homogenates irradiated with ultraviolet light. Photochem. Photobiol. **65**: 355–365.
7. THIELE, J.J. et al. 2001. The antioxidant network of the stratum corneum. Curr. Probl. Dermatol. **29**: 26–42.
8. PEHR, K. & R.R. FORSEY. 1993. Why don't we use vitamin E in dermatology? Can. Med. Assoc. J. **149**: 1247–1253.
9. RICCIARELLI, R. J.M. ZINGG & A. AZZI. 2001. Vitamin E: protective role of a Janus molecule. FASEB J. **15**: 2314–2325.
10. BURTON, G.W. & K.U. INGOLD. 1989. Vitamin E as an *in vitro* and *in vivo* antioxidant. Ann. N.Y. Acad. Sci. **570**: 7–22.
11. BEIJERSBERGEN VAN HENEGOUWEN, G.M., H E. JUNGINGER & H. DE VRIES. 1995. Hydrolysis of RRR-alpha-tocopheryl acetate (vitamin E acetate) in the skin and its UV protecting activity (an in vivo study with the rat). J. Photochem. Photobiol. B. **29**: 45–51.
12. THIELE, J.J., S.U. WEBER & L. PACKER. 1999. Sebaceous gland secretion is a major physiologic route of vitamin E delivery to skin. J. Invest. Dermatol. **113**: 1006–1010.
13. VERALDI, S., A.L. FRASIN & R. SCIANCHI. 2004. Allergic contact dermatitis from topical vitamin E. Contact Dermatitis. In press.
14. DARMSTADT, G.L. et al. 2002 Impact of topical oils on the skin barrier: possible implications for neonatal health in developing countries. Acta Paediatr. **91**: 546–554.
15. KURIYAMA, K. et al. 2002. Vitamin E ointment at high dose levels suppresses contact dermatitis in rats by stabilizing keratinocytes. Inflamm. Res. **51**: 483–489.

Appendix: Vitamin E and Health

Background and Objectives

KAREN HOPKIN

BIOAVAILABILITY AND BIOKINETICS OF VITAMIN E

Vitamin E is actually the generic name for a group of eight plant-derived, lipid-soluble substances, including four tocopherols and four tocotrienols. During the 1990s, studies using deuterium-labeled vitamin E advanced our understanding of how these various forms are handled by the human body.

Attention has focused on how chemical differences between vitamin E isomers dictate how they are processed and handled. In addition, this work has confirmed that, together with dietary fat, all forms of vitamin E are absorbed in the digestive tract, incorporated into chylomicrons, and transported in the lymphatic system. Part of the absorbed stereoisomers are taken up into extrahepatic tissues by the action of lipoprotein lipase, and the remainder is delivered in chylomicron remnants to the liver.

Vitamin E is Assimilated from the Diet and Directed to Target Tissues, but How?

It is also now clear that a hepatic cytosolic α-tocopherol transfer protein (α-TTP) regulates the distribution of vitamin E into the circulation. α-TTP is selective for α-tocopherol in its RRR or 2R forms. The protein shows much less affinity for other tocopherols and tocotrienols, including 38% for β-tocopherol, 9% for γ-tocopherol, 2% for δ-tocopherol, and 12% for α-tocotrienol.

In the liver, vitamin E is incorporated into very-low-density lipoprotein (VLDL) and released into the systemic blood circulation. Excess amounts of α-tocopherol, along with the other absorbed forms of tocopherols and tocotrienols, are metabolized or eliminated by the biliary tract.

VLDL is converted into low-density lipoprotein (LDL), and excess surface components including α-tocopherol are transferred to high-density lipoprotein (HDL). Delivery of α-tocopherol to peripheral tissues takes place through binding of LDL to specific receptors and subsequent cellular uptake. These advances and the question of how vitamin E is assimilated from the diet and directed to target tissues were covered in Session I.

Karen Hopkin as a freelance writer in Somerville, Massachusetts, She holds a Ph.D. in Biochemistry and, with Bruce Alberts *et al.*, is a coauthor of the textbook *Essential Cell Biology* (2003. Garland Publishing Company. New York).

ANTIOXIDANT FUNCTIONS OF VITAMIN E

All natural isoforms and synthetic stereoisomers of vitamin E exhibit to varying degrees the ability to inhibit lipid peroxidation as a "chain-breaking" antioxidant. Vitamin E primarily destroys peroxyl radicals and thus protects polyunsaturated fatty acids (PUFA) from oxidation.

Additionally, vitamin E scavenges a variety of oxygen-derived free radicals, including alkoxyl radicals, superoxide, and other reactive oxygen species, such as singlet oxygen and ozone, and it reacts with nitrogen species. Vitamin E is extremely effective at all these, and one reason is that it does not work alone.

Vitamin E is Effective: It Does Not Work Alone

Since 1989, Lester Packer and his colleagues have shown that vitamin E participates in an *antioxidant* network, and so vitamin E radicals can be recycled or regenerated back to their native form, for example, by vitamin C.

When vitamin C radicals form as a result, they may be regenerated by thiol or polyphenol antioxidants in the body. These interactions between redox antioxidant substances and enzymes form the basis for the body's underlying antioxidant defense system.

All naturally occurring analogues and synthetic stereoisomers of vitamin E exhibit redox cycling activity to varying degrees in the system of antioxidant defense against oxidative stress. When vitamin E interacts with lipid peroxyl and other lipid radicals in cell membranes or lipoproteins, a tocopheroxyl or tocotrienoxyl radical is formed.

However, like other natural antioxidants such as vitamin C or polyphenols, vitamin E radicals are not as dangerous species as the ones they have destroyed, because the free electron is delocalized around their chemical ring structure. This is the unique feature of biological antioxidants, such as vitamin E.

Given these various properties, vitamin E appears to play a central role in regulating cellular oxidative stress. In addition, vitamin E has been shown to modulate the concentrations of nitric oxide, a chemical that regulates the relaxation of blood vessels. All these aspects of vitamin E metabolism were reviewed in Session II, providing a basis for a new understanding of the range of the functions of vitamin E.

CELL REGULATORY FUNCTIONS OF VITAMIN E

One of the major questions relating to vitamin E is how tissue concentrations are regulated. Recently, cytosolic tocopherol-associated proteins (TAPs) have been reported showing α-tocopherol-specific binding characteristics and also nuclear translocation and transcriptional activation in various mammalian cell types and organs. A further cytosolic vitamin E regulatory protein, tocopherol-binding protein (TBP), has been reported with yet unknown functions. All this provides a basis for understanding the range of new functions that are now ascribed to vitamin E.

Vitamin E Appears to Play a Central Role in Regulating Cellular Oxidative Stress

In the early 1990s, Angelo Azzi and his colleagues suggested inhibition of protein kinase C (PKC) activity by vitamin E as the crucial factor for inhibition of cell proliferation in smooth muscle cells. Importantly, the inhibition of PKC appeared to be independent of its antioxidant activity of vitamin E, suggesting that the biological role of vitamin E goes beyond its antioxidant function.

PKC plays a major role in cell signaling and modulates gene expression during cell growth, proliferation, and differentiation. Its activity contributes to such disorders as vascular disease, cancer, diabetes, and other age-related degenerative diseases.

Confirmed in a variety of animal studies, vitamin E has subsequently been shown to inhibit PKC activity in many cell types including smooth muscle cells, monocytes, macrophages, neutrophils, fibroblasts, and mesangial cells. Inhibition of PKC activity by vitamin E occurs indirectly via activation of a phosphatase that cleaves the active, phosphorylated form of PKC, or by modulating diacylglycerol kinase activity.

Several lines of evidence suggest a cell-signaling role for vitamin E. For example, advances in molecular biology and availability of microarray techniques for studying effects of vitamin E on gene expression have revealed vitamin E–sensitive genes and signal transduction.

At the transcriptional level, vitamin E regulates the expression of several genes, including collagen-α1 and α1-TTP in liver, collagenase in skin, adhesion molecules and chemokines such as VCAM-1 and MCP-1 in endothelial cells, different integrins in erythroleukemia cells, α-tropomyosin in smooth muscle cells, and scavenger receptors class A (SR-A) and CD 36 in macrophages and smooth muscle cells.

Several Lines of Evidence Suggest a Cell-Signaling Role for Vitamin E

At the post-translational level, vitamin E regulates the expression of cyclooxygenase in monocytes, leading to a decrease in prostaglandin E_2 levels. As this effect was also observed with other vitamin E homologues compatible with antioxidant activity, this function of vitamin E may involve redox signaling.

These newly discovered actions of vitamin E are reviewed in Session III. These actions may help to explain vitamin E's beneficial effects in the chronic and degenerative diseases that occur late in life.

PROTECTION FROM OXIDATIVE STRESS AND INJURY

Vitamin E is the body's major lipid-soluble antioxidant protecting lipoproteins and membranes where it resides. It prevents free radical–mediated lipid peroxidation, which, if not prevented or interrupted, causes widespread oxidative molecular damage and pathology. All natural isoforms and synthetic stereoisomers of vitamin E exhibit varying degrees of ability to inhibit lipid peroxidation as a "chain-breaking" antioxidant.

Oxidative Stress is an Important Factor in Cell Injury

Oxidative stress is recognized as an important factor in a range of conditions involving cell injury. Strenuous exercise, excessive lipid oxidation in atherosclerosis, and UV injury to the eye are just a few conditions in which vitamin E is thought to play a beneficial role. Each of these conditions and the underlying role of vitamin E are explored in Session IV.

VITAMIN E AND VASCULAR NETWORKS

Vitamin E Disturbances Have Been Implicated in Vascular Diseases

Vitamin E primarily destroys peroxyl radicals and thus protects polyunsaturated fatty acids (PUFA) from oxidation. Additionally, vitamin E scavenges a variety of oxygen-derived free radicals, including alkoxyl radicals, superoxide, and other reactive oxygen species such as singlet oxygen and ozone, and it reacts with nitrogen species.

As a consequence of these functions vitamin E disturbances have been implicated in a range of diseases that involves the vascular system. In Session V the unique functions of vitamin E are considered in the regulation of blood vessel function, inflammation, and diabetes.

PREVENTION, PROTECTION, AND TREATMENT OF DISEASES

Indications of vitamin E deficiency have been found in premature babies and children suffering from an inability to absorb vitamin E, as in abetalipoproteinemia, chronic cholestatic liver disease, cystic fibrosis, and short-bowel syndrome. In contrast, a mutation in the α-TTP gene, as found in familial isolated vitamin E deficiency, results in a failure to deliver α-tocopherol to the systemic circulation.

Early Diagnosis and Treatment are Crucial to Ameliorate Neurologic Symptoms

In these cases, clinical vitamin E deficiency is recognized in babies showing symptoms of retrolental fibroplasia and intraventricular hemorrhage, as well as in children suffering from muscular dystrophy, ataxia, and other disorders. High-dose vitamin E supplementation can reduce or eliminate clinical symptoms in these patients. However, to achieve amelioration of neurological symptoms early diagnosis and early start of treatment are crucial.

More frequently, a chronic suboptimal supply in vitamin E (i.e., theoretically an intake below RDA levels) occurs in some individuals in all age groups. This may cause impaired defense against oxidative stress and increased susceptibility to oxidative injury and adverse health effects. In most diseases that have been examined with any degree of scrutiny, evidence for "oxidative stress" and oxidative damage has been observed in some stage of disease initiation or progression.

Can Vitamin E Given for Just a Fraction of Our Lifespan Prevent or Delay Disorders?

It has thus always seemed obvious that vitamin E, like other antioxidants, may prevent or delay disease progression. However, it is still unclear whether vitamin E at dietary levels or as supplements given over a short period relative to our lifespan effectively prevents chronic disease or delays age-related degenerative disorders.

Although some supportive evidence is available from observational, clinical, and experimental studies, results are eagerly awaited from several small clinical trials and six large human intervention studies that are ongoing. Session VI summed up the puzzle and looked ahead to potential results.

EPIDEMIOLOGICAL AND INTERVENTION STUDIES

In recent years, four large, prospective clinical trials have tested the ability of α-tocopherol supplementation to prevent cardiovascular events in different populations—the Alpha-Tocopherol Beta-Carotene (ATBC) Study; the Cambridge Heart Antioxidant Study (CHAOS); the Gruppo Italiano per lo Studio della Supervienza nell'Infarto miocardico (GISSI) Study; and the Heart Outcomes Prevention Evaluation (HOPE) study. In addition, two smaller prospective clinical trials have been completed—the Secondary Prevention with Antioxidants of Cardiovascular Disease in Endstage Renal Disease (SPACE) and the Antioxidant Supplementation in Atherosclerosis Prevention (ASAP) study.

Clinical Trials to Date Are Not Easily Compared

Each of these trials has inherent problems, and collectively they are not easily compared. Major differences include the selection criteria of individuals, the geographical (and hence the dietary) differences of the study, the stage of the disease, the selected endpoints, and the dosage, mode, and chemical form of vitamin E application.

Taken together, it is not surprising that the results are inconsistent. Collectively, these studies have brought confusion to vitamin E research. The results of these trials are reviewed in Session VII and strategies to move forward are discussed.

Overview: New Roles for a Familiar Nutrient

KAREN HOPKIN

Fifteen years ago, the New York Academy of Sciences sponsored a symposium dedicated to the science of vitamin E; the proceedings of that symposium, *Vitamin E: Biochemistry and Health Implications*, were published in 1989 as Volume 570 of the *Annals*. This conference in turn took place 40 years after the Academy's first meeting on vitamin E.. Since then, researchers have learned a great deal about this family of fat-soluble vitamins. They have seen how the different forms are metabolized, which is preferred by the body, and how it gets whisked from the liver by a specialized protein that ferries it to the blood and to vital organs such as the brain. What remains unclear is what exactly vitamin E does in the body and how it does it.

At this most recent conference—and as reflected in the papers in this volume—researchers reviewed the role that vitamin E plays in human health. Participants discussed whether vitamin E supplements can prevent or treat a variety of disorders from cancer to the common cold and reviewed the conflicting studies on vitamin E and heart disease.

FROM BASIC BIOLOGY TO DISEASE PREVENTION

The meeting covered a variety of topics, from the basic biology of vitamin E to clinical studies of its effectiveness in thwarting disease. The topics included discussions of how humans obtain, metabolize, and absorb vitamin E; how vitamin E controls the production of key cell signaling molecules; how vitamin E regulates the activity of genes; how vitamin E protects the body from oxidative stress; the role that vitamin E plays in inflammation; how vitamin E can prevent illness, including respiratory infection and Alzheimer's disease; and the results of clinical trials and observational studies that examine vitamin E's role in cardiovascular disease. A pair of roundtable discussions considered future directions in both pre-clinical and clinical research.

A Lively Debate

The most lively debate centered around the mechanism by which vitamin E carries out its biological role. Scientists have long believed that vitamin E acts as an antioxidant, disarming the toxic molecules produced as a byproduct of metabolism. Left to their own accord, these free radicals disrupt cells destroying DNA, lipids, and

---

Karen Hopkin as a freelance writer in Somerville, Massachusetts, She holds a Ph.D. in Biochemistry and is a coauthor, along with Bruce Alberts *et al.*, of the textbook *Essential Cell Biology* (2003. Garland: New York).

other key components. Now researchers are finding that vitamin E appears to have additional capabilities.

Molecules in the vitamin E family act as anti-inflammatory agents and prevent the clumping of platelets. And they regulate gene activity, cell proliferation, and the production of important cell-signaling molecules such as nitric oxide. Given this surfeit of skills, some participants wondered whether vitamin E acts as an antioxidant at all.

The new functions are exciting because they suggest how vitamin E might help to prevent disease. Sticky platelets are associated with atherosclerosis and a reduction in arterial nitric oxide correlates with an increased risk of heart attacks. So vitamin E's ability to reduce platelet aggregation and elevate nitric oxide production suggests that the molecule should help stave off heart disease and atherosclerosis.

Indeed, a number of observational studies suggest that vitamin E might do just that. Unfortunately, the large-scale clinical trials have so far been disappointing. Only one study suggested that vitamin E could affect the course of disease.

Dissecting the Discrepancy

Much of the conference was devoted to dissecting this apparent discrepancy and why the clinical trials turned up negative results. Perhaps researchers tested the wrong combination of vitamins or the wrong population. Most of these trials failed to collect data that might have indicated why vitamin E fell short of expectations. To avoid this shortcoming, conferees suggested that future studies include measurement of subjects' vitamin E concentrations along with biomarkers for oxidative stress or inflammation.

The good news is that vitamin E does show some demonstrated benefits in disease prevention. Speakers presented data indicating that vitamin E can thwart respiratory infections and the common cold in seniors, slow Alzheimer's disease, and prevent pre-eclampsia in pregnant women. Trials are also under way to investigate whether vitamin E might help to prevent prostate cancer.

Until then, one participant concluded that taking vitamin E "can't hurt." And maybe 15 years from now, researchers will know more about how it can help.

VITAMIN E AND HEALTH

Introduction

Back in the 1950s a nutritionist named Max Horwitt wanted to determine the daily requirement for vitamin E. At the time, Horwitt was working at Elgin Hospital, a state-run mental institution, where he had ready access to "volunteers," in an experiment that would no longer be feasible under today's ethical guidelines.

For two years, the doctor fed a handful of patients a diet low in vitamin E. But the deprivation had no noticeable effect, so Horwitt added rancid fat to the patients' meal plan to further enhance destruction of the fat-soluble vitamin. A few years later, the doctor discovered that his subjects' red blood cells were more fragile than those of well-fed patients, breaking more readily when doused with hydrogen peroxide.

With those results in hand, Horwitt set out to determine how much vitamin E it would take to make his subjects' red blood cells as resilient as those of patients who were dining on standard hospital chow. He arrived at a value of 30 international units (IUs) per day, which in 1968 became the recommended dietary allowance for vitamin E. And everyone seemed satisfied.

More Than an Antioxidant

Or were they? True, as far as we know, Horwitt's patients suffered no permanent damage from their participation in the experiment. But their robust physical condition raised a question that has perplexed researchers for 50 years— what role does vitamin E play in human health and disease?—a question still asked at the current conference, where researchers discussed whether vitamin E supplements can prevent or treat a variety of disorders, from cancer to the common cold, and reviewed the conflicting studies on vitamin E and heart disease. The previous Academy-sponsored meeting dedicated to vitamin E was held 15 years ago. Since then, researchers have discovered that vitamin E is more than an antioxidant. Molecules in the vitamin E family act as anti-inflammatory agents and prevent the clumping of platelets, suggesting that they should help to stave off atherosclerosis.

And they regulate gene activity, cell proliferation, and the production of important cell-signaling molecules. Unfortunately, what these activities have to do with human health remains somewhat elusive.

BIOAVAILABILITY AND ANTIOXIDANT FUNCTION

Buttered Toast and Zebrafish

"We still don't know what exactly vitamin E does in the body," says Maret G. Traber of Oregon State University in Corvallis. Vitamin C, for example, is known to be a cofactor for an enzyme that modifies collagen so that it can assume the shape needed to build strong bone. "But we have yet to show in any enzyme system that vitamin E does anything," she says.

What researchers do have are "intriguing clues that vitamin E is critical," says Traber, perhaps the most interesting of which is the tocopherol transfer protein (TTP). This protein salvages α-tocopherol—the form of vitamin E that our bodies prefer—grabbing it from the liver and whisking it into the blood before it gets degraded and excreted. Even zebrafish have TTP.

So our need to hoard α-tocopherol "goes back to the days when we were all fish," says Traber. "If nature has chosen α-tocopherol out of all the thousands of antioxidants in the environment for us to sequester, there must be a reason," adds Angelo Azzi of the University of Bern.

α-Tocopherol can be hard to come by. "If you eat a lot of spinach and nuts and sunflower seeds, you might get 30 IUs," says Traber. But a person would need to drink two quarts of corn oil to get the 400 IUs in a typical vitamin E capsule.

Even taking supplements is no guarantee. Traber finds that vitamin E washed down with a glass of skim milk barely shows up in plasma, whereas the same supplement taken with a bowl of cereal raises plasma tocopherol concentrations by 500%. And John Lodge of the University of Surrey has shown that breakfast cereal can't hold a candle to buttered toast when it comes to boosting blood levels of vitamin E.

What's more, the ability to hold onto vitamin E might depend on one's genes. Frank J. Kelly of King's College in London noted that individuals vary widely in their ability to absorb vitamin E. Those who are good at taking up vitamin E wind up with decent amounts of tocopherol coursing through their veins. while others are not as fortunate. "It shows that you can't just take a group of individuals and give them a supplement and think that they're all doing the same thing with it," Kelly concludes.

Renegade Molecules and Molecular Signals

Some 70–80% of the American public is not getting the required amount of vitamin E, Traber estimates. And though, like Horwitt's patients, we might not appear ill, the deficiency could make us more prone to atherosclerosis or diseases that involve an enhanced production of oxygen radicals.

These renegade molecules can rampage throughout cells, destroying lipids, proteins, and DNA. By disarming oxygen radicals, vitamin E might act as "an insurance policy against oxidative stress," says Traber.

But vitamin E might do more than sop up excess radicals. John Keaney of Boston University Medical Center has shown that, in animals and humans, α-tocopherol reduces platelet aggregation and elevates production of nitric oxide (NO), a signaling molecule that regulates the relaxation of blood vessels.

The results could have implications for people prone to cardiovascular disease: sticky platelets are associated with atherosclerosis and a dearth of arterial NO correlates with an increased risk of heart attacks.

CELL REGULATION AND OXIDATIVE STRESS

An Important Regulatory Molecule?

Vitamin E also appears to regulate the activity of genes involved in cell adhesion, cell division, and cell signaling. Angelo Azzi goes one step further, insisting that vitamin E doesn't act as an antioxidant at all. He finds that tocopherol phosphate, a molecule with no known antioxidant properties, works just as well as α-tocopherol. "Just because a molecule acts as an antioxidant in a test tube does not mean it acts the same way in cells, tissues, organs, or animals," he says. Besides, why would the body use a special molecule for such a mundane task? "If it has unique regulatory functions, you don't use it for menial work," says Azzi, who likened such a waste to washing dirty dishes with top-of-the line facial cleanser.

Where Is the Duck?

Others argue that vitamin E does have demonstrated antioxidant effects in humans. Maret Traber, for example, has found that in marathon runners, vitamin E prevents lipid oxidation and cuts isoprostanes, a molecule that the body generates under oxidative stress. "There's good rationale for using vitamin E to treat atherosclerosis," as well, said Roland Stocker of the University of New South Wales School of Medical Sciences in Sydney. Vitamin E reduces cell adhesion and minimizes the concentrations of the molecular markers associated with the disorder.

Perhaps vitamin E is both an antioxidant and an important regulatory molecule, says Joseph Lunec of the University of Leicester. He studies the ability of vitamin E to protect cells lining the colon from becoming cancerous.

In cell cultures, he finds, vitamin E inhibits lipid oxidation, a chemical event that might drive tumor initiation and promotion. At the same time, vitamin E also speeded up DNA repair and slowed cell proliferation, activities that have nothing to do with its antioxidant properties. Lunec's conclusion: "If it looks like a duck and quacks like a duck, it may or may not be a duck."

VASCULAR NETWORKS AND DISEASE PREVENTION

Atherosclerosis, Adenovirus, and Alzheimer's Disease

Vitamin E could also dampen inflammation, which plays a major role in atherosclerosis. Ishwarlal Jialal of the University of California, Davis Medical Center, has found that patients with heart disease given high doses of α-tocopherol for two years have decreased concentrations of C-reactive protein (CRP), a marker of inflammation.

Much of the remainder of the conference was devoted to discussing the use of vitamin E in preventing or treating disease. Simin Nikbin Meydani at Tufts University showed that vitamin E prevents upper respiratory infections and the common cold in the elderly.

Anatol Kontush of INSERM in France described studies showing that vitamin E could slow the functional deterioration in patients with mild Alzheimer's disease (AD). A combination of vitamins E and C also reduced the prevalence of AD in an elderly population.

In one small study of pregnant women, vitamins E and C reduced the risk of preeclampsia, a leading cause of maternal death and premature births. The outcome most likely rests on vitamin E's nonantioxidant properties, particularly its ability to retard inflammation, says Lucilla Poston of King's College, one of the study's authors. She found that, compared to women who received a placebo, those treated with vitamin E produced fewer pro-inflammatory molecules. Poston hopes that larger clinical trials currently under way will support the positive results of the smaller study.

EPIDEMIOLOGY AND FUTURE DIRECTIONS

To E or Not To E

But not all the news was good or as straightforward. In the final session of the conference, participants tried to make sense of the conflicting studies about whether vitamin E can stall atherosclerosis and cardiovascular disease. The discussion panels turned their attention to the future directions both in clinical and preclinical vitamin E research.

Observational studies indicate that high blood levels of vitamin E go hand in hand with a low risk for cardiovascular disease and heart attacks. But so far the large-scale clinical trials have been disappointing: only one study has suggested that vitamin E could affect the course of disease.

Why the apparent discrepancy? First, observational studies that simply track volunteers' dietary and exercise habits are not good for nailing down which individual factors track with disease or with health. People who report taking vitamin E supplements probably also follow healthier diets, eat fruits and vegetables, exercise regularly, take multivitamins, and don't smoke.

All of these things could reduce the risk of heart attack "so it is hard to tease out vitamin E's effects from those of lifestyle," says Maret Traber.

And perhaps the trials were testing the wrong compounds. Ishwarlal Jialal suggests that more studies try, for example, vitamins E and C in combination. "Just taking one vitamin and assuming that it's going to do everything for you is a mistake in my view," says Jialal.

Changing the Subject

Another problem is that large-scale trials often use a population with a higher risk of disease. We need to perform similar studies on a healthier population, says J. Michael Gaziano of the Brigham and Women's Hospital in Boston. "Once a lesion has formed, it might be hard to get rid of" adds Mohsen Meydani of Tufts. So perhaps vitamin E will be better at disease prevention than cure.

At the very least, Jialal suggested, researchers should run clinical trials to measure their subjects' vitamin concentrations and look at biomarkers of oxidative stress and inflammation, such as isoprostanes and CRP. "If [previous trials] had done this, it would have told us a lot about these studies, why some were positive and others were not," he says.

Additional trials using healthier patients are ongoing and might provide more welcome results. Until then, Gaziano added, there's no need for despair: "We studied cholesterol for a century and a half before we got the story straight."

In the meantime, Traber says that we might be expecting vitamin E to do too much: "It does not make sense to eat a poor diet, be a couch potato, and take a vitamin E pill to solve your problems." She advocates eating right and staying in shape. "Along with that, if you want to take vitamin E," says Traber, "it can't hurt."

And 15 years from now, perhaps researchers will know more about how it can help.

Index of Contributors

Adelwöhrer, C., 344–347
Adolfsson, O., 96–101
Ahmed, T., 412–414
Ahuja, K.C., 387–390
Aisa, C., 348–351, 391–394
Aksoyek, A., 352–356
Ambra, R., 143–157
Ames, B.N., 399–400
Atkinson, J., 324–327, 330–331, 332–333
Azzi, A., 86–95, 305–312, 405–411

Bando, N., 415–417
Barella, L., 102–108, 334–336
Basu, S., 339–340, 352–356
Belisle, S., 418–421
Bergmann, A.R., 378–380
Bermudez, O.I., 385–386
Blumberg, J., 313–323
Bray, T., 357–360
Brigelius-Flohé, R., 40–43
Bronson, R., 418–421
Bruno, R.S., 357–360
Buoncristiani, U., 348–351
Burton, G.W., 1–12

Campbell, S.E., 223–233
Canali, R., 143–157
Cangemi, R., 292–304
Cardinault, N., 381–384
Carpentier, Y.A., 432–434
Chen, C.S., 395–398
Chung, H., 412–414
Conte, C., 348–351, 391–394
Cross, C.E., 109–126, 328–329
Cuddihy, S.L., 428–431
Curtis, V., 324–327

De Leeuw, I., 439–442
Ducart, A., 432–434
Dugan, L.L., 428–431
Dunster, C., 339–340

Eichhorn, J.C.P., 339–340
Ekanayake-Mudiyanselage, S., 184–194

Fischer, A., 102–108
Floridi, A., 348–351, 391–394
Frahm, G., 324–327
Frank, J., 365–367

Galli, F., 348–351, 391–394
Gao, X., 385–386
Gay, R., 418–421
Gaziano, J.M., 280–291
Gianello, R., 405–411
Gille, L., 341–343, 344–347
Godzdanker, R., 109–126
Gohil, K., 109–126, 328–329
Goldman, J.D., 387–390
Grabner, G., 344–347
Gregor, W., 341–343, 344–347
Gysin, R., 86–95

Hacquebard, M., 432–434
Hall, W.L., 60–73
Halligan, E., 169–183
Hamer, D.H., 214–222
Hamilton, R.L., 1–12
Han, S.H., 418–421
Han, S.N., 96–101, 214–222, 422–424
Hayakawa, M., 368–375
Hayton, S.M., 263–270
Heller, R., 74–85
Hiller, D., 381–384
Hopkin, K., 449–453, 455–460
Hoppe, P.P., 435–438
Huber, B., 412–414

Igarashi, M., 401–404

Jackson, M.J., 158–168

Jeanes, Y.M., 60–73
Jialal, I., 195–203, 313–323
Jiang, Q., 399–400
Johnson, A., 337–338

Kaini, R.R., 109–126
Kamal-Eldin, A., 365–367
Karakoula, K., 169–183
Katircioglu, S.F., 352–356
Kelly, F.J., xi–xiii, 22–39, 242–248, 339–340
Kempná, P., 86–95
Khanna, S., 127–142
Khassaf, M., 158–168
Khoschsorur, G., 361364
King, G.L., 204–213
Klein, E.A., 234–241
Koch, W., 435–438
Kontusha, A., 249–262
Kraemer, K., 184–194, 305–312, 435–438
Krishnan, K., 223–233

Lee, C.-K., 96–101
Lee, R., 22–39, 339–340
Leonard, S.W., 328–329, 357–360
Libinaki, R., 405–411
Lim, Y., 328–329
Liu, L., 425–427
Lodge, J.K., 60–73
Lunec, J., 169–183, 313–323

Manor, D., 324–327, 330–331, 332–333, 337–338
Manuel-y-Keenoy, B., 439–442
Maras, J.E., 385–386
Maritschnegg, M., 361–364, 381–384
Marko, M., 412–414, 418–421
Marktfelder, E., 381–384
McArdle, A., 158–168
McArdle, F., 158–168
McCormick, C.C., 13–21
Meinitzer, A., 361–364
Meydani, M., xi–xiii, 271–279, 422–424, 425–427
Meydani, S.N., 96–101, 214–222, 313–323, 412–414, 418–421, 422–424, 425–427

Mistry, N., 169–183
Miyazawa, T., 401–404
Morley, S., 330–331, 332–333
Morrow, J.D., 428–431
Moshfegh, A.J., 387–390
Mudway, I.S., 22–39
Muller, D.P.R., 263–270
Munteanu, A., 86–95, 405–411
Musiek, E.S., 428–431

Nakagawa, K., 401–404
Nava, P., 324–327, 330–331
Negis, Y., 86–95
Nesaretnam, K., 143–157
Niki, E., 305–312, 368–375
Nishio, K., 368–375
Nohl, H., 341–343

O'Roark, E., 109–126
Ogru, E., 405–411
Ordovas, J., 96–101
Ozer, N., 305–312
Ozkan, M., 352–356

Packer, L., xi–xiii, 109–126, 328–329, *Moderator*: 305–312, 313–323
Panagabko, C., 332–333
Panin, G., 443–447
Parker, R.S., 13–21, 376–377
Pignatelli, P., 292–304
Piroddi, M., 391–394
Poston, L., 242–248
Preinsberger, M., 381–384
Prolla, T., A., 96–101
Proteggente, A.R., 60–73

Qian, J., 330–331
Qui, M., 223–233

Radhakrishnan, A., 143–157
Raijmakers, M., 242–248
Ramakrishnan, R., 357–360
Resch, U., 378–380
Ribalta, J., 40–43, 361–364, 381–384
Rimbach, G., 102–108, 334–336

INDEX OF CONTRIBUTORS

Rock, E., 40–43, 361–364, 381–384
Roob, J.M., 40–43, 361–364, 378–380, 381–384
Rosenau, T., 344–347
Rota, C., 334–336
Roy, S., 127–142

Sabatino, G., 292–304
Saito, Y., 368–375
Schekatolina, S., 249–262
Schmartz, D., 432–434
Schock, B.C., 109–126, 328–329
Scott, J.A., 204–213
Selvaduray, K.R., 143–157
Sen, C.K., 127–142
Sies, H., 305–312
Singh, U., 195–203
Sontag, T.J., 13–21, 376–377
Sprinz, G., 381–384
Staniek, K., 341–343
Stocker, A., 44–59, 332–333
Stöcklin, E., 334–336
Stoecklin, E., 102–108
Stone, W.L., 223–233
Strumia, R., 443–447
Sundl, I., 361–364, 378–380, 381–384
Swanson, J.E., 13–21

Tembo, N., 432–434
Terao, J., 415–417
Thiele, J.J., 184–194
Tiran, B., 40–43, 361–364, 381–384
Traber, M.G., 1–12, 109–126, 328–329, 357–360, 365–367
Tsuzuki, T., 401–404
Tucker, K.L., 385–386

Ulus, A.T., 352–356

Ursini, F., 443–447

Van Campenhout, A., 439–442
Van Gaal, L., 439–442
Vasilaki, A., 158–168
Vatassery, G., 305–312
Vertommen, J., 439–442
Vessby, B., 352–356
Villacorta, L., 86–95
Violi, F., 292–304, 305–312, 313–323
Virgili, F., 143–157
Visarius, T., 86–95
Vitage Study Group, 361–364, 381–384

Wells. P.G, 395–398
Werner, E.R., 74–85
Werner-Felmayer, G., 74–85
West, S., 405–411
Whaley, S.G., 223–233
Wilde, P.E., 385–386
Willett, W., 313–323
Wilson, K., 330–331
Winklhofer-Roob, B.M., 40–43, 361–364, 378–380, 381–384
Wong, J., 399–400
Wonisch, W., 361364
Wu, D., 412–414, 422–424, 425–427
Wuga, S., 40–43, 361–364, 381–384

Yamamoto, M., 415–417
Yamanishi, R., 415–417
Yang, H., 223–233
Yoshida, Y., 368–375

Zingg, J.-M., 86–95, 405–411